The Managed Health Care Handbook Series

Best Practices in Medical Management

The Managed Health Care Handbook Series

The Managed Health Care Handbook, Third Edition
Peter R. Kongstvedt

The Managed Health Care Handbook, Third Edition, on CD-ROM
Peter R. Kongstvedt

Essentials of Managed Health Care, Second Edition
Peter R. Kongstvedt

**Readings in Managed Health Care:
A Companion to Essentials of Managed Health Care, Second Edition**
Peter R. Kongstvedt

Best Practices in Medical Management
Peter R. Kongstvedt and David W. Plocher

The Managed Health Care Handbook Series

Best Practices in Medical Management

Edited by

Peter R. Kongstvedt, MD, FACP
Partner
Ernst & Young LLP
Washington, DC

David W. Plocher, MD
Partner
Ernst & Young LLP
Minneapolis, Minnesota

AN ASPEN PUBLICATION®
Aspen Publishers, Inc.
Gaithersburg, Maryland
1998

This publication is designed to provide accurate and authoritative information in regard to the Subject Matter covered. It is sold with the understanding that the publisher is not engaged in rendering legal, accounting, or other professional service. If legal advice or other expert assistance is required, the service of a competent professional person should be sought. (From a Declaration of Principles jointly adopted by a Committee of the American Bar Association and a Committee of Publishers and Associations.)

Library of Congress Cataloging-in-Publication Data

Best practices in medical management/
edited by Peter R. Kongstvedt, David W. Plocher.
p. cm.—(The managed health care handbook series)
Includes bibliographical references and index.
ISBN 0-8342-1090-8
1. Managed care plans (Medical care)—Quality control.
2. Managed care plans (Medical care)—Standards.
3. Medical care—Standards. 4. Medical protocols.
I. Kongstvedt, Peter R. (Peter Reid)
II. Plocher, David W. III. Series.
[DNLM: 1. Managed Care Programs—organization & administration. 2. Delivery of Health Care—organization & administration. 3. Practice Management, Medical—organization & administration. W 130 AA1B56 1998]
RA413.B475 1998
362.1′04258′068—dc21
DNLM/DLC
for Library of Congress
98-19519
CIP

Copyright © 1998 by Aspen Publishers, Inc.
All rights reserved.

Aspen Publishers, Inc., grants permission for photocopying for limited personal or internal use. This consent does not extend to other kinds of copying, such as copying for general distribution, for advertising or promotional purposes, for creating new collective works, or for resale. For information, address Aspen Publishers, Inc., Permissions Department, 200 Orchard Ridge Drive, Suite 200, Gaithersburg, Maryland 20878.

Orders: (800) 638-8437
Customer Service: (800) 234-1660

About Aspen Publishers • For more than 35 years, Aspen has been a leading professional publisher in a variety of disciplines. Aspen's vast information resources are available in both print and electronic formats. We are committed to providing the highest quality information available in the most appropriate format for our customers. Visit Aspen's Internet site for more information resources, directories, articles, and a searchable version of Aspen's full catalog, including the most recent publications: **http://www.aspenpublishers.com**

Aspen Publishers, Inc. • The hallmark of quality in publishing
Member of the worldwide Wolters Kluwer group.

Editorial Services: Jane Colilla
Library of Congress Catalog Card Number: 98-19519
ISBN: 0-8342-1090-8

Printed in the United States of America
1 2 3 4 5

To my family:
my late father, Gerald Nicholas Kongstvedt;
my mother, Elizabeth Pearson Kongstvedt;
my sister, Chris Lieberman;
and especially my wife, Sheryl, and my son, David

Peter R. Kongstvedt

To my understanding family:
Michelle and our children, Jessica, David, and Joseph;
and my parents, Edward and Paula

David W. Plocher

Table of Contents

Contributors xxi

Preface xxv

Chapter 1—Introduction to Advanced Care Management and Its Implementation 1
David W. Plocher, Jacqueline A. Lutz, Wendy Wilson, and Ann Huston

    The Context for Advanced Care Management 1
    Defining Advanced Care Management 3
    Integrating the Components of Care Management 4
    Defining the Future of Care Management 7
    The Role of Physicians in Care Management 8
    Building an Advanced Care Management System: A Typical Process 9
    Conclusion 13
    Appendix 1–A: Description of the Components of the Advanced
        Care Management System 15

PART I—MEMBER HEALTH RISK ASSESSMENT 19

Chapter 2—Introduction to Health Risk Appraisals 21
Walter S. Elias

    Introduction 21
    HRA Models 22
    HRA Technologies 24
    Target Populations 25
    The Future 26

Chapter 3—Choosing and Using a Health Risk Appraisal Instrument 29
Walter S. Elias

    Introduction 29
    Why? 29
    Who? 31
    How? 31
    When? 32
    What Action? 32
    Methodology Issues 32
    Evaluating Instruments 32
    Conclusion 33

PART II—PRIMARY PREVENTION 35

Chapter 4—Prevention in Managed Care 37
Leif I. Solberg

    Introduction 37
    Why Should an MCO Do Prevention? 37
    A Typology of HP/DP Activities 39
    A Framework for Action 39
    Community Outreach Programs 40
    Public Policy Initiatives 42
    Prevention Section Overview 42

Chapter 5—Taking Advantage of the Clinical Setting for Prevention 45
Leif I. Solberg and Gail Amundson

    Introduction 45
    Direction and Energy 47
    The How of Change 49
    Other Considerations 51
    Primary Versus Secondary Prevention 51
    Facilitating Change from the Outside 52
    Conclusion 52

Chapter 6—Outreach from the Managed Care Organization to the Population 55
Nicolaas P. Pronk

    Introduction 55
    Population Health Cycle 56
    Framework for Action 57
    Conclusion 61

Chapter 7—Delivering Clinical Preventive Services to Underserved and Immigrant Populations 63
Thomas E. Kottke, Mary Alice Trapp, and Milo L. Brekke

Introduction 63
Establishing Contact 66
Community Assessment 67
Program Design and Development 67
Fostering Commitment 69
Progress Evaluation 69
Expanding the Role of Nurses To Increase Program Access and Acceptability 69
Against, and For, Interpretation 70
What Makes a Preventive Services Program Culturally Sensitive? 72
Conclusion 72

PART III—SPECIAL PREVENTIVE PROGRAMS FOR SELECTED HIGH-RISK BEHAVIORS 75

Chapter 8—Smoking Cessation: New Approaches Blend Marketing Theory with Emerging Technologies 77
Neal Sofian, Daniel L. Newton, and Joan DeClaire

Introduction 77
State of the Art in Cessation Therapies 78
New Approaches to Reaching Larger Populations 79
Taking Our Lessons from Marketing 81
Using Technology To Treat Populations One Person at a Time 85
The Dynamic Relationship among Impact, Reach, and Cost 88
A Shared Responsibility 88

Chapter 9—Preventing Unwanted and Unplanned Pregnancies 91
David Share

Introduction 91
Health Plan Perspective 91
Behavioral Factors 91
Role of Public Health Agencies 92
Education 93
Removing Barriers to Contraceptive Care 94
Associated Risk Factors 94
Service Coverage and Reimbursement Policies 94
Religion 95
Conclusion 96

PART IV—SELF-CARE AND HEALTH ADVISORY SERVICES ... 97

Chapter 10—Medically Directed, Delegated Self-Care ... 99
Gary Montrose

Introduction ... 99
History and Benefits of Self-Care ... 100
Physician Involvement in Medical Self-Care ... 101
Physician Obstacles ... 101
Separate Domains of Care ... 103
Self-Care as Part of Standard Practice ... 104
Delegated Self-Care ... 105
Contact Management ... 109
Enabling Technologies ... 111
Broader View of Managed Care ... 111

Chapter 11—Nurse Advice Services ... 117
Barry W. Wolcott

Introduction ... 117
Historical Incentives and Services ... 117
Incentives in Today's Marketplace—The Changing Face of Nurse Advice Services ... 119
Importance of Clinical Knowledge Systems ... 120
Technology Factor ... 121
Process Engineering—The Hidden Motor ... 121
Toward an Integrated Future—Redefining Medical Management Services ... 122

PART V—EMERGENCY DEPARTMENT SERVICES ... 125

Chapter 12—Efficient Use of Emergency Medicine Services ... 127
Casey J. Jason

Introduction ... 127
Prehospital Triage ... 128
Emergency Department Triage ... 129
Site and Staff Selection for Immediate Care ... 132
Site and Staff Selection for Continuing Care ... 133
Conclusion ... 133

Chapter 13—The Fast Track Emergency Department ... 135
Angela Zotos

Introduction ... 135
Observation Unit ... 135
Staffing the Fast Track ... 136
Best Practices ... 136

Key Considerations when Designing a Fast Track Program in the ED 137
Results Achieved 137

Chapter 14—Chest Pain Centers **139**
Suzanne K. White

Introduction 139
Traditional Approaches to Managing Chest Pain 139
Drivers for Change in the Management of Chest Pain 140
The Chest Pain Center Approach 140
Clinical and Economic Benefits of a Chest Pain Center Approach 146
Chest Pain Center Development 148
Conclusion 149

PART VI—ACUTE INPATIENT CARE **151**

Chapter 15—Managing Basic Medical-Surgical Utilization **153**
Peter R. Kongstvedt

Introduction 153
Administrative Costs Versus Medical Costs 153
Demand Management 154
Specialty Physician Utilization Management 156
Institutional Utilization Management 161
Conclusion 176

Chapter 16—The Hospitalist Model: A Method for Managing Inpatient Care **179**
David W. Plocher, Jean Stanford, and Bruce Meltzer

Introduction 179
The Hospitalist Model 179
The Hospitalist Model and Clinical Outcomes 181
The Hospitalist Model and Community Physicians 182
Hospitalists and the Continuum of Care for Patients and Families 183
Some Potential Pitfalls 183
Recruiting and Managing Hospitalists 184
Conclusion 184

Chapter 17—Case Management and Managed Care **187**
Catherine M. Mullahy

The Case Manager's Role 187
Patient Profile: Not Every Case Needs a Case Manager 188
On-Site Versus Telephone-Based Case Management 190
Case Managers in Managed Care 191
The Case Management Work Format and Process 192
Utilization Review: Preadmission and Concurrent Review and Case
    Management 200
Preadmission and Concurrent Review Case Management Reports 205

Red Flags: Indicators for Case Management 205
Timing Case Management Intervention 213
Beyond the Case Management Basics 213
A Long-Term Solution to a Long-Term Problem 216

Chapter 18—Critical Paths: Linking Care and Outcomes for Patients, Clinicians, and Payers 219
Richard J. Coffey, Janet S. Richards, Susan A. Wintermeyer-Pingel, and Sarah S. LeRoy

Background and Terminology 220
Scope and Uses of Critical Paths 220
Environment for Critical Paths 221
Approach to Developing Critical Paths 223
Use of Critical Paths 226
Alternative Formats and Sample Uses 227
Resource Formats 228
Calculate and Use Float/Slack Time Information 233
Results 233
Conclusion 235

PART VII—AMBULATORY CARE 239

Chapter 19—Management of Clinical Services in the Clinician's Office 241
Gordon Mosser

Introduction 241
Finding the Clinicians' Points of Engagement 241
Clinical Practice Guideline Development as an Engagement Strategy 242
Planning the Guideline Program 242
Guideline Development 243
Fostering Improvement of Clinical Care Through Collaboratives 245
Holding Practices Accountable 247
The Necessity for Trust 248

Chapter 20—Clinical Services Requiring Authorization 249
Peter R. Kongstvedt

Definition of Services Requiring Authorization 250
Definition of Who Can Authorize Services 250
Claims Payment 252
Point of Service 252
Categories of Authorization 253
Staffing 255
Common Data Elements 256
Methods of Data Capture and Authorization Issuance 257
Authorization System Reports 258
Open Access HMOs 259

		Specialty Physician–Based Authorization Systems 260
		Non–Physician-Based Authorization Systems 260
		Conclusion 260

Chapter 21—Guideline Use for Ambulatory Procedures 261
	Victoria P. Haulcy

		Introduction 261
		Guideline Products in Ambulatory Care 263
		Guidelines for Managing Financial Risk 265
		The Future of Guidelines in Ambulatory Care Decisions 265

PART VIII—POST–ACUTE CARE SETTINGS 267

Chapter 22—Home Health Care 269
	Peggy H. Rodebush, Kathleen M. L. Popper, and Barry K. Morrison

		Introduction 269
		What Is Home Care? 270
		History of Home Care 270
		Update 270
		Indicators and Predictors of Home Care Demand 271
		Home Care Services 273
		Professional Home Care Disciplines 274
		Regulations Guiding Home Care 275
		Financing Home Care Services 277
		Regulatory Issues Impacting Home Care 278
		Measuring Quality in Home Care Services 279
		Examples of Advanced Clinical Practices in Home Care 280

Chapter 23—Subacute Care 283
	Kathleen M. Griffin

		Introduction 283
		Subacute Care Defined 283
		Subacute Care Categories 283
		Subacute Patients 284
		Subacute Providers 286
		Subacute Care Within a Continuum of Care 289
		Payment for Subacute Care 290
		Selecting a Quality Subacute Care Provider 291
		Conclusion 294

Chapter 24—Hospice Care in the United States: Issues and Emerging Trends 295
	Anne C. Dye, Peggy H. Rodebush, and Geri Hempel

		Hospice Overview 295
		Financing and Reimbursement 297
		Size of the Hospice Industry in the United States 298

Major Policy Issues 300
Program Development 301
Budget Development 302
Future Integration and Affiliation Strategies 304

PART IX—ANCILLARY SERVICES 307

Chapter 25—Ancillary Diagnostic and Therapeutic Services 309
Peter R. Kongstvedt

Introduction 309
Ancillary Services 309
Physician-Owned Ancillary Services 310
Data Capture 311
Financial Incentives 311
Feedback 311
Control Points 312
Contracting and Reimbursement for Ancillary Services 313
Conclusion 315

Chapter 26—Pharmaceutical Services in Managed Care 317
Henry F. Blissenbach and Peter Penna

Cost of Drugs 318
The Pharmacy Benefit 318
The Providers 321
Determining Pharmaceutical Benefit Costs 323
Managing the Pharmacy Benefit 324
Ingredient Cost 326
Quantitative Drug Utilization Review 329
Audits 330
Management of Quality 330
Qualitative Drug Utilization Review 333
Measurement of Success 334
Pharmacy Benefit Management: Next Phase 335
Conclusion 336

PART X—DISEASE MANAGEMENT AND SELECTED CLINICAL CONDITIONS IN DISEASE MANAGEMENT 337

Chapter 27—Fundamentals and Core Competencies of Disease Management 339
David W. Plocher

Definition 339
Definition Clarification 339
Barriers and Drivers for Disease Management 341
Business Plan 342

Survey of Disease Management Programs 342
Important Linkages 344
Case Study 345
Conclusion 346

Chapter 28—Disease Management of Congestive Heart Failure 349
George Mayzell

Background 349
Disease Management Programs 350
Disease Care Continuum 350
Population-Based Identification and Confirmation 351
Validation and Confirmation 353
Stratification and Prioritization 353
Interventions 354
Cardiac Nurses/Case Management 355
ACE Inhibitors 356
The Role of the Cardiologists 356
Education 356
Telemonitoring 357
Home Visits 357
Outpatient CHF Clinics 358
Cardiac Rehabilitation 358
Acute Care 358
Incentives 358
Measurement and Evaluation 359
Cost Benefit Analysis 360
Conclusion 360

Chapter 29—Diabetes Disease Management 363
David K. McCulloch

Introduction 363
A Population-Based Approach to Diabetes Care 364
Practical Changes Necessary To Have More Effective Diabetes Care 371
Future Directions 374

Chapter 30—Asthma Disease Management 377
Benjamin Safirstein, Joan Kennedy, and Barbara Barton

Disease Management: An Innovative Concept 377
The Suitability of Asthma for Programmatic Disease Management 378
A Framework for Setting Program Objectives 379
Nine Critical Components in the Oxford Health Plan 380
The Four Most Critical Steps 385
Industry Alternatives to a Comprehensive Disease Management Program ... 392
Barriers to Program Implementation 393
Conclusion 394

Chapter 31—Disease Management and Return on Investment 397
David W. Plocher and Robert S. Brody

Introduction 397
Economic Concept of Cost and Observation on Its Measurement in
    Disease Management 397
Basic Evaluation Issues in Disease Management 398
Benefits 401
Costs 403
Conclusion 405

Chapter 32—Managed Behavioral Health Care and Chemical Dependency Services 407
*Donald F. Anderson, Jeffrey L. Berlant, Danna Mauch, William R. Maloney,
Terri Goens, and Katherine Olberg Sternbach*

Introduction 407
Key Treatment Principles 408
The Ideal Continuum of Care 412
Treatment Services 413
Benefit Plan Design 417
Utilization Management 419
Channeling Mechanisms 420
Behavioral Health Provider Networks 422
Provider Structures for Integrated Delivery Systems To Meet Managed Care
    Objectives 423
Quality Assurance 425
Information Systems 427
Public/Private Systems Integration 429
Emerging Issues 430
Conclusion 431

PART XI—CLINICAL QUALITY AND OUTCOMES MEASUREMENT AND MANAGEMENT 433

Chapter 33—Quality Management in Managed Care 435
Pamela B. Siren and Glenn L. Laffel

Traditional Quality Assurance 435
Components of a Quality Management Program: Building on Tradition 438
A Process Model for a Modern Quality Management Program 439
Setting the Improvement Agenda 456
Conclusion 456

Chapter 34—Introduction to the Measurement of Clinical Outcomes 461
Michael Pine

Introduction 461
Domains of Clinical Outcomes Measurement 461

Goals of Clinical Outcomes Measurement 462
Six-Step Process for Measuring Comparative Risk-Adjusted Clinical
    Outcomes 463

Chapter 35—Crafting Valid, Relevant Measures of Clinical Performance 479
Michael Pine

Introduction 479
Creating Cost-Effective Databases To Monitor Risk-Adjusted Clinical
    Outcomes 485
Using Control Charts To Obtain a Dynamic View of Performance 487
Integrating Information about Health Care Services To Identify
    Providers of Choice 489
Risk-Adjusted Functional Status 493
Monitoring Clinical Outcomes of Ambulatory Care 498

Chapter 36—Introduction to the Management of Clinical Outcomes 501
Michael Pine

Introduction 501
Components of Clinical Processes 501
Characterization of Clinical Processes 502
Relating Clinical Outcomes to Processes of Care 504
Conclusion 509

PART XII—USE OF INFORMATION IN CARE MANAGEMENT 511

Chapter 37—Using Data in Medical Management 513
Peter R. Kongstvedt

Introduction 513
General Requirements for Using Data To Manage the Health Care
    Delivery System 513
Focus 516
Hospital Utilization Reports 517
Outpatient Utilization 520
Provider Profiling 522
Conclusion 523

Chapter 38—Provider Profiling 525
Peter R. Kongstvedt and David W. Plocher

Introduction 525
What To Measure? 526
Episodes of Care 527
Adjusting for Severity and Case Mix 527
What Specialty *Is* the Physician? 528
What Constitutes the Group? What Linkages Exist? 529

Incorporation of Other Data 529
Comparing the Results of Profiling 529
Selection of a Profiling Vendor 530
Conclusion 531

PART XIII—CHANGING BEHAVIOR IN MANAGED CARE 533

Chapter 39—Physician Behavior Change in Managed Care Plans 535
Peter R. Kongstvedt

Introduction 535
Inherent Difficulties in Modifying Physician Behavior 536
General Approaches to Changing Behavior 540
Programmatic Approaches to Changing Physician Behavior 541
Changing the Behavior of Individual Physicians 543
Conclusion 546

Chapter 40—Member Behavior Change 549
Nancy W. Spangler

Introduction 549
They Know Better, So Why Don't They Just Stop? 549
Models for Affecting Patient Behaviors 553
Tools for Enhancing Change 558
From Theory into Practice: Humana's CHIP Program 561
Conclusion 564

PART XIV—COMPLEMENTARY AND ALTERNATIVE MEDICINE 567

Chapter 41—Complementary and Alternative Medicine 569
Alan Dumoff

Growth in Alternative Practices 569
The Modalities 570
Prevention and Wellness 575
Efficacy of CAM Approaches 575
Growth in Professional Development 576
Growth in Coverage 577
Structuring CAM Caregiving 578
Understanding CAM Philosophy: Guidance for Inclusion in MCO Settings 583
Conclusion 583

Chapter 42—Structure for CAM Integration 587
John Weeks

Introduction 587
Motivators for CAM Integration and Coverage 588
Challenges to CAM Integration 590
Credentialing 593
Selecting and Defining the CAM Benefit 597
Discounted CAM Services Through Credentialed Networks 597
The CAM Rider 598
Conclusion 601
Appendix 42–A: Case Studies 603

PART XV—CLINICAL MANAGED CARE IN GOVERNMENT PROGRAMS 611

Chapter 43—Medicaid Managed Care 613
Donna M. Henderson

Introduction 613
What Is Medicaid? 613
Medicaid Enrollment and Expenditures 615
Barriers to Care for Medicaid Beneficiaries 616
Preventive Care and Medicaid Beneficiaries 617
Health Risk Factors for Medicaid Beneficiaries 617
Medicaid Managed Care Initiatives 618
Capitation Rates for Medicaid Managed Care 618
Characteristics of an Effective Medicaid Managed Care Plan 619
Successful Interventions for Improving Member Access and Compliance 620
Conclusion 621

Chapter 44—Medical Management in the Medicare Population 623
Rita Petty Manninen and Barry K. Baines

Introduction 623
Unique Characteristics of Medicare Managed Care 623
Conceptual Model for Program Development in Managed Care 625
Managing Acute Care 626
Population Management 633
Where To Start in Developing a Medicare Managed Care Program 634
Conclusion 635

Glossary of Terms and Acronyms 637

Index 659

About the Editors 675

Contributors

Gail Amundson, MD
Associate Medical Director
Quality and Utilization
HealthPartners
Minneapolis, Minnesota

Donald F. Anderson, PhD
Principal
William M. Mercer, Inc.
San Francisco, California

Barry K. Baines, MD
Associate Medical Director
Centralized Patient Care Services
HealthPartners
Minneapolis, Minnesota

Barbara Barton, RN
Clinical Manager
Disease Management
Oxford Health Plans
Milford, Connecticut

Jeffrey L. Berlant, MD, PhD
Assistant Clinical Professor
Department of Psychiatry
University of Washington School of Medicine
Seattle, Washington

Henry F. Blissenbach, PharmD
Former President
Diversified Pharmaceutical Sevices
Minneapolis, Minnesota

Milo L. Brekke, PhD
President
Brekke Associates
Minneapolis, Minnesota

Robert S. Brody, MPH
Epidemiologist
Ernst & Young LLP
Phoenix, Arizona

Richard J. Coffey, PhD
Director
Program and Operations Analysis
University of Michigan Hospitals and Health Centers
Ann Arbor, Michigan

Joan DeClaire
Content Development Manager
Lexant
Seattle, Washington

Alan Dumoff, JD, MSW
Executive Director
LifeTree Medical Center, Inc.
Rockville, Maryland

Anne C. Dye, MHSA
Senior Consultant
Ernst & Young LLP
Tampa, Florida

Walter S. Elias, PhD
Chief Executive Officer
Kosmeo, Inc.
Minneapolis, Minnesota

Terri Goens
Consultant
Mental Health and Substance Abuse Services
William M. Mercer, Inc.
San Francisco, California

Kathleen M. Griffin, PhD
National Director
Post Acute and Senior Services
Health Dimensions Consulting Group
Scottsdale, Arizona

Victoria P. Haulcy, RN, BSN, MPH
Director of Marketing
Health Risk Management, Inc.
Minneapolis, Minnesota

Geri Hempel
Manager
Ernst & Young LLP
Tampa, Florida

Donna M. Henderson, RN
Director
Resource and Case Management
Alexian Brothers Hospital
San Jose, California

Ann Huston, MHS
Senior Manager
Ernst & Young LLP
Cleveland, Ohio

Casey J. Jason, MD, FACEP, FAAP
Vice President
Cove Hospitalist Program, MidAtlantic Region
Alexandria, Virginia
Assistant Clinical Faculty
Internal Medicine
Georgetown University
Washington, DC

Joan Kennedy, MIM
Director
Disease Management and Behavioral Health
Oxford Health Plans
Milford, Connecticut

Peter R. Kongstvedt, MD, FACP
Partner
Ernst & Young LLP
Washington, DC

Thomas E. Kottke, MD, MSPH
Professor of Medicine
Mayo School of Medicine
Consultant
Department of Medicine
Mayo Clinic
Rochester, Minnesota

Glenn L. Laffel, MD, PhD
Principal
Clinical Solutions, Inc.
Newton Center, Massachusetts

Sarah S. LeRoy, MSN, RN
Clinical Nurse Specialist
Pediatric Cardiology
C.S. Mott Children's Hospital
University of Michigan Hospitals and Health Centers
Ann Arbor, Michigan

Jacqueline A. Lutz, MBA
Assistant Director
Ernst & Young LLP
Chicago, Illinois

William R. Maloney, MBA
Principal
William M. Mercer, Inc.
Phoenix, Arizona

Rita Petty Manninen, RN, MPH, MBA
Manager
Geriatrics Programs
HealthPartners
Minneapolis, Minnesota

Danna Mauch, PhD
President
Magellan Public Solutions
Boston, Massachusetts

George Mayzell, MD, MBA
Medical Director
Blue Cross and Blue Shield of Florida
Jacksonville, Florida

David K. McCulloch, MD, FRCP
Diabetologist
Group Health Cooperative of Puget Sound
Seattle, Washington

Bruce Meltzer, MD
Center for Health Care Emerging Technology
Ernst & Young LLP
Boston, Massachusetts

Gary Montrose
President
Ashby * Montrose & Co.
Denver, Colorado

Barry K. Morrison
Senior Consultant
Health Care Business Transformation
Ernst & Young LLP
Charlotte, North Carolina

Gordon Mosser, MD
Executive Director
Institute for Clinical Systems Integration
Minneapolis, Minnesota

Catherine M. Mullahy, RN, CRRN, CCM
President
Options Unlimited
Huntington, New York

Daniel L. Newton, PhD
Principal
The NewSof Group
Redmond, Washington

Peter Penna, PharmD
Vice President of Managed Pharmacy
CIGNA HealthCare
Hartford, Connecticut

Michael Pine, MD, MBA
President
Michael Pine and Associates, Inc.
Research Associate
Department of Medicine
University of Chicago
Chicago, Illinois

David W. Plocher, MD
Partner
Ernst & Young LLP
Minneapolis, Minnesota

Kathleen M. L. Popper, PhD
Senior Manager
Health Care Strategy
Ernst & Young LLP
Washington, DC

Nicolaas P. Pronk, MA, PhD
Director
Center for Health Promotion
Associate Investigator
HealthPartners Research Foundation
Minneapolis, Minnesota

Janet S. Richards, MS, RN, CNAA
Director
Mercy Health Telemanagement
Mercy Health Services
Ypsilanti, Michigan

Peggy H. Rodebush, RN, MSN
Senior Manager
Health Care Business Transformation
Ernst & Young LLP
Tampa, Florida

Benjamin Safirstein, MD, FACP, FCCP
Vice President
Medical Affairs
Oxford Health Plans
Associate Clinical Professor of Medicine
Mount Sinai Medical Center
New York, New York

David Share, MD, MPH
Clinical Director
Center for Health Care Quality
Blue Cross and Blue Shield of Michigan
Detroit, Michigan
Medical Director
The Corner Health Center
Ypsilanti, Michigan

Pamela B. Siren, RN, MPH
Senior Health Care Consultant
ML Strategies, Inc.
Boston, Massachusetts

Neal Sofian, MPH
Principal
The NewSof Group
Redmond, Washington

Leif I. Solberg, MD
Clinical Director of Research
HealthPartners Research Foundation
Minneapolis, Minnesota

Nancy W. Spangler
President
Spangler Associates, Inc.
Prairie Village, Kansas

Jean Stanford
Associate Director, Health Care Consulting
Ernst & Young LLP
Washington, DC

Katherine Olberg Sternbach, MEd, MBA
Principal
Behavioral Health Care Practice
William M. Mercer, Inc.
San Francisco, California

Mary Alice Trapp, RN
Project Director and Trainer
Mayo Cancer Center
Mayo Clinic
Rochester, Minnesota

John Weeks
Principal
Integration Strategies for Natural Healthcare
Executive Editor
Alternative Medicine Integration and Coverage
Seattle, Washington

Suzanne K. White, MN, RN, FAAN, FCCM, CNAA
Senior Vice President, Patient Services
Chief Nursing Officer
Saint Thomas Health Services
Nashville, Tennessee

Wendy Wilson, MD, MSE
Senior Manager
Ernst & Young LLP
Cleveland, Ohio

Susan A. Wintermeyer-Pingel, MSN, RN, OCN
Clinical Nurse Specialist
University of Michigan Hospitals and Health Centers
Ann Arbor, Michigan

Barry W. Wolcott, MD
Chief Medical Officer
Access Health
Broomfield, Colorado
Associate Professor
Military and Emegency Medicine and Internal Medicine
Uniformed Sevices University
Bethesda, Maryland

Angela Zotos, RN, MS
Senior Manager
Ernst & Young LLP
Detroit, Michigan

Preface

Medical management, or as some prefer, care management, is the constellation of activities that surround the provision of care to members in a managed care organization. This may mean preventive care to well members, the identification of health risks or latent clinical disease, or the provision of self-care. Medical management also entails the more traditional functions of utilization and quality management, but even those activities have evolved significantly in recent years. Beyond those traditional functions, medical management also encompasses what happens outside the acute care setting and considers health care provision longitudinally. Medical management even is involved in alternative forms of health care, forms that are not always accepted by traditional medical practitioners.

The purpose of this book is to provide a comprehensive overview of many best practices in medical management as they are applied in managed health care. There are fine books and articles that go into great depth about narrowly defined subjects within medical management, but few that cover all the topics in medical management as comprehensively as possible. This book fulfills that function, giving readers reasonable depth about these best practices, but not necessarily an exhaustive discussion about each one. It is our intent to demonstrate the wide range of activities within the field and to give the reader a strong sense of the richness of thought and the high level of professionalism that exist within best practices in managed care today.

This book focuses solely on clinical care management in a managed care setting. Except for occasional references to aid understanding, there is little or no discussion about networks or network development, reimbursement, medical group management, human resource issues, and so forth.

In order to illustrate certain concepts and activities such as disease management, it was necessary to select a few clinical conditions and highlight those conditions in their own chapters. Only a textbook of medicine could cover all possible diseases in one book. Therefore, while there are very good approaches to diseases such as human immunodeficiency virus, chronic pain, low back pain, and so forth, space constraints do not permit them to be included in this book.

Similarly, this book does not attempt to discuss every type of care setting (eg, managed care organizations, integrated medical delivery systems, medical groups, public health initiative clinics, teaching hospitals) because settings are not the focus of this book. The focus is on how, not where, care is delivered in a managed care setting so as to constitute a best practice.

The book is divided into parts and then chapters. If readers are particularly interested in the topic of one chapter, they will benefit from reading the other chapters in the part. Where appropriate, we have indicated in the body of a chapter which other parts or chapters the reader may want to read.

This book is part of *The Managed Health Care Handbook Series,* and its most immediate parent is *The Managed Health Care Handbook,* 3rd Edition, Aspen Publishers, 1996. In this book, there are a few chapters that originally appeared in that parent text; here, they have been updated and modified as appropriate. There are also in-text references to *The Managed Health Care Handbook,* 3rd Edition, for topics that are closely related but out of the scope of this book.

Everything changes, and the information presented here will change too, so readers must constantly be aware of recent developments. In other words, what is defined as a best practice today may no longer be a best practice tomorrow. To put an even finer edge on that statement: this book is not a substitute for a textbook of clinical medicine; it is a book about managerial concepts embedded in best practices of clinical care in a managed care setting.

We hope that you find this book helpful as you develop, evaluate, or simply learn about medical management. Even more, we hope that some of you create new best practices that advance the body of knowledge in the clinical aspects of managed care. In an industry such as managed care, and in the broader field of medicine, evolution is rapid; best practices in medical management will evolve at the same speed.

We thank Jack Bruggeman, who initiated the creation of this book, and Kalen Conerly and Jane Colilla for their help with the editorial process. We thank Susan Wiebenga and Paulette Land for their excellent work in manuscript preparation. We also thank Joanne Allport, MD, Senior Manager in Ernst & Young's Washington, DC, office, for her contribution toward sourcing and beginning the work on Chapters 41 and 42.

Preface xxvii

Interventions in Care Management

```
                                                    Resource
                                                    Use
                                                    Targets
                                                      |
                                                      v
  Member Risk Assessment                    Inpatient              Outcome
                                            Critical               Data
  Primary Prevention                        Path and   ─────►      and
                                            Redesign              Practice
  Demand          Service                      ▲                  Profiling
  Management      Necessity  ──►  Utilization   │
                  Criteria       Management    │
         │                            │        │
         └──► Triage ◄────────────────┘        │
              ERT                              │
                ▲                       Ambulatory
                │                       Critical ──────►
           RN Protocols                 Path
                                           ▲
                                           │
                                   Practice Guidelines
                                           and
                                   Specialty Referral Guidelines
```

| Disease Management | Post-Acute Care | End of Life Care |

| Conventional Case Management |

This figure enables the reader to review at a glance the series of initiatives necessary for a comprehensive care management program. The chapters in this book supply detail within each of these intervention categories. The emphasis in this book is clinical; each chapter may only mention the requirements for information technology, finance, or operations.

Courtesy of Ernst & Young LLP.

CHAPTER 1

Introduction to Advanced Care Management and Its Implementation

David W. Plocher, Jacqueline A. Lutz, Wendy Wilson, and Ann Huston

Chapter Outline

- The Context for Advanced Care Management
- Defining Advanced Care Management
- Integrating the Components of Care Management
- Defining the Future of Care Management
- The Role of Physicians in Care Management
- Building an Advanced Care Management System: A Typical Process
- Conclusion

THE CONTEXT FOR ADVANCED CARE MANAGEMENT

Managed care dynamics motivate many organizations to assemble historically fragmented components of the health care system—hospitals, physicians, managed care organizations (MCOs) and health maintenance organizations (HMOs), postacute services, and so forth, into integrated delivery systems (IDSs). Integration can be defined as the optimization of interactions among components of a system to provide health services of high value to those served.[1] It is predicated on economic theory that suggests that an organization achieves a competitive advantage by controlling or managing, through ownership or contract, as large a span of the health care value chain as possible.

As markets evolve, developing more aggressive forms of managed care, clinical delivery systems come under greater pressure to reduce and manage costs. However, future success in this environment cannot be achieved by simply cutting costs; rather, a cost-competitive position must be reached through effective clinical integration and resource management. A number of common initiatives—advanced care management, process and system redesign, change management—are complex efforts aimed at reducing costs and increasing quality and value by transforming organizational processes, resource utilization, and service delivery.

A recent *Hospital & Health Services Administration* article on clinical integration notes that simply forming an IDS, even one with all the needed components, while necessary for integration, is not sufficient to actually achieve it.[2] However, progress toward integration can be assessed according to the following four criteria:[3]

1. coordination of clinical activities and services among operating units
2. avoidance of unnecessary duplication of clinical facilities and services
3. appropriate sharing of clinical services among operating units
4. integration of clinical services and facilities to achieve cost-effective patient care

Considerable effort has gone into trying to define the functional requirements and competencies for successfully meeting these criteria. Since

---

This chapter is courtesy of Ernst & Young LLP.

the ability to accept and manage capitated or fixed risk for medical costs is a common goal for MCOs and IDSs, advanced care management invariably appears as one of the critical success factors for MCOs and IDSs. The term *advanced care management* is used to differentiate these new types of management from more basic forms of utilization management, quality management, and medical management. (See Appendix 1–A for a description of the components of advanced care management.) As demonstrated in this book, advanced care management is clearly focused on issues of utilization and quality (as distinct from other administrative or clinical activities involved in the provision of health care), but in a far more comprehensive manner than ever before.

Advanced care management refers to a comprehensive, integrated program that allows an organization to effectively assess and manage (1) the clinical performance of its providers and (2) the health status of the insured population. In this context, care management refers to the program components, competencies, processes, and infrastructure necessary to manage and deploy the clinical resources within the system.

The rationale for adoption of an advanced care management system extends far beyond the economic advantages. Excellence in clinical quality and consumer satisfaction will probably become significant market drivers in the near future and have already shaped health care in advanced markets. An advanced care management system allows for optimization of outcomes on several axes, all of which are important outcomes in the future success of large systems.[4,5] These key outcomes are well described in the clinical value compass as developed by Batalden et al. Those outcomes include the following[6]:

- business/financial outcomes, discussed here as "total costs"
- classical medical outcomes, typically morbidity and mortality, discussed here as "clinical outcomes"

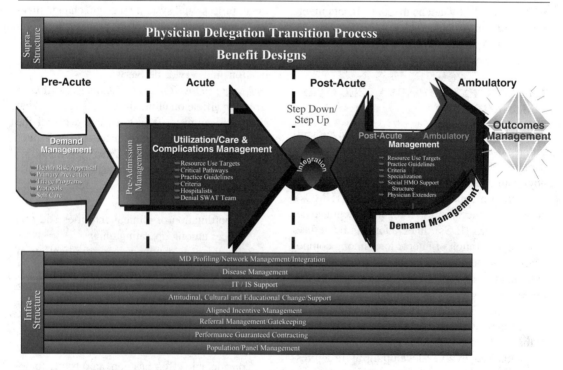

Figure 1–1 Care Management Components, Payer-System Perspective

- recently developed outcomes systems, including a broad variety of functional, health status, quality of life, and patient-referenced outcomes, depicted here as "functional health status"
- patient/member satisfaction, driving member retention, employer purchasing, and market trends that are impacted by member choice and consumerism, depicted here as "satisfaction against need" (this can encompass multiple customers' and providers' satisfaction as well)

DEFINING ADVANCED CARE MANAGEMENT

The primary objective of advanced care management is to ensure each enrollee receives the appropriate level of care (including preventive services), at the lowest cost, with appropriate outcomes.

Advanced care management goes beyond traditional utilization or stand-alone case management programs by evaluating care in all settings against a more comprehensive set of criteria (eg, quality, cost, patient satisfaction, and health promotion) and within more aggressive time frames (eg, prospective as opposed to retrospective review). Figures 1–1 and 1–2 outline a single model for advanced care management seen from two different perspectives. The model provides a framework for developing and structuring comprehensive care management systems.

As illustrated in Figures 1–1 and 1–2, advanced care management comprises various

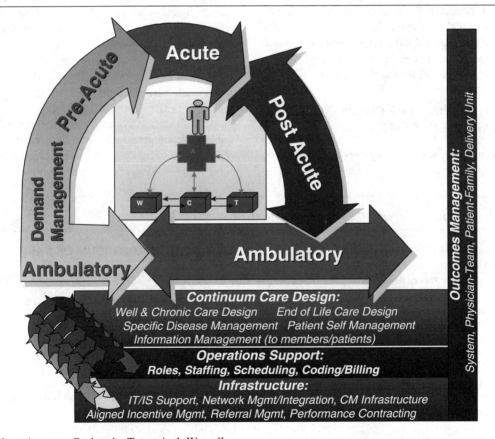

Note: A, acute; C, chronic; T, terminal; W, well.

Figure 1–2 Care Management Components, Patient/Member-Population Perspective

program elements that are designed to move patients to the most appropriate setting for their health care services. In this way, care management programs reflect the full continuum of care, in terms of settings and scope of services. Two program elements—disease management and case management—seek to coordinate activities across various elements of the broader program. Conventional case management typically addresses inpatient cases and attempts to streamline activities associated with a particular inpatient admission. Disease management encompasses a broader spectrum of health care settings and focuses on integrating services for a particular disease state, such as asthma, congestive heart failure, or diabetes.

There are other components of care management that help transform the program from a series of independent elements to a truly integrated system capable of managing care and resources. These components include information technology and systems, network management, and the integration model for the delivery system.

INTEGRATING THE COMPONENTS OF CARE MANAGEMENT

In many health care systems, current care management activities are predominantly insurance focused. The various components are designed to respond to external demands for utilization controls and retrospective review. As a result, the system and processes do not encourage sharing information among providers, caregivers, utilization management staff, social workers, discharge planners, and so on. In addition, the focus of the activities is typically the inpatient arena. Care management, under this scenario, is a support function for patient care.

Care management models typically evolve from insurance-focused programs, to care delivery models, and eventually to continuum of care models. This evolution is outlined in Exhibit 1–1. What truly differentiates the continuum of care model from the other models is that care management *drives* patient care. It is no longer a support function but a core business of the health system. This is a subtle but significant difference.

The evolution of care management systems is neither simple nor linear. Organizations must invest in the core program elements, develop the supporting infrastructure (eg, disease management, information systems), and determine the appropriate integration model to convert the program elements into an integrated care management system. Program development requires

Exhibit 1–1 The Evolution of Care Management Models

INSURANCE MODEL	CARE DELIVERY MODEL	CONTINUUM OF CARE MODEL
• Utilization review and quality assurance functions	• Development and use of standard tools such as critical pathways and care plans	• Focus on appropriate provider and optimal care site
• Inpatient focus	• Inpatient focus with some attention given to preadmission and postadmission service requirements	• Continuous quality improvement (CQI)
• Compliance and access orientation		• Driven by promotion of wellness and community health status
• Driven by insurance benefit parameters and national practices	• Exception-based review	• Balances cost, access, and quality by managing across the continuum
• No integration among components or patient care providers and settings	• Driven by medical staff buy-in and system integration efforts (eg, PHO)	• Multidimensional
	• One dimensional (linear)	

Courtesy of Ernst & Young LLP.

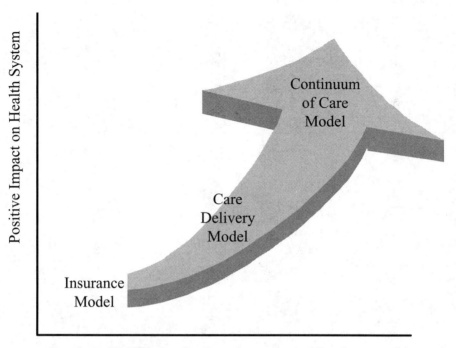

Figure 1–3 The Impact of Care Management Models on Integrated Systems

consistent and continuous effort over a significant period of time. However, as illustrated in Figure 1–3, the more advanced models have significantly more impact on the ability of the health system to manage resources and health status, thereby providing an appropriate "return on investment." Care management initiatives result in significant reductions in *utilization*. The net revenue impact depends on (1) current utilization levels, (2) scope of care management programs, (3) level of centralized administration, (4) scope of clinical services and settings, (5) method of reimbursement, (6) portion of premium dollar controlled, and (7) overhead expended.

In order to truly appreciate Figure 1–3, one simply has to consider the theory and practice of the IDS. The theory driving organizational integration is that controlling all inputs to the health care process can produce improved quality and service and lower cost structure, and achieve the critical mass necessary to remain a dominant player in the market. Yet in practice, results to date appear less than stellar. For most IDSs, clinical integration has not yet been achieved. Systems have not realized anticipated cost reductions. The market does not yet recognize significant improvements in quality and health status.

Yet systems are still investing time and resources into integration. Accordingly, Figure 1–4 defines the evolution of integrated systems. Most IDSs are in the early stage of collecting assets. These systems are trying to build a continuum of care in a market region through vertical and horizontal integration. The transition stage requires systems to define and develop new competencies—many of which were not required in traditional fee-for-service markets. These competencies—which include care management—are complex, multidisciplinary processes. During the transition stage, an organization begins to develop an understanding and definition of "systemness."

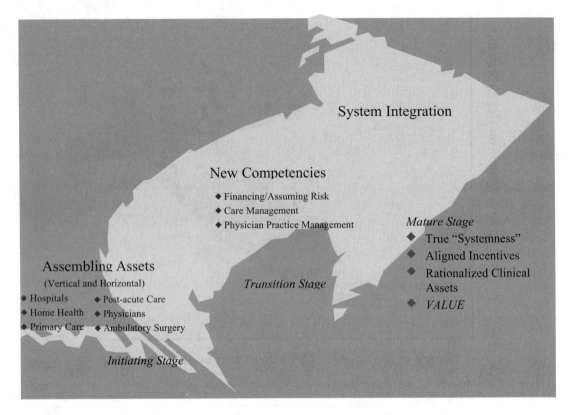

Figure 1–4 The Evolution of Integrated Delivery Systems

The four criteria for assessing progress towards integration (discussed previously) may be incorporated into a number of key characteristics for integrated care management. In this way we can differentiate between the components or program elements, and an advanced care management system.

Key Characteristics of Advanced Care Management

- Multidisciplinary teams (eg, physicians, nurse managers, members of the hospital administration) drive the development and ongoing operation of the care management system. Physicians are well integrated into these teams.
- Communication and documentation are enhanced throughout the system.
- Patient care and service across the different settings and departments are well coordinated.
- Processes are streamlined and resources are effectively managed to improve service and reduce costs.
- There is a marked reduction in the duplication of clinical and administrative efforts.
- Services are redesigned to allow departments and operating units to share resources, as appropriate.
- Internal and external customer satisfaction improves throughout the health system.
- Within the health care organization, care management is functionally and structurally situated as a core business.

DEFINING THE FUTURE OF CARE MANAGEMENT

In the future, care management is expected to reclaim some of the personal touches and advantages that were present in the fee-for-service (FFS), non-risk-bearing environment. Physicians and caregivers moving into an advanced care management model sometimes complain that it feels "impersonal" to treat an individual patient as a "member of a population" with "defined population-based outcomes." The n:1 model lacks the 1:1 touch (Figure 1–5).

In migrating to an advanced care management system, there will be significant shifts in provider roles and the nature of care delivery. Inevitably, there will be a radical increase in the numbers of nonphysician providers. There will also be increased intrageneralist specialization of physicians along new lines, creating the role of the hospitalist, among others. Postacute services will move to expanded coverage, with many patients directly admitted, 7 days a week, to the subacute environment for what was previously acute care (stroke, heart failure, diabetes). Observation units will stabilize another group of patients who were previously admitted to the acute environment (encompassing such diagnoses as diabetic ketoacidosis, congestive heart failure, pyelonephritis, and so forth). These patients will be rapidly stabilized and their exacerbations treated in as little as 10 to 12 hours.

In the future, care management will most likely garner greater control and extension across the continuum of care. It will extend beyond its current continuum to encompass the health and well-being of the community. Systems will begin to rationalize programs and services relative to community need. The continuum services will also expand beyond what has been considered conventional and strictly medical, to encompass holistic and alternative medicine and nonmedical interventions in the community. And perhaps most pivotally, the nature

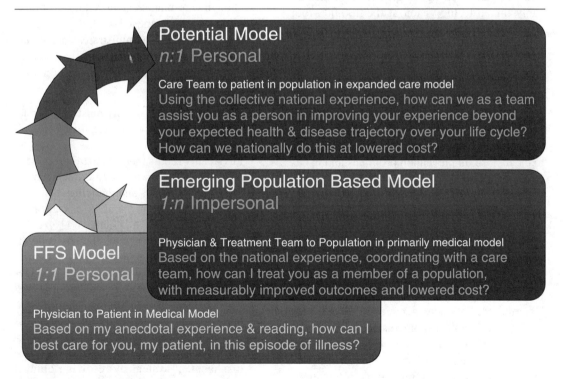

Figure 1–5 Models of Care Delivery and Targeted Aims

of relationships within the system will be substantially altered as provider/patient relationships deepen, perhaps even to the point of expanding accountability—formerly transitioned from the payer to the provider—to the patient/customer.

In order to move across these radically extended boundaries, philosophically and physically, care management design will demand new tools and new implementation depths. Systemwide care management design has often been considered "high level" or "lofty," existing above the care environment itself. To meet the future, care management will of necessity be designed at the level of the smallest replicable unit of care,[6,7] efficiently and effectively leveraging advantage across the system. A corresponding infrastructure will be needed at the system or multisystem level. Bilevel design (at the level where the work occurs and at the level where system integration occurs) will allow for true clinical integration and system transformation, with design and change at ground level inextricably linked to the vision at the 200,000-foot level, delivering communitywide, yet very personalized care.

Provider/patient relationships will be altered substantially, moving as leadership has moved in the last decade to being principle centered, for the purpose of incorporating patients/members as partners. In disease management, we do something *to* the patient, and the patient stands as host to the disease. In prevention programs and in demand management, we do something *for* the patient, generally delivering educational materials. To shift a portion of responsibility to patients, we must do something *with* our patients, and enter into true partnerships at a systemwide level: patient self-management or comanagement.

Similarly, in conventional managed care relationships, physicians are managed from above. External forces make decisions, set requirements, and establish protocols for these physicians based on data that the physicians do not hold or originate. Future care management systems will likely provide infrastructure, relationships, and processes to allow physicians and teams to self-manage in alignment with multiple priorities (individual, system, regulatory, and managed care)—the system operating in partnership, *with* them.

THE ROLE OF PHYSICIANS IN CARE MANAGEMENT

The successful development and administration of a care management system is highly dependent on a "partnership" between the health system and its affiliated physicians. Currently, physicians remain the primary providers of patient care services and, as such, manage the overall health of their patients; are a critical element in providing patients with information related to wellness programs; and determine diagnoses, care settings, treatment plans, and follow-up. As providers, therefore, physicians largely drive the use of clinical resources within the health system.

Although care management requires a multidisciplinary team composed of physicians, other clinical practitioners, administrative personnel, and external (eg, payer) representatives, physicians perform a number of critical roles in care management.

- As providers, physicians must collaborate with patient care teams regarding overall care plans.
- Physicians retain the technical knowledge needed to develop many care management tools (eg, pathways and guidelines).
- Physicians are primary users of care management information systems.
- Physicians document care, thereby generating a considerable amount of data that should be retained within the care management system. Ongoing management and improvement of the care management system depends, in part, on information access and information management.
- Physicians act as advisors within the care management system by resolving clinical practice issues and serving as a technical re-

source for case managers and other care management providers.
- Physicians are primary intermediaries with payers, providing clinical information critical to resolving care and benefit issues.
- Finally, physicians have clinical leadership and administrative roles within the health system. In these roles, physicians help define the direction and priorities of the health system.

The following section of this chapter broadly outlines a typical process for developing a care management system. Because of the many roles physicians play within this system, it is critical that they provide leadership and input throughout the development process.

BUILDING AN ADVANCED CARE MANAGEMENT SYSTEM: A TYPICAL PROCESS

Building an advanced care management system is typically a four-phase process.

1. mission and vision, current state assessment
2. benchmarking and future state design
3. construction of the model and long-term plan
4. staged implementation

Classically, such a system is built sequentially. With the rapid evolution of corporate change processes, nonlinear design/implementation processes are becoming popular, leading to a variety of accelerated process methods. A classical design/implementation process is described below, contrasted with examples of accelerated methods.

Phase 1: Mission and Vision, Current State Assessment

Early in the building process, it is important to relate the emerging care management model to the overall mission and vision of the integrated system. Unique priorities and structures would be built, for example, if the primary current developmental aim of the integrated system were to achieve access and care for vulnerable and disadvantaged populations rather than to build components of the system to serve an affluent population that demands alternative/complementary medicine and wellness programs from its providers of care.

It is also important to define the current state of the system. Overall system maturity, financial health, market pressures, population served, and position in the evolution of care management systems should be evaluated.

- A very mature system may have little need for length of stay reductions and remodeling of inpatient care management, and much more need to refine its delivery of care to capitated populations across the continuum at multiple sites of care.
- An integrated system that is new or economically fragile may choose to focus on care management initiatives that improve quality while concurrently reducing cost with a rapid rate of return on investment (by, for example, implementing a congestive heart failure management program, which may yield up to a 10% cost reduction in 90 days). By contrast, a very solvent and mature system may choose to implement care management initiatives (such as extended health risk assessment and outreach among well populations) that are "the right things to do," that attract and retain key populations but require an investment that may or may not yield a financial benefit in the short term.
- A large system that has recently been integrated may have a profound need to achieve clinical integration among various sites, ramifying best practices within the overall system and facilitating the formation of a learning organization.

Depending on what aspects of care management are being redesigned and implemented, it may be important to complete a very detailed current state assessment, as explained below.

Assessment of Hospital-Based Processes

- discharge planning
- infection control
- social service
- quality management
- risk management
- guest relations
- points of access
- scheduling
- ancillary services
- regulatory requirements

Assessment of Ambulatory Practice and Extended Continuum Processes (Figures 1–6 and 1–7)

- processes that are general across the system and affect all patient populations (access, scheduling, documentation, etc)
- care of specific populations along the continuum (well care, chronic care, terminal care)
- care of patients/members with specific diseases (disease management)
- current state of attempts to reduce demand in the system (demand management including nurselines and self-care education)

Assessment of Current Infrastructure Design and Current Organizational Change Processes

- information systems and technology
- outcomes measurement and feedback
- care management infrastructure, roles, responsibilities, and organization of providers
- facilities: physical configuration and geographic proximity
- approach to organizational change: organizational structure and alignment of incentives

This phase is typically completed through a series of interviews and facilitated sessions, and data analysis. It may be abbreviated and consolidated considerably in accelerated delivery by combining some of its aspects with later phases in accelerated sessions. For example, there are

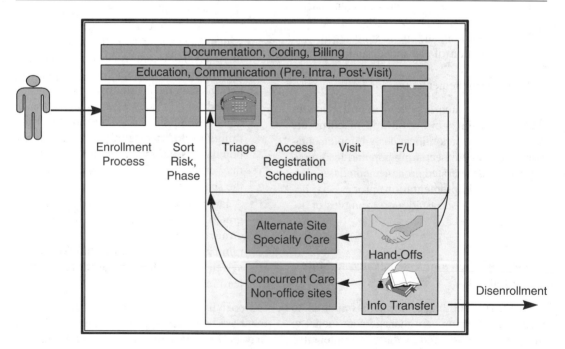

Figure 1–6 Processes Affecting All Patients

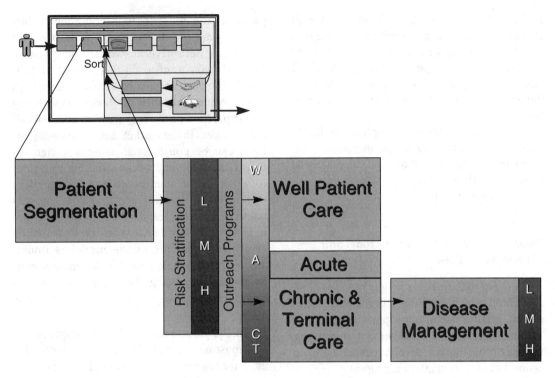

Note: H, high; L, low; M, medium.

Figure 1–7 Detail Risk Stratification Process Population/Disease Management

methodologies for facilitating this phase with small (ie, fewer than 20 or so) and large (ie, up to 200) numbers of participants. Very large group facilitation (up to 1,000 to 2,500 organizational participants) is useful for full-scale change in large organizations and is applicable to a variety of needs (eg, strategic planning, business planning, process redesign/transformation).

Phase 2: Benchmarking and Future State Design

Taking into account key aspects of organizational mission and vision and opportunities as defined in the current state assessment, this phase further defines the initiatives to be undertaken based on where the strongest opportunities lie. Both internal and external systems and information should be used to develop an analysis of leading practices. The elements typically targeted include

- cost: length-of-stay data, resource utilization, per member per month (PMPM) and procedure costs (defined across key populations and diseases)
- classical medical outcomes: morbidity and mortality data (complications, deaths, etc)
- functional and health status outcomes
- multiple customer satisfaction and retention rates

The possible opportunities are contrasted against the organizational "gaps." For instance, where do significant deviations from best practice lie? Where do these deviations correspond to areas in which improvement is relatively easy to achieve? Again, a very mature and financially healthy organization on the leading edge of change may well decide to undertake initiatives that do not have a defined return on investment and are relatively experimental but are either "the right thing to do" or the next logical, although unproven, step in the organization's evolution.

This phase is typically completed in facilitated sessions and workgroups in classical design/implementation methods and can readily be combined with aspects of other phases in accelerated change design.

Phase 3: Construction of the Model and Long-Term Plan

Design of the care management model will include both a high-level design to achieve clinical integration across multiple sites and key "ground-level" care management initiatives, with key infrastructure development and organizational change management support.

The infrastructure design, tailored to the organization's market, maturity, and approach, includes designing where support personnel (such as case managers and physician extenders) will be positioned and how they will be paid.

- Will such disease-specific case managers function at the corporate level and be funded by "corporate moneys" or will they inhabit individual physician practices and be paid by those practices?
- Will the system have, for a given geographic area, a "practice without walls" of leading providers managing its diabetic population, for example, or will it have a common protocol to be implemented through numerous primary care providers who then refer to key specialists?

Infrastructure development also includes definition of key areas such as information support, outcome measurement and dissemination, and incentives alignment design.

In addition to infrastructure, design and implementation must include components targeted toward physician/clinical team behavior change. A definitive answer to the question "Why do you want to do this?" must be provided. The answer must be compelling enough to overcome resistance to change. Depending on the position of the organization and individual providers in the market, a motivational platform can be constructed using a variety of "push-and-pull" approaches: the burning platform versus the manifestation of a compelling vision. Once the message is defined, a systemwide communication program must be put in place, with key data and outcomes delivered at critical moments as the model is implemented. Development and/or dissemination of an approach to change behavior and a process that is relatively easy to implement must follow closely.

Finally, ground-level design and implementation must be planned. The key preventive, disease management, and demand management programs to be implemented are prioritized and defined, as are key population and panel management programs. The organization must answer the following questions:

- What do we want and need to achieve in 1 year?
- What do we want and need to achieve in 5 years?
- What will we achieve this quarter?

The system will need to incorporate tools for some process standardization, outcomes measurement, reporting, and variance documentation, including

- interdisciplinary clinical guidelines
- outcomes measurements
- variance tracking documentation tools
- methods for variance analysis and reporting
- methods for data feedback and communication of progress relative to need

Measurements will need to be developed to provide feedback on the integrated care management program. Examples of these include patient functional status, patient clinical indicators, patient satisfaction survey results, physician satisfaction survey results, return on investment, and resource consumption or utilization.

The new care management system will create new skill and resource requirements within the health system. Clearly, a key element of the future transition is that we will develop a variety of new positions and responsibilities. Staffing, operations support, and roles and responsibilities are key elements of ground-level redesign.

A long-term plan becomes essential at this stage. The probable initiatives to be undertaken in the next 3 to 6 months are defined in the overall context of the long-term plan. This plan will need to be revised periodically, as it applies to a rapidly changing target.

This phase is typically conducted through the formation of work teams under the purview of a steering committee. Again, this phase can be effectively consolidated with the previous phases through any variety of accelerated methods. Such methods typically combine members of the steering committee with ground-level employees for very effective and rapid design sessions, typically spanning 3 to 5 days for a defined initiative, followed by the implementation phase (which can be conducted in classical or accelerated form).

Phase 4: Staged Implementation

During implementation, the staff members who will take on new roles within the organization are trained and other personnel learn about the changes in their roles and in work processes. Transition to these changed roles and processes is often very challenging, and the training and communication make it easier for staff members to meet the new expectations.

The training and communication program for physicians, case managers, and new physician extenders as well as those whose current roles will be directly affected by the new model should be developed during the design phase of the process. Typically, a number of initiatives are selected for design and implementation in a given quarter. For example, an organization might choose to develop the following program in a given quarter:

1. system coordination
   - key aspects of care management infrastructure: development of specialty case manager "pods"
   - key aspects of information systems development
   - key aspects of incentives alignment/design
2. organizational change and communication
   - physician/clinical team motivational platform construction and communication
   - definition of key organizational and clinical team outcomes and ongoing reporting/communication
3. care process redesign/implementation
   - development of coordinated systemwide disease management pilot
   - development of selected Medicare health risk assessment pilot

This program could be accomplished—in part—with classical methods, and probably in full with accelerated methods.

CONCLUSION

In summary, the development of a comprehensive, integrated care management system requires a significant and essential investment. The requirements of the managed care marketplace are clear and unavoidable: the ability to efficiently and effectively manage health care resources will determine the viability and success of today's health care organizations. With these necessary investments will come benefits (Exhibit 1–2). Many of the benefits can be quantified, once current and target levels of resource utilization are determined.

Exhibit 1–2 Value Proposition for Care Management—Inpatient Case Management

INVESTMENTS	BENEFITS

• *People*
  1. Project manager
  2. Staff support for design/implementation
  3. Medical and other clinical leadership
  4. Training in redesigned job areas
    –Role
    –Technology
• *Technology*
  1. Laptop computers for care coordinators
    –Information systems interface—financial data
  2. On-line clinical documentation
  3. On-line interface with payers/providers
  4. On-line interface to claims payment system
  5. Software support
    –Clinical practice guidelines
    –Case finding
    –Case tracking and monitoring
    –Best practice measurement
• *Capital*
  1. Software/hardware to support operations
	• Significant decrease in clinical resource use
	  1. Decreased length of stay/equivalent dollars
	  2. Decreased cost per member per month
	• Full-time equivalent reductions realized through elimination of duplication of effort within and among facilities
	• Savings related to process improvement
	  1. Dollar reduction through skill mix changes
	  2. Savings through capacity management
	  3. Increased provider/patient satisfaction
	• Ability to deliver and manage care under a fixed payment system

Courtesy of Ernst & Young LLP.

REFERENCES

1. Berwick D. Continuous improvement as an ideal in health care. *N Engl J Med.* 1989;320(1):53–56.
2. Young D, Barrett D. Managing clinical integration in integrated delivery systems: a framework for action. *Hosp Health Serv Adm.* 1997;42(2):255–279.
3. Gillies R, Shortell S, Anderson D, Mitchell L, Morgan K. Conceptualizing and measuring integration: findings from the health systems integration study. *Hosp Health Serv Adm.* 1993;38(4):467–489.
4. Nelson EC, Mohr JM, Batalden PB, and Plume SK. Improving health care: part 1, the clinical value compass. *Joint Commission J Quality Improvement.* 1996;22(4):243–258.
5. Nelson EC, Batalden PB, Plume SK, and Mohr JM. Improving health care: part 2, clinical improvement worksheet and users manual. *Joint Commission J Quality Improvement.* 1996;22(8):531–548.
6. Batalden P, Mohr J, Nelson E, et al. Continually improving the health and value of health care for a population of patients: the panel management process. *Quality Manage Health Care.* 1997;5(3):41–51.
7. Quinn JB. *The Intelligent Enterprise.* New York: Free Press; 1992.

JACQUELINE A. LUTZ, MBA, is an assistant director for Ernst & Young's Health Care Consulting Practice. In her current role for strategic services, she is responsible for service line infrastructure development, knowledge deployment, thought leadership, and the development and deployment of strategy products and services. Ms. Lutz started her health care career as a product development engineer in the medical device industry. After receiving her MBA from Wharton, she entered consulting, specializing in partnering strategies and the development of integrated systems.

WENDY WILSON, MD, MSE, is senior manager for Ernst & Young LLP in Cleveland, Ohio.

ANN HUSTON, MHS, is a consultant with Ernst & Young's national health care practice. Prior to consulting, she served as a senior executive officer of an integrated system. Ms. Huston's areas of focus include strategy formation, partnering, and integrated system design and development.

APPENDIX 1–A

Description of the Components of the Advanced Care Management System

Following are brief descriptions of the components of the advanced care management system. Far more detailed discussions and examples of these components (as well as additional components that some organizations will want to consider) are provided elsewhere in this book. For now, consider the following components as basic to any advanced care management program.

PROGRAM ELEMENTS OF MEDICAL MANAGEMENT

Health risk assessment (HRA) is designed to identify individuals who could benefit from targeted health promotion programs or appropriate interventions, thus helping them become aware of the risks of their unhealthy habits and motivating them to change. The HRA can also be used to track the progress of members who have taken steps to change their behavior.

Primary prevention refers to wellness programs and other interventions/screenings (eg, yearly exams, well-baby care, immunizations, regular screenings, etc) typically provided, in a managed care setting, by the primary care physician. Within a care management program, primary prevention involves the development of appropriate recommendations for the type and frequency of these primary care services.

This appendix is courtesy of Ernst & Young LLP.

Demand management is designed to encourage the appropriate utilization of health services by offering triage programs and providing patients with information about their diseases, disease processes, and desired outcomes, thereby enabling them to participate in self-care and the selection and utilization of health services. Demand management programs, in addition to increasing member and physician satisfaction, typically reduce the nonurgent cases at emergency rooms, urgent care settings, and primary care facilities.

Triage refers to the process of sorting out member requests for services into those who need to be seen right away, those who can wait a little while, and those whose problems can be handled with advice over the phone. Because of the military origins of the term "triage," many managed care organizations and integrated delivery services use alternate terms for the same activity.

Basic utilization management is the coordination of the various tools capable of managing resource utilization (eg, length of stay for inpatients) within specific care settings. Tools that support utilization management include the following:

- *Protocols* specify the care that is to be provided to a patient undergoing a particular treatment. Protocols are often used in clinical research. They are strict management directives and more binding than clinical guidelines.

- *Resource use targets* facilitate optimum resource use and outcomes by outlining "leading practice" patterns of resources that should be consumed during the treatment of inpatients and outpatients.
- *Referral guidelines* indicate the appropriateness of referral to or consultation with a specialty physician by a primary care physician, or other specialty physician managing the patient.
- *Practice guidelines* are systematically developed statements to assist practitioner and patient decisions about appropriate health care for specific clinical conditions.
- *Pathways* are plans that suggest an optimal sequencing and timing of interventions by physicians, nurses, and other staff members for a particular diagnosis or procedure. Pathways help to minimize delays, resource utilization, and unit costs, and to maximize the quality of care.

Outcomes reporting improves the effectiveness of health care services by examining measures of health care quality, utilization, and cost, including underutilization, readmission, and recidivism rates; levels of improvement in clinical status; functional performance; morbidity; mortality; and satisfaction.

Provider profiling uses a denominator-based population to help develop measurements to monitor the impact of the care management system on provider practice patterns.

SUPPORTING INFRASTRUCTURE

Conventional case management is a collaborative multidisciplinary process designed to manage an individual's care for a specific illness or episode. Case management streamlines all of the services provided and focuses on the achievement of quality outcomes within a defined time frame using appropriate resources in a cost-effective manner.

Disease management is designed to produce optimal clinical outcomes in a cost-effective manner through a system-based, proactive, disease-specific approach to delivering health care services. This process spans the entire continuum of care and focuses on the natural course of chronic diseases (eg, patients with asthma, diabetes, congestive heart failure, etc).

Conventional case management and disease management can be differentiated as shown in Table 1–A–1.

ADDITIONAL PROGRAM ELEMENTS BEYOND MEDICAL MANAGEMENT (EXHIBIT 1–A–1)

Premium management refers to the development of specific financial services relating to contracting and risk adjustment across the system, between internal and external entities.

Practice management refers to the development of support structures and practices that optimize physician coordination and effectiveness across the system, provide for aligned incen-

Table 1–A–1 Conventional Case Management Versus Disease Management

	Case Management	*Disease Management*
Goal	Streamline components	Integrate components
Emphasis	Treatment of sickness	Prevention and education
Setting	Inpatient	All settings
Timing	Concurrent	Prospective
Guidelines	Generic	Customized to diagnosis
Caregivers	Nurse	Multidisciplinary team

Courtesy of Ernst & Young LLP.

Exhibit 1–A–1 Comparison of Premium, Medical, and Practice Management

PREMIUM MANAGEMENT	MEDICAL MANAGEMENT	PRACTICE MANAGEMENT
• Payer contracting • Provider contracting • Risk adjustment • Reinsurance • Actuarial services • Premium allocation/risk sharing • Legal services • Financial services	• Disease management • Demand management • Utilization and referral management • Outcomes management • Case management • Health risk appraisal • Practice profiling and credentialing • Population-based management • Critical pathways • Clinical/practice guidelines	• Organization/governance • Faculty practice • Physician leadership and training • Physician productivity • Physician compensation • Incentive alignment • Documentation redesign • Billing, accounts receivable

Courtesy of Ernst & Young LLP.

tives, and support the practice effort of the physician enterprise.

Network management refers to the development and management of the overall clinical delivery system. The intent is not only to acquire the clinical services necessary to provide a full continuum of care, but also to build the administrative and organizational infrastructure to manage the strategic and operational activities ongoing within the system.

Information system (IS) and information technology (IT) refer to a comprehensive system capable of accessing, integrating, and processing data, real-time, throughout the delivery system. IS and IT are critical elements of advanced care management. Typical technology enablers include automated clinical information systems, automated medical records, clinical decision support systems, health maintenance surveillance systems, comparative databases, and technology-based education tools.

Integration model refers to provider organizational structure and processes that help transform individual program elements into a truly integrated care management system. A very simple example is a physician-hospital organization (PHO).* The PHO attempts to integrate providers for the purpose of accepting risk-based managed care contracts. If under capitated contracts the hospital and physicians now share financial risk, the PHO frequently encourages development of more sophisticated medical management programs. The structural link of the PHO provides the health system with an opportunity to share information critical to managing contracts negotiated by the PHO.

---

*The authors recognize that many PHOs have not been successful, and do not intend by the example in this chapter to necessarily endorse one structure over another.

PART I

Member Health Risk Assessment

Health risk assessments, sometimes called health risk appraisals, have been with us for several decades. These tools generally have not been used effectively—some physicians might administer them, some individual citizens might self-administer an appraisal, but for the most part, they remained neglected. The world of health risk assessments has changed dramatically in the past decade. Where there was once a generalized approach, these assessments have evolved into much more sophisticated tools not only for the identification of high risk behaviors, but for identification of members who are not yet seriously ill but have serious potential to become significantly sicker. The potential to have a positive effect on health outcomes and to better manage health care resources has grown along with the evolution of these tools. In Part I, you will read about how health risk assessments have changed and improved and how to use them more effectively than has been done in the past.

CHAPTER 2

Introduction to Health Risk Appraisals

Walter S. Elias

Chapter Outline

- Introduction
- HRA Models
- HRA Technologies
- Target Populations
- The Future

INTRODUCTION

Health risk appraisal (HRA) is a procedure that uses epidemiological data to project the mortality or morbidity risk of an individual over some future period, usually 10 years. An HRA has three parts.

- the instrument—a questionnaire that gathers current health, health history, family health history, and health-related behavior information about the individual
- the risk projection calculation—a formula (usually a computerized model) that uses the information provided in the instrument to calculate the user's risk, commonly expressed as "health age"
- the message or report—a means of informing the user of his or her current risk and suggesting behavioral changes that could mitigate that risk

The use of health history to diagnose disease and/or health risk dates to Hippocrates in the fourth century BC. However, the formal linking of an HRA instrument and risk projection is credited to Drs Lewis C. Robbins and Jack H. Hall at Methodist Hospital in Indianapolis. Their instructional book for physicians, *How to Practice Prospective Medicine*, was published in 1970.[1] It provided a procedure for recording patient health habits and family and personal health history, calculating risk of mortality due to chronic disease or accident, and then working with the patient to modify risk factors (eg, lose weight or lower cholesterol) and thereby lower risk of death.

The practice was slow to catch on because physicians were not yet ready to incorporate preventive medicine into their everyday practice. The HRA concept was given an enormous boost in the late 1970s when the Canadian government made the HRA process part of its national public health policy. Shortly thereafter, the Centers for Disease Control (CDC) computerized the Robbins and Hall methodology. Several entrepreneurial organizations, recognizing the potential benefit of the HRA concept, built on the CDC computerized model and integrated it into their corporate wellness products as an assessment tool. HRAs were widely used as a planning tool for corporate health promotion as well as for raising individual awareness and motivation.

Early HRAs computed patient mortality risk. Later, methodology was developed to incorporate morbidity risk as well. The Risk Factor Update project and a Canadian initiative improved the accuracy of risk prediction.[2]

Under the Robbins and Hall model, risk of death was seen as a motivator for behavior change. This philosophy gradually fell into disfavor, as it became apparent that most people recognized the health dangers of smoking and other risky behaviors but needed help to change their behavior. Thus, the HRA evolved to a more habit-based model. New technology has supported this evolution, using interactive voice technology, the Internet, and tailored messages via digital printing to deliver user-specific support for behavior change.

As the medical community undergoes change and managed care organizations (MCOs) begin to dominate the care delivery scene, health assessment is changing as well. New tools no longer calculate morbidity and mortality risk. These tools are really data collection instruments and sometimes overlook member feedback, although some still offer feedback reports to members. The new emphasis is on utilization prediction rather than health risk, with MCOs segmenting the population and targeting "demand management" or care management efforts for specific groups as a means of both delivering appropriate care and managing costs under a capitated payment structure.

HRA MODELS

The basic structure of the traditional HRA model has changed little from the Robbins and Hall procedure. It begins with a questionnaire, which may be administered directly by a physician or nurse practitioner or be filled out by the patient as a paper form, in a telephone interview, using an automated interactive telephone questionnaire, on a computer, or over the Internet. The core questionnaire may be as brief as 25 questions or as long as 100 or more. Each question attempts to capture an important piece of information regarding the patient's current health status, health history, family health history, or habits and behavior.

The information from the HRA instrument is input into a predictive/analytical model, which uses known cause and effect factors to determine probable outcomes for this patient. The model makes it possible to estimate the patient's risk of death from disease or accident. In early HRAs, the person scoring the instrument would calculate scores for particular sections of the questionnaire and then look them up in an actuarial table to determine the probable risk. Now scoring is done by a computer, allowing more sophisticated analysis of factors and results.

Results are compiled in a report that identifies the patient's risk factors and that may suggest lifestyle changes. As HRAs become more sophisticated, more specific instructions and messages based on population segmentation and comorbidity may be delivered.

When the same HRA tool is used for large groups of people, it is possible to aggregate data for planning purposes. This is particularly useful in commercial populations, where it is possible to assemble a variety of screening and health education programs to help individuals stay healthy or modify their behavior. Managed care populations need to be able to predict the utilization of health services in the short term. Often, screening tools that no longer incorporate the Robbins and Hall methodology serve this purpose best, supplemented by physician referrals, claims analysis, or input from utilization review.

Various health assessment models concentrate on measuring risk of disease or death, likelihood of changing health behavior (incorporating the Prochaska readiness-to-change model,[3] as discussed below), and utilization of health care services.

Risk-Based HRAs

The earliest HRAs, based on the Robbins and Hall methodology, were risk-based. They were designed to measure mortality risk factors and have demonstrated acceptable validity in measuring and predicting risk on a group basis. A major study of predictive validity of 41 HRA scoring systems found acceptable validity coefficients of .65 to .79, although some HRAs overestimated mortality risk.[4] All studies addressed risk validity at the group level. No research to date suggests that any traditional HRA accurately predicts individual risks.

As risk-based HRAs evolved, they embraced morbidity risks as well as mortality factors, with approximately the same level of accuracy. Projections of group results are based on average probabilities of highly variable risk distributions, as developed by the CDC. Thus, while the averages hold for large populations, for any given individual the outcome can be anywhere within a sizable range.

Early HRAs projected mortality risk in terms of health age. That is, given the specific health behavior characteristics of an individual, he or she had the same life expectancy as a person of a specific age, based on national mortality statistics. For example, a 36-year-old man who was 65 pounds overweight, smoked two packs of cigarettes per day, drank six alcoholic beverages per day, and never wore his seat belt might have a health age of 51. The individual's "achievable" age, the normative age-equivalent that could be attained if all controllable risk factors were at optimum levels, was also projected.

While this method was expected to capture individuals' attention and motivate them, it proved ineffective. First, the "age impact" of improving a risky behavior could usually be measured in months, not years. The impact was not dramatic enough to motivate people to change. Second, most people were already aware that some behaviors put them at risk. They needed help and support in effecting behavioral change; the "scare factor" of health age projections was not sufficient.

Habit-Based HRAs

As use of HRAs grew in the workplace, the shortcomings of the mortality-based risk model became apparent. The tool was insufficient to support the behavior-change goals of workplace health promotion programs. Designed as one-on-one counseling tools for physicians, the risk-based HRAs lacked sophisticated behavior change methodology.

A habit-based model emerged. This model focused on feedback on modifiable behaviors rather than mortality risk. Instead of telling an employee to just stop smoking to modify cancer risk, it put much more emphasis on how to change smoking behavior. It reduced the reliance on clinical measurements, simplified quantitative feedback, and prioritized change recommendations, providing the individual with comparisons over time. This model was much more sensitive to small behavior changes.

Habit-based HRAs incorporated the principles of behavioral science and adult education. As health promotion goals became more refined, these instruments attempted to help move the individual up the Prochaska readiness-to-change continuum,[3] rather than effect an immediate and complete behavior change. Questionnaires have been refined to include behavioral intentions, barriers to change, organizational factors, and attitudes toward health. And the model has utilized emerging "mass customization" technologies to individualize messages.[5] Instead of a one-size-fits-all report, participants receive newsletters, pamphlets, or books containing personalized guidance based on these individuals' specific risks and their willingness to address them. No longer does the marathon runner receive a report advising him or her to start a walking program.

Although HRAs were once administered as both a measurement tool and an intervention, the habit-based model clearly separates the two functions. There is no evidence that feedback from the instrument itself produces behavioral change.[6] Therefore, the focus has shifted to more precise definitions of target populations and their segments.

Utilization-Based HRAs

There is a growing trend in the managed care industry to look to traditional HRAs as predictors of health-care utilization. However, there is no evidence that these tools are particularly effective in predicting who will use health care services. To the contrary, research has concluded that

- One HRA model accounted for only 6% to 8% of the variance in health care costs.[7]

- Most HRA-identified variance was accounted for by psychosocial variables and not traditional physiological risk factors.[8]
- Mortality and morbidity risk is not a good predictor of health care services utilization.[9]

Often, a small percentage of employees or members will account for a large percentage of utilization. This so-called Pareto group (named for the Italian economist who noted a similar pattern in the concentration of wealth) is the key to successful utilization prediction. Table 2–1 shows how health care costs of $300,000 might be distributed in a company with 100 employees.

As shown in Table 2–1, the most expensive five employees accounted for almost three quarters of the total health care expenditures. To date, no instrument has successfully predicted when individuals will move from the general low utilization group to the Pareto group, nor do we know which risk factors predict utilization behavior. However, this is a fertile area of research and new product development.

HRAs can be valuable tools for determining intervention strategy and for helping individuals change, but they are of little value in screening for high utilizers. Some screening tools not using HRA methodology have the capability to identify potential high utilizers accurately. A simple eight-question tool developed at the University of Minnesota for seniors has proved valid in several test populations.[10] A screening questionnaire enables a provider to know that a member will become a high utilizer of health care services, but further assessment is necessary before it is known which health resources will be used and any treatment plan can be put into place.

HRA TECHNOLOGIES

Health risk assessments have taken advantage of virtually all available technologies with some degree of success. A physician or nurse, either in the office or over the phone, directly administered the earliest HRAs (interestingly, after 30 years, this method of use is again in favor, as noted in Chapter 3). As soon as the HRA moved from the "one-on-one" physician-patient environment to the mass commercial market, companies supplying HRA tools moved to the best available technologies.

The first escalation was to machine-scorable paper-and-pencil surveys. As in many standardized examinations, users marked their multiple-choice selections in an appropriate box. Their questionnaires were read by mark-sense equipment and computer scored. Some early HRAs were structured for self-scoring or were designed for computerized instant feedback.

Businesses with local area networks can put HRAs on the network and let employees fill them out during work hours. This remote processing strategy allows for instant compilation and permits interactivity as well. With the proliferation of home computers, the HRA can also be provided as "take-home" software. Today, the Internet is also a viable delivery strategy. All of these interactive computer-based systems provide for instant compilation and response.

Where computers are not available, the telephone network can serve nearly the same purpose. Interactive voice response technology allows the HRA to be administered by a computer over the telephone with the user signaling choices using the touch-tone pad.

Response rates for HRAs vary not so much by technology as by surveyed population. Some populations, such as the elderly, respond in high numbers to any survey dealing with their health and/or their health care provider. Other popula-

Table 2–1 Distribution of Health Care Costs in Example Company

Number of Employees	Average Cost per Employee ($)	Total Cost ($)
20	100	2,000
60	500	30,000
15	3,000	45,000
5	44,600	223,000

Source: Copyright © 1993, Bruce Barge.

tions, such as young adults who are most prone to risky behavior, respond in low numbers unless the health care organization or employer provides a rich incentive. Expect participation rates of 20% to 50% in commercial populations and 50% to 90% in Medicare risk groups.

This technology has allowed a more individualized approach to HRA administration and reporting, while also making it easier to analyze groups and compare them with norms from similar populations. The individualization follows the habit-based model and provides direct support to individuals in effecting changes to modifiable behavior patterns. The compilation capabilities allow the HRA to become a key input tool for developing health promotion programs and, in some cases, disease management strategies.

TARGET POPULATIONS

Capitation and other forms of performance-based reimbursement or risk sharing in the U.S. medical system (see *The Managed Health Care Handbook, 3rd Edition* for an in-depth discussion of these forms of reimbursement) have created a demand for more appropriate utilization of health resources within specific population groups. And, while HRAs are poor predictors of individual utilization of health resources, they do provide valuable population data and can be used as one part of a strategy for more effective health management.

HRAs originally came into prominence as key tools for helping businesses manage health care costs. By surveying their employee populations, businesses were able to identify groups that represented higher risk and implement health promotion programs to reduce the risk. This might take the form of smoking cessation and weight loss clinics, antidrug programs, campaigns to promote the use of seat belts, and educational programs to make people more aware of their health and smarter consumers of health services. MCOs often administer HRAs and run health promotion programs as part of their marketing strategy to attract and keep large commercial clients.

HRAs in the commercial population are frequently coupled with cholesterol tests, blood pressure checks, and other types of health screenings. These tools become part of a campaign to make employees more aware and more responsible for their own health.

More recently, health care organizations have been serving Medicare and Medicaid populations on a capitated basis. The dollar limitations require better management of services delivered. Both the Medicare and Medicaid populations use many health care services. Both populations are subject to chronic diseases such as diabetes and asthma. If not managed, these chronic diseases can lead to catastrophic costs. But these diseases can be managed within a relatively low-cost model that actually provides higher quality of life for patients.

Recently, tiers of screening tools have been used to help manage these populations. At the top level, all group members are given a questionnaire that is designed for the specific population. (For Medicare populations, it will focus on issues for seniors; for Medicaid populations, it may focus on issues of concern to many single parents—family violence, basic nutrition, and so on.)

Individuals who state that they have a disease or are at risk due to their living environment are given a more specific questionnaire (often administered on the telephone) that identifies disease- or condition-specific situations that may increase the individual's risk. The results of these disease-specific HRAs are input for case managers or other providers assigned to help these individuals adjust their lifestyle to reduce their risk and to help train the individuals in relevant self-care.

Follow-up questionnaires may be administered as frequently as every 3 months. Results of these programs indicate that they are effective in reducing the number of emergency room visits, physician visits, hospital stays, and sick days.[11]

This multitiered strategy that first segments specific populations for more intense treatment, then develops very specific information about their needs, has delivered both lower cost and better care. It is the disease management model

Exhibit 2–1 Methods for Identifying and Intervening with High Utilizers of Health Care: Comparison of Next-Generation and Traditional HRAs

Next-Generation Instrument	**Traditional Health Risk Appraisal**
• Collects a broader scope of health information than traditional HRAs. Measures the major risks for high utilization. • Assesses the behavioral sources of total employee benefit costs. • Is integrated with a telephone-based health consultation service. • Offers built-in longitudinal follow-up to support behavior change and motivation. • Is linked with system providing analysis of medical claims. Analysis suggests targeted interventions.	• Is narrowly focused on risk for disease and death: cancer, heart disease, and stroke. • Is focused on less than 15% of total benefit costs: the contribution of cancer, heart disease, and stroke to group health costs. • Is not integrated with toll-free nurseline for employee use. • Uses episodic and short-term follow-up. • Has almost no claims analysis capacity.

Source: Courtesy of Elias & Associates, Inc, St Louis Park, Minnesota.

that promises to be the major focus for future health assessment tools.

THE FUTURE

The HRA of the future will reflect the needs of managed care to identify and manage high utilizers of health care resources (Exhibit 2–1). It will be integrated into a suite of products and services that allows intervention throughout the continuum of risk. For low- and medium-risk groups, interventions will be administered through nurselines, self-care books, on-line services, and targeted newsletters. The high-risk population will see a new generation of psychosocially oriented case managers, counselors, and call nurses working to remove barriers to more appropriate use of health care services.

REFERENCES

1. Robbins L, Hall J. *How To Practice Prospective Medicine.* Indianapolis, IN: Methodist Hospital; 1970.
2. Schoenbach VJ, Wagner EH, Beery WL. Health risk appraisal: review of evidence for effectiveness. *Health Serv Res.* 1987;22:553–580.
3. Prochaska J, Norcross J, Di Clemente C. *Changing for Good.* New York: William Morrow; 1994.
4. Smith KW, McKinlay SM, Thorington BD. The validity of health risk appraisal instruments for assessing coronary heart disease risk. *Am J Public Health.* 1987;77:419–424.
5. Strecher VJ, Kreuter M, DenBoer DJ, et al. The effects of computer-tailored smoking cessation messages in family practice settings. *J Fam Prac.* 1994;39:262–270.
6. Anderson DR, Staufacker MJ. The impact of worksite-based health risk appraisal on health-related outcomes: a review of the literature. *Am J Health Promo.* 1996;10:499–508.
7. Golaszewski T, Lynch W, Clearie A, Vickery D. The relationship between retrospective health insurance claims and a health risk appraisal–generated measure of health status. *J Occupational Med.* 1989;31:262–264.
8. Yen L, Edington D, Witting P. Associations between health risk appraisal scores and employee medical claims costs in a manufacturing company. *Am J Health Promo.* 1991;6:46–54.
9. Lynch WD, Vickery DM. The potential impact of health promotion on health care utilization: an introduction to demand management. *Am J Health Promo.* 1993;8:87–92.
10. Boult C, Pacala JT, Boult LB. Targeting elders for geriatric evaluation and management: reliability, validity, and practicality of a questionnaire. *Aging Clin Exp Res.* 1995;7:159–164.
11. Fries JF, Carey C, McShane FJ. Patient education in arthritis: randomized controlled trial of a mail-delivered program. *J Rheumatol.* 1997;24:1378–1383.

WALTER S. ELIAS, PHD, is currently chief executive officer of Kosmeo, Inc, a St Paul, Minnesota, based company specializing in product and business development in prevention, disease, and demand management. He has over 20 years of experience in marketing and applied research in health care cost containment and corporate wellness programs. His PhD is in anthropology and sociology, and he has combined his research background in health care cost containment with solid sales/marketing and program development skills.

CHAPTER 3

Choosing and Using a Health Risk Appraisal Instrument

Walter S. Elias

Chapter Outline

- Introduction
- Why?
- Who?
- How?
- When?
- What Action?
- Methodology Issues
- Evaluating Instruments
- Conclusion

INTRODUCTION

Implementing a health risk appraisal (HRA) represents a substantial expense. Therefore, most organizations do not begin using an HRA without specific goals and a desire for a return on investment through improved health, more targeted care, and lower cost.

An organization looking to purchase an assessment tool must select from a bewildering number of vendors, types of instruments, delivery systems, and analytical engines.[1] There are tools specifically designed for certain population groups, specific diseases, and demand management. It is fair to say that whatever an organization's health goals, there is at least one health assessment product available to serve those needs, or there is an organization that will custom-design one to fit the need.

Despite the vast array of available products, leaders of many organizations choose to build their own, sometimes from scratch and sometimes building on an existing platform. This decision may be based on a belief that no one knows their organization and/or populations as well as they do. As shown in Exhibit 3–1, the driving motivation is often that the process of designing an assessment tool is an excellent team building exercise and a perfect excuse to bring together personnel from all the organizations that will team to serve the target population. Even where an organization chooses to design and administer the questionnaire, it may look to outside agencies for analysis and reporting. It is clear, however, that a vendor-purchased instrument will be in use far sooner than one built in-house.

In this chapter we will look at the key decision points relative to selecting or designing an instrument and provide references that will aid readers in finding information about specific HRAs and HRA vendors. The key questions are:

- Why?
- Who?
- How?
- When?
- What Action?

WHY?

Organizations employ HRAs for different reasons. As depicted in Figure 3–1, employers

Exhibit 3–1 Build Versus Buy Analysis for a Health Risk Appraisal Instrument

Build	Buy
• Long time to market	• Quick to market
• Reliability and validity testing is time- and labor-intensive	• Testing complete
	• Instrument dropped in
• Development process brings together functional units of organization into a functioning team	• Need vendor to consult on integration process (typically not their expertise)
• Better integration into care process	

Courtesy of Elias & Associates, Inc, St Louis Park, Minnesota.

have traditionally used this mechanism to identify the prevalence of high-risk behavior. Then, based on the aggregate data, they developed or purchased behavior modification programming. Low- and medium-risk employees are offered maintenance programs.

Managing escalating health care cost is certainly one motivation for using HRAs, but businesses also believe that there is a payoff in increased employee productivity and job satisfaction. Repeated use of the HRA provides an easy mechanism for measuring the progress achieved with health promotion programming.

Health care organizations are more interested in targeting and segmenting populations. Some managed care organizations (MCOs) embed satisfaction surveys into health assessment questionnaires to satisfy the National Commit-

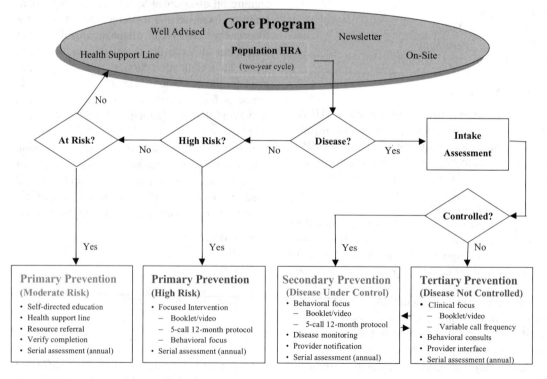

Figure 3–1 "At Risk" Interventions. Courtesy of Staywell, Inc, St Paul, Minnesota

tee for Quality Assurance (NCQA; see Chapter 33) and the Health Plan Employer Data and Information Set (HEDIS; see Chapter 37) requirements. Administration of HRAs has been part of health care plan marketing programs to commercial customers.

With the increase in capitated health care payment systems, targeting and stratification approaches have been applied to help health care providers plan and deliver services more cost-effectively and encourage health care users to use the system's resources more appropriately. At the highest level, the tool may be used to stratify the plan's members into the well, worried well, persons with chronic conditions, and the very ill. This may be refined to target groups within the population that exhibit specific behavior patterns that increase health risk—such as smoking, driving without a seat belt, and so on. The plan then provides information and access to programs that will educate members and/or help them change their behavior.

Stratification and targeting can become more refined. Many employers and health care providers escalate to the next step, demand management. Rather than wait for individuals identified as high risk to call in for services, those individuals are approached via telephone counseling services or targeted print messages.

More organizations—both health care providers and specialized disease management firms—are using health assessment tools to enhance disease management. At the highest level, members with chronic conditions are identified by a general questionnaire. Then, these members receive disease-specific instruments that zero in on their behavior relative to their specific medical condition—such as asthma, diabetes, or hypertension. Answers to the disease-specific tool guide intervention via targeted messages, nurseline counseling (see Chapter 11), or case management (see Chapter 17).[2]

WHO?

Who should be surveyed with a health assessment instrument depends on what the organization wants to achieve. Some businesses survey only their employees. Others, recognizing that a higher percentage of health care cost is associated with dependents than with employees themselves, try to incorporate every covered life in the process.

Health care organizations often apply the tool to identifiable capitated groups such as Medicare, Medicaid, and commercial users. Some try to segment further, surveying teenagers and young adults where there is an immediate need for and potential payoff from education regarding risky behavior, sexual practices, and parenting.

In the disease management model, the instrument is used with specific chronic disease groups, such as persons with diabetes (see Chapter 29), asthma (see Chapter 30), osteoarthritis, or hypertension.

HOW?

Traditional pencil-and-paper surveys still dominate health assessment administration. People are handed surveys at work, receive surveys in their mailboxes, or are given surveys while in their physician's waiting room. The second most popular survey method is the in-person survey. Questions are posed, either over the phone or in the physician's office, by a trained interviewer. Both of these methods are costly and slow. Data must be converted from the manual entry to a computer-readable format.

Modern technology is catching on. Two technologies show the most promise.

- interactive voice response (IVR), where the questionnaire is administered over a touch-tone telephone by a computer and the respondent enters responses using the touch-tone pad
- the Internet, where the respondent accesses the survey at a Web site and answers the questions using the computer keyboard

These two methods allow for a more interactive and directed questionnaire that can be refined in real time in response to the answers given. They also allow for immediate scoring and instant feedback, if desired.

WHEN?

HRAs may be administered annually by most employers. MCOs usually administer a health assessment when individuals enroll. Some follow up with an annual or biannual survey.

There is a growing practice within MCOs to administer a senior health assessment whenever there is a significant change in health state, such as a hospitalization or diagnosis of a chronic condition.

WHAT ACTION?

While the information gathered via an HRA has value, the real value is in the action precipitated by the HRA response. The type of response varies by the intent of the process. Most commercial population HRAs result in a health risk profile that is given to the individual and that suggests behavioral changes. A few commercial organizations screen for very high risk people and then engage proactively in direct counseling to assist in behavior change.[3] This level of concern and willingness to challenge privacy issues are still rare.

Generic health information has proven to be worth little in actually causing behavior change. However, better results have been garnered with messages tailored to individuals' specific situations and needs.[4] Some health questionnaires focus on the interests of both the health care organization and the member. They output customized newsletters or telephone messages specific to individuals' needs. Generally, they focus on a single high-priority issue and attempt to move individuals at least one more step up the readiness-to-change[3] ladder.

Under the demand management model, individuals receive information that will help them get appropriate care using minimal health care resources. This care may include a self-help book focused on a specific situation, such as parenting. It may include specific instructions for a condition, such as a prenatal nutrition plan and schedule for obstetrical visits. Often, a special helpline is identified, where the individual can be counseled over the phone.

Output from disease-management-focused instruments is the most specific. Under this model, the individual is provided a detailed self-care plan (or the provider is supplied with a medical management plan) that is tailored to the individual's disease state.[5] This approach is discussed in several chapters in Part X.

METHODOLOGY ISSUES

HRAs are built around probability models. Most instruments have been designed using the same risk tables that are based on decades of data captured and published by the Centers for Disease Control. The predictive value of these instruments is at the group level. No instrument—be it an HRA, a paper-and-pencil health assessment tool, or a claims-based product that attempts to estimate future utilization—predicts with high accuracy on the individual level. These instruments still require the expertise of the health educator, psychologist, nurse, or physician to round out the picture. Thus, HRA data at the aggregate level is useful for planning resource requirements but cannot accurately predict what it will cost a health care organization to cover a specific individual.

There is a danger in the HRA process that must be considered when using even aggregate data for resource planning. Most HRAs are self-administered. Persons willing to complete an HRA may be different from the general population. They may, for example, be persons referred to as the "worried well," that is, healthy people who are concerned about their health. Historically, persons with chronic lifestyle[6] disorders, such as obesity, depression, or chemical dependency, are least likely to fill out the survey, or, if they do fill it out, are most apt to lie. Thus HRAs tend to undersample the most at-risk individuals and oversample the healthiest.

EVALUATING INSTRUMENTS

Some commercially available HRA instruments are high-quality products that use sound probability analysis based on nationally reported disease incidence and, most recently, outcome data. Vendor selection should be based in part on vendors' medical and scientific credibility. Since health assessment is used to satisfy a variety of needs, look to see how well the particular type of instrument meets your organization's goals.

Of course, targeting and segmentation of populations can be accomplished through the analysis of medical claims.[7] Various organizations use medical claims, pharmacy, and membership data to predict which members will utilize the most resources. Many plans combine claims analysis with HRAs.[8]

The instrument can be tested for ease of use and comprehensibility with focus groups of people that mirror the organization's demographics and psychographics. The focus groups can rate the time involved—too much, too little—and the method of administering. New technologies should also be tested with focus groups. Some groups have a level of technophobia that precludes using computers or even telephones as a delivery method. Other groups embrace the new technologies.

Health assessment instrument vendors typically do not know what effect their instrument has had on behavioral or disease outcomes. It is often too administratively difficult and costly to conduct research that is able to separate the effects of the HRA from subsequent interventions.

CONCLUSION

HRAs have two principal values: (1) they gather data for statistical analysis of groups, allowing effective planning of resources; and (2) they encapsulate an individual's health history, providing a basis for one-on-one counseling. Questionnaires and statistical reports by themselves do not constitute an effective intervention. However, the process is effective for preparing an individual for intervention.

Historically, HRAs have more accurately reflected the general population than the Pareto group (ie, those individuals who will consume the most system resources). Members of the Pareto group tend to avoid filling out the questionnaire or fill it out inaccurately.

A hierarchical HRA structure that first identifies a population subgroup with a particular condition, then drills down to the specific risks of individuals within the subgroup, can be effective in managing a chronic disease.

For any HRA to be effective, it must result in an individualized, actionable plan based on both what the health plan wants the member to do as well as what the member is prepared to do. Surveys that leave out member feedback lose the opportunity to affect member retention and involve the member in self-management practices.

REFERENCES

1. Peterson KW, Hilles SB, eds. *Handbook of Health Risk Appraisals*. Omaha, NE: Society of Prospective Medicine; 1996.
2. Montgomery EB, Lieberman A, Singh G, et al. Patient education and health promotion can be effective in Parkinson's disease: a randomized controlled trial. *Am J Med*. 1994;97:429–435.
3. Russell C. A new model for demand and disease management services. *Managing Employ Health Benefits*. Fall 1997;35–41.
4. Strecher VJ, Kreuter MW. The psychosocial and behavioral impact of health risk appraisals. In: Croyle RT, ed. *Psychosocial Effects of Screening for Disease Prevention and Detection*. New York: Oxford University Press; 1995.
5. Wehrwein P. Can health plans change behavior? *Managed Care*. 1997;6:23–38.
6. Lynch WD, Gilfillan LA, Jennet C, et al. Health risks and health insurance claims costs: results for health hazard appraisal responders and nonresponders. *J Occupational Med*. 1993;35:28–33.
7. Allen J. Electronic clinical logic revamps medical management. *Data Strat Benchmarks*. January 1998: 1–4.
8. Fletcher J, Hoggard Green J. Population health planning and management: two case studies from benchmarking organizations. Presented at the National Chronic Care Consortium National Conference; September 22, 1997; Minneapolis, MN.

WALTER S. ELIAS, PHD, is currently chief executive officer of Kosmeo, Inc, a St Paul, Minnesota, based company specializing in product and business development in prevention, disease, and demand management. He has over 20 years of experience in marketing and applied research in health care cost containment and corporate wellness programs. His PhD is in anthropology and sociology, and he has combined his research background in health care cost containment with solid sales/marketing and program development skills.

PART II

Primary Prevention

The very term *health maintenance organization* was predicated on the concept that health could be maintained through early detection and prevention. This has proven to be a central part of most managed care organizations, though this has not always been acknowledged. Further, some plans have not concentrated on this aspect of medical management, placing far more focus on the management of acute care. There are many arguments that prevention is cost effective, and there are an equal number of arguments that prevention costs money that is never recouped. To argue prevention in economic terms completely misses the point—prevention should be done when it is effective and can improve the health of the population. In Part II, you will read about how prevention is carried out in sophisticated managed care organizations and how special attention is given to proactively reaching out to members of a health plan, as well as to the underserved and immigrant population, who are increasingly showing up in managed health care plans.

Chapter 4

Prevention in Managed Care

Leif I. Solberg

Chapter Outline

- Introduction
- Why Should an MCO Do Prevention?
- A Typology of HP/DP Activities
- A Framework for Action
- Community Outreach Programs
- Public Policy Initiatives
- Prevention Section Overview

INTRODUCTION

Mary Jones was already favorably inclined toward health maintenance organization (HMO) X because she had heard about its goal of reducing heart attacks by 25% and its success in reducing preterm births and had seen its clever television counter-advertising discouraging teenage smoking. Therefore, when her employer offered HMO X as one of the alternatives for her health care, she chose that plan. And she was pleasantly surprised when she was given the opportunity to complete the plan's health risk assessment survey (see Chapters 2 and 3) at work. She was even more pleased when a health education counselor called from HMO X to discuss how HMO X could help Mary with the weight and exercise concerns she had identified in the survey. The counselor told her about the relevant health promotion programs they had developed at her workplace and about other community resources. The counselor also explained that the HMO provided various counselors who could assist her over the telephone. And when staff at the primary clinic she had chosen took advantage of her visit to identify her disease prevention needs and to recommend specific services for Mary and her family, she knew she would never willingly go anywhere else for care.

Corny? Impossible? Such a scenario is occurring daily at HealthPartners, and various elements of it are a growing part of other leading managed care organization (MCO) programs around the country. HealthPartners is a 750,000-member MCO with one third of the members served by a staff model medical group and two thirds served through contracts and partnerships with 47 primary care medical groups and about 2,500 consultants. It is concentrated in the Minneapolis-St. Paul metropolitan region of Minnesota, where about 80% of the population is covered by managed care. This chapter is designed to encourage the spread of health promotion and disease prevention (HP/DP) activities by explaining why they are increasingly prevalent in MCOs, to provide conceptual frameworks for these activities, and to describe examples of them. Although most examples are drawn from the experience of HealthPartners, many other MCOs are doing similar things.

WHY SHOULD AN MCO DO PREVENTION?

Because It Is Possible

When HMOs were first conceived, Ellwood et al called them health maintenance organizations because they thought that the prepaid economics and the integrated care system would make it both attractive and feasible to shift health care from an illness-based approach to one that emphasizes preventing disease and maintaining health.[1] Although they didn't foresee the high turnover of members, which makes it less obvious that prevention services will pay off financially, MCOs still have the advantages of a large defined population and an integrated comprehensive care system. They also have data about the health and health care of that population. These elements make it possible to address prevention in a way that was nearly impossible in a fragmented fee-for-service (FFS) marketplace.

Unfortunately, it has become a common joke to ridicule the term "health maintenance organization" as if these plans provide no more prevention actions than a typical FFS does. Studies comparing members of HMOs with those in indemnity insurance plans have mostly confirmed that HMO members receive more clinical preventive services, even when (as in the classic Rand study) those services are free for FFS members.[2-4] However, there have been no good studies comparing other types of HP/DP services. Nevertheless, there is reason to doubt that this potential has been very widely exploited, and some of the HMO advantage may have been due to selection bias.

Because It Is Becoming Necessary

Although there is a growing proportion of the population that, like Mary Jones above, values prevention, we have still not reached the point where prevention activities determine the choices of most potential MCO members. However, the purchasing decisions are still being made largely by employers, employer groups, and governments, and they are increasingly wanting evidence of effective prevention programs. This is evidenced by the Health Plan Employer Data and Information Set (HEDIS; see Chapter 37) measures, many of which are prevention indicators.

Rundall and Schauffler have suggested that the ability, necessity, and extent of managed care prevention activities will depend upon the evolutionary stage of the local health care marketplace.[2] Table 4–1 illustrates their ideas about this association between market stage and prevention for MCOs. In the Twin Cities, we are well into Stage 4, expecting that the next stage

Table 4–1 Market Stage and Prevention

Stage	Description	Prevention
1	Largely fee-for-service and provider groups that are not allied.	Prevention gets little attention and is limited to clinical preventive services.
2	Prepaid care and mergers develop.	There is more concern about appropriateness of preventive services and with development of health data systems and some health promotion activities.
3	Prepaid care covers 30% to 50% of the population; purchaser alliances may develop.	MCOs are being held accountable for quality, service, and access, including prevention. This requires plans to improve, to collect data about health status and risks, and to address community health and collaborative actions.
4	Most of the population is covered by prepaid care, and purchaser alliances demand both cost reduction and quality.	Population-based and public policy aspects of HP/DP become increasingly important along with much more active attention and accountability for all aspects of prevention.

Source: Data from TG Rundall and HH Schauffler, Health Promotion and Disease Prevention in Integrated Delivery Systems: The Role of Market Forces, *American Journal of Preventive Medicine*, Vol 13, pp 244–250, © 1997, American College of Preventive Medicine, Association of Teachers of Preventive Medicine.

will only increase the need to devote attention and resources to prevention. Where is your marketplace in this picture?

A TYPOLOGY OF HP/DP ACTIVITIES

Regardless of the stage of your marketplace, it is useful to have a conceptual typology when establishing your plan's prevention activities. A modification of Rundall and Schauffler's typology[2] seems as good as any, building on the same evolutionary sequence shown in Table 4–1.

Clinical Preventive Services

These are services provided primarily in the clinical care setting, essentially all of the screening, counseling, and immunization activities considered by the U.S. Preventive Services Task Force.[5–6] They include efforts to reduce risks for both asymptomatic individuals and those with existing diseases.

Health Data Systems

This involves taking advantage of existing administrative, financial, and utilization data systems as well as creating and integrating systems that capture population-based health-related information such as outcomes, risks, use of preventive services, and various epidemiologic data.

Population-Based (Member) Programs

Here, HP/DP services are provided to individuals and groups in schools, workplaces, and other venues. These services include health education classes, group behavior change programs, and direct MCO outreach to members through the mail or phone systems. They often involve relationships with nonmembers of the MCO and with various community organizations.

Community Programs

These programs are aimed at the entire community and are intended to influence health or health behaviors of large numbers of people, regardless of whether they are members of the MCO. Most involve media campaigns or public information and may require partnerships or collaborations, sometimes with competitors.

Public Policy

This covers the advocacy for public policies aimed at protecting or improving the health of the entire population. It requires policy analysis and participation in the political process, usually in collaboration with other organizations.

A FRAMEWORK FOR ACTION

Being able to categorize prevention activities is a necessary but insufficient foundation for carrying them out. The other and more important precondition is a strong commitment to prevention from senior leadership. In the absence of such leadership desire, active support, and commitment of major resources, it may not be possible to achieve very much.

Berwick has identified leadership as a key element in a new, more effective approach to prevention.[7] The other keys are process and system knowledge, reliance on data and information, fundamental changes in the work system, and innovation testing. His agenda is a good summary of what an MCO needs to do for prevention (Exhibit 4–1).

In keeping with that agenda, once MCO leaders decide to make prevention an organizational priority, they should establish specific public objectives and designate authority, responsibility, and resources to achieve those objectives. Ideally, those objectives should be information based and measurable, and they should require such a large effort that many will doubt they can be accomplished. The eight goals established at HealthPartners to be accomplished within 4 years are listed in Table 4–2. When these goals were established, HealthPartners announced them in a very public way, making it very hard to avoid trying its best to reach them.

Exhibit 4–1 A Prevention Agenda

1. Refine general aims into specific, measurable goals for care systems. These goals are needed to focus improvement energies but must be locally sensible and modified over time as needed.
2. Develop new designs for the delivery of preventive services, designs that break the current molds of encounters, location, job descriptions, financing, and schedules.
3. Develop and ensure mechanisms for the prompt dissemination of effective new prevention designs, both locally and generally.
4. Link improving preventive practice to improving the capabilities of leaders in health care systems and communities. These leaders must have the skills necessary for managing prevention, including skills in conflict resolution, experimentation, data collection and analysis, systems thinking, and change management.

Source: Data from DM Berwick, From Measuring to Managing the Improvement of Prevention, *American Journal of Preventive Medicine,* Vol 11, No 6, pp 385–387, © 1995, American College of Preventive Medicine, Association of Teachers of Preventive Medicine.

In order to accomplish these goals and to increase our ability to promote health, many separate programs and initiatives have been developed. Most of these efforts have relied on continuous quality improvement (CQI) concepts and techniques, using a variation of the well-established PDSA (Plan-Do-Study-Act) approach to developing new processes and improving existing ones. The approach at HealthPartners involves an interdisciplinary team following an organized process improvement approach with seven steps.

1. Identify the problem (opportunity).
2. Collect the data required to understand the problem and process.
3. Analyze the data to understand root causes.
4. Develop alternatives and choose an approach.
5. Generate recommendations and methods.
6. Implement the changes.
7. Evaluate and improve.

This approach is based on using data as much as possible for making decisions and on repeated evaluation of whether changes are being implemented and are producing the desired effects. However, it is important to stick to small samples and to avoid the tendency to study problems to death. The CQI approach is also based on iterative cycles, using repeated test and measure cycles where possible, like those described by Nolan and Batalden et al.[8,9] This cyclic process is illustrated in Figure 4–1.

However, the biggest challenge is not proving that changes can work in small tests, but disseminating successful models of new systems widely throughout one's organization. This is the real test of an organization's leadership and its ability to implement the changes needed to deal with challenging times.

COMMUNITY OUTREACH PROGRAMS

At HealthPartners, we have taken very seriously the fact that tobacco use is by far the most important preventable cause of death and disease (see also Chapter 8). In order to reach beyond our membership to try to influence the entire community's attitude about tobacco, we have undertaken some major counter-advertising initiatives.

- A dragon-themed smoking cessation calendar with encouragement and quit tips for each day after quitting was distributed throughout the state as a supplement in newspapers.
- A version of this very popular calendar is being developed for similar distribution to teenagers.
- Television and radio ads were developed with extensive teen input. These ads, called "Garbage-face," feature a smoking teen girl's face being morphed into a variety of garbage collages as she talks about the ap-

Table 4–2 HealthPartners Prevention Goals for a 4-Year Period

Goal	Topic	Specifics
1	Heart disease	Reduce by 25% the number of heart disease events (eg, heart attacks).
2	Breast cancer	Reduce by 50% the number of cases that reach an advanced stage before detection and increase to 85% the number of women ages 50–74 who are screened at least biennially.
3	Diabetes	Reduce by 25% the progression from high-risk to active disease and reduce by 30% the onset and progression of eye, kidney, and nerve damage resulting from diabetes.
4	Childhood injuries	Reduce by 25% the number of childhood (ages 0–14) injuries severe enough to require medical attention and by 10% the number of those requiring hospitalization.
5	Childhood immunization	Increase from 75% to 95% the number of children fully immunized by the age of 2.
6	Pregnancy	Reduce by 30% the infant and maternal complications of pregnancy.
7	Dental caries	Reduce by 50% the number of new dental caries in all age groups among dental members.
8	Abuse	Increase by 50% the screening for domestic violence among women seen for preventive services or relevant presenting symptoms.

Courtesy of HealthPartners, Minneapolis, Minnesota.

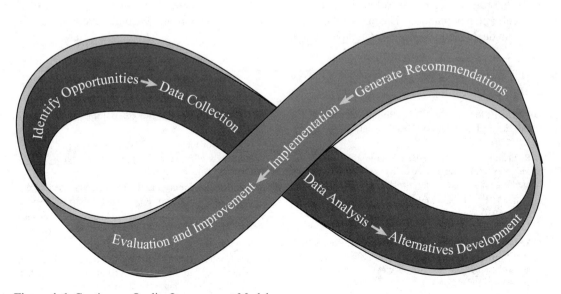

Figure 4–1 Continuous Quality Improvement Model

proach of a boy she idolizes, only to be spurned by him as he tells her to get breath mints. These ads have garnered a lot of favorable attention.

PUBLIC POLICY INITIATIVES

HealthPartners has long been an active sponsor of the Minnesota Coalition for a Smoke-Free 2000. In the past two years, however, we have made antitobacco legislation one of our lobbyists' highest priorities. In addition, a phone tree of employee volunteers has been used at several critical points in the legislative process to generate large numbers of legislator contacts on short notice. These efforts have been fairly successful and have generated both favorable attention for the company and important health promotion changes for the community.

PREVENTION SECTION OVERVIEW

Chapter 5 describes the many ways that clinical preventive services can be improved. Ideas and programs implemented at HealthPartners are used as examples.

Chapter 6 describes the innovative concepts and programs that can be developed for the entire health plan population. They go well beyond the usual health education classes and pamphlets that are typically found in MCOs or care delivery systems. We think that they represent the future and a real opportunity for an MCO to distinguish itself in quality generally and in prevention in particular. Since we know that the advice and support of one's personal clinician are critically important to a member's motivation to make health behavior change, Chapter 6 also emphasizes the various linkages that are being developed between population programs and clinical care.

Chapter 7 covers an issue that will become increasingly important to the efforts mentioned above as MCOs become responsible for the health and health care of disadvantaged and underserved populations. These populations generally have both lower rates of preventive services and higher rates of health risk factors and diseases. MCOs will need to be able to address these problems in culturally sensitive ways as they work to correct the multiple reasons for those lower rates and higher risks.

Overall, we hope that Part II of this book will heighten the interest and increase the capabilities of managed care plans to address disease prevention and health promotion issues. They are the future, and although some regions might still be in earlier market stages (see Table 4–1), farsighted plans will start to work now on what will increasingly become a necessity.

REFERENCES

1. Ellwood PM, Anderson NN, Billings JE, Carlson RJ, Hoagberg EJ, McClure W. Health maintenance strategy. *Med Care.* 1971;9:291–298.
2. Rundall TG, Schauffler HH. Health promotion and disease prevention in integrated delivery systems: the role of market forces. *Am J Prev Med.* 1997;13:244–250.
3. Miller RH, Luft HS. Managed care plan performance since 1980—a literature analysis. *JAMA.* 1997;271:1512–1519.
4. Manning WG, Leibowitz A, Goldberg GA, Rogers WH, Newhouse JP. A controlled trial of the effect of a prepaid group practice on use of services. *N Engl J Med.* 1984;310:1505–1510.
5. US Preventive Services Task Force. *Guide to Clinical Preventive Services.* 2nd ed. Baltimore: Williams & Wilkins; 1996.
6. US Department of Health & Human Services. *Clinician's Handbook of Preventive Services.* Washington, DC: US DHHS; 1994.
7. Berwick DM. From measuring to managing the improvement of prevention. *Am J Prev Med.* 1995;11:385–387.
8. Nolan T. Accelerating the pace of improvement: an interview with Thomas Nolan. *Joint Commission J Qual Improvement.* 1997;23:217–222.
9. Batalden PB, Mohr JJ, Nelson EC, Plume SK. Improving health care, part 4: concepts for improving any clinical process. *Joint Commission J Qual Improvement.* 1996;22:651–659.

SUGGESTED READINGS

Centers for Disease Control and Prevention. Prevention and managed care: organizations, purchasers of health care, and public health agencies. *JAMA*. 1996;275(1):26–29.

Schauffler HH, Rodriguez T. Managed care for preventive services: a review of policy options. *Med Care Rev*. 1993;50:153–198.

Schoenbaum SC. Implementation of preventive services in an HMO practice. *J Gen Int Med*. 1990;5(suppl): S123–S127.

Thompson RS, Taplin SH, McAfee TA, Mandelson MT, Smith AE. Primary and secondary prevention services in clinical practice: twenty years' experience in development, implementation, and evaluation. *JAMA*. 1995;273:1130–1135.

LEIF I. SOLBERG, MD, is the associate medical director for care improvement research at HealthPartners Research Foundation and a practicing family physician in the HealthPartners Medical Group. His research interests include disease prevention (especially tobacco cessation), chronic disease management, and quality improvement. He has published more than 69 peer-reviewed journal articles and 17 book chapters. Dr. Solberg is particularly interested in conducting research that addresses care delivery concerns and in translating research lessons back into patient care.

CHAPTER 5

Taking Advantage of the Clinical Setting for Prevention

Leif I. Solberg and Gail Amundson

Chapter Outline

- Introduction
- Direction and Energy
- The How of Change
- Other Considerations
- Primary Versus Secondary Prevention
- Facilitating Change from the Outside
- Conclusion

INTRODUCTION

It is both logical and important to start planning managed care prevention interventions in the clinical care setting. Members are already present for face-to-face interventions, often at times when they are particularly ready to make changes in their health risks. Moreover, members are more likely to pay attention to recommendations for preventive services or behavior changes if the recommendations come from their personal clinician. For example, the most common reason given by women for not having had a mammogram is that their physician has not encouraged them to do so.

On the other hand, there are also factors that make it difficult to use these prevention opportunities. The most important barriers are clearly time constraints and the need to focus on the presenting problem.[1] In addition, both physicians and patients have traditionally regarded the routine "physical," not other types of visits, as the time for prevention, even though many patients do not schedule routine physicals and physicals center on an examination that has been found to be of little preventive value. Thus, patients who need important clinical preventive services usually do not receive recommendations for them during acute care visits and are only somewhat more likely to receive them during physicals.[2] This is especially true for identifying behavioral risk factors and for providing counseling to modify those behaviors.

Much research has been done on this problem over the last 10 years, resulting in a gradually developing consensus that the main way to improve the above problems is to institute the systematic, organized prevention approaches that are typically absent from clinical settings. Most existing clinic systems are designed to support only acute care, in part because most physicians have not considered care for populations to be their responsibility. A recent report by the American Cancer Society Advisory Group on Preventive Health Care Reminder Systems came to this conclusion, recommending office systems and extensive delegation to office staff.[3] Solberg et al have summarized the supporting literature and described the major features of such an office prevention system[4] and have also

---

Material in this chapter was supported in part by the Agency for Health Care Policy and Research, grant RO1HS08091.

documented that those system features are currently absent in most primary care practices.[5]

It is helpful to think of an overall prevention system as a single system composed of separate processes. Each of these processes is a series of step-by-step actions designed to accomplish a particular overall task (eg, summarizing information about the current status of many preventive services for each patient). However, as with any system, those individual processes must be well integrated, and if they are not designed to serve the needs of all preventive services, they will not result in patients receiving needed services consistently. Exhibit 5–1 describes 10 of the main processes in the prevention system.

These processes describe only the supports needed for providing preventive services, not who needs to actually recommend and perform those services. It is increasingly clear that the more that nonclinician staff can be involved in recommending and performing preventive services (through standing orders), as well as in handling all other processes, the more likely it is that the system will work consistently. The trick is to increase delegation where possible without losing the valuable re-

Exhibit 5–1 Processes in a Prevention System

> **1. Guidelines:** The process by which a clinical organization develops, obtains broad buy-in, and updates a specific uniform set of preventive services for defined age/gender/risk groups. Without organizational agreement on the recommended services, effective and efficient prevention systems cannot be developed.
>
> **2. Screen:** The process of obtaining health risk and previous preventive service information in a standard way about all patients of a clinic in order to identify their specific prevention needs.
>
> **3. Summarize:** The process of organizing and updating the information obtained in the screening process so that it is all in one place and can easily be reviewed by those needing to know the current prevention status of a particular patient. Without a continuously updated summary of each patient's preventive service status, it is not possible to keep members up to date on the recommended services.
>
> **4. Cue/Remind:** The process of reminding clinic staff and clinicians about their need to undertake necessary prevention system tasks.
>
> **5. Follow-Up:** The process of communicating to patients the results of preventive services along with appropriate explanations and recommendations.
>
> **6. Resources:** The process of selecting, gathering, organizing, and maintaining patient education and referral information needed by both patients and clinic personnel.
>
> **7. Counsel:** The process of assisting patients and their families to make needed changes in their behavior.
>
> **8. Track and Recall:** The process of reminding patients, especially those patients without acute care visits, about their needs for specific preventive services.
>
> **9. Patient Activation:** The process of encouraging patients to take greater responsibility for their own preventive services and behavior changes.
>
> **10. Prevention Visits:** The process of providing all of the preventive services needed by a patient during a single visit designed and organized for that purpose. This special visit may not be necessary in the future for many patients who have their preventive service needs met during other visits.
>
> *Source:* Reprinted with permission from LI Solberg et al, Delivering Clinical Preventive Services Is a Systems Problem: The Paradigm Shift of Improvement, *Annals of Behavioral Medicine,* Vol 19, No 3, pp 271–278, © 1998, Society of Behavioral Medicine.

inforcing role of the clinician-patient relationship.

The real challenge for a managed care plan that wishes to improve the delivery of clinical preventive services in its care delivery settings is how to facilitate the development, implementation, and maintenance of such prevention systems. This is no small challenge. Nevertheless, the task is so important that it requires substantial attention. For example, routine physicals fill 20% of the appointment schedule in our staff model medical group, and nationally physicals are the most common medical visits, despite the fact that routine physicals do not address preventive needs very well.

Creating such systematic new ways to support the provision of preventive services appears to require that certain conditions be present. The conditions, which overlap with Berwick's prevention agenda from Chapter 4, are listed in Exhibit 5–2. Some might add another condition to this list—minimal distracting turmoil or financial pressure. However, turmoil can also force a medical group to change, and waiting for tranquil times may be as futile as waiting for Godot.

If these conditions are present in an individual medical group or clinical site, they will be able to greatly improve preventive services delivery. However, if a managed care organization (MCO) wants consistent preventive services delivery to be implemented in all its delivery settings and for all its members, then the MCO itself will need to have these conditions as well. It will also need to work hard at facilitating the development of these conditions in its care delivery sites.

Let us move now from theory to a case study of the actions that can be and are being taken in one MCO to facilitate the improvement of preventive services in its care delivery system. Although this process begins with the MCO's choices of clinical partners and systems that support prevention in the first place, the next sections will focus on how to improve preventive services in any mix of staff, group, and individual practice sites.

DIRECTION AND ENERGY

If prevention is to become a meaningful priority, it must be an important part of the organization's mission. HealthPartners' mission is "to improve the health of our members and our community." That mission is taken very seriously, and all organizational activities are assessed for their alignment with and contribution to achieving the mission. Our commitment of resources and other actions confirms to participating provider groups that we truly intend to follow our mission.

As noted in Chapter 4, we have laid out a set of explicit prevention goals in the Partners for Better Health Program. Those goals are reinforced in the program initiatives we undertake, but more important, they are reinforced with financial incentives for provider groups, with specific resources to support improvement efforts, and with collaborative actions.

The financial incentives are contained in the Outcomes Recognition Program. This program identifies selected performance targets for those contracting medical groups with sufficient HealthPartners membership to make them care about our initiatives (arbitrarily set at 2,500 people). Seventy percent of the financial bonus associated with this program is paid for technical quality of care, and 30% is for patient satisfaction.

A limited number of topics were selected for this program, because an organization can focus on only a few areas at one time. The actual numerical targets for these topics were selected af-

---

Exhibit 5–2 Environmental Preconditions for Prevention Success

1. Prevention is identified as a high priority for the organization.
2. Effective, strong leadership is present and supports that priority.
3. There are knowledge and the ability to facilitate organizational change.
4. Leadership has a clear systems-oriented vision.
5. Measurement and data are recognized as crucial to the identification of needs and the improvement of the process.
6. Creativity and innovation are valued and rewarded.

ter baseline measurements told us the current performance levels of all medical groups. We believe that making the performance levels public for peer comparison among the medical groups was also an important stimulant for the groups to care about these rates. Like the Partners for Better Health goals, the target levels were set to require a considerable effort while still being attainable. The 1997 and 1998 topics and targets are listed in Table 5–1. Each year,

Table 5–1 Outcomes Recognition Program Targets

1997

Service	Criteria	Target (%)
Pap smear	In the past 3 years for women 18–65	82
Mammography	In the past 2 years for women 50–75	85
Immunization	Up to date for children at age 2	95
Tobacco	Identification of use* for adults at last visit	80
	Advice to quit if a user*	80
Satisfaction	Those *very satisfied* with "overall quality of care and service"	49

Shadow Criteria

Low density lipoprotein (LDL) rate and level in patients with identified coronary artery disease		TBD
HbA1c rate and level in patients with diabetes		TBD

1998

Service	Criteria	Target (%)
Mammography	In the past 2 years for women 50–75	85
Immunization	Up to date for children at age 2	95
Tobacco	Identification of use* at last visit	80
	Advice to quit if a user*	80
LDL	In the past year for patients with known coronary artery disease	60
	Level at or below 130	60
HbA1C	In the past 6 months for patients with diabetes	75
	Level at or below 8	75
Satisfaction	Those *very satisfied* with the "overall quality of care and service"	49

Shadow Criteria

Preventive services		TBD
Tobacco prevalence		TBD

*Tobacco use is defined as exposure to a passive smoking environment for the age cohort 0–12 years or as personal use for the age cohort 13+ years.

TBD = to be decided.

Courtesy of HealthPartners, Minneapolis, Minnesota.

other topics are being measured as "shadows" likely to be added to the program in the future.

Besides this direct financial incentive, there are several other spurs to action on the prevention agenda. One comes from the HealthPartners Consumer Choice Program, which provides consumers with computer kiosk or Internet access to comparative performance information about individual medical groups on various parameters, including selected preventive services. Consumers can use these data in their decision of which group to choose as their source of primary care, thus stimulating groups to take actions that will retain or enlarge their patient base.

Another spur comes from a parallel incentive by the Buyers Health Care Action Group (BHCAG), consisting of 25 of the largest employers in the Twin Cities. BHCAG has announced the provision of Excellence in Quality Awards to be given for the first time in 1998 to recognize care systems that have made particularly outstanding achievements in quality and service. Potentially there will be one $100,000 award, three $50,000 awards, and additional special recognition awards for care systems that meet a threshold level of patient satisfaction, achieve a targeted high rate of patients who are up to date with complete preventive services, and fully implement a specified number of clinical guidelines. While this incentive is specifically for this market, there is always the potential for this concept to expand to other markets.

Finally, provider groups are spurred to action by being involved collaboratively in the development and implementation of clinical guidelines and improvement efforts. When HealthPartners was being established through the merger of two health maintenance organizations (HMOs) in 1993, it decided to fund a separate organization that would be run by the participating medical groups. This nonprofit organization, called the Institute for Clinical Systems Integration (ICSI), is directed by a board consisting of physicians from the three major medical groups (Mayo Clinic, Health System Minnesota, and the HealthPartners staff medical group) as well as representatives of the (now 17) smaller groups.[6] There are also representatives on the board from the BHCAG to help ensure that ICSI continues to address the needs of its customers.

ICSI believes that if medical groups are actively involved in the creation and oversight of evidence-based guidelines, they will take the tasks seriously. Thus far, ICSI has developed 47 guidelines, 10 of them addressing preventive services. This has clearly had a reinforcing effect on the desire of medical group leaders to improve preventive services.

THE HOW OF CHANGE

Just as guidelines are a necessary but insufficient platform for quality improvement efforts, financial and cultural incentives to improve preventive services are necessary but insufficient ingredients in improvement. If the medical groups focused on outdated and relatively ineffective ideas about how to produce significant change, little would happen. Exhortation by leaders, education, research, and even changes in individual clinician financial incentives will not produce much change if the barriers noted above are not addressed and effective system supports are not established. The practice environment must be changed so that it makes it more difficult to avoid than to provide preventive services during the course of *all* encounters with patients.

An increasing number of medical group leaders, especially those involved in ICSI, are learning this lesson. Thus, they are developing the necessary systems vision and are learning how to transform their organizations so that these environmental changes are possible. Several factors have been helpful in this regard.

ICSI—An Improvement Collaborative

First, ICSI recognized from the beginning that measurement was a key to improvement, so each guideline developed was accompanied by a measurement plan to assess implementation. Before long, these measurements made it clear that there was not a lot of change going on in many guidelines. This conclusion was reinforced by measurements generated by a series of ICSI-sponsored "impact studies." These studies also identified success stories[7] and features of guidelines and implementation that were more likely to lead to improvement.

As a result of these findings and the medical groups' frustration with having to work on all guidelines at once, ICSI made a sharp change in direction in 1997. It shifted emphasis from development to implementation and separated participating medical groups (by their own choice) into two implementation programs. The first was designed to facilitate the development or strengthening of organizational change skills among groups that needed to have a stronger foundation for improvement efforts. Exhibit 5–2 highlights many of these skills.

Those groups with such a foundation already in place joined four "Action Groups." An Action Group was patterned in part on the Breakthrough Series improvement collaboratives sponsored by Berwick's Institute for Healthcare Improvement. Each Action Group was made up of medical groups that wanted to focus their efforts on a particular guideline. Preventive Services has been one of the most popular Action Groups. The Preventive Services Action Group meets bimonthly to share information and strategies and has adopted a group aim of improving each medical group's rate of overall preventive services being up to date by 50% over 18 months. Almost all of this group's meetings are devoted to ways to build office systems, though there is also some attention to how to achieve buy-in from clinicians.

IMPROVE—A Learning Research Trial

Another activity that has helped the medical groups learn how to produce organizational change around the delivery of preventive services has been a large research trial funded by the Agency for Health Care Policy and Research. This project—IMPROVE (IMproving PRevention through Organization, Vision, and Empowerment)—was designed to test whether an intervention based on continuous quality improvement (CQI) and from a managed care sponsor could lead medical groups to implement office systems and to a resulting improvement in the rates of important adult preventive services.[8]

Although the outcomes from this trial are not known yet, the 22 clinics randomized to the intervention arm of the trial valued the experience it gave them enough that most (17) of the comparison clinics chose to obtain the same help at the end of the trial. The two sponsoring HMOs (HealthPartners and Blue Plus) also chose to learn this training, facilitation, and networking approach and to use it with many of their other medical group partners.

The Data Tool

Both of the above experiences have reinforced the importance of basing improvement efforts on the collection and analysis of relevant data. Many of those lessons about data have been incorporated in an article on the three types of measurement: measurement used for improvement, measurement used for accountability, or measurement used for research.[9] Although Solberg et al concluded that it is difficult and dangerous to confuse these different uses for data, each of them also has a clear and valuable place in the effort to improve preventive services delivery.

For example, accountability data have been an invaluable aid in spurring action, as noted above. The Outcomes Recognition Program financial incentives are based on accurate accountability data, as is the information used by members to choose providers and that used by BHCAG in recognizing excellence. These data also help each medical group to know its baseline performance and what has been achieved by other groups, thus providing clinicians with facts about their performance gaps. A recent measurement approach that has identified a large gap is the percent of members seen who are up to date on an entire set of selected guideline recommendations (this proportion is usually quite low). This measurement also encourages medical groups to approach preventive care as a system.

Research data from the ICSI impact studies, the IMPROVE Project, and the literature have been critical to understanding what is needed to make real improvements. However, it is the data collected by each medical group for improvement purposes that are really the guide to those efforts. These types of data do not need to be of the same reliability and validity as the other types, since they are needed only for a group's own use in identifying areas needing attention, disabusing clinicians and staff of false assumptions about their problems, and assessing the success of any changes made.

The MCO can also supply population-based data to facilitate improvement. The names of MCO members at each medical group who are in need of certain preventive services are provided to the groups from our administrative data sets. We call these "at risk" lists. They are currently being provided to support mammography, diabetic control, Pap smears, childhood immunizations, and low density lipoprotein (LDL) tests in coronary heart disease patients. Some medical groups have found these lists useful for focusing their efforts to reach patients in particular need of services, although much needs to be done to learn how to make the best use of this information.

Yet another way for the MCO to facilitate prevention actions at the medical group level is to supply care providers with data about services other than those in the Outcomes Recognition Program. At HealthPartners, there are another eight clinical indicators of prevention that are measured annually and reported publicly by medical groups beyond those in Table 5–1. We are also in the process of developing an on-line computer set of member data that can be accessed by medical groups to help them perform their own audits and analyses more easily.

OTHER CONSIDERATIONS

Although the main focus for improving preventive services in clinical settings should be on helping those settings to use effective internal systems to build prevention into every encounter with patients, there are other ways that an MCO can help to make these clinic systems more effective. For example, patient education materials and risk behavior change programs and classes can be made available to the clinics or on referral from them.

Special member outreach prevention programs (like those discussed in Chapter 6) should also be integrated with clinic-based efforts, because synergy can be developed between them. For example, if the MCO identifies risk behaviors through outreach at the work site, it can pass this information on (with member permission) to the member's clinic site so that change efforts can be supported there as well. Alternatively, when the clinic identifies patients ready to make changes in risk factors like smoking, it can make use of follow-up or phone-line counseling run from the MCO.

HealthPartners also has training classes in CQI techniques to help personnel from medical groups learn how to manage organizational improvements more efficiently and effectively. It also has a major research organization committed to public domain research (HealthPartners Research Foundation) that conducts studies relevant to implementing guidelines and improving care. Medical group members often participate in these research projects (notably IMPROVE and the similar IDEAL [improving diabetes through empowerment, active collaboration, and leadership] project for improving care for patients with diabetes) and learn from that participation.

PRIMARY VERSUS SECONDARY PREVENTION

Traditionally, textbooks of disease prevention have distinguished between primary and secondary prevention activities.

- primary = efforts to prevent the occurrence of conditions in individuals without them (eg, smoking cessation to prevent cancer)
- secondary = efforts to detect a condition

early enough or to manage it so well as to improve the likelihood of a good outcome (eg, Pap smears to detect early cervical cancer or lipid reduction treatment in patients with known heart disease)

There is little practical reason for an MCO to separate these activities, either conceptually or programmatically. Both will occur predominantly in the primary care setting, although secondary prevention activities will often involve some coordination with specialty consultants. Those patients who have conditions that are complicated enough to require ongoing care supervision exclusively in specialty clinics will need to have their overall prevention needs addressed there as well. This means that those clinics will also need to have supportive office systems, since subspecialists are traditionally even less likely to address preventive needs that lie outside their area. The same is true for disease management programs.

FACILITATING CHANGE FROM THE OUTSIDE

Even when there is an environment in which the health plan and most of its contracting medical groups want to improve prevention and are working at doing so, there are still challenges. We have learned some lessons from attempting to facilitate change.

- It's not easy!
- It will take time and considerable effort to get past the initial suspicion that many clinicians and medical groups have about the motives and capabilities of the MCO with which they contract.
- It is not necessarily easier to make change in a large group than in a small one. Although the larger group may have more resources, it may have more inertia and making changes may be more complicated.
- It is not necessarily any easier to make change in an "owned" staff clinic than in a contracted one.
- Clinician leaders with the skills and vision identified in Exhibit 5–2 are rare—treasure and support them.
- Data knowledge and skills are as rare as they are important—work to provide training and support for their development.
- Training, consulting, and networking with peers in other medical groups are each valuable—provide or facilitate them.
- The medical groups that seem to be making the most progress are those that have at least one skilled staff person dedicated to making progress happen.

CONCLUSION

The examples described above are not necessarily unique to HealthPartners. Similar approaches to improve prevention in the clinical setting have been described by other MCOs, particularly Group Health of Puget Sound, the various Kaiser plans, and Harvard Pilgrim. Nevertheless, most MCOs still have not gotten very involved in these efforts, and all MCOs have a lot to learn about how to best facilitate the necessary changes.

The real question is whether you want to wait until the local market requires such efforts, or whether you want to get ahead of the pack and thereby stimulate the creativity and energy that comes from being on the cutting edge. All the prevention activities described in Chapter 4 are accessible to this commitment, but the heart of it is what happens in the care delivery setting.

REFERENCES

1. Kottke TE, Brekke ML, Solberg LI. Making "time" for preventive services. *Mayo Clin Proc*. 1993;68:785–791.
2. Kottke TE, Solberg LI, Brekke ML, Cabrera A, Marquez M. Preventive services rates in 44 Midwestern primary care clinics: room for improvement. *Mayo Clin Proc*. 1997;72:515–523.
3. Leininger LS, Finn L, Dickey L, et al. An office system for organizing preventive services. *Arch Fam Med*. 1996;5:108–115.
4. Solberg LI, Kottke TE, Brekke ML, Conn SA, Calomeni CA, Conboy KS. Delivering clinical preventive services is a systems problem: the paradigm

shift of IMPROVEment. *Ann Behav Med.* 1998;19(3). In press.

5. Solberg LI, Kottke TE, Brekke ML. The case of the missing clinical preventive services delivery systems. *Effective Clin Pract.* In press.

6. Reinertsen JL. Collaborating outside the box: when employers and providers take on environmental barriers to guideline implementation. *Joint Commission J Qual Improvement.* 1995;21(11):612–618.

7. O'Connor PJ, Solberg LI, Christianson J, Amundson G, Mosser G. Mechanism of action and impact of a cystitis clinical practice guideline on outcomes and costs of care in an HMO. *Joint Commission J Qual Improvement.* 1996;22(10):673–682.

8. Solberg LI, Kottke TE, Brekke ML, Calomeni CA, Conn SA, Davidson G. Using CQI to increase preventive services in clinical practice—going beyond guidelines. *Prev Med.* 1996;25:259–267.

9. Solberg LI, Mosser G, McDonald S. The three faces of performance measurement: improvement, accountability, and research. *Joint Commission J Qual Improvement.* 1997;23(3):135–147.

LEIF I. SOLBERG, MD, is the associate medical director for care improvement research at HealthPartners Research Foundation and a practicing family physician in the HealthPartners Medical Group. His research interests include disease prevention (especially tobacco cessation), chronic disease management, and quality improvement. He has published more than 69 peer-reviewed journal articles and 17 book chapters. Dr. Solberg is particularly interested in conducting research that addresses care delivery concerns and in translating research lessons back into patient care.

GAIL AMUNDSON, MD, practices general internal medicine and geriatrics and serves as associate medical director of quality and utilization management at HealthPartners. Dr. Amundson has extensive experience in systems development, information systems applications, quality measurement, and clinical quality improvement. She led the analysis and design of a systems approach to delivering preventive services within HealthPartners Medical Group. She has participated in preventive service guideline development and led the development of a supporting health risk assessment instrument. She was instrumental in the development of the innovative outcomes recognition program for HealthPartners' network medical group partners.

CHAPTER 6

Outreach from the Managed Care Organization to the Population

Nicolaas P. Pronk

Chapter Outline

- Introduction
- Population Health Cycle
- Framework for Action
- Conclusion

INTRODUCTION

This chapter outlines various approaches that may serve as examples around which managed care organizations (MCOs) and integrated delivery systems (IDSs; in this chapter, the term MCO will be used to refer to both MCOs and IDSs) can organize themselves to effectively reach out to their membership and the communities they serve. As in Chapters 4 and 5, examples will be taken from experiences of the HealthPartners MCO to illustrate this chapter's points. At HealthPartners, several population health improvement models have been developed and implemented as part of the Partners for Better Health (PBH) Program. PBH is a unique, highly proactive program designed to reduce the incidence of disease and health risks in eight categories, which cover heart disease, childhood immunization, breast cancer, diabetes, infant and maternal health, dental health, childhood injuries, and domestic violence (see Chapter 4 for all 8 goal definitions).

The first step in reaching out to the population is an assessment and evaluation of the health status and risks of the entire membership. Then the individuals needing to be reached with health improvement opportunities must be identified. Subsequently, interventions must be provided systematically and via appropriate channels to optimize the chances for success. As a reassessment of the health status and risks of the population is completed to evaluate the effect of the intervention, the steps are repeated with appropriate adjustments to the programs and the selected population. This approach is outlined in Figure 6–1.

Two additional conceptual models have been helpful in focusing our resources on the identified high-risk groups. First, a population health cycle outlines the relationship among several key population health concepts. Second, a risk-interaction-change model, designed to organize departments dedicated to health improvement program delivery, outlines steps around which a proactive health improvement system may be developed. One of the critical and most unique features of PBH is its closed loop, systems thinking approach. In such a model, various linkages are developed that allow information to be shared appropriately with key stakeholders in health improvement and disease prevention. Hence, clinicians may refer their patients into programs outside the clinic setting but receive updates on how well the patient is doing. Employer groups receive aggregate reports on their employees' health status, their program participation, and program impact. Individual members re-

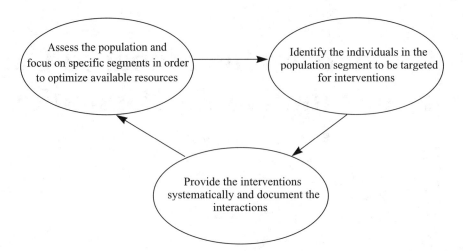

Figure 6–1 Assess-Identify-Intervene Model. Courtesy of HealthPartners, Minneapolis, Minnesota.

ceive information regarding their opportunities for health improvement and, once they decide to participate, become actively engaged in the process.

POPULATION HEALTH CYCLE

The population health cycle (Figure 6–2) is initiated by the public announcement of population health improvement goals.[1] On February 21, 1994, HealthPartners publicly announced PBH to its membership and the larger community via local media, an open letter to the community, and articles in widely read news sources such as the *Wall Street Journal*. This public announcement committed the MCO to take a bold step toward successful population-based disease prevention and health improvement programs by establishing a joint accountability with its members for improving their health. The goals were designed to address important health issues and align as much as possible with local, state, or national health agendas to create partnerships, synergy, and momentum.

When initiating a program, partnerships should be forged among purchasers of health coverage, medical practitioners, care systems administrators, public health officials, MCO members, and the general community. All these parties are critical to the success of the program. Furthermore, the goals should be specific, measurable, and designed to force the traditionally acute care–oriented medical delivery system to address prevention from a different perspective. The goals should be set as "stretch goals," forcing people and systems to work differently, thereby coming up with innovative approaches that allow groundbreaking improvements to occur. For example, PBH defines one of its eight population health improvement goals as follows: Reduce by 25% the number of heart disease events (eg, heart attacks) among members. This goal will not be achieved by merely working harder; it may be achieved only if the system changes to work "smarter" by optimizing its own resources and the resources of all key partners in this process.

The next three steps in the population health cycle outline an approach to understand the receptivity of the membership to health improvement programs, measure the health status of the population, and understand the membership's readiness to change lifestyles and behaviors. A survey of HealthPartners' membership revealed that 85% reported being very willing to participate in two-way communications with the health plan to improve their health.[2] In such an environment, the health status assessment of the population can be initiated, individuals at risk may be

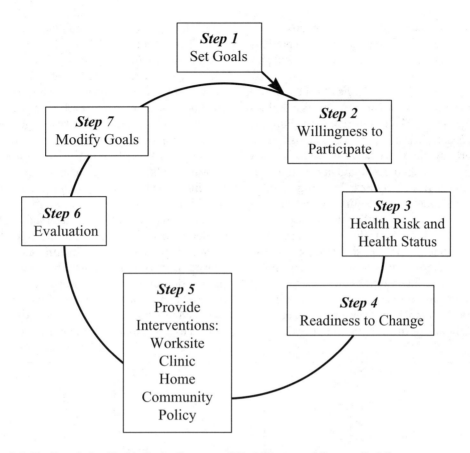

Figure 6–2 The Population Health Cycle. Courtesy of HealthPartners, Minneapolis, Minnesota.

identified, and interventions may be provided following an assessment of individuals' readiness to change specific behaviors. This approach is successfully implemented in a worksite-based model where health risk assessment surveys (see Chapters 2 and 3) are directly linked to both proactive outbound telephone counseling services and clinical linkage via electronic data systems, a program described below. The steps outlined above are necessary to organize an infrastructure that provides ongoing interventions. In addition, they provide a thorough understanding of what the degree of participation and anticipated outcome of interventions may be.

Step 5 denotes the systematic provision of interventions in various settings. Based on the evaluation of the intervention programs (Step 6), Step 7 represents a time of reflection where modification of the program and its goals may be considered prior to cycling through the population health cycle once again. This population health cycle provides a focused approach to initiate and organize population health improvement efforts.

FRAMEWORK FOR ACTION

The risk-interaction-change model is a three-dimensional conceptual framework (Figure 6–3) around which the Center for Health Promotion at HealthPartners has organized itself. This model provides an organizing principle to guide the substantial challenges of program design, development, and implementation. It differs from the population health cycle in that this model is entirely focused on the interventions (the programs) rather than on the population. The floating dot represents stage-matched, risk-sensitive, and site-specific interventions.

The first axis denotes the health risk continuum from both a behavioral as well as a biological perspective. The health risk continuum includes 5 categories: no/low risk, at risk, high risk, early symptoms, and active disease. PBH is designed to help move members from higher risk to lower risk categories. The program also strives to prevent people from moving from less serious to more serious risk categories.

The second axis of the risk-interaction-change model concerns the site where the member becomes engaged in the intervention. Topic-specific interventions may vary widely depending on the place where they are delivered. For example, a message promoting a physically active lifestyle that is provided at a clinic during a routine health maintenance visit will differ from one delivered to the general community as part of a marketing campaign. The former message may be tailored to the patient by his or her physician, while the latter may be based on social marketing techniques designed to reach and influence a large segment of the population. Both approaches may present identical messages focused on, for example, increasing walking among members by increasing enrollment in mall walking programs during the winter.

The third axis on the risk-interaction-change model refers to the readiness of the individual to change behavior so that health may be improved. Behavior change may be viewed as the progression through a series of stages of readiness (precontemplation, contemplation, preparation, action, and maintenance) that are directly related to the individual's intent to change. This

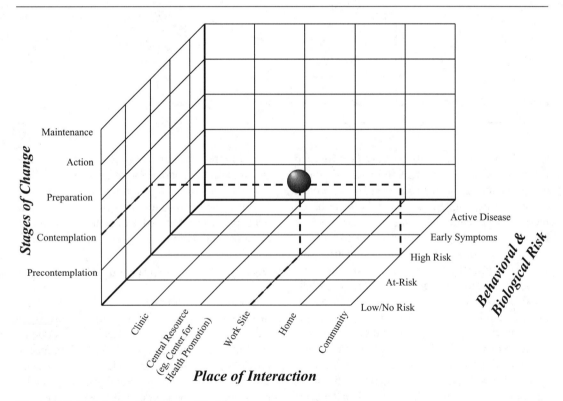

Figure 6–3 Risk-Interaction-Change Model

"state of change" approach is the central construct of the transtheoretical model developed by James Prochaska and colleagues.[3] This construct has been shown to reveal consistent patterns across 12 different behaviors relating to how individuals weigh the pros and cons of change.[4] It provides a theoretical framework within which individual change may be viewed as a process involving progress through a series of stages. Further, at each stage there are specific steps to guide practitioners in helping a person advance to the next stage. Thus, stage-matched messages provide an actionable approach to reach out to individuals at various levels of behavioral and/or biological risk in a variety of settings.

The PBH Employer Initiative (PBHEI) is an example of how this model is brought to life using an integrated approach to health management. In this program, the MCO develops partnerships with the employers to achieve a common goal of health improvement. To do this effectively, optimizing available resources, a needs assessment is completed first. This needs assessment includes a review and analysis of the company's claims experience, an analysis of these claims to outline the preventable portion of medical care expenses incurred, an environmental and cultural audit of the worksite, and a health risk assessment (HRA) of the employee population (see Part I). After identifying the needs, the employer and the MCO agree on the focus of the program to be implemented. This approach allows for a targeted effort that optimizes both program goal achievement and use of resources.

The HRA process is telephone based. An employee receives a calling card in the mail, dials an access number, and is asked a set of health risk and demographic questions. The answers are entered using the telephone keypad and stored electronically in a computer database. Upon completion of the survey, the employee's calling card is credited with 20 minutes of free long-distance telephone time (to encourage participation). As employees voluntarily participate in the HRA process, the collected data are presented back to them in a format that outlines their health risks and steps they can take through the HealthPartners system to reduce these risks. While this is an approach typically associated with HRA feedback reports, the more unique part of PBHEI is that the same data are also presented to the employee's physician, are documented in the medical record, and are used proactively by both clinical and health education staff to follow up on identified health risks. This is achieved by closing the loop with all those employees who answer a "preapproval to notify" question in the survey. Once the health plan receives preapproval to contact, follow-up telephone calls are initiated from a centralized lifestyle and behavior change support service called the PBH Phone Line, which is staffed by registered dietitians and health educators. This proactive outreach allows the health plan to engage employees in programs that directly address their individual risk factors. Given the stage of readiness to change and health risks present, the counselor and member identify together which behavior to address first. In case of elevated risk factors, the physician or clinic nurse is the one who signs off on the most appropriate follow-up based on the clinical care plan for that particular patient. Once this follow-up is outlined, the clinic staff may schedule the employee for a clinic visit or refer back to the PBH Phone Line counselors for behavioral follow-up. All counseling provided by PBH Phone Line staff is documented in the medical chart so that the clinic staff may use this information at the next scheduled patient visit.

Does this proactive outreach actually reduce health risk? Weight management results of this telephone-based program, designed around behavioral approaches to health improvement, indicate that participants lose an average of 6.1 kg (13.3 lbs) over 6 months as a result of receiving an average of 9.9 counseling sessions that are approximately 15 minutes in duration. Considering the relatively short duration of the counseling intervention (about 2.5 hours over 6 months), these results appear to be similar in magnitude to some of the most prominent university-based, cognitive, behavioral weight control programs in the nation.[5]

Table 6–1 HRA Follow-Up According to Level of Risk

	Category or Follow-Up Action Step	Number	Percentage
1	Total number of employees who completed an HRA. This number represents a 48% response rate of the entire employee population of this employer group (all received individual feedback reports outlining their health risks and providing them with health education materials and resources).	2,975	100%
2	Employees who were members of a different MCO but participated in the HRA. These employees received only an individual feedback report package and a letter encouraging them to share their results with their primary care physician.	685	23%
3	Employees identified to be at low risk. These employees received immediate follow-up via the PBH Phone Line if they provided preapproval for follow-up.	387	13%
4	Employees identified to be at moderate risk. These employees received immediate follow-up via the PBH Phone Line if they provided preapproval for follow-up.	655	22%
5	Employees identified to be at elevated risk. The reports of these employees were first triaged into the clinics where clinic provider staff (physician or nurse) would review their health risks and prescribe follow-up action steps.	1,250	42%

Clinic action taken for elevated risk reports—steps initiated by the clinic staff for 42% (n = 1,250) of the reports that were identified as elevated risk

6	Report was reviewed but based on review no additional follow-up was needed.	575	46%
7	Report was reviewed and based on review of health risks an immediate referral back to PBH Phone Line Health Educator was thought to be most appropriate (eg, counseling on physical activity, smoking, or stress management was recommended).	250	20%
8	Report was reviewed and based on review of health risks an immediate referral back to PBH Phone Line Dietitian was thought to be most appropriate (eg, counseling on eating patterns or weight management was recommended).	137	11%
9	Report reviewed and based on review of health risks an immediate referral back to PBH Phone Line Health staff was made in order to send out risk-specific information and, if appropriate, stage-matched behavior change materials.	238	19%
10	Report reviewed and based on review of health risks a follow-up visit at the clinic was scheduled. This may be the case if an employee with a previous diagnosis of diabetes and hypertension has not been seen by his or her physician for over 6 months.	50	4%

Courtesy of HealthPartners, Minneapolis, Minnesota.

The PBH Phone Line interventions are also successful at increasing the number of participants who are in "action" or "maintenance" stages of readiness to change for physical activity behavior (ie, those stages associated with the performance of at least 30 minutes of physical activity on most days of the week). In a recent analysis of 100 randomly selected counseling charts on physical activity, 38% of individuals who indicated they were in "contemplation" or "preparation" stages for physical activity moved into action or maintenance by the end of 6 months of counseling. On average, individuals received 8.3 sessions that were 15 minutes long. Moreover, no participants in the action or maintenance stages relapsed into a stage of physical activity below recommended levels. Hence, the proportion of individuals who were in the action or maintenance stages increased from 55% at baseline to 91% at the end of 6 months of counseling.

To indicate the process flow of the worksite-based HRA program and the subsequent linkage of the health risk–related information to behavior change and clinical care processes, Table 6–1 outlines the proportion of employees from a large employer group who participated in the HRA and the immediate steps that were taken to provide them with the most appropriate follow-up on the risk factors they reported. In the case of elevated self-reported risks, feedback reports were sent to the clinics where the employees were seen. On the other hand, if the risks identified were moderate or low, immediate follow-up was provided via the health educators or dietitians on the PBH Phone Line. Regardless, all those who provided preapproval to be notified of programs designed to improve their health were contacted. Hence, using a stage-matched behavior change approach, interventions are provided to the employee at the worksite, the clinic, the home, and via the Center for Health Promotion that are tailored to their individual behavioral and biological health risks. Only 4% of the elevated risk individuals were scheduled for a follow-up clinic visit (1.7% of the total number of employees who completed an HRA).

CONCLUSION

The approach outlined in this chapter is highly proactive, reaches a large number of people, and facilitates a behavior change process designed to improve health while providing information linkages to the various stakeholders involved in this program. As long as the overall objective is health improvement, partnerships are formed among key stakeholders in the process. The interaction with members is respectful, sensitive to privacy and confidentiality issues, and focused on long-term relationships. The potential for this program to bring about dramatic improvements in a population's health status is enormous.

REFERENCES

1. Pronk NP, O'Connor PJ. Systems approach to population health improvement. *J Ambulatory Care Manage.* 1997; 20:24–31.
2. O'Connor PJ, Rush WA, Rardin KA, Isham GJ. Are managed care members willing to engage in two-way communications to improve health? *HMO Pract.* 1996; 10:17–19.
3. Prochaska JO, DiClemente CC. Stages of change in the modification of problem behaviors. *Prog Behav Modif.* 1992;28:184–218.
4. Prochaska JO, Velicer WF, Rossi JS, et al. Stages of change and decisional balance on twelve problem behaviors. *Health Psychol.* 1994;13:47–51.
5. Pronk NP, Wing R. The role of physical activity in the long-term maintenance of weight loss. *Obes Res.* 1994; 2:587–599.

NICOLAAS P. PRONK, MA, PHD, is director of health risk measurement and worksite programs at the Center for Health Promotion, and he is associate investigator in the HealthPartners Research Foundation. He received his PhD in exercise science from Texas A&M University and completed a postdoctoral research fellowship in behavioral medicine at the University of Pittsburgh School of Medicine. Dr. Pronk's work is focused on bridging the gap between research and application of health improvement efforts for defined populations.

Chapter 7

Delivering Clinical Preventive Services to Underserved and Immigrant Populations

Thomas E. Kottke, Mary Alice Trapp, and Milo L. Brekke

Chapter Outline

- Introduction
- Establishing Contact
- Community Assessment
- Program Design and Development
- Fostering Commitment
- Progress Evaluation
- Expanding the Role of Nurses To Increase Program Access and Acceptability
- Against, and For, Interpretation
- What Makes a Preventive Services Program Culturally Sensitive?
- Conclusion

INTRODUCTION

As managed care becomes more widespread throughout the United States and as states look to managed care organizations (MCOs) to provide services to Medicaid populations, MCOs will increasingly find themselves responsible for providing health care services to historically underserved and immigrant populations. Effective program development will require both meeting the biological needs of the populations and designing programs that address those needs in a manner that the client population accepts.

Defining Biological Needs

The infectious disease burden can be expected to be far higher for immigrant populations than for populations historically served by MCOs. In 1996, 9% of all refugees arriving in Minnesota were positive for hepatitis B surface antigen, and 43% had at least one parasite identified by screening.[1] Tuberculosis in the United States is concentrated in two populations, homeless persons and recent immigrants. In response to this burden, the Minnesota Department of Health recommends that recent immigrants be screened for tuberculosis, hepatitis B, intestinal parasites, sexually transmitted diseases, and malaria (Table 7–1). Any MCO will need to educate itself about the epidemiology of diseases in the populations it plans to serve. State health departments, the Centers for Disease Control and Prevention (CDC), and World Health Organization documents are sources of epidemiological background material.

The actual causes of death in the client population may be different from expectations. For example, the three leading causes of death for Alaskan Natives in 1994 were heart and cerebrovascular disease (24.2% of all deaths), cancer (17.6% of all deaths), and accidents and adverse ef-

---

Material in this chapter was supported by Agency for Health Care Policy and Research grant R01HS08091, Centers for Disease Control and Prevention Cooperative Agreement U57/CCU510175, and National Institutes of Health grant CA15083.

Table 7–1 Minnesota Department of Health (MDH) Initial Health Screening Tests Recommended for All Refugees/Immigrants

Disease or Condition	Screening Recommendations
Updating of immunizations	Assess and update immunizations for each individual. Immigrants may not have records of previous immunizations. If no dates of previous immunization are found, begin a primary series for age-appropriate immunizations. Always update the personal immunization record card.
Tuberculosis (TB)	Perform a Mantoux skin test for all individuals (regardless of bacillus Calmette-Guérin [BCG] history), unless medically contraindicated. A chest X-ray should be performed for all individuals with a positive Mantoux skin test, for those classified as TB Class A or TB Class B during the immigration medical screening, and for those who have symptoms compatible with TB disease, regardless of Mantoux results. MDH recommends TB screening of high-risk children at three stages of childhood and adolescence that coincide with routine health appraisals or immunizations, including 12–15 months, 4–6 years (ie, at school entry), and 14–16 years (ie, once during adolescence). However, TB screening may be appropriate as soon as 6 months of age, when cell-mediated immunity of a degree sufficient for a significant skin test reaction has developed.
Hepatitis B	Administer a hepatitis B screening panel including hepatitis B surface antigen (HBsAg), hepatitis B core antibody (anti-HBc), and hepatitis B surface antibody (anti-HBs) for all individuals. Screen appropriate household contacts if possible and immunize those who are susceptible.
Intestinal parasites	Conduct stool examinations for ova and parasites; three stool specimens should be obtained at intervals more than 24 hours apart. If parasites are identified, one stool specimen should be submitted 2–3 weeks after completion of therapy to determine response to treatment.
Sexually transmitted diseases	If symptomatic, administer venereal disease research laboratory (VDRL) or rapid plasma reagin (RPR) for those 14 years old or older. Confirm positive VDRL or RPR by FTA-ABS/MHATP or other confirmatory test. Repeat VDRL/FTA in 2 weeks if lesions typical of primary syphilis are noted and person is seronegative on initial screening.
Malaria	If symptomatic, obtain blood for malarial parasites.
Other health problems: hematologic disorders (eosinophilia, anemia, microcytosis), dental caries, decreased weight for age and height, thyroid disease, otorhinologic and ophthalmologic problems, dermatologic abnormalities.	Complete medical and dental examinations (height, weight, blood pressure, vision and hearing evaluation, complete blood count [CBC], serum chemistry profiles, urinalysis) to detect other health problems. Perform pregnancy test when indicated. Pay special attention to suspected signs of Hansen's disease. Assess mental health needs. Refer to health programs as indicated.

Source: Reprinted from Refugee Health Screening in Minnesota: Current Status and Recommendations, *Minnesota Department of Health Disease Control Newsletter,* Vol 25, pp 37–48, 1997, Minnesota Department of Health.

fects (18.8% of all deaths).[2] A significant number of the deaths from cancer are due to lung cancer.

Defining Cultural Needs

Health care providers who are working to develop preventive services programs for underserved populations can expect to hear requests for "culturally sensitive" programs. However, through trial and error they will have to discover what qualifies as culturally sensitive; they can expect that no two people will provide the same definition.

Although a comprehensive definition of culture is elusive, the following definition may be useful: "A society's culture consists of whatever it is one has to know or believe in order to operate in a manner acceptable to its members."[3(p11)] This definition emphasizes that societies have a set of knowledge and beliefs that translate into rules about how to live life appropriately. As Hall describes in *Beyond Culture*, individuals tend to consider their own culture to be innate.[4] And, just as individuals in one culture consider their own culture to be innate (and therefore *correct*), they consider the practices of different cultures to be more or less misdirected attempts to deal with the same problems of life. This tendency applies to both members of client populations and MCO employees.

Just as individuals consider their culture to be innate, people find it almost impossible to describe or offer insight into their own culture's beliefs. Most people are not accustomed to thinking this way. Hall suggests that, to develop a sensitivity to differences in cultural expectations, the program developer has to remain alert for situations in which he or she wants to "escalate"—in other words, to act on frustration or anger. In health care, situations that trigger the urge to escalate would include noncompliance with instructions or repeatedly missed appointments. A program developer's or clinician's urge to escalate suggests that a difference in cultural expectations is present. Recognizing an urge to escalate creates an opportunity to analyze the situation, learn of one's own and another's cultural assumptions, and develop appropriate programmatic responses.

A sense of befuddlement or confusion—that is, saying to oneself, "I just can't understand what _____ is thinking"—is also a sign of differences in cultural expectations. When the program planner has these thoughts, it is time to back up and try different assumptions until one seems to explain why the client believes he or she is behaving rationally. It is helpful for the program planner to keep in mind that his or her behavior probably seems confusing or offensive to clients as well.

From working in international settings and with American Indians, Alaskan Natives, Southeast Asians, and East Africans, we have concluded that most cultural clashes are not due to what many people would consider cultural (eg, cosmology, traditions of clothing, or religious practices), because these differences are obvious. Rather, misunderstandings arise from beliefs about how day-to-day life ought to be led—how time, space, or other resources should be used. For example, we have been socialized to consider an unreturned telephone call as a sign of disinterest or of rebuke. In some client cultures, however, the message "Tom called with a question" simply does not evoke a sense of need to respond; it is assumed that Tom will call again if he still needs his questions answered.

The differences in cultural assumptions that cause frustration and nonadherence can be even more difficult to discern when the historically underserved or immigrant population speaks English or has been in the geographic vicinity of the MCO for a long time. In these situations the cultural origins of the differences are less obvious, and it may be assumed that the population should have "learned" how to use the health services system. Although the cultures employ the same vocabulary, they may use words differently. For instance, physicians and Native Americans have very different definitions of the expression "to practice medicine." The doctor would say, "Practicing medicine is what I do; of course I wouldn't do it if I weren't good enough." On the other hand, many of our Native American patients have told us that they believe it is called *practicing* medicine on the reservation because "a doctor practices treating Native Americans until she becomes good enough to treat Caucasian patients." The Native American experience reinforces their definition—young physicians just out of training come to the reservation, become increasingly competent over a period of 1 or 2 years, and then go back to practice in a Caucasian population. Thus, it can be useful to avoid the verb "practice" in certain cross-cultural interactions. "Experiment" can, in a similar fashion, have very negative connotations. If members of the client population react in an unexpected fashion to the use of a particular word or phrase, it is best to ask an individual knowledgeable about both cultures about what that word or phrase might mean to those members.

Many populations do not share the health care culture's highly acute (to some, overly acute) sense of time. In our projects at the Mayo Clinic, members of the population to be served seemed to show up any time they wished, even though they were given what the authors thought were clear instructions to present themselves at a specific time, on a specific day, and on a specific date. From the patients' perspective, however, transportation and child care were scarce resources, the availability of which determined when they could come to the clinic. Since they knew the hours when their health care providers would be at work, and they had limited transportation resources and could not leave children unattended, it seemed most reasonable to them to present for care when they had transportation and child care rather than at a time that seemed to be arbitrarily selected by the health services organization.

Trying to address cultural assumptions and differences before developing programs is difficult; as stated by Hall, we discover that our cultural assumptions are different from our patients' only when the two cultures fail to mesh.[4] We have no pretensions that we have written a complete guide to error-free cross-cultural program development; cultural analysis and program development are both broad fields in themselves. We encourage readers to explore the Suggested Readings section at the end of the chapter and, in particular, to develop a habit of reflecting on their own assumptions about the "right" approach to program implementation and then ask if that "right" way is the only right way. Program developers should try to understand the feeling of "right" from the patient's perspective, attempting to view his or her own culture and the culture of the client community from the same perceptual distance. When members of the client community make a request, the program developer ought to ask, "Do we do the same thing but in a somewhat different form or format?" Frequently, the answer is "Yes." The willingness of health care providers to examine their own cultural assumptions and make allowance for others' assumptions forms the foundation for cross-cultural program development and enriches the lives of health care professionals through increased self-understanding.

ESTABLISHING CONTACT

Wilson et al[5] suggest a series of steps in developing cross-cultural programs (Exhibit 7–1). These steps are very similar to the steps described in Chapter 6. The authors' experience with Vietnamese, Cambodian, and Somali women in Rochester, MN, corroborates the advice that initial contact with a previously under-

---

Exhibit 7–1 Steps in Program Implementation Suggested by the Centers for Disease Control and Prevention

Step 1: Involve your community.
Step 2: Assess your community.
Step 3: Design your program.
Step 4: Foster commitment by matching your program to the community.
Step 5: Evaluate your progress.

Source: Reprinted from R Wilson et al, *Creating Physical Activity Programs in American Indian Communities,* 1995, Centers for Disease Control and Prevention.

served or immigrant population needs to take place in the community, not the clinic. As a sign of respect for the established cultural institutions of the population, initial contacts should be with community leaders and community organizations. The goals of these meetings are to explain how the population will benefit from the program and to gain permission to work in the community.

Remember that health care professionals work to meet many needs. While these needs include the delivery of services to others, professional growth, and personal satisfaction, few would work if they were not paid for their services. Therefore, individuals from the community should be *hired* to serve as program development liaison workers; members of the client community should not be expected to volunteer when the program developer is paid for the same work. Just because someone in the client community is unemployed does not mean he or she likes it that way.

Most communities will have nurses who understand the belief systems of both Western medicine and the community. These nurses tend to make very good liaison workers. There may also be immigrant physicians in the community who cannot practice in the United States. When available, their knowledge of both the medical culture and their personal culture is invaluable.

COMMUNITY ASSESSMENT

Although community assessment activities should include an estimate of the number, ages, and gender of individuals in the community, the burden of disease, and the health services needs, community assessment must be much richer. Community assessment should also attempt to elucidate the formal and informal leadership structure, communication channels, and belief systems related to disease causality and prevention. Interviews, meetings with groups of community leaders, and focus groups are three ways to collect this information. Table 7–2 describes information collected in focus groups with Cambodian women living in Rochester.[6] A list of the responses to the barriers is also presented.

While the program developer may receive advice that reliable data can be collected only through the use of structured questionnaires, structured questionnaires simply do not work in some situations, even if administered by native speakers of the language. One of our medical students was working with a population that spoke an oral language without a written counterpart. Even though the surveyors were bilingual and the questionnaire had been translated into phonetic text, the surveyors never were able to learn to read the survey instrument in a conversational tone. Thus, respondents would not answer their questions. After the surveyors were allowed to translate the survey in their own words from English, the collection of reliable data progressed at a nice pace.

PROGRAM DESIGN AND DEVELOPMENT

The program developer must expect that the resources required to lay the foundation for design and development of a cross-cultural preventive services program will be significantly greater than the resources required to develop the same program for long-term users of the MCO's services. In one of our breast and cervical cancer screening programs for Vietnamese immigrant women, for example, initial telephone contact between an interpreter (a Vietnamese nurse) and participants being recruited for focus groups required 30 minutes per call.[6] The three most frequently asked questions were: "Will men be at the meeting?" "Will there be an examination at the first meeting?" and "What will the examination cost?" Yet most of the time was spent reassuring the women that the intentions of the clinic were appropriate and legitimate.

Table 7–2 Barriers to Cancer Screening Identified Through Focus Groups with Cambodian Women and Responses To Overcome the Barriers

Barrier	Response
1. Lack of understanding of purpose of cancer screening	1–4. Videotaped educational program was presented and summarized by staff member.
2. Belief that cancer cannot be treated successfully	
3. Belief that cancer is contagious	
4. Fear of rejection by community if cancer is diagnosed	
5. Misunderstanding of English or technical language	5. Videotape was translated into Cambodian; interpreters were present at educational programs and clinics.
6. Suspicion of authority figures	6. Mall group educational meetings were scheduled, time for social interchange with staff was allowed, and screening clinic sessions were held in a place with an informal atmosphere.
7. Shyness over physical examination by male physician	7. Female physician performed examination.
8. Disregard for punctuality	8. Custom transportation was provided and appointment times were flexible.
9. Lack of transportation or parking funds	9. Transportation was provided.
10. Expense of examination	10. Not addressed; all women but one were covered by Medicare.
11. Fear of a large medical facility	11. Screening clinic sessions were held in a seldom-used area; staff members accompanied patients everywhere.
12. Fear of technical equipment	12. Staff member and interpreter explained directions and findings.
13. Discomfort at individual appointments	13. Group appointments were arranged.

Source: Reprinted with permission from AW Kelly et al, A Program To Increase Breast and Cervical Cancer Screening for Cambodian Women in a Midwestern Community, *Mayo Clinic Proceedings*, Vol 71, pp 437–444, © 1996, Mayo Clinic.

In this project, women were convened in groups of no more than 15 so that the basic concepts of cancer causality and cancer screening could be presented, the women could have their questions answered, and the women could be reassured that the suggested activities were safe and appropriate. As a result of the information collected in focus groups (Table 7–2), the women who chose to participate were provided with specific appointment times, transportation, and an escort to the screening site within the hospital where the screening took place. Ethnically desirable foods were served at the community meetings and after screening. By the end of the project, 75% of the married women from the client community were up to date on breast and cervical cancer screening.

FOSTERING COMMITMENT

Rogers[7] provides useful analyses about how a new program can be packaged to be most acceptable to the client community. Studying more than 3,000 reports of innovations, both within cultures and across cultures, Rogers defined five properties that are associated with adoption of an innovation by a client community (Exhibit 7-2). Although an MCO does not have the option of choosing *among* services when it is developing a preventive services program, it should strive to package the program to optimize each of the five qualities listed in Exhibit 7-2. Rogers has also observed that maximizing these factors *from the perspective of the client community* rather than the perspective of the MCO is critical.

PROGRESS EVALUATION

Without evaluation, neither the MCO nor the community can recognize the progress that is occurring. In fact, they may reach false conclusions about the program's success or failure. The goal of preventive services is to reduce morbidity and mortality—in other words, to try to make things *not* happen. Unfortunately, the products of this goal—the absence of events—are not directly observable. Therefore, surrogate endpoints that are observable must be established (eg, the number of people up to date on screening and immunizations or the number of people who are exercising regularly and eating a healthy diet).

Process evaluation is also important for both the MCO and the client community. Process evaluation tells the MCO which program attributes need to be changed and which attributes need to be retained. Process evaluation also gives the client community an opportunity for input into ongoing program development. Exhibit 7-3 lists the results of a process evaluation we conducted with Vietnamese women who had attended a breast and cervical cancer screening clinic.[8] As a result of this evaluation, we learned which program elements needed to be retained to ensure that women in this population would participate in the screening program.

Exhibit 7-2 Properties of Innovations Associated with Innovation Adoption

> 1. *Relative advantage:* Innovations that offer perceptible benefit to the adopter are more likely to succeed than innovations that offer no perceptible benefit.
> 2. *Compatibility:* Innovations that are perceived as consistent with the existing values, past experiences, and needs of the potential adopters are more likely to diffuse than innovations that are not compatible.
> 3. *Complexity:* Simple innovations are more likely to be adopted than complex innovations.
> 4. *Trialability:* Innovations that can be tried or sampled without a commitment to adopt are more likely to be adopted than innovations that require an all-or-none decision.
> 5. *Observability:* Innovations that produce an observable positive effect on the adopter are more likely to diffuse than innovations that have no observable effect.
>
> *Source:* Data from EM Rogers, *Diffusion of Innovations*, 3rd ed, © 1983, Free Press.

Exhibit 7-3 Top Five Reasons for Attending a Breast and Cervical Cancer Screening Clinic (Responses Given by Vietnamese Women)

> 1. the guaranteed presence of a female interpreter
> 2. presence of a female clinician
> 3. free transportation
> 4. prearranged appointments
> 5. availability of a person to guide them through the building

EXPANDING THE ROLE OF NURSES TO INCREASE PROGRAM ACCESS AND ACCEPTABILITY

In 1993, the Mayo Clinic was asked to develop a program to make women health care professionals available to provide breast and cervical cancer screening services for American Indian women. Because physicians in general and women physicians in particular are in short supply at sites that serve American Indian women, we elected to expand the role of nurses so that nurses provided examinations. The nurses work in a team with physicians and the entire clinical service unit. The high quality of the Pap test specimens collected by the nurses has been documented,[9] and the program has been well accepted by the women in the client communities.

We see no reason not to give nurses the central role in the delivery of clinical preventive services for all adults. The services recommended for the periodic health examination for adult women and men can be carried out by nurses in collaborative practice with a physician (Exhibit 7–4).[10] If nurses are not already available in the client population, nurses can be trained *de novo* within 2 or 3 years (versus 10 years or more for physicians), and we have found that there are usually women in the client populations who have already been trained as nurses. We have also found that nurses enjoy providing preventive services and, because they are compensated at a lower rate than physicians, program costs are reduced.

AGAINST, AND FOR, INTERPRETATION

> "Once again, I was reminded why I can't stand anthros and archies and socios—they make snap judgments based on superficial observations."
>
> —*Russell Means*[11]

> "The trick is not to achieve some inner correspondence of spirit with our informant; preferring, like the rest of us, to call their souls their own, they are not going to be altogether keen about such an effort anyhow."
>
> —*Clifford Geertz*[12]

The health care professional working to establish an MCO preventive services program for previously underserved or recent immigrant populations may, in an attempt to display empathy and understanding, be tempted to interpret a custom or behavior exhibited by clients. As suggested by the quotations from both Russell Means and Clifford Geertz, such a display of knowledge is not likely to be greeted with enthusiasm and will drive a wedge between the program developer and the client community. As Geertz also intimates, this reaction is not unique to immigrant or underserved communities. None of us like to be told what we are thinking or told the "real reason" why we do what we do.

While interpreting the meaning of other cultures' rituals is not fruitful, reflecting on the rituals of the health care culture can be productive. The health care environment is loaded with rituals, some of which may stand in the way of good patient care.

The *American Heritage Dictionary of the English Language* gives five definitions for "ritual" used as a noun.[13 (p1121)] The first, "the prescribed form or order of conducting a religious or solemn ceremony," probably comes to our minds first and may not be considered applicable to health care, but the fifth definition, "any detailed method of procedure faithfully or regularly followed," clearly encompasses the delivery of some health services. At a meeting in Minneapolis in 1997, Dr. Donald Berwick recounted his run-in with a health services ritual: He was scheduled to have arthroscopic knee surgery and, because he was to have a spinal anesthetic, his surgeon had agreed to let him watch the surgery on the video monitor. Even so, on multiple occasions, nurses, doctors, and other health care workers tried to take his glasses from him for no apparent reason other than dictionary definition number 5. The health services system has a multitude of rituals to be examined and questioned. The authors encourage reading Miner's essay "Body Ritual among the Nacirema"[14] as an introductory text on ritual in the United States.

Rather than interpreting rituals of client cultures for members of the client population, program developers should try to demonstrate respect for and interest in communities and

Exhibit 7–4 United States Preventive Services Task Force: Recommended Periodic Health Examination for Adults

WOMEN

Screening: Measure blood pressure, height, weight, total cholesterol (age 45–64); obtain Pap test, fecal occult blood (age 50+), mammogram and breast exam (age 50–69); screen vision and hearing (age 65+); assess for problem drinking, rubella serology, or rubella vaccination history
Immunizations: Tetanus/diphtheria (all), rubella (childbearing years), flu and pneumonia (age 65+)
Chemoprophylaxis
Multivitamins (women planning or capable of pregnancy)
Hormone prophylaxis (peri- and postmenopausal women)
Counseling:
- Substance use—tobacco cessation, avoid alcohol/drug use while driving, swimming, boating, etc
- Diet and exercise—limit fat and cholesterol; maintain caloric balance; emphasize grains, fruits, vegetables, and adequate calcium intake; obtain regular physical activity
- Injury prevention—lap/shoulder belts, helmets, smoke detectors, firearm safety, hot water <120–130°F, cardiopulmonary resuscitation (CPR) training for household members
- Sexual behavior—sexually transmitted disease (STD) prevention, contraception
- Dental health—regular visits to a dental care provider; floss and brush with fluoride daily

MEN

Screening: Measure blood pressure, height, weight, total cholesterol (age 35–64); obtain fecal occult blood (age 50+); screen vision and hearing (age 65+); assess for problem drinking
Immunizations: Tetanus/diphtheria (all), flu and pneumonia (age 65+)
Counseling
- Substance use—tobacco cessation, avoid alcohol/drug use while driving, swimming, boating, etc
- Diet and exercise—limit fat and cholesterol; maintain caloric balance; emphasize grains, fruits, vegetables; obtain regular physical activity
- Injury prevention—lap/shoulder belts, helmets, smoke detectors, firearm safety, hot water <120–130°F, CPR training for household members
- Sexual behavior—STD prevention, contraception
- Dental health—regular visits to dental care provider, floss and brush with fluoride daily

Source: Reprinted with permission from *United States Preventive Services Task Force Guide to Clinical Preventive Services*, 2nd ed, © 1996, Williams & Wilkins.

cultures by participating in cultural events when invited and showing interest when community members initiate conversations about communities. However, the authors also believe that involving the community members in a truly collaborative effort to develop an effective preventive services program is the most effective way for the MCO and its employees to gain the respect and confidence of the community it is seeking to serve.

WHAT MAKES A PREVENTIVE SERVICES PROGRAM CULTURALLY SENSITIVE?

The MCO program developer needs to imagine being asked to go for an unknown exam in a strange place by strange people for some abstract and unclear reason. Explanatory brochures are available, but they are in a language that the program developer can't read, the people in the pictures don't look or dress like most people the program developer knows, and the colors of the brochure seem garish or unpleasant. This is the experience of many members of historically underserved or immigrant populations coming into a health care arena.

We would define a culturally sensitive program as "a program in which the goal is to orient even the smallest details of the program, whenever possible, to satisfy the wants and needs of the client community rather than the wants and needs of the health care provider." When the program developer finds himself or herself explaining that details can't be changed or details don't need to change, it is time to stop and ask, "Do things really have to stay the same?"

We have had no trouble recruiting women for breast and cervical cancer screening once we have oriented the "little details" of our programs as the client community requested. In one population, the women asked that they not be made to disrobe entirely for a breast examination and Pap test. Therefore, the women were allowed to partially disrobe for the breast examination, rerobe, and then disrobe below the waist for the Pap test.

This change in procedure did not diminish the quality of the exam, and it took no extra time for the health care professionals. Yet it made the participants far more comfortable. It seems that attending to the little issues will make the big issues care for themselves.

CONCLUSION

In this brief chapter on the development of preventive services programs for historically underserved and recent immigrant populations, we have tried to balance theory with specific examples from our experience with American Indians, Alaskan Natives, Southeast Asians, and East Africans. For the MCO, there is no way to develop these programs except through repeated cycles of listening, trial, error, repeated listening, and improvement—in other words, a conventional continuous quality improvement cycle. Errors will be made, but if the program developers are willing to listen to the members of the client community and act on their suggestions whenever possible, we expect that these errors will be forgiven and program development will progress.

The benefits to providing preventive services to historically underserved and immigrant populations extend beyond these communities. It is a common experience among health care professionals that many of our patients who look just like us, dress just like us, and perhaps even are related to us, do not accept our offerings of preventive services—and we do not understand why. The same analytic and program development techniques that we suggest for work with previously underserved and immigrant populations are appropriate for use with these other patients. When health care providers develop the skills to detect differences in cultural expectations, they learn to tailor their services to account for different patient expectations. Tailoring services to account for different cultural expectations holds the promise of helping both the MCO and the patients it serves achieve their respective goals with increased levels of satisfaction.

REFERENCES

1. Refugee health screening in Minnesota: current status and recommendations. *Minn Department Health Dis Control Newsletter.* 1997;25:37–48.
2. Alaska Bureau of Vital Statistics. *1994 Annual Report.* Juneau, AK: State of Alaska Department of Health and Social Services, Division of Public Health, Bureau of Vital Statistics; 1996.
3. Geertz C. *The Interpretation of Cultures.* New York: Basic Books; 1973.
4. Hall ET. *Beyond Culture.* Garden City, NY: Anchor Books; 1977.
5. Wilson R, Leonard B, Martin M, Sterling TD, Schmid TL. *Creating Physical Activity Programs in American Indian Communities.* Atlanta, GA: Centers for Disease Control and Prevention; 1995.
6. Kelly AW, del Mar Fores Chacori M, Wollan PC, et al. A program to increase breast and cervical cancer screening for Cambodian women in a Midwestern community. *Mayo Clin Proc.* 1996;71:437–444.
7. Rogers EM. *Diffusion of Innovations.* 3rd ed. New York: Free Press; 1983.
8. Tosomeen AH, Marquez MA, Panser LA, Kottke TE. Developing preventive health programs for recent immigrants: a case study of cancer screening for Vietnamese women in Olmsted County, Minnesota. *Minn Med.* 1996;79:46–48.
9. Kottke TE, Trapp MA. The quality of Pap test specimens collected by nurses in a breast and cervical cancer screening clinic. *Am J Prev Med.* 1998;14:196–200.
10. US Preventive Services Task Force. *Guide to Clinical Preventive Services.* 2nd ed. Baltimore: Williams & Wilkins; 1996.
11. Means R. *Where White Men Fear to Tread.* New York: St. Martin's Press; 1995.
12. Geertz C. From the native's point of view: on the nature of anthropological understanding. In: Rabinow P, Sullivan WM, eds. *Interpretive Social Science.* Berkeley, CA: University of California Press; 1979:225–241.
13. Morris W, ed. *The American Heritage Dictionary of the English Language.* Boston: Houghton Mifflin Company; 1969.
14. Miner H. Body ritual among the Nacirema. In: Lessa WA, Vogt EZ, eds. *Reader in Comparative Religion: An Anthropological Approach.* 2nd ed. New York: Harper & Row; 1965:414–418.

SUGGESTED READINGS

Berger PL, Luckmann T. *The Social Construction of Reality.* Garden City, NY: Doubleday and Co; 1966.

Goodenough WH. *Cooperation in Change.* New York: Russell Sage Foundation; 1963.

Hall ET. *The Hidden Dimension.* Garden City, NY: Anchor Books; 1969.

THOMAS E. KOTTKE, MD, MSPH, is professor of medicine in the Mayo School of Medicine and a consultant in the Mayo Clinic Division of Cardiovascular Diseases. He received his MD from the University of Minnesota and his MS in public health from the University of North Carolina at Chapel Hill. He has 25 years of international experience in comprehensive heart disease prevention programs and cancer prevention programs.

MARY ALICE TRAPP, RN, is project director and trainer at the Mayo Cancer Center. She coordinates and conducts the on-site training for the Nurses Providing Annual Cancer Screening program. She traveled to 10 states and 1 US territory to train health care providers. She is also a MammaCare specialist and director.

MILO L. BREKKE, PHD, is a licensed psychologist and president of Brekke Associates, a partnership providing services and consultation in research and evaluation design, data management and analysis, and change management related to higher education, religion, and delivery of health services. He is currently a consultant for the Institute for Clinical Systems Integration and is evaluation director for Project IMPROVE, a randomized controlled trial of continuous quality improvement and systems to improve preventive services in primary care.

Part III

Special Preventive Programs for Selected High-Risk Behaviors

Related to the topics discussed in Part II, Part III focuses on some selected high-risk behaviors. There are obviously more high-risk behaviors than are represented here, but smoking and unwanted pregnancy are two common high-risk behaviors that illustrate well the concepts of focused prevention. Similar programs can be found for the prevention of human immunodeficiency virus infection, drug and alcohol abuse, physical abuse, and more. The two conditions represented in Part III are highly common in all health plans. Readers are encouraged to research preventive programs for whatever high-risk behaviors are prevalent in their own plan, medical group, or health care facility.

CHAPTER 8

Smoking Cessation: New Approaches Blend Marketing Theory with Emerging Technologies

Neal Sofian, Daniel L. Newton, and Joan DeClaire

Chapter Outline

- Introduction
- State of the Art in Cessation Therapies
- New Approaches to Reaching Larger Populations
- Taking Our Lessons from Marketing
- Using Technology To Treat Populations One Person at a Time
- The Dynamic Relationship among Impact, Reach, and Cost
- A Shared Responsibility

INTRODUCTION

Despite significant strides in the past quarter century to curb smoking in the United States, tobacco use remains a leading cause of preventable illness and death in our society. Linked to diseases such as cancer, heart disease, stroke, chronic obstructive pulmonary disease, hypertension, asthma, and diabetes, smoking continues to be implicated in more than 400,000 deaths in the United States each year. With one in five deaths attributable to smoking-related illness, tobacco kills more Americans than acquired immune deficiency syndrome (AIDS), heroin, alcohol, fire, automobile accidents, homicide, and suicide combined.[1]

Tobacco use continues to take a financial toll as well. Americans now spend $50 billion annually on medical costs for problems attributed to smoking. In addition, our society loses another $47 billion to smoking-related disability each year.[2] Many studies show smokers accrue higher health care costs, have higher rates of hospital utilization, and miss more days from work than nonsmokers do.[3] One study found hospital admission rates among smokers to be 50% higher than nonsmokers' rates, with smokers spending 25% more time in the hospital.[4] In addition, smokers' outpatient payments were 60% higher; their overall health care costs were higher by 50%. Conservative estimates show that each smoker costs his or her employer an extra $900 to $1,100 per year when compared to nonsmokers.[5] The extra costs are attributable to higher health care expenditures, increased absenteeism, and increased workers' compensation claims.

Such costs remain high at a time when our society appears stalled in its progress toward helping smokers quit. While the adult smoking rate fell dramatically for a time, from 40% in 1965 to 29% in 1990, it has remained stable since the beginning of this decade. One cause of this plateau is the recent alarming growth in the teen smoking rate—a number that had been declining throughout the 1980s. According to the University of Michigan's national Monitoring the Future project,[6] the proportion of eighth graders who reported smoking daily has recently increased by almost 50%—from 7% in 1992 to 10.4% in 1996. At the 12th-grade level, daily smoking among young people has increased 43% over the past 5 years. In 1997, nearly one in four high school seniors admitted to smoking every day. As a result of such growth in teenage smoking, the millions of adults who quit each year are replaced by millions of younger people who are smoking as teens and then age into the ranks of nicotine-addicted adults. Studies show that most smokers start in their teens.[7] Also, early initiation is associated with heavier use, longer duration of smoking, and stronger nicotine dependence. Unless the growth in youth smoking rates is stopped, it portends a disturbing picture of tomorrow's prevalence of smoking-related illness and death.

What can be done? With 3,000 children becoming regular smokers each day, has our culture exhausted its capacity to dissuade children from starting to smoke in the first place? With nearly 50 million adults still smoking, has our society hit some invisible ceiling? Have we already reached all those who can be influenced to quit?

We don't think so. Indeed, we propose that new developments in information and communication technology, coupled with society's growing understanding of how people change health behaviors, provide new opportunities for breakthroughs in smoking cessation.

We also believe preventive efforts are key. Although we will not provide an in-depth discussion of smoking prevention in this chapter on cessation, we believe more can be done to prevent young people from adopting the smoking habit. We also believe recent legislative efforts to curb tobacco marketing to teens are encouraging. Over the past several years, various local and state governments have passed laws to limit tobacco advertising aimed at youth, decrease teenagers' access to tobacco products, increase tobacco education, and obtain tobacco excise taxes to support prevention activities. Tobacco marketing is also facing significant challenges on a national level. In 1997, tobacco companies and the states discussed settlements that call for the industry to drastically alter marketing campaigns, to submit to regulatory control by the US Food and Drug Administration, and to reimburse the states for public funds spent on smoking-related illnesses.[8,9] While many in the antitobacco forces feel such settlements would not go far enough, others believe they would be steps in the right direction.

In the meantime, our society is looking for new ways to help those already addicted to tobacco. That search is leading to the development of interventions that apply state-of-the-art marketing and motivational techniques to delivery channels such as telephone call centers, the Internet, interactive voice response, and tailored print communications. Through such developments, health professionals are discovering cost-effective ways to reach and assist large populations of smokers—including those for whom traditional cessation approaches have not worked. Before we explore these innovations, however, it may be helpful to review individual smoking cessation strategies currently proven to work best, as well as the limitations of such approaches.

STATE OF THE ART IN CESSATION THERAPIES

To help individual smokers, traditional smoking cessation therapies are varied, differing by location, frequency, duration, facilitator training, and cost. Formats range from self-help booklets, to group classes, to one-on-one advice offered during physician visits. Most one-on-one and group programs report cessation rates after one year of between 15% and 40%.[10]

Many programs offer help through pharmacological approaches such as nicotine replacement therapy. Pharmaceutical company studies show that the transdermal nicotine patch combined with counseling can result in 1-year quit rates of about 25% among smokers who have expressed an interest in quitting, although most of these studies report just 3 months of data.[2] Quit rates with nicotine gum can be comparable, but some patients have problems with its taste and with understanding how to use it in appropriate dosages.

The antidepressant buproprion (Zyban) is demonstrating initial results that it can be an effective aid to smoking cessation. In a recent double-blind, placebo-controlled trial, researchers from the Mayo Clinic found that 44% of patients who took buproprion while attempting to quit were smoke-free after 7 weeks of treatment, compared to just 19% in the placebo group.[11]

With or without drug therapy, the smoking

cessation programs that have been studied and show the highest rates of success typically involve physicians delivering one-on-one advice in a clinical setting. One study demonstrated that such physician sessions can double the likelihood that a smoker will make a quit attempt.[12] Another study of the physician's role in cessation efforts indicated that the most effective programs involve physicians and other health care workers using various methods to deliver individual advice on multiple occasions.[13] This study also suggested that cessation rates would be further improved by increasing the number and intensity of contacts through follow-up visits or other contact. In addition, experience shows that such additional contacts can happen in conjunction with clinical care, but do not necessarily have to be delivered by clinical staff in order to be effective.[14]

While intensive one-on-one and group programs have been shown to help many smokers quit,[15] such programs are hindered in their ability to reach large populations. Health care providers in accredited managed care organizations are now required by the National Committee on Quality Assurance to track how many smokers are urged to quit during patient visits, but few clinicians have the time, resources, and/or skills to do in-depth individual smoking cessation therapy in this setting. Those who do address smoking may refer their patients to group programs, but a majority of smokers find such groups unacceptable for reasons ranging from inconvenient times and locations to discomfort learning in a group setting.[16] According to a 1997 report from the Agency for Health Care Policy and Research (AHCPR), only 5% of smokers are willing to enroll in group programs.[15] And even if they do enroll, they may find their instructor's one-size-fits-all approach lacking relevance to their individual needs, interests, motivations, and barriers.

The cost of group programs can be another disincentive, especially for the growing proportion of smokers with low incomes. Many programs are compelled to charge sizable fees to cover expenses such as registration, instructor salaries, training, travel expenses, materials, and facilities.

And finally, many group programs are limited by decentralized delivery methods that inhibit instructor supervision and peer review, quality assurance, the ability to replicate effective intervention models, and the ability to create efficiencies of scale. Such programs often are inaccessible to small groups or groups in isolated areas. In addition, most lack the organization necessary to track participants over time—a deficiency that inhibits outcomes measurement.

NEW APPROACHES TO REACHING LARGER POPULATIONS

Given the limitations of traditional face-to-face formal cessation programs, many authorities are calling for the development of new self-help intervention techniques. Such strategies make sense when you consider that some 85% to 90% of smokers who quit do so on their own.[16] Still, the number of successful quitters is so small that it's clear more people need more help. According to the 1986 Adult Use of Tobacco Survey, more than 30% of people in the United States (17 million) who had smoked during the preceding year said they had tried to quit during that period.[17] Of those who tried, just 1.3 million—less than 10%—were successful (Figure 8–1).[1,14,18,19] Michael Fiore, director of the Center for Tobacco Research and Intervention at the University of Wisconsin Medical School, describes the problem this way: "Smoking relapse is markedly slowing the overall potential decline in smoking prevalence in the United States. The important question is whether anything can be done to improve this low success rate."[18(p2760)]

We believe that the answer lies in developing highly effective mass-customized programs. Such programs must reach large populations while addressing the full diversity of learning styles, health beliefs, interests, and barriers that exist among people they intend to reach. Rather than simply providing smokers with information, programs need to place greater emphasis on the timing of interventions and the continuity of follow-up. Such efforts need to be cost-effective and their outcomes need to be measurable on both an individual basis and a population basis. If all of this sounds like a tall order, that's because it is.

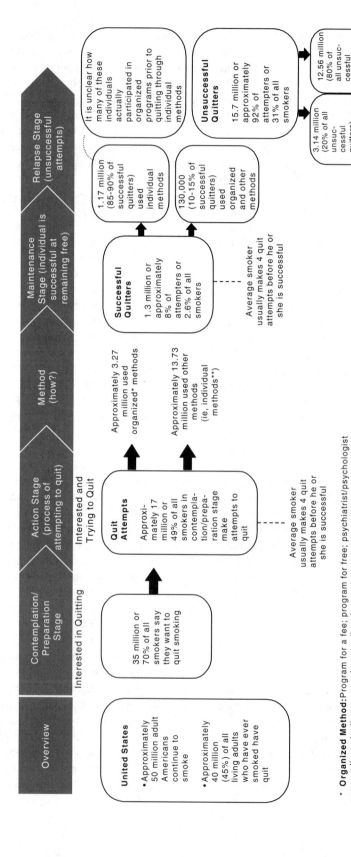

Figure 8–1 Quantifying How People Quit. Courtesy of Lexant, Seattle, Washington.

But we predict such breakthroughs are possible by applying proven theories of behavior change to a broad range of new information technologies.

TAKING OUR LESSONS FROM MARKETING

Perhaps no field understands better how to motivate large populations of people to change their behavior than marketing. American marketers, advertisers, and public relations practitioners achieve an amazing degree of sophistication and efficacy as they work to persuade the public to try new products or to switch brands. Most people would like to believe that marketing and advertising rarely affect their behavior, but the facts are quite to the contrary. This has been all too evident in the tobacco industry, which has been credited with (or blamed for) inventing our society's modern concept of public relations. Beginning in the 1920s, when the American Tobacco Company used publicity stunts that successfully linked women's rights to images of smoking, the industry has used its marketing and public relations machine to seduce millions into nicotine addiction and premature death from smoking-related illness.

"Decades of saturation cigarette advertising and promotion continued into the 1950s via billboards, magazines, movies, TV and radio," write John C. Stauber and Sheldon Rampton, editors of the quarterly *PR Watch: Public Interest Reporting on the PR/Public Affairs Industry*. "Thanks to . . . early pioneers of public relations, cigarettes built a marketing juggernaut upon an unshakable identification with sex, youth, vitality, and freedom."[20(p26)]

How can health professionals counter such powerful messages? How can they help smokers break free of their addiction and adopt lifestyles that truly deliver more vitality and better health? We believe it can be done only by using many of the marketing tools and strategies that the tobacco industry has used to the detriment of public health.

Frequency, Intensity, and Duration

Imagine if tobacco companies relied only on in-house newsletters and an occasional public service announcement to persuade people to use their products. Forget the flashy billboards, magazine advertisements, and rock concert promotions that cigarette manufacturers have used in the past to peddle their products. There is no fancy promotional gear, no carefully maintained mailing lists. In this scenario, the only way you hear the tobacco companies' message is by signing up for an 8-week class offered twice a year on Thursday nights at the hospital across town. Ridiculous? Perhaps. But that's all the marketing most traditional smoking cessation programs have ever done. The problem, of course, is that such low-key strategies ignore a fundamental principle of commercial advertising: To influence a potential buyer, you must ensure that your message is heard frequently, with high intensity, over an extended period of time.

Multiple studies of smoking cessation program efficacy prove that this commonsense approach is valid. In 1988, for example, Thomas Kottke published a meta-analysis of 108 interventions in 39 smoking cessation trials.[13] Kottke found that the most effective programs were those that "employed more than one modality for motivating behavior change, involved both physicians and non-physicians in an individualized face-to-face effort, and provided motivational messages on multiple occasions over the longest possible period of time."[13(p2888)]

What advice for future program development can be taken from Kottke's work? "Program development and program delivery will probably be most fruitful if focused on how the nonsmoking message can be given clearly, repeatedly, and consistently through every feasible delivery system," Kottke wrote in 1988.[13(p2889)] At that time, he was calling for personalized advice, printed materials, the mass media, and smoke-free medical, school, and home environments. With growth in new communications technology over the past 10 years, that list can be expanded to include media such as the Internet and interactive voice response. But the principle of frequency, intensity, and duration remains the same.

Segmentation and Resource Optimization

Another primary strategy of modern marketing is segmentation—that is, dividing a large population into smaller niches in order to appeal more closely to individuals' needs and desires. The tobacco industry has used this strategy for years, identifying the desires of their targeted audiences and then delivering images and messages that resonate with those specific groups. Consider how young women who want to lose weight and gain power identify with the chic, independent models in Virginia Slims ads; or how the young man who wants to look cool, macho, and adventurous relates to the Marlboro cowboy or the semi-defunct Joe Camel.

Contrast this approach to the traditional stop-smoking campaign, which often is based on messages related to the health hazards of tobacco ("stop smoking or you'll die of cancer," "stop smoking and you'll be healthier"). What such campaigns fail to do—and what tobacco marketing has done so well—is to link subliminally the concept of a smoke-free life to people's most cherished dreams and desires ("stop smoking and you'll look good," "stop smoking and you'll have more romance," "stop smoking and you'll have more influence at work, better relationships with your family, more fun on weekends").

Of course, different individuals are driven to change by different factors. For example, a 55-year-old male cardiac patient and a 21-year-old female college student would both do well to quit smoking. But the two smokers' attitudes and beliefs about smoking are probably different. While one might feel vulnerable to life-threatening disease as a result of smoking, the other does not. Weight gain may be of tremendous concern to one, but the other couldn't care less. To be most effective, smoking cessation programs must be tailored to address such differences. By studying what motivates people in certain segments of the population to change, targeted interventions can be designed to address the most common concerns of that particular age group, risk group, ethnic group, and so on. Then programs must track the effectiveness of their interventions to determine impact. This will allow continual matching and refinement for each smoker, extending the relationship until the sale (effectively quitting smoking) is consummated and brand loyalty (a smoke-free lifestyle) is established.

Such targeting can be done in broad strokes—designing separate interventions for seniors and younger people, for example. Or it can be done at a very detailed level, using computer-based tailored-messaging systems to design thousands of customized interventions addressing the many idiosyncrasies of an individual's health beliefs, level of self-efficacy, social support system, emotional state, and more.

These messages can be delivered in what might be considered the ultimate level of customization—the face-to-face counseling intervention. Or they can be delivered through combinations of new technologies, such as tailored print, the Internet, and interactive voice response. The advantage of using new technologies, of course, is the ability to maintain high impact while significantly reducing costs and increasing reach.

Segmentation is integral to the highly regarded transtheoretical model proposed by Prochaska and DiClemente.[21] Their theory categorizes a smoker into one of five distinct groups (precontemplation, contemplation, preparation, action, and maintenance) based on his or her stage in the change process. Using this theory, a facilitator can determine which therapeutic processes will be most effective in helping that individual move closer to cessation.

"The intensity, duration, and type of intervention should be responsive to the client's stage of change," DiClemente and Prochaska wrote.[22(p302)] "Later-stage subjects may benefit from more intense, shorter, action-oriented types of interventions. Subjects earlier in the process of change may need less intense and more extensive types of programs to be able to follow them through a quitting cycle and move them to successful action."[22(p302)]

Prochaska's studies show that cessation strategies tailored to stage of change can double quit rates over standard approaches.[23] As a result, programs now are beginning to incorporate stage-of-change theories into their interventions. One hospital corporation, for example, offers employee smokers in the action stage a fairly intensive telephone-based counseling program with referral to nicotine replacement therapy. Meanwhile, smokers in the precontemplative and contemplative stages are enrolled in a less expensive but highly tailored newsletter program intended to increase awareness of their own risks, barriers, and solutions. Based on their growing awareness, these smokers eventually advance to the action stage where they enroll in the telephone program, if needed. This approach allows the client to reach out to all smokers in its population, offering all of them opportunities to move on to the next stage in the cessation process. But only those who are truly ready to quit receive the more intensive, more expensive intervention. In essence, an integrated continuum of behavioral care is established, much like a medical continuum of care or clinical care path might be established for a given disease state.

Developing targeted cessation programs based on stages of change is just the beginning. As researchers continue to discover the various psychosocial and physiological factors that predict success with specific cessation strategies, organizations can improve their ability to match the right people to the right interventions at the right times.

The rewards of matching the right person to the right program were recently explored by Lexant, a population-based behavior change organization, and the Health Communications Research Laboratory at Saint Louis University.[24] As Figure 8–2 shows, there is an opportunity to investigate whether smoking cessation efforts are more successful when people can choose one of a variety of smoking cessation programs based on their individual situation and specific needs. When smokers were matched to programs with features they cared about, they were willing to be recruited at a significantly higher rate (38%) than the control group (18%). Cessation rates were also higher for the matched group compared to the controls.

As the Lexant research project shows, organizations can optimize limited resources by proactively recruiting specific smokers into intervention modalities that will be most beneficial to the individual and most cost-effective for the payer.

Organizations can also achieve resource optimization by stratifying their smoking populations based on expected costs. This strategy gives organizations the opportunity to be more selective in determining approaches to population intervention at an individual level.

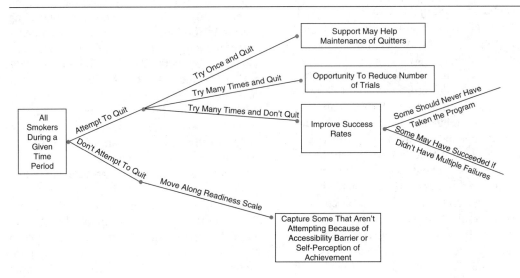

Figure 8–2 Identifying Opportunities for Improved Cessation Through Enhanced Personalization and Program Matching. Courtesy of Lexant, Seattle, Washington.

Dee Edington, dean of the University of Michigan's Health Management Research Center, has been a leader in researching the relationship between health risks and costs. His work has led to stratification models that use algorithms to identify potential high utilizers based on lifestyle-related data.[25] With such knowledge, payers can assign health cost trends to each individual and then determine intervention strategies accordingly. Edington's projections can be based on the integration of health habit and lifestyle data with information from medical claims and pharmacy claims, and other organizational performance measures such as absenteeism and participation in health programming.

To demonstrate how Edington's work might be applied, we can use our earlier examples of a 55-year-old male cardiac patient and a 21-year-old college student who are both smokers. It is reasonable to guess that the pair will cost the health care system different amounts over the next 3 years. The cardiac patient is likely to be expensive and to stick with his health plan because of the care he is receiving. The 21-year-old is another story. While she may have increased utilization because of upper respiratory infection, she probably will not be a major user of health care, nor is she likely to be loyal to her current health plan. If the payer's goal is strictly cost containment (as opposed to creating a better overall population health status), the payer might want to limit the intensity, frequency, and variety of modalities available to the low utilizer, while offering a wide range of integrated services to the high utilizer. Without a system like Edington's, all of these decisions are based on guesswork related to what we might know about these two individuals or data from population segments to which they belong. But by focusing on individual data within a segment, one can eliminate the guesswork and establish an individually generated intervention based on future cost. In other words, such systems allow a payer to make well-informed intervention investment decisions on an individual basis.

This is not to say that such cost-benefit analysis should always drive this type of decision making about behavioral care. Segmentation can be based upon psychodemographics (readiness, self-efficacy, etc), cost, or a combination of the two. But whatever segmentation approaches health plans or employers choose, they now have a highly refined tool that makes it possible to create the most effective outcome for the lowest possible cost.

Pricing and Demand

Another fundamental tenet of marketing is that products must be priced at a level consumers find acceptable. The right price point is crucial. Unfortunately, experience tells us most individuals or payers will not pay much money out of their own pockets for preventive services such as smoking cessation therapy. This is true despite a 1997 study by AHCPR that found that all the types of smoking cessation programs it reviewed are cost-effective in the long term.[15] Therefore, it would make good financial sense for health care payers (employers and care delivery systems) to pick up the tab for smoking cessation therapy, eliminating cost as a barrier to individual enrollment.

Managers at Group Health Cooperative of Puget Sound recently learned this lesson in setting copayment amounts for Free & Clear, the health maintenance organization's (HMO's) highly successful smoking cessation program, which is offered in both telephone counseling and group formats.[26] In 1991, the HMO had a goal of reducing the prevalence of smoking in its population by half—from its 1985 level of 25% to 12.5% by the year 2000. Unfortunately, fewer than 200 smokers annually were signing up to participate in the HMO's smoking cessation programs. Suspecting that smokers were inhibited from enrolling by a substantial out-of-pocket fee, the organization conducted a pilot study in 1992 in which participants had to make only a minimal copayment. If the participant was deemed an appropriate candidate for nicotine replacement therapy (patch or gum), the pharmaceutical support would be included at no cost. The results were dramatic: Registration increased from 175 individuals in 1992 to more than 2,800 in 1993. Among the 1993 participants, 33% were still not smoking 12 months after they finished participating in the program. Unfortunately, close to 800 individuals who signed up for the program that year never made their copayments and were thus eliminated from the program. Nonetheless, participation had increased by more than 1,000% without significantly changing cessation outcomes.

In 1996, Group Health began a controlled study to see how different copayment levels would affect utilization, satisfaction, and outcomes in the smoking cessation program.[26] The study confirmed that reducing cost barriers results in far more individuals successfully quitting smoking. When copayments were totally eliminated, participation increased 2,000%. In addition, Group Health found that in groups with a $42 Free & Clear copayment, approximately 30% of smokers who signed up initially dropped out before they paid their portion of the program fee. In cohorts with no copayments, only 1% of smokers who registered failed to participate.

Removing financial barriers was just one effort Group Health made to achieve its impressive cessation results. Other strategies involved providing both telephone-based and group-based programs, allowing nicotine replacement therapy as appropriate, and developing more effective marketing and advertising methods, including a significant physician education component. But there is no doubt that eliminating the financial burden for individuals played a significant role in the program's success.

Prevalence of tobacco use at Group Health *has* dropped from 25% in 1985 to 20% in 1990 to 15.5% in 1994. These figures are in sharp contrast to the much slower rate of decline during the same period in the state of Washington's general population: from 23% in 1987 to 21% in 1993.[26]

Based on 1996 figures from Group Health, the total cost for intensive telephone counseling or group programming is approximately $150 to $175 for behavioral change intervention plus an average of an additional $152 for nicotine replacement therapy, which is used by 50% to 60% of participants. This makes the average cost for the comprehensive program, which includes three complementary modalities of intervention (telephone, group, and nicotine replacement therapy), $238 to $254 per participant. When taking into account the costs of providing services both to successful quitters and relapsers, the entire program costs $582 per successful quitter. Based on these figures, a cost-effectiveness calculation model used by the state of Washington[27] shows that intervention is valued at $366 per year of life saved. Meanwhile, even the most conservative estimates identify savings of more than $500 per year in direct excess health care costs.[5] Additionally, when absenteeism and workers' compensation are included in the equation, savings equal more than $900 per year per successful quitter. In contrast, hypertension and cholesterol treatment and cervical, breast, and colon cancer screening—preventive care services now routinely included in medical coverage—average $10,000 to $100,000 per year of life saved.

USING TECHNOLOGY TO TREAT POPULATIONS ONE PERSON AT A TIME

Improving smoking cessation by adopting state-of-the-art marketing principles is only half the story. We believe that cessation programs become exponentially more powerful when they employ and integrate new communications channels such as telephone call centers, the Internet, tailored newsletters, and interactive voice response. Connected to powerful computer systems that can organize and store large amounts of psychodemographic data from individual smokers, these channels can deliver highly personalized interventions that zero in on each smoker's stage of change, health beliefs, motivations, barriers, and more. Whether the resulting intervention is delivered via a telephone counselor, an interactive voice response phone system, a Web site, or a newsletter, it is designed to meet the individual smoker's needs. Such integrated programs also make it possible to reach smokers anywhere at any time.

What outcomes can be anticipated with the type of integrated new technologies we have proposed? Although it is too soon to tell, we expect answers to emerge over the next 2 to 3 years through innovations under way nationwide. In the meantime, we can look to the success of preventive health programs that have employed discrete components of more integrated programs. Many such discrete programs are described below.

The Internet

Use of computers and the Internet has grown at a dizzying pace over the past 5 years. As more people go on line, they will gain access to a broad range of health information and interactivity. While health professionals have much to learn about promoting smoking cessation via the Internet, the power of computerized health education programs has been proven in dozens of studies.

In July 1997, the *Journal of Family Practice* published a review of 22 randomized clinical trials evaluating the acceptability and usefulness of such interventions.[28] The study looked at 13 instructional programs, 5 information support networks, and 4 systems for health assessment and history taking. Researchers concluded that "computerized educational interventions can lead to improved health status in several major areas of care, and appear not to be a substitute for, but a valuable supplement to, face-to-face time with physicians."[28(p25)] The reviewers found that computers are often the preferred educational method for patients with chronic diseases that require a high degree of self-management. Computerized health education programs frequently helped patients better understand their disease and helped them gain a greater sense of control and confidence in their ability to improve their health, the reviewers wrote. They also found that the patient's age did not appear to affect his or her acceptance of the computerized educational methods. Furthermore, they reported that in some studies, patients seemed more willing to confide in computers than in human interviewers. The reviewers speculated that the patients perceived the computers as nonjudgmental, evoking less embarrassment on sensitive subjects. (Telephone smoking cessation and diabetes counselors who compared their work to previous experiences counseling in face-to-face intervention services have made similar observations. The counselors reported being highly surprised that callers were willing to provide so much more intimate information over the phone than they had been willing to offer in group or one-on-one sessions.)

With the number of health-related Web sites growing substantially, many health care providers express reasonable concern over the quality of health information their patients gather from the Web. But as the *Journal of Family Practice* reviewers emphasize, providers can make their own jobs easier by becoming familiar with credible Web sites and pointing their patients to them.

High-quality preventive health information on the Web has many advantages over traditional print materials in that it can be updated instantly to reflect the latest medical research. On-line chat groups can be a good source of social support—proven to be an important benefit to people who are quitting smoking. Internet users also can get quick access to information from on-line experts and counselors. And finally, the interactivity of the Web provides an excellent format for cost-effectively delivering personally tailored questionnaires and advice.

Tailored Print

Letters, newsletters, magazines, and self-help guidebooks are familiar forms for health education. But research shows they take on added impact when customized to fit the individual reader's concerns. Studies have proven the effectiveness of tailored print interventions for a variety of health issues including smoking,[29] mammography,[30] nutrition,[31] and exercise.[32] In a North Carolina study, for instance, health psychologists Victor Strecher and Matthew Kreuter and their colleagues collected information on individuals' cigarette consumption, interest in quitting, and perceived benefits and barriers to quitting, as well as other characteristics relevant to smoking cessation.[29] They then created newsletters with messages individually tailored by computer to match the smokers' interests and concerns. Smokers were randomly assigned to two groups, one that received the tailored newsletters and one that received a generic smoking cessation newsletter. After 6 months, 30.7% of the moderate to light smokers who got the tailored newsletter had quit, compared with 7.1% in the control group.

Another study to determine whether printed physicians' recommendations regarding breast cancer screening would be more effective if they were tailored to individuals' perceptions showed similar results.[30] Tailored letters that addressed each woman's specific beliefs about breast cancer and mammography's ability to detect it, as well as the individual's barriers (cost, fear of radiation, fear of finding cancer), were more likely to be thoroughly read and remembered than generic letters.

Telephone Call Centers

The efficacy of outbound telephone programs for smoking cessation was first addressed in a 1991 study conducted by the National Cancer Institute.[33] In this investigation, University of North Carolina researcher C. Tracy Orleans and her colleagues used the Free & Clear program at Group Health to produce 16-month abstinence rates of 23%. This compares with a national average of 10% to 12% for self-help cessation programs and 30% for high-quality group programs. Free & Clear's results were achieved by trained counselors delivering up to four brief personalized phone calls over a period of 60 weeks. The counselors focused on behavior modification techniques and nicotine fading, a process of brand switching that moves smokers to lower tar and nicotine cigarettes prior to quitting. Further research using the same program in cooperation with GTE Northwest demonstrated 12-month quit rates of 34% by expanding the intervention to include six calls over a 12-month period.[34]

A 1996 study of a telephone-based effort at the University of California San Diego produced similar results.[35] This study compared three groups of smokers. One group received a self-help quit kit and up to six phone calls from counselors, one group received the kit and just one phone call, and the third group received the kit only. After 12 months, among those who attempted to quit, only 14.7% in the kit-only group made it. The group with one phone call had a 19.8% success rate. The group with up to six phone calls had a rate of 26.7%.

Smoking cessation studies generally show that the more frequently smokers are contacted, the higher their success rate. Still, even one brief intervention call often has a significant impact on smokers' success. Indeed, researchers in the Free & Clear study got such positive results among smokers after just two phone calls that they concluded four calls may not have been necessary. As health professionals learn more about tailoring interventions, they can determine which individuals need only one call and which need six or more calls in combination with other modalities.

Interactive Voice Response

Adding interactive voice response (IVR) technology to their repertoire of communication channels may allow smoking cessation programs to increase their effectiveness even further while reducing cost.

Automated IVR systems, which allow patients to enter and receive information via the touch-tone pad on their telephones, have already proven to be an effective assessment, monitoring, and education tool in a variety of preventive care and disease management programs.[36-38] Robert Friedman, an internist at Boston University Medical Center who has pioneered the use of IVR for patients with hypertension and hypercholesterolemia, proved that this technology can help patients adhere to medication regimens and manage their illnesses.[36]

IVR has also proven to be a valid tool for assessing and monitoring patients with mental disorders and alcoholism. A recent Wisconsin study compared diagnoses of primary care patients' mental disorders obtained via IVR to those obtained by a trained clinician over the telephone using a structured clinical interview.[37] Researcher Kenneth Kobak and his colleagues concluded that IVR "allows for increased availability and provides primary care physicians with information that increases the quality of patient care without additional physician time and at minimal expense."[37(p905)] As with other forms of computerized health assessment, Kobak and others found that patients tend to disclose more about sensitive behavioral issues when they use an IVR assessment than when they are being interviewed by clinicians. Kobak discovered, for example, that patients using IVR reported rates of alcohol abuse that were twice as high as rates reported to their physicians. He concluded that the IVR assessment's "high levels of sensitivity, specificity, and accuracy"[37(p910)] can help clinicians make better treatment decisions, thus improving quality of patient care. Given that IVR improves the assessment and treatment of problems like alcohol abuse, one can assume that it will prove efficacious in assessing and treating smoking behavior as well.

THE DYNAMIC RELATIONSHIP AMONG IMPACT, REACH, AND COST

Although it is still too early to reliably predict outcomes from the integrated use of new marketing approaches and emerging technologies, we believe such programs can positively affect the ability to reach large populations, lower costs, and impact health behavior. We also anticipate that such outcomes will depend on how the sponsoring organizations choose to define the dynamic relationship that exists among impact, reach, and cost.

To understand this dynamic, imagine a health plan with a limited budget for smoking cessation. If administrators decide that *impact* ought to be their top priority, they might invest in a smoking cessation program that promises to deliver the highest quit rates. Smokers would be invited to participate in a high-intensity program that would include several in-depth phone calls and tailored self-help materials. They would be contacted repeatedly, receiving all forms of psychological support and education, as well as nicotine replacement therapy. In the end, long-term quit rates might be as high as 40%. But because of cost, access might be limited to a small percentage of the plan's smoking population.

If, on the other hand, the health plan decides to place its emphasis on *reach*, administrators might choose a low-impact, low-cost intervention that includes just one supportive phone call and generic (not tailored) health education materials. While the long-term quit rates of such a program most certainly will be lower (say, 10%), the program's lower cost could ensure its availability to a much larger audience, ultimately resulting in more smokers quitting.

Other alternatives include stratifying the smoking population and offering a variety of programs. For example, those with the highest risk, cost, or level of readiness could get the more intense, more expensive interventions. Those with lower risk, lower cost, or less motivation could get the less expensive, less intense interventions. These types of stratification could also be based on factors such as self-efficacy, learning style, geography, and so on. Such approaches can ensure that the right people get just the right amount of help at the right time and the right cost.

A SHARED RESPONSIBILITY

However sponsors choose to balance the forces of reach, impact, and cost, we believe the advent of new technologies brings about more choices in designing smoking cessation programs and a greater potential for significantly lowering smoking rates in the near future.

The current trend for managing the health of large populations is to choose from a variety of modalities (print, telephone, Internet, IVR, etc). Organizations that are particularly progressive are optimizing resources through market segmentation—for example, designing interventions in ways that present a different mix of modalities for groups with different needs. We believe the next challenge is to create "segments of one," determining the most appropriate intervention for each individual in a given population.

This approach can be applied effectively not only to smoking cessation and prevention, but to all areas where personal behavior is critical to people's health and well-being. Whether the goal is to reduce a diabetic's hemoglobin A1C percentages or to manage the complicated drug regimen of an AIDS patient on a protease inhibitor "cocktail," such individualized approaches play a critical role in managing health risk and disease within large populations.

Responsibility for our society's success in this venture must be shared with a variety of stakeholders, including health care providers, health plans, employers, lawmakers, and smokers themselves. Research shows that most smokers want to quit. It also shows that physicians have a tremendous, yet unrealized, power to help their patients through individual consultation during routine visits. But given today's demand on physician time and resources, health care systems must use new techniques to leverage physicians' power to help smokers. As Michael Fiore writes, "Just as every clinician has a professional responsibility to assess and treat tobacco users, so health care administrators, insurers, and purchasers have responsibility to craft policies, provide resources, and display leadership in fostering smoking cessation efforts."[14(p525)]

Through new advances in technology and our growing understanding of how to change behavior, health care systems and employers will be able to provide effective interventions for smoking cessation and other lifestyle-related issues. As leaders in preventive care have stated, heart disease and cancer are not the leading causes of death in our country. Rather, millions face death prematurely as a result of smoking, lack of activity, excess weight, and other personal health behaviors. Now is the time for health care systems and employers to make high-quality behavior change programs part of our society's standard of care. Nothing less is acceptable.

REFERENCES

1. US Department of Health and Human Services. *Reducing the Health Consequences of Smoking: 25 Years of Progress: A Report of the Surgeon General.* DHHS pub no. (CDC) 89-8411. Atlanta, GA: Centers for Disease Control, National Center for Chronic Disease Prevention and Health Promotion, Office on Smoking and Health; 1989.
2. Rothenberg R, Lewis N, Honchar P. Smoking cessation in the clinical setting. *The 1998 Wellness and Prevention Sourcebook.* New York: Faulkner & Gray; 1997: 62–78.
3. Sofian N, McAfee T, Doctor J, Carson D. Tobacco control and cessation. In: O'Donnell MP, Harris JS, eds. *Health Promotion in the Workplace.* 2nd ed. Albany, NY: Delmar; 1994:343–366.
4. Penner M, Penner S. Excess insured health care costs from tobacco-using employees in a large group plan. *J Occup Med.* 1990;32(6):521–523.
5. Sofian NS, Graff W. Myths of smoking in the workplace. *Compensation Benefits Manage.* 1987;3(2):31–36.
6. University of Michigan News and Information Service. *Monitoring the Future Study Press Release.* December 20, 1997.
7. Breslau N, Peterson EL. Smoking cessation in young adults: age at initiation of cigarette smoking and other suspected influences. *Am J Public Health.* 1996;86: 214–220.
8. Smolowe J. Sorry, pardner: big tobacco fesses up and pays up. *Time.* June 30, 1997:24–29.
9. Carey J. Big tobacco's hidden war. *Business Week.* November 10, 1997:139–140.
10. Schwartz JL. Methods of smoking cessation. *Med Clin North Am.* 1992;76(2):451–476.
11. Hurt RD, Sachs DP, Glover ED, et al. A comparison of sustained release buproprion and placebo for smoking cessation. *New Engl J Med.* 337(17):1230–1231.
12. Manley MW, Epps R, Glynn T. The clinician's role in promoting smoking cessation among clinic patients. *Med Clin North Am.* 1992;76(2):477–494.
13. Kottke T, Battista R, DeFriese G, Brekke M. Attributes of smoking cessation interventions in medical practice. *J Am Med Assoc.* 1988;259(19):2883–2889.
14. Fiore M. Smoking cessation: a clinical guideline from AHCPR. *Drug Benefit Trends.* 1996;8(9):29–32, 35.
15. Cromwell J, Bartosch WJ, Fiore M, Hasselblad V, Baker T. Cost-effectiveness of the clinical practice recommendations in the AHCPR guideline for smoking cessation. *JAMA.* 1997;278:1759–1766.
16. Schwartz J. Methods for smoking cessation. *Clin Chest Med.* 1991;12(4):737–753.
17. Schwartz J. *Review and Evaluation of Smoking Cessation Methods: United States and Canada, 1978–1985.* National Institutes of Health publication 87-2940. Bethesda, MD: US Department of Health and Human Services; 1987.
18. Fiore M, Novotny T, Pierce J. Methods used to quit smoking in the United States: do cessation programs help? *JAMA.* 1990;263(20):2760–2765.

19. Glynn TJ, Boyd GM, Gruman JC. Essential elements of self-help/minimal intervention strategies for smoking cessation. *Health Educ Q.* 1990;17(3):329–345.

20. Stauber J, Rampton S. *Toxic Sludge Is Good for You: Lies, Damn Lies, and the Public Relations Industry.* Monroe, ME: Common Courage Press; 1995.

21. Prochaska J, DiClemente C. Stages and processes of self-change of smoking: toward an integrative model of change. *J Consult Clin Psychol.* 1983;51:390–395.

22. DiClemente C, Prochaska J. The process of smoking cessation: an analysis of precontemplation, contemplation, and preparation stages of change. *J Consult Clin Psychol.* 1991;59(2):295–304.

23. Prochaska J, DiClemente C, Velicer WF, Rossi JS. Standardized, individualized, interactive, and personalized self-help programs for smoking cessation. *Health Psychol.* 1993;12:399–405.

24. Brennan L, Kreuter M, Newton D, et al. Using assessment-based matching to link smokers to appropriate cessation programs: results from a randomized trial. Presented at the American Public Health Association Annual Meeting; November 1, 1997; New York.

25. Edington D, Tze-ching YL. The financial impact of changes in personal health practices. *J Occupational Environ Med.* 1997;39(11):1037–1046.

26. McAfee T, Sofian N, Wilson J, Hindmarsh M. The role of tobacco intervention in population-based health care: a case study. *Am J Prev Med.* 1998;14(2):46–52.

27. State of Washington Department of Public Health. *Tobacco and Health in Washington State.* Olympia, WA: State of Washington Department of Public Health; 1990.

28. Krishna S, Balas E, Spencer D, et al. Clinical trials of interactive computerized patient education: implications for family practice. *J Fam Pract.* 1997;45(1):25–33.

29. Strecher V, Kreuter M, DenBoer DJ, et al. The effects of computer-tailored smoking cessation messages in family practice settings. *J Fam Pract.* 1994;39(3):262–270.

30. Skinner C, Strecher V, Hospers H, et al. Physicians' recommendations for mammography: do tailored messages make a difference? *Am J Public Health.* 1994;84(1):43–49.

31. Brug J, Steenhuis I, Van Assema P, DeVries H. The impact of a computer-tailored nutrition intervention. *Prev Med.* 1996;25:236–242.

32. King A, Carl F, Birkel L, Haskell W. Increasing exercise among blue-collar employees: the tailoring of worksite programs to meet specific needs. *Prev Med.* 1988;17:357–365.

33. Orleans CT, Schoenback V, Wagner E, et al. Self-help quit smoking interventions: effects of self-help materials, social support instructions, and telephone counseling. *J Consult Clin Psychol.* 1991;59(3):439–448.

34. McAfee T, Sofian N. Smoking cessation at GTE Northwest. Presented at the Wellness in the Workplace Conference; 1998; Long Beach, CA.

35. Zhu SH, Strecher V, Balabanis M, Rosbrook B, Sadler G, Pierce T. Telephone counseling for smoking cessation: effects of single-session and multiple-session interventions. *J Consult Clin Psychol.* 1996;64(1):202–211.

36. Friedman RH, Kazis L, Jette A, et al. A telecommunications system for monitoring and counseling patients with hypertension: impact on medication adherence and blood pressure control. *Am J Hypertens.* 1996;9:285–292.

37. Kobak KA, Taylor L, Dottl S, et al. A computer-administered telephone interview to identify mental disorders. *JAMA.* 1997;278(11):905–910.

38. Searles JS, Perrine MW, Mundt JC, Helzer JE. Self-report of drinking using touch-tone telephone: extending the limits of reliable daily contact. *J Stud Alcohol.* 1995;56(4):375–382.

NEAL SOFIAN, MPH, is a principal of the NewSof Group, which offers strategic/business planning, marketing, and consulting related to initiatives in health behavior change, disease management, health promotion, and outcome assessment. Previously, he was vice president of intervention development for Lexant, a health management company, and he has managed worksite and community health promotion programs at Group Health Cooperative of Puget Sound. He has also been assistant director of the Bureau of Community Health Education in the Missouri State Division of Health.

DANIEL L. NEWTON, PHD, is a principal of the NewSof Group. Previously, he was vice president of operations for Lexant, and he was a senior consultant with the Benfield Group, a national health care consulting firm. Dr. Newton has more than 13 years of experience in the design, implementation, monitoring, and evaluation of comprehensive, integrated health risk management programs for large health care, corporate, and government organizations.

JOAN DECLAIRE is a content development manager for Lexant. She has worked for 20 years as a writer and editor of health materials for print and online media. She has a BA in journalism.

CHAPTER 9

Preventing Unwanted and Unplanned Pregnancies

David Share

Chapter Outline

- Introduction
- Health Plan Perspective
- Behavioral Factors
- Role of Public Health Agencies
- Education
- Removing Barriers to Contraceptive Care
- Associated Risk Factors
- Service Coverage and Reimbursement Policies
- Religion
- Conclusion

INTRODUCTION

Though most people consider pregnancy and childbearing life-affirming acts that should be consciously chosen, the reality is very different. Sadly, most pregnancies are unintended and many are unwanted. About two thirds of premenopausal adult women and 4 in 10 teenage girls are at risk of unintended pregnancy.[1] At any age, unintended pregnancies are about as likely to end in induced abortion as they are to end in live birth.[1] Pregnancies that are terminated are clearly unwanted and mostly unplanned. Many pregnancies that result in live birth are unplanned, and some of these are unwanted as well.[1] This is especially true for teens; 85% of all teen pregnancies are unplanned.[2]

HEALTH PLAN PERSPECTIVE

Health plans are concerned with the costs and volume of maternity and newborn care, which are proportionately and absolutely large for all plans. However, plan administrators usually assume a passive attitude toward this aspect of health care, assuming that a plan's maternity and newborn care costs and volume are immutable, driven solely by demographics.

Programs designed to improve the quality and efficiency of reproductive care, and related member satisfaction, are almost always focused on postconception care. Common efforts include programs to prevent premature labor and promote healthy pregnancy outcomes, decrease rates of Caesarean section, and decrease postpartum length of stay. However, it is rare for health plans to explicitly acknowledge or attempt to address the fact that most pregnancies are unplanned and many pregnancies are unwanted.

BEHAVIORAL FACTORS

Over half of all women who become pregnant are not actively trying to conceive. Yet they have engaged in sexual intercourse without regular use of effective contraception. When questioned, while denying a clear intent to conceive, most of these women acknowledge an awareness that they were at risk of becoming pregnant.[3]

This reflects the complex emotional nature of the act of procreation. For some, making a conscious choice to bear a child is overwhelming, and a passive, subconscious choice is far easier. For others, risking unplanned pregnancy is more a statement of wanting to sustain an intimate relationship than it is an expression of a desire to have a child. Risk taking also may occur when a person has strong and conflicting attitudes and emotions about sustaining intimate relationships, raising a child, affording a child, and changing his or her life to accommodate a child. These emotions can yield profound ambivalence.

People's feelings about a pregnancy can also be complex. Often, they depend on the nature and tone of the relationship with the conception partner and the partner's expectations regarding the relationship and child rearing. Other key factors include employment, financial obligations, and maternal age and educational status.

Some women wish they had prevented an unplanned pregnancy, and others, on balance, are glad that they did not. It is often difficult to clearly differentiate wanted from unwanted pregnancies. The ambivalent attitudes and motivations of many pregnant women also make it difficult to rigorously delineate planned from unplanned pregnancies.

In contrast, a minority of women clearly have negative, unambiguous feelings regarding unplanned pregnancy. This attitude is most common for women at the extremes of the reproductive age range: teens and women in their 40s.

Unwanted pregnancies can occur because of contraceptive failure or failure to contracept. They can also occur because of physical or emotional coercion. Whatever the causes or motivations, unwanted pregnancies represent a large personal and societal cost.

Given the complex set of issues and the highly charged emotions and motivations pertaining to childbearing, it is not surprising that health plans have shied away from addressing the problem of unwanted and unplanned pregnancies. Procreation issues tend to engender the same passivity and ambivalence in health plans that they do in people. In fact, throughout our culture, acquiescence and passivity tend to surround procreation concerns.

ROLE OF PUBLIC HEALTH AGENCIES

Unwanted and unplanned pregnancies represent a major challenge that health plans, historically, have left to public health agencies. However, as more health care resources are directed to the private sector, especially managed care plans, the financial base of public health agencies has been eroded. At the same time, the mission of public health is being redefined in most regions of the country.

This new definition is quickly reducing or eliminating direct service provision from the public health agenda, which is now focusing on community health assessment and planning. This change in focus has created a relative vacuum; there are few community efforts to address the problem of unwanted and unplanned pregnancies.

Health plans, which have benefited indirectly from public health efforts in this regard, now must directly address the problem in collaboration with other health and social service agencies. Failure to rise to this challenge will erode community well-being and lead to higher plan costs associated with the medical consequences of social problems. As plan administrators take on this challenge, they should keep a key public health principle in mind: Ensure the acceptability, accessibility, and affordability of care.

To ensure access to contraceptive services, and to successfully contracept, sexually active women need information about contraception and ready access to contraceptive services and supplies. Efforts to create and disseminate information about contraception have been primarily carried out by local and state public health departments and their family planning programs, Planned Parenthood affiliates, and teen health centers. Health plan administrators should recognize and affirm the depth of experience and effectiveness of these programs. Rather than trying to replace such efforts, plans should take advantage of this expertise by sponsoring and supporting this work or collaborating with these agencies. Examples of community-based family planning education include school- and youth group–based peer education efforts, teen theater troupes, and community center health fairs. Health departments, in collaboration with other agencies, are beginning to disseminate information about contraception through the Internet and interactive computer kiosks. These efforts, in the aggregate, achieve results. Condom use, for example, has increased threefold in the last 10 years as a result of widespread education regarding human immunodeficiency virus (HIV) transmission and sexually transmitted disease (STD) prevention.[1] This success contributes to decreasing the incidence of unplanned and unwanted pregnancy.

EDUCATION

In addition to fostering and enhancing such community-based educational efforts, plans can use existing, internal lines of communication to share additional information with members about the nature and availability of contraception. Such vehicles include plan newsletters and magazines, and community or medical center health fairs. Creative activities could include focused marketing efforts to groups, such as teenagers, at high risk of unwanted and unplanned pregnancies.

Information about contraception should be included in member educational materials. In addition to providing general contraceptive information, plans could actively work to ensure that all adult women know where they can find covered contraceptive services and supplies. Unlike teens, adults are a diverse group without strong peer identification. Adults are more independent than teens and not likely to be receptive to highly directive family planning intervention. As a result, it is most appropriate to focus efforts for adults on providing them with factual information regarding contraception and access to contraceptive services and supplies.

Teens are different. They are a readily identifiable, discrete subgroup with a powerful peer group association. They are somewhere between the dependence of childhood and the relative independence of adulthood. As a result, they are more open than adults to services designed to help educate them about important life choices.

Teens are at particularly high risk of unplanned and unwanted pregnancies. The social, financial, and emotional consequences of unplanned pregnancies among teens are profound and life changing. Though an unwanted pregnancy can be problematic at any age, it can be especially devastating for teens, because they have not completed their education and probably lack adequate employment, social support, and earning potential.

Teen health centers offer adolescent-oriented services in culturally sensitive, comfortable, accessible settings. Often, teens will make use of teen health centers for services that they would not readily seek in traditional health care settings. Teen health centers, and adolescent medicine practitioners in general, routinely engage in assessment and education with a prevention focus. They address many issues surrounding maturation, including sex, during encounters for other services such as school and sports physicals and visits for common illnesses. Plans should take advantage of this experience, expertise, and prevention focus by including such providers in the plan network, and actively recommending these providers to adolescent members and their parents.

Unfortunately, teens aren't known for their long-term planning skills. They don't readily and independently assess their potential health needs, their alternative sources of health care, and the steps necessary to access such services in a managed care system. Creative, proactive efforts are needed to maximize teens' access to services that are specially designed to be culturally and geographically accessible and acceptable.

For example, a marketing effort could include a two-sided letter sent by the plan. One side could be addressed to parents on plan letterhead, encouraging them to be actively involved in helping their teens lead healthy lives and informing them about the plan network's teen health center services. The other side of the letter, on the letterhead of the teen health center, could be addressed to the teens, informing them of the teen health center and its inclusion in the plan network and inviting them to make use of the center's services.

A program could also be designed to educate adult members about communicating with their preadolescent and teen children about sex, responsibility in relationships, and other behaviors and issues associated with maturation and health. Again, such programs are most likely to succeed if they are conceived and implemented in cooperation with community-based social service and public health agencies.

REMOVING BARRIERS TO CONTRACEPTIVE CARE

Managed care plans could establish policies allowing teens to receive covered care from teen health centers without the need for gatekeeper authorization. Independent, confidential access to teen-oriented services will measurably increase the proportion of sexually active teens in a plan's membership who successfully seek care.[4] Hopefully, this will prevent unwanted pregnancy, STDs, and other problems associated with common adolescent health risk behaviors. While the potential impact of the primary care physician may be diminished by such a policy, many teens are uncomfortable going to their family doctor or the doctor assigned to them by the health plan or their parents. If there is a strict requirement that all services must be provided by or referred by the primary care gatekeeper, these teenagers may avoid seeking services altogether.

ASSOCIATED RISK FACTORS

Plans should recognize that some teen health risks are associated with other teen health risks. That is, teens who engage in unsafe sex, without contraception, often are experimenting with alcohol, cigarettes, and other drugs, or with drinking and driving.[5] Providers specializing in adolescent health routinely assess and intervene on all such health risk behaviors. This practice, and expertise in communicating with this unique group, can positively affect many aspects of teen health, not just pregnancy prevention.[6]

Support of community-based services might be groundbreaking for a plan, especially an integrated health system with its own providers. It is especially difficult for plans to approve prevention strategies that lead to resources going outside of the traditionally defined system. However, in selected instances, such investments are well rewarded. When it comes to maternity and newborn care for unwanted pregnancy, an ounce of prevention is worth a pound of care services. Investment in teens' access to community-based adolescent health expertise is a wise long-term investment in plan financial success, community support, and community well-being.

Plans should recognize and foster an awareness of the fact that women of all ages, especially younger women, experience partner violence and substance abuse in conjunction with unprotected sex. Health plans should actively educate participating providers about the high prevalence of these problems and the likelihood that if one of these problems is identified, others are also present. Much can be accomplished by establishing programs that address these issues, training clinicians and nurses to routinely screen for and assist clients with these concerns, and to educate members about the need for and availability of care. Substance abuse, partner violence, and unplanned pregnancy education efforts represent excellent opportunities for collaboration between health plans and community social service agencies.

SERVICE COVERAGE AND REIMBURSEMENT POLICIES

Plan policies should be consciously crafted to eliminate barriers to access to preventive services. Reimbursement strategies must incorporate nuances pertinent to the unique circumstances of contraceptive services providers. This is especially important in capitated plans. For example, plan administrators should recognize that traditional means of assessing clinician productivity are not applicable to adolescent medicine. Adolescent medicine specialists and teen health centers generally serve teens who are self-selected, or who seek care on referral, because they have specific health problems. Standard adolescent capitation rates will simply not cover the costs of providing care to a group of teens who disproportionately need contraceptive services and supplies; have STDs, eating disorders, depression, and school problems; or are pregnant. This adverse selection should be viewed positively; it indicates that such specialists and teen clinics are attracting clients most in need of services. Plans should take this expected adverse selection into account when crafting reimbursement policies. Failure to do so will diminish the availability of such services and their ability to help plans prevent the costly consequences of high-risk behavior.

It is unrealistic to expect that health plans, and the traditional medical practices with which they usually contract, will be successful in attracting and serving all clients who historically have used community-based programs sponsored by public health departments, Planned Parenthood clinics, or teen health centers. Just because contraceptive services are available in primary care physicians' offices doesn't mean that plan members will avail themselves of the services in these settings. Access to contraceptive services in community-based agencies should be fostered, not restricted by overly zealous adherence to gatekeeper requirements. This approach to maximizing access will encourage teens, especially, to seek care earlier and address problems more effectively, which will increase the likelihood of preventing unwanted pregnancies and other serious problems commonly faced by adolescents.

Plan policies should be crafted to carefully avoid barriers to access created by policies that make contraceptive supplies unaffordable. For example, pharmacy benefits that do not cover contraceptive supplies, or that cover only selected, low-cost supplies, are counterproductive in the long run. Most plans do not cover the cost of or encourage access to emergency contraceptive pills. Yet this method prevents unintended pregnancy cost-effectively.[7] While many women will pay out of pocket for supplies associated with their preferred contraceptive method, many will not, often because of competing demands for their limited income. Yet these women are disproportionately likely to perceive an unplanned pregnancy as stressful and undesirable.

To increase profitability, some hospitals require provision of contraceptive supplies to patients on an outpatient basis following discharge. For example, some hospitals refuse to offer Depo-Provera injections or Norplant implants during a maternity stay. This shifts the service provision and reimbursement to the outpatient setting. The result is decreased pharmacy costs associated with a diagnosis-related group (DRG) payment. This practice saves the hospital money, but it costs the health system and society much more if more women engage in intercourse without contraception during the first weeks postpartum. A managed care organization may choose to negotiate an add-on to its rate to accommodate this practice.

The peculiarities of benefit policies also affect reimbursement restrictions for devices such as the Norplant implant. Some plans will cover the cost of the Norplant implant only if the claim is submitted by the provider responsible for inserting the device. Since the acquisition cost nears $400, many community clinics and private physicians can't afford to stock these implants. Yet, in such instances, pharmacies will not dispense the implants directly to patients, since patients will not be reimbursed by the plan. This leads to a paradox for the patient, who must go to another provider who both stocks and inserts the device. Some patients faced with this challenge are willing to make this extra effort, but many are not. For them, unplanned and undesired pregnancy is often the result.

RELIGION

Finally, health plans and health systems with religious affiliations often are reluctant to establish policies and practices that ensure access to contraceptive services. This attitude can take form in many ways. For example, a hospital might refuse to provide surgical sterilization or intrauterine devices (IUDs).

Some health systems and health plans find ways around religious proscriptions. One approach is to contract with a third-party administrator that, in turn, handles insurance premiums or reimbursements for contraceptive services and independently contracts with providers to offer contraceptive services to consumers.

CONCLUSION

Most pregnancies are unintended and many unwanted. Health plans have not, historically, addressed this problem. Yet each year the cost of more than 150,000 teen pregnancies is borne by the managed care industry.[8]

While it will never completely go away, the problem is remediable. For example, each year publicly funded contraceptive services help women avoid 1.3 million unintended pregnancies, which would have resulted in 534,000 births; 632,000 abortions; and 165,000 miscarriages. For every dollar spent on publicly funded contraceptive services, the public saves an estimated $3 in Medicaid costs for pregnancy-related and newborn care.[9]

Health plans are encouraged to ensure that contraceptive services are accessible, affordable, and acceptable to members. Teens are a population of special concern. Resources should be devoted to addressing the problem of teen pregnancy in partnership with community health agencies, especially those with a mission to serve adolescents. Health plan efforts to address this problem will be rewarded by improved member satisfaction and positive community perception of the plan. The savings achieved by averting unplanned and unwanted pregnancies will more than offset the costs of such services.[9]

REFERENCES

1. US Department of Health and Human Services. *Guide to Clinical Preventive Services*. Report of the US Preventive Services Task Force. Washington, DC: US Department of Health and Human Services; 1989.
2. Hatcher R, Stewart F, Trussell J, et al. *Contraceptive Technology 1990–1992*. 15th ed. New York: Irvington Publishers; 1990.
3. Forest JD. Epidemiology of unintended pregnancy and contraceptive use. *Am J Obstet Gynecol*. 1994;170(suppl 2):1485–1489.
4. Ford CA, Millstein SG, Halpern-Felsher BL, Irwin CE. Influence of physician confidentiality assurances on adolescents' willingness to disclose information and seek future health care: a randomized controlled trial. *JAMA*. 1997;278:1029–1034.
5. Dryfoos JG. *Adolescents at Risk*. New York: Oxford University Press; 1991.
6. American Medical Association. *Guidelines for Adolescent Preventive Services (GAPS): Recommendations and Rationale*. Chicago: American Medical Association; 1994.
7. Trussel J, Koenig J, Ellerston C, Stewart S. Preventing unintended pregnancy: the cost-effectiveness of three methods of emergency contraception. *Am J Public Health*. 1997;87:932–937.
8. Teen Birth-Control Coverage Could Save Money. *AHA News*. 1997;33(30):3.
9. Forest JD, Samara R. Impact of publicly funded contraceptive services on unintended pregnancies and implications for Medicaid expenditures. *Fam Plann Perspect*. 1996;28:188–195.

DAVID SHARE, MD, MPH, is the clinical director of the Center for Health Care Quality at Blue Cross and Blue Shield of Michigan. He has served as the medical director at The Corner Health Center in Ypsilanti, Michigan, since 1981. The Corner is a nonprofit, community health center for teens and their children.

Part IV

Self-Care and Health Advisory Services

In a book such as this one, there is emphasis on health care delivered by professionals in direct encounters with patients, but health care usually begins well before that. Even the best prevention does not prevent everything, and people may be afflicted with any number of symptoms, many of which represent acute but self-limited medical conditions. For these symptoms, self-care, which generally refers to health care services that one provides to oneself, is a far more common occurrence than most of us think. Uncertainty may accompany a symptom of a medical condition, and the afflicted person may not have a clear idea what to do. A major step up from self-care, then, is the health advisory service, often provided through (though certainly not limited to) nurse advice lines available 24 hours a day, 7 days a week. In Part IV, you will find an overview of these forms of health care delivery that occur without the hands-on participation of physicians or hospitals.

Chapter 10

Medically Directed, Delegated Self-Care

Gary Montrose

Chapter Outline

- Introduction
- History and Benefits of Self-Care
- Physician Involvement in Medical Self-Care
- Physician Obstacles
- Separate Domains of Care
- Self-Care as Part of Standard Practice
- Delegated Self-Care
- Contact Management
- Enabling Technologies
- Broader View of Managed Care

INTRODUCTION

Discussions and evaluations of medical care delivery focus almost exclusively on the capabilities, decisions, and systems of professional health care providers. Metrics used to compare health plans focus mostly on relative frequency and cost of services delivered. Perceived problems in the delivery system are often translated into inconsistencies among providers.[1] Some recent reviews of the impact of standardized protocols and guidelines on delivery and outcomes in primary care report inconsistent and disappointing results.[2,3] Not surprisingly, poor results lead to proposals for how to better disseminate and enforce standardized practices among noncompliant or ineffective providers.[4] As such, the blame and the credit for health care quality and outcomes fall squarely on the shoulders of the provider.

Using the broadest definition of health care, the overwhelming majority of one's care occurs outside the professional setting.[5] Most behaviors and decisions people choose and apply in response to health issues occur without the input of a health care professional.[6,7] For new symptoms, consumers choose where, when, and whether to seek professional care.[8] For existing problems, consumers decide whether they will follow a medical regimen, change a lifestyle behavior, or monitor their condition.[9] Although it may appear obvious, often ignored in discussions of delivery, quality, or outcomes is the fact that patients influence strongly virtually every aspect of care and recovery.

Despite large bodies of literature on both professional care delivery and self-care delivery, discussion of the overlap between the two areas is polite and informal. Advocates of each domain certainly acknowledge the value and importance of the other's. Recent reviews of programs in demand and disease management present arguments that ideal care delivery involves both clinical management and self-management components.[10,11] Yet, despite such supportive acknowledgment, the two areas generally remain functionally separate; physicians do what they do, and patients do what they do.

Professionals are encouraged to educate and engage the patient.[12,13] Patients are coached to ask questions and request involvement with providers' decisions. Some helpful dialogue may occur during a medical encounter, but once the patient leaves the office there is little formal accountability on either part for what happens before the next visit.

This chapter explores the implications of making self-management a prescribed part of medical care, for which providers assume responsibility for delegating and monitoring a self-care plan, and for which patients assume explicit accountability for executing a plan using appropriate monitoring and self-care behaviors. Delegated self-care makes formal the known and acknowledged need for a collaborative effort between patients and providers.[11] Delegated self-care also makes a clear request for patient involvement in care, reinforcing that medical treatment (in most cases) is not the sole determinant of successful health outcomes.

To make the case for delegated self-care, this chapter will review evidence regarding the benefits of self-care, past barriers to physicians' participation in self-care, and successful models integrating self-care and medical care. This chapter will also propose steps that could be used to formalize the delegation process, with the least disruption to current standard practice. Finally, there will be examples of how advances in information technology make patient participation in and responsibility for self-care more feasible than ever.

HISTORY AND BENEFITS OF SELF-CARE

Self-care occurs whenever individuals initiate responses to symptoms and manage an acute condition or illness process on their own or with the assistance of other laypeople. Since the 1970s, those interested in initiating and managing their own care gained access to an ever-increasing supply of information and support services to help guide their efforts. Kemper et al and Lorig et al reported on the effectiveness of self-initiated interventions from the research literature.[14,15] Taken as a whole, longitudinal studies, general studies, and symptom-specific studies all pointed to the "widespread use of self-care, the effectiveness of self-care education in reducing health care utilization, and the safety of self-care."[14(p37)] Similar findings have been reported by a number of other researchers.[16–18]

Although aspects of medical self-care can be traced to the beginnings of civilization, at least some of the current interest in self-initiated responses to medical problems comes out of the 1960s cultural drive for self-reliance, minimizing one's dependence on the "medical establishment." The self-care movement had as its defining moment the publication of *Our Bodies, Ourselves* by the Boston Woman's Health Book Collective in 1971,[19] followed in 1976 with release of the now-classic self-care guidebooks, titled the *Healthwise Handbook*[20] and *Take Care of Yourself*.[21] Distribution of such books by economically minded health plans has resulted in safely reducing avoidable office and emergency department visits.[14,22,23]

The benefits of self-care have not been limited to situations involving self-assessment and treatment of acute, minor symptoms. Evidence accumulates in virtually each new edition of chronic disease journals, demonstrating improved outcomes and appropriateness of care as a result of patient self-management.[24] Whether for chronic diseases that produce discomfort and disability, such as arthritis,[25] or chronic conditions with life-threatening complications, such as hemophilia[26] or asthma,[27] active self-management improves outcomes.[10] Patients have fewer hospitalizations, improve function, require fewer medical visits, adhere better to medication schedules, and report better health status as a result of self-management training.[28]

Implementation of self-help programs has expanded from traditional written materials to include audio phone text libraries, fax on demand, live nurse support lines, e-mail "ask your doc" contact, local support groups, and virtual support and chat groups.[29] In some cases, all-hours information and support are available by telephone, beeper, or the Internet for people with high-risk conditions (eg, the human immunodeficiency virus [HIV], diabetes, and pregnancy). Most often, sponsors of support services are those responsible for financing health care, not those delivering care.[30] Nurse call centers have emerged as tools commonly used by employers, health plans, or pharmaceutical companies to provide information and encourage behaviors that will promote health and produce economic benefits.[31,32] Despite a growing market for these services, few have involved, let alone integrated, providers into the information or service loop. Most operate separately from and out of contact with providers. Many of these consumer communication and demand management systems have been deployed as a means to bypass providers because physician interest in ongoing care support, extensive information support, and self-care training is simply not a part of standard clinical practice.

The immense popularity of on-demand information services, daily television news magazines, over-the-counter self-care products, and publications sold at the supermarket and through mail order catalogs demonstrates the public's insatiable interest in medical self-care. Patients seem to be asking for more information and involvement, and receiving them—for the most part—outside their physicians' offices.

PHYSICIAN INVOLVEMENT IN MEDICAL SELF-CARE

Missing from the frenzy of demand for self-care information and support is much of the medical profession. The cynical reason sometimes given for this lack of physician interest is economic self-interest: Why should physicians encourage people to take care of themselves if self-care reduces a physician's personal income? The reasons are, of course, far more complex than simple economics. They deserve thoughtful consideration by those interested in promoting the incidence and effectiveness of medical self-care. Changes in financial incentives, it is often said, will stimulate interest in medical self-care. But sudden changes in payment arrangements are not sufficient to result automatically in an effective transformation of traditional medical practices. To implement effective self-care in partnership with their patients, physicians face significant challenges. More than a simple addition of information to the medical encounter, effective medical self-care will require practice redesign, as discussed below.

PHYSICIAN OBSTACLES

There are a number of obstacles to physician support for self-care. These obstacles involve factors beyond the control of most practicing physicians. A curriculum involving the behavioral sciences, from which expertise in patient self-care strategies might be derived, is absent from the medical school, internship, and subsequent training experiences of most physicians. Only within the past two decades have the behavioral sciences produced a sufficient body of research to provide a credible basis on which physicians might recommend alternative self-care strategies. Because of the dearth of training, physicians report not feeling qualified or confident[33,34] in their ability to assess the behavioral factors that indicate the need for behavioral interventions and the types of interventions to recommend.

Physician–patient communication style has also received a great deal of attention in recent years. Yet much of the emphasis on style has come as messages of warning about the potential legal consequences of a poor bedside manner.[35,36]

From an operational perspective, modern medical practice evolved during a time when treatment of acute illness and urgent medical events predominated. Primary prevention, secondary prevention, and chronic condition management were beyond the scope of hard medical sciences. Performance and payment incentives to motivate and reward physicians in private or group practice were designed to compensate providers for performing a diagnosis and responding with a prescription, treatment, or referral within 15 to 20 minutes. Complex chronic conditions, and the even more complex behavioral factors associated with causing and controlling such conditions, require appointment times and repeat visits that far exceed the decade-old performance measures used to compensate physicians in clinical practice today. In addition to long office visits, patients with such conditions require repeat visits to a number of allied health professionals, some having expertise in behavioral fields.[11]

Traditionally, physicians have needed minimal knowledge of (and received little training in) health behavior and have had limited professional contact with behavior experts. Not knowing what to do in the behavioral domain of health care, not knowing enough about behavioral specialists to whom they can and should refer, and not receiving compensation for involvement in such matters, practicing clinicians are rightfully at a loss about how best to manage their patients' behavioral needs.[37]

Without a clear structure to guide behavioral change, or an understanding of behavior change theory, efforts to support behavior change can appear futile to physicians. In one study where physician intervention increased smoking cessation rates from 4% to 8%, public health officials emphasized the tremendous impact of "100% improvement in sustained cessation."[38(p142)] Physicians, the study implied, were not impressed with the impact of the intervention, given that people failed to quit in more than 9 out of 10 cases.[38]

Because behavior change occurs through a cycle of trials, failures, and relapses,[39,40] a patient's progress does not follow the traditional medical sequence of treatment followed by cure. Processes for engaging patients in self-care behaviors, as well as measures of their success, cannot focus on full and complete adherence as the only positive outcome. Rather, steps and measures must focus on incremental improvements in awareness, readiness, and self-efficacy. Given a 90% likelihood of failing (in the smoking example), there is little wonder providers doubt the efficacy of behavioral counseling. Notably, in instances where the goals are to demonstrate changes in awareness, intention, or readiness—not to achieve full adherence—success becomes less immediate, less tangible, and less visible. In most settings, physicians receive little reinforcement and there are few support services to help manage such complex behavioral factors. Without a clear understanding of the behavior change process or resources to support an ongoing change process, physicians have limited ability to make a meaningful impact on the motivational, behavioral, or kinesthetic prerequisites of behavior change and effective medical self-care.

The possibility of negative reactions by patients may also discourage physicians from recommending self-care. In an era where both health outcomes and patient satisfaction carry great value in distinguishing a health plan or group practice, physicians may be reluctant to pass on potentially unwanted self-care responsibilities to their patients. Physicians have been trained to give answers and heal the sick, not tell patients to try harder. The mixed message of (1) treating patients as customers while (2) empowering them to take charge of their own care can appear to be a no-win situation. Too much effort in one direction can sabotage efforts in the other direction.

Concerns that asking for personal involvement in care alienates patients appear to be exaggerated. Although individuals differ considerably in the amount of information and decision-making power they desire, patients seem to react positively to collaborative decisions.[41,42] In one study, patients who rated their physicians low in participatory style (not encouraging and including the patient in decisions) were twice as likely to change physicians as those giving their physicians high ratings.[43] In a large consumer survey, four of the top six most frequently reported complaints about office visits dealt with either insufficient involvement (not being asked their opinion or encouraged to ask questions) or insufficient information (about what they could do for themselves, or detailed information about medication).[44] Indeed, the degree to which patients understand the information they receive from their physicians correlates with both their satisfaction with care as well as their adherence to treatment regimens.[45]

Thus, patients seem to respond positively to information and involvement. However, studies indicate that the manner with which a physician delivers the message may count as much as the message itself. Patients value empathy and reassurance most,[46] demonstrated through use of both verbal and nonverbal cues.[47,48] Indeed, patients who experience the most empathy and interaction (being asked to give ideas and express concerns) report getting the most information from their doctors[49]; patients who rate their doctors as good communicators also rate those doctors highest in technical competence.[50]

Given the complexity of health behavior change and the importance of patient perceptions, delivery of high-quality health care can become a daunting and seemingly impossible task for a physician. Evidence reviewed above indicates that a patient's perception of "good care" depends not only on delivery of the appropriate clinical and technical care, but also on the degree to which the patient plays a sufficient role in decision making, has a voice in the interaction, knows enough about the situation, and likes the communication style of the provider. The patient wants a healer, a technician, a social worker, a librarian, and a confidant, rolled into one. With few exceptions, physicians rarely have the training, experience, time, or resources to meet such an unrealistic expectation. To a great extent, these ancillary skills are even considered unnecessary by the medical profession.[51] Rather than having to serve as the all-in-one doctor, educator, and counselor, perhaps physicians should instead be asked to delegate and orchestrate behavioral services, to complement their specialized medical skills.

SEPARATE DOMAINS OF CARE

The literature contains many illustrations of behavioral models, cost-effective support services, and clinical trials demonstrating efficacy of aggressive self-care practices.[24,52,53] However, few, if any, examples involve the integration of self-care into the foundation of care delivery—the physician–patient encounter. Instead, self-care remains separate from "real" medical treatment.

Figure 10–1 illustrates the typical cycle that occurs in the physician's and patient's respective roles when self-care has no explicit place in the dialogue or care plan. Without clear, shared expectations about self-care, results can be uncoordinated, even harmful. Where physicians lack training in, knowledge of, and referral options for self-care support services; lack confidence in the efficacy of self-care; and fear negative consequences for the patient and themselves, they will be reluctant to promote aggressive medical self-care. When patients look to physicians to promote or endorse self-care efforts and lack the knowledge, skills, training, and self-confidence to engage in medical self-care, patients too are reluctant to engage in meaningful self-care efforts. This mutually reinforcing lack of confidence becomes a nonproductive cycle that ignores the body of evidence supporting consumer satisfaction and positive clinical outcomes resulting from effective self-care.

Despite good intentions on both parts, opportunities for endorsing and reinforcing self-care efforts can easily be missed. The clinician may stay away from potentially uncomfortable—and presumed ineffective—efforts to improve patient behavior and stick to medical "knowns." The patient listens for what the doctor thinks is important and receives little guidance about recommended self-care. As a result, the opportunity to begin or continue the process of self-management passes by.

The impact of these lost opportunities is significant and alarming. Literature suggests that less than half of diabetic patients receive coun-

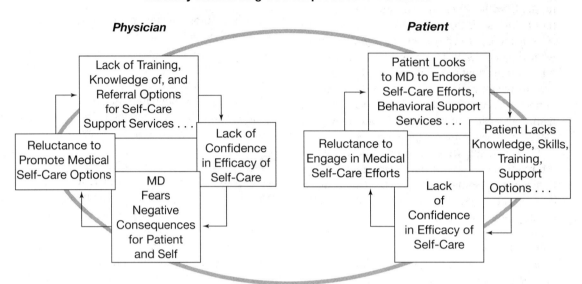

Figure 10–1 Lack of Physician and Patient Confidence in Medical Self-Care. Courtesy of Ashby * Montrose & Co, 1998, Denver, Colorado.

seling on critical clinical issues such as weight loss and diet.[54] (An in-depth discussion of diabetes care management may be found in Chapter 29.) Over a third miss, or stop entirely, taking required medication.[55] As many as one quarter of diabetics do not monitor their blood glucose levels.[56] The disregard for behaviors so essential to well-being presents a serious challenge to effective diabetic management. As disease management (see Part X) becomes an increasingly visible goal for health plans, failures also become more troubling and noticeable. Consequently, blame gets placed on physicians for not following practice guidelines, and then placed on patients for their blatant noncompliance, despite impressive compliance rates and positive clinical outcomes for patients receiving appropriate behavioral self-care support under clinical trial conditions where the efficacy of medical self-care is reported for a variety of disease conditions.[10,11]

Although it may provide little consolation, neither the provider nor the patient has sole culpability for failures in chronic disease management. Neither has the training, skills, or support needed to be successful. The solution does not come from pointing fingers at the various parties, or from mass education of either patients or providers to assume full responsibility for behavior change. Instead, a systematic set of strategies is needed to move toward a model of shared responsibility, facilitated by outside resources and supportive technology.

SELF-CARE AS PART OF STANDARD PRACTICE

Within the traditional medical profession, there is little training and virtually no qualifying standards concerning human psychology, competency in counseling, or communication skills. Though very important, communication skills remain more of an intangible aspect of care; they rarely become an issue in daily practice until they result in provider switching,[43] disciplinary action, or litigation.[12] The ability to engage patients, garner their shared commitment to healthy practices, and support them through the process of behavior change are all competencies considered essential in the training and delivery of effective self-care. Notably, these are also competencies that other health care professions (some aspects of nursing, health promotion, health education) use regularly in behavioral aspects of patient care.

To best use the combined skill sets of different health professions, it would seem most reasonable to maximize the effect of each of their strengths. Toward this end, this chapter describes two practice intervention strategies. The first involves restructuring the patient encounter process to "standardize" a formal role for physicians in assessing need and assigning responsibilities for medical self-care. This process will be called *delegated self-care*. The second strategy relies upon information technology to support physician and patient involvement to maintain a high level of medical self-care activities over time. This technology-based strategy will be called *contact management*. Terms and definitions for this discussion are shown in Exhibit 10–1.

Medical self-care, as used in this chapter, describes formal efforts toward bringing practicing physicians and their patients into closer alignment for those preventive, acute, and chronic conditions that require effective collaboration between provider and patient to achieve optimum patient outcomes. Professional involvement in medical self-care implies active support from trained health care providers (when required) to carry out appropriate performance of self-assessment, self-treatment, or self-management of personal health conditions.

Effective self-care occurs when an individual demonstrates that he or she is ready, willing, and able to assert a sufficient measure of control over symptoms, with an appropriate level of dependence on professional service providers. Individuals will each have a different range of actual and perceived need for professional support relative to what they are able to do for themselves. The objective of medical self-care is to increase wherever possible the motivation, self-confidence, and ability of individuals to perform the highest level of self-care they wish to assume in their own care management.

To achieve this objective in a variety of different clinical circumstances, this chapter describes a strategy for improving the incidence and effectiveness of *physician* involvement at a level far greater than that practiced for decades under traditional practice models. Increasing physician involvement in proactive promotion of self-care, especially for hard-to-manage chronic conditions, is an essential component of any population health management strategy. Advances in the behavioral sciences over the past decade, along with the availability of information technology, play a pivotal role in the support of complex behavior management efforts. Improvements in the structure, practice, and incidence of medical self-care will be necessary for the next wave of "managed care" efforts toward improving the appropriate use of medical services, controlling costs, and ameliorating patient outcome measures.

DELEGATED SELF-CARE

What differentiates *delegated self-care* from other descriptions of self-care is explicit, confident acknowledgment—by physicians—of value, expectations, and responsibilities. Delegated self-care identifies the patient's role in care and healing through a sequence of familiar medical routines: assessment, referral, prescription, and follow-up.

Delegated self-care embeds the patient's role into expected standards of practice. The new responsibilities of the physician mirror those in traditional care. The clinician determines or confirms the existence of a condition. Medical treatments are discussed and prescribed. Next, the clinician, an appointed staff member, or outside specialist assesses the patient's degree of knowledge, confidence, skills, and readiness for self-management through standard, validated tools available for most common medical conditions. Depending upon each patient's unique responses, the clinician or support staff devise a care plan that includes all aspects of medical,

Exhibit 10–1 Terms and Definitions

Medical care: Medical care describes the cognitive, procedural, or prescriptive actions taken by an individual who is regarded as a "professional" because of medical school training, professional board qualifications, state licensure, hospital credentials, and community standing among peers to engage in certain medical practices. With multiple, third-party recognition of expertise, a medical care professional attains the authority to assess a patient's condition, render a diagnosis, assume sole responsibility for the patient's care, refer to other professionals, or engage in certain invasive procedures. In short, qualification as a medical professional recognizes the knowledge and technical skills necessary to practice science-based medical tasks on behalf of patients. In the medical care paradigm, the physician makes decisions and takes actions on behalf of the patient, typically with the patient's implied or explicit consent.

Self-care: Self-care describes what individuals decide and do for themselves. It refers to that series of steps "lay" individuals take to assess and treat an illness or injury, typically without the benefit of higher levels of training in the theory or science of medicine and with little or no consultation with a medical professional. Self-care has been practiced since the beginning of civilization. In modern times, advocates of self-care from many walks of life have provided oral advice and written guidelines intended to pass along the accumulated knowledge of others. Such information would provide the individuals with enough information to take certain actions on their own, and to assess and treat certain health care situations. Self-care implies taking specific steps in response to a health-related event, with or without a deep understanding of the underlying causal theory, biological, or other causal factors affecting the condition or knowledge about the probable impact of alternative actions.

Self-management: Self-management implies a level of knowledge, motivation, skill, and confidence sufficient to properly assess and manage acute or permanent, chronic health conditions, with minimum involvement from health care professionals, except on a routine or ad hoc review or urgent need basis. Self-management implies a high level of ability and responsibility in the day-to-day management of these conditions, especially over a prolonged period of time. Self-management means that the individual has a higher level of knowledge, exercises discretion, establishes priorities, and generally assumes overall daily responsibility. Under the rubric of self-management, a person is presumed competent to choose between certain alternatives, set priorities, involve others or not, establish rewards and punishments for him- or herself and others, and live with the consequences of the decisions. Self-management involves more complex decision making, a scope of authority to act or not act within certain parameters (based upon certain policies and procedures) and the use of reason and prior experience within the scope of one's authority and expertise.

Self-care guidelines: To assist a person with self-care, narrow vignettes of situation-specific information may be presented on a single page of a self-care guide, with immediate action steps arranged in an algorithmic order. The individual conducts a self-assessment, decides on his or her own which decision path to follow, and applies self-care at home or is directed to seek care from a health care provider immediately, or at a later time. Self-care may involve use of special learned skills, often provided by a health care professional, in assessing and treating a specific condition, usually at one specific point in time to meet one particular need.

pharmacological, and behavioral interventions designed to maximize the likelihood of optimum health outcomes. A written self-care action plan identifies those care management components and, more important, who takes responsibility for each. If the results of the self-care assessment indicate inadequacies in skill or knowledge, the plan may include referral to educators or courses. As shown in Figure 10–2, responsibility may be kept by the primary care physician (PCP), delegated to the patient or caregiver, or referred to other resources inside or outside the

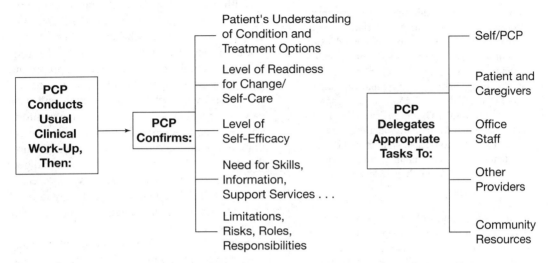

Figure 10–2 Principles of Delegated Self-Care. Courtesy of Ashby * Montrose & Co, 1997, Denver, Colorado.

office setting. The components of the self-care assessment are shown in Exhibit 10–2.

The behavioral assessment contains three key elements: knowledge, readiness, and self-efficacy. All three are well documented in the health promotion literature as the foundation for behavior change and medical self-care.[59,60] The assessment can be administered outside, and prior to, the actual medical encounter, so that the physician can simply review a profile of the patient's self-care abilities and respond with appropriate delegation. The physician does not have to address the deficiencies directly, just identify them, acknowledge the need to improve them, and let the patient know how he or she is expected to participate.

Choices for devising the plan remain flexible, depending on the preferences of the physician, medical specialty, resources available, and patient motivation and capabilities. However, the standards for delegated self-care would have two requirements: (1) a clear, measurable understanding by the physician, the patient, and any other delegated provider of the desired self-care behavior and who accepts responsibility for components of achieving the desired goal; and (2) data of sufficient specificity, taken at appropriate intervals to document progress in medical care and self-care practices.

The adoption of delegated self-care as a standard of practice does not impose huge new requirements on providers. Nor does it necessitate redesigning clinics to house a new combination of health professionals. Rather, the differences are subtle but powerful shifts in the messages physicians deliver to patients about how to and why they should try to get better.

In the days when physicians treated mostly acute problems and infections, "modern" medicine was focused on magical pills that caused discomfort to disappear. In addition, just by their presence and reassurance, physicians delivered a demonstrable and powerful placebo effect. For chronic conditions, physicians can no longer deliver a magic pill or healing touch that can cure or comfort the patient after he or she leaves the office. Yet, patients continue, to everyone's frustration, to seek hope and answers from professionals only. Here is where delegated self-care shifts expectations by forming a collaborative relationship with explicit assignment of roles and responsibilities to physi-

Exhibit 10–2 Self-Care Assessment Components

> *Basic knowledge:* Although not sufficient to produce behavior change, a certain level of knowledge is necessary to perform self-care. Essential knowledge includes a basic understanding about the causes and irritants associated with the condition and symptoms. Patients should also understand appropriate responses to changes in their condition (eg, when emergency care is warranted or when self-care can help). Patients should also understand key metrics that indicate how well their condition is under control (eg, blood glucose levels or blood pressure).
>
> *Readiness*[39]: Stages of readiness indicate the likelihood of successful adoption of new behaviors. Tools for assessing readiness have been validated repeatedly (see Chapter 40). Readiness indicates the type of information and support that will move the patient toward sustained self-management. Those not ready to take action are poor candidates for a skills management or smoking cessation class. Low readiness indicates a need for awareness building, possibly through a video or counseling program. Patients at low readiness need reasons from their physicians why they should see their behaviors as a potential threat. A clear message from the physician that their current responsibility is to learn more about this topic can help advance readiness.[57]
>
> *Self-efficacy*[58]: Self-efficacy is the confidence one has that he or she can actually perform a specific task or skill. A person may understand the seriousness of a condition and feel ready to take an active role in self-care but not feel confident in his or her ability to do so. Low self-efficacy indicates a need for coaching, skills training, and periods of "trying on" a new behavior. A patient may not feel confident that he or she would recognize if a certain exercise were harmful. A patient might worry that he or she could not read a monitor accurately. With explicit instructions about whom to contact, and guidance as patients try to implement their new skills, self-efficacy improves.

cians, patients, and other behavioral support services.

With delegated self-care the physician delivers a clear message: "Science tells us that a combination of approaches brings the best results. Some of these things I am responsible for providing to you: the best medicine and appropriate tests. I am also responsible for making sure you understand your options. Some tasks only you can perform, and we can help you feel comfortable and competent doing them: monitoring your symptoms, taking your medicine, avoiding things that make your condition worse, and getting the rest, nutrients, and activity you need to thrive. Let's talk about what support you need and when we will meet again to reassess our progress."

As closely as possible, delegated self-care follows a sequence familiar to both physicians and patients. First, using input from the patient as well as diagnostic tools, the physician diagnoses the medical condition. The problem is labeled, and potential solutions are jointly identified and discussed. Solutions that require seeing a specialist or applying or taking a curative substance are provided following specific instructions by the physician and an explicit referral to the appropriate resource. Then, at some specified interval, the physician and patient revisit progress made thus far. The only difference is that the patient becomes one of the explicitly named providers, responsible for the delivery of, or receipt of, some aspect of care or training.

Upon completion of the standard clinical work-up, assessment of readiness, self-efficacy training requirements, and task delegation, the provider may elect to complete the medical self-care delegation process with the cosigning of a self-care informed consent form. This formality would codify mutual understandings and agreed-upon expectations and responsibilities. It would encourage full disclosure of treatment options, risks of action or inaction, treatment limitations, and the range of possible outcomes. The process would furnish primary care providers with a tool equivalent to that used routinely by surgeons to help clarify issues, options, and expectations, positive and potentially adverse. Such a statement would be helpful as a postvisit instruction guide for the patient, office staff, case managers, and other behavioral support staff. In it, providers would customize their roles and responsibilities to assist as needed and appropriate, while outlining the limitations of their responsibilities for follow-up care and outcomes that are beyond providers' reasonable control.

CONTACT MANAGEMENT

The continued evolution of medical information systems from paper-based to electronic will facilitate medically delegated self-care, as it already has for commercial self-help vendors. Whether simple or sophisticated, accessible information collection and feedback systems are essential to making delegated self-care feasible for providers and usable for patients. Information technology also widens the spectrum of possible media through which behavioral support can be delivered. Information can be accessed by telephone, fax, or computer channels. Feedback can be delivered verbally, in scannable written form, or transmitted automatically from monitoring devices through cellular technology. Appointments can be scheduled by people or computers. Reminders can be delivered by pager, automated voice mail, e-mail, talking pillboxes, or other forms of communication.

With currently available information technologies, coordinated delivery among various professionals and lay caregivers no longer requires excessive labor costs or additional time on the part of the physician. Systems that collect information from diverse sources can conveniently monitor and quickly plot a patient's progress, alerting providers when problems arise, and print and aggregate performance metrics on an individual or group basis. Systems have begun to take the place of the need for humans to schedule routine appointments, remind patients to attend individual or group sessions, collect and transcribe information, and provide results to the physician on a regular basis.

As an example, automated voice systems have been used successfully to collect glucose values from patients, record symptoms and biometric measures, and record the degree to which patients followed self-care guidelines over the past week.[53] These systems can call patients at any time or number convenient for them and are smart enough to prompt a call to the patient from the physician in cases of an abnormal reading or urgent situation. Optional, customized instructional messages can be added to the outbound and inbound calling algorithms where appropriate. Over 80% of all calls in this diabetes study were successfully completed.[53] More important, 98% of patients found the calls helpful and easy to complete, and 77% reported that such a system of calls—reminding them about self-care and self-monitoring—would make them more satisfied with care.

Examples demonstrating the use of such technology as a mechanism for behavioral support dispel the myth that such approaches will be rejected by patients, especially seniors or minority populations,[61] as too impersonal and unmanageable. The majority of the patients in the diabetes study cited above were over 55 years old, and 40% were from non-Caucasian ethnic groups. Older participants were twice as likely to listen to preventive messages as their younger counterparts. The information collected by the automated system provided explicit feedback about the ongoing management of their condition and the degree to which patients reported following the practices "recommended by their doctor."

Successful medical self-care requires behavioral support from a range of allied health practitioners and a high degree of contact management among all parties to ensure that each medical self-care program is executed optimally. Yet, even within the most highly evolved integrated delivery systems, the principal care coordinator and service delivery integrator is typically the individual patient. For a small percentage of high-cost managed care patients, case managers and informatics specialists devise programs to help track scheduled appointments and care management processes.

Certain disease management companies also use software programs with telephonic nurse counselors to help meet the challenge in an economical and feasible way. Some combination of such efforts will emerge as proposed solutions to the challenges posed by medical self-care. The coordination tasks for this are illustrated in Figure 10–3.

Contact management is a construct designed to blend the best of physician-focused medical management practices with the best of consumer-focused demand management practices. Its basic tenet is that both the physician and patient will benefit in their dealings with each other through automated systems that serve to remind all parties about the decisions and behavioral prerequisites of longitudinal care management involving complex behavioral change and management of chronic conditions. Both physicians and patients do relatively well managing acute care diagnostic and treatment activities. It is the more complex series of behaviors over time, involving changes in behavior, where standard acute care practice modalities produce suboptimal results.

Given the alarming statistics regarding the number of patients who do not follow recommended standards of self-care (eg, glucose monitoring or diet[54,56]), contact management suggests that significant improvements are possible—without placing unreasonable new demands on health care providers. Physicians should be expected to identify (or have staff members counsel patients about) prudent self-care practices. Patients should be expected to make reasonable efforts to engage in those practices. Information should be available to all parties about how the patient is feeling and progressing. Certainly, expectations should be higher. Information and communication technologies can and will make those expectations manageable.

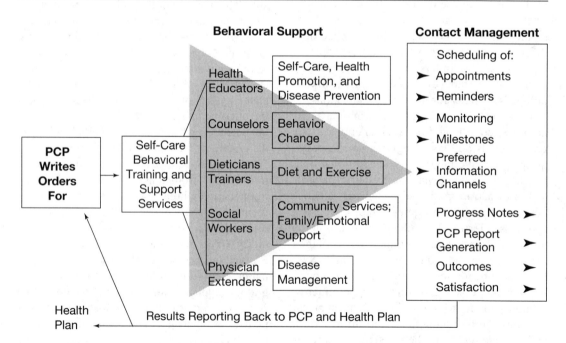

Figure 10–3 Medical Self-Care Coordination Tasks by Case Managers and Informatics Specialists. Courtesy of Ashby * Montrose & Co, 1998, Denver, Colorado.

ENABLING TECHNOLOGIES

Numerous contact management technology solutions are in various stages of development. Fortune 500 companies in the fields of financial services, entertainment, telecommunications, pharmaceuticals, and physician practice management, and smaller entrepreneurs, are exploring ways to deploy information and call center technologies designed to help bridge the gap between physicians and patients. Examples of such efforts, pieces of which are already commercially available, include the following.

One large health plan has built a nurse call center system that includes licensed psychologists and social workers available 24 hours a day to respond to inbound calls. Another health plan has designed a comprehensive program of in- and outbound calls where patients are stratified according to their health problem and readiness to change. The plan identifies people at risk, notifies the assigned PCP, attempts to register targeted patients in appropriate personal change and self-care programs, conducts phone assessments, refers to basic education classes as needed, schedules monthly mailings and personal phone calls, and advises the provider of progress and plan completion. This "automated system" provides the contact management needed to coordinate behavioral support services for those individuals requiring longitudinal reminders, progress tracking, and results reporting that few individual physicians could manually administer.

A variety of Internet, telephone triage, and disease management software programs are available as stand-alone or integrated telephony solutions for small and large practice settings that help staff in physicians' offices track calls, register patients in education programs, and schedule appointments as ordered by the physician. Office staff nurses or service bureau call center nurses are alerted to call patients according to schedule to track patient adherence to assigned care protocols. Some pharmaceutical companies have developed elaborate prescription- and disease-specific telephonic protocols designed to track medication refill patterns, respond to questions, and launch outbound reminder calls at refill time or to monitor behavior change for patients enrolled in specific health promotion and disease prevention programs. Many of these programs now incorporate tailored messages designed to address personal needs, demographic criteria, attitudinal differences, and physician practice preferences. These and other programs will continue to evolve as innovative ways to automate the complex demands of physician-delegated self-care programs that require ongoing monitoring, behavioral support, and results reporting back to the attending physician and health plan.

Several pharmaceutical companies have established strategic relationships with nurse call center vendors that will provide physicians and their patients with round-the-clock inbound and outbound calling capabilities. Outbound calls are made to remind patients of drug dosing and biometric monitoring requirements according to agreed-upon schedules. These calls are made by nurses but can and may increasingly include automated, prerecorded messages reminding patients about diet and exercise commitments, insulin or allergy injection times, self-monitoring requirements, and scheduled appointments. The patient can respond by voice or touch-tone dialing to confirm understanding of and adherence to the self-management orders. Inbound calls from the patient can be directed to automated recording devices to track behavioral compliance or to a live nurse, social worker, or physician responding to inquiries, problems, or requests for confirmation and encouragement. The patient's own physician or other emergency resources can always be contacted as necessary.

BROADER VIEW OF MANAGED CARE

Changing reimbursement systems from fee-for-service to risk-based reimbursement has not and will not automatically help physicians cope with the changing demands of today's medical practice. (For an in-depth discussion of various forms of reimbursement methodologies in managed care, the reader is referred to *The Managed*

Exhibit 10–3 Competing Paradigms

Medical Management: Managed care's practice of influencing or even "micromanaging" the decisions of physicians in order to control avoidable, costly service utilization, referred to as medical management (see Parts VI and VII), has resulted in financial successes along with a significant loss of public goodwill.* As a cost and care management strategy, medical management is encountering increased resistance from providers, patients, and public policy makers because it is thought to alter individual decision making in a way perceived to be coercive, and many physicians and patients feel that it does not add any value to the physician–patient encounter. Managed care, especially risk-based managed care of seniors, continues to grow each year because employers and governmental payers require control over health care costs in a way not realized under fee-for-service indemnity payer arrangements. Medical management enjoyed economic success as a way to regulate the suppliers of high-cost hospital admissions, procedures, and tests ordered by physicians that appeared to be avoidable. The negative impact associated with "denying" or restricting consumers' access to specialty physicians and services on the growing volume of ambulatory office and emergency department visits led to the rise of a new business strategy known as demand management.

Demand management: Demand management evolved as an alternative or adjunct to medical management (see Chapter 11 for a discussion of one prevalent form of this: the nurse advice line). It represents a way to increase the consumer's ability to engage in self-care at home and to more appropriately direct patients to the most cost-effective providers for those needs that could not be self-managed over the telephone by a nurse counselor. Toward this end, managed care organizations have purchased millions of self-care guidebooks and contracted with nurse call center service providers in an attempt to control avoidable service utilization from the consumer (demand) side. These self-care interventions made sense from an economic and marketing perspective by adding something of value to their members in the form of 24-hour urgent care support and a sense of personal control over minor, acute situations. Such consumer-focused strategies were purchased by health plans as a way to reduce avoidable ambulatory encounters, resulting in a positive return on investment for the sponsoring health plans. However, an inability or unwillingness of providers to properly integrate the principles and tools of demand management into their clinical practices has made some health care industry participants think poorly of demand management service providers.

Contact management: Both medical management and demand management may be perceived as unable to fully deliver the type of impact on individual and population management hoped for. Each strategy attempts to reduce inappropriate, or avoidable, service utilization, from opposite ends of the supply-and-demand spectrum. Medical management is designed to control the decisions and behaviors of service providers on the supply side, while demand management aims to influence the decisions and behaviors of patients from the demand side. Medical management attempts to influence the behavior of physicians without directly involving patients, while demand management attempts to influence the behavior of consumers without effectively engaging the physician in that series of interactions.

Contact management is designed to bridge the communication gap between the two domains. Automated connectivity solutions available through information technology, using service delivery programs implemented in other industry sectors, will help physicians keep track of patient compliance and self-care behaviors in ways not previously feasible. Consumers have generally demonstrated their ability and willingness to use automated voice response, Internet, and other technologies for banking, entertainment, and other services. Health care connectivity solutions will make medical self-care technically and financially feasible.

*The reduction in public approval of managed care is certainly more complex than focusing on only this issue would imply. However, for purposes of this discussion, it is not necessary to widen that discussion.

Health Care Handbook, 3rd Edition.) To play a more effective role in managing the care of defined "managed" patient populations, especially high-risk, high-utilization patients, physicians need new practice tools and support services. Changes in economic incentives, demographics, and communications technology make it increasingly necessary and feasible for physicians to improve the scope and quality of their interactions with their patients without increasing burdens on their practice. Acting as team captains, with support services at their disposal, primary care providers and specialists can play a meaningful role in assessing and recommending behavioral interventions necessary to support clinical interventions.

Medical self-care as described here is designed to improve physician interactions with patients, and to motivate and support patient self-care practices for individuals who would otherwise turn to third-party vendors and alternative care providers that may or may not meet their health and medical needs. Moral and financial responsibility to patients should dictate interest in ensuring that they receive the best possible care, whether obtained from within or outside of the formal delivery system.

The rise of commercial, Medicare, and Medicaid risk-based compensation managed by new provider service organizations and an aging population with complex chronic conditions necessitates a renewed focus on the effectiveness of the physician–patient encounter. Chronic conditions related to lifestyle, inappropriate care-seeking practices, and behavior can be affected only by the actions of each individual. Appropriate types of medical *and behavioral* support not designed into the current health care delivery system will be required to realize improvements in health status measures called for by the National Committee for Quality Assurance and other performance-measuring bodies.

The paradigms described in Exhibit 10–3 illustrate how self-care has sometimes been treated as an either/or proposition, rather than a strategy to be embedded into standard practice. Medical management and demand management proponents have often been at odds over how

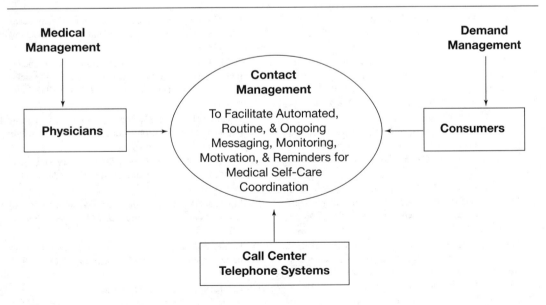

Figure 10–4 Call Center Telephone Systems Make Contact Management for Medical Self-Care Feasible. Courtesy of Ashby * Montrose & Co, 1998, Denver, Colorado.

each might get in the other's way. Inherent in the battles has been the ultimate question of who assumes eventual responsibility for the health of the patient. Consumer activists believe the individual has ultimate responsibility. Providers often argue that, regardless of the patient's beliefs, it is the physician who ends up legally and ethically responsible when something goes wrong. Given the new systems available to help coordinate joint efforts, perhaps it is reasonable to consider a combined approach. Figure 10–4 illustrates how the paralysis that keeps these two domains effectively separate can and is being bridged through use of numerous and creative communication technology systems.

To accomplish better connectivity, the medical and demand management paradigms must recognize the value of the other. Regrettably, organized medicine has paid remarkably little attention to the potential of medical self-care as a serious clinical and business discipline. The reasons for this lack of interest are deeply rooted in tradition, including the structure of clinical practice and role expectations between patients and physicians designed to respond to acute rather than chronic medical conditions. There is a convergence of market forces calling for a concerted effort to respond to medical self-care as a strategic, economic, and ethical imperative.

The elevation of medical self-care as a productive managed care strategy requires entirely new management and operational constructs.[62] It requires expertise from epidemiologists, behavioral counselors, psychologists, patient educators, nurse specialists, physician practice managers, and data management and information technology specialists. Finally, the practice of medical self-care requires leadership to overcome perceptions that professional and lay involvement in the practice of medical self-care will have minimal clinical impact and financial rewards. The evidence and need are now compelling enough to warrant institutional and professional leadership in this area.

REFERENCES

1. Cave DG. Profiling physician practice patterns using diagnostic episode clusters. *Med Care.* 1995;33(5):463–486.
2. Davis DA, Taylor-Vaisey A. Translating guidelines into practice: a systematic review of theoretic concepts, practical experience and research evidence in the adoption of clinical practice guidelines. *Can Med Assoc J.* 1997;157(4):408–416.
3. Worrall G, Chaulk P, Freake D. The effects of clinical practice guidelines on patient outcomes in primary care: a systematic review. *Can Med Assoc J.* 1997;156(12):1705–1712.
4. Harsha DM, Saywell RM Jr, Thygerson S, Panozzo J. Physician factors affecting patient willingness to comply with exercise recommendations. *Clin Sports Med J.* 1996;6(2):112–118.
5. Stoller PE. The dynamics and process of self-care in old age. Presented at National Invitational Conference on Research Issues Related to Self-Care and Aging; May 26, 1994; Washington, DC.
6. Dean K. Self-care responses to illness: a selected review. *Soc Sci Med.* 1981;15(5):673–687.
7. Kart CS, Dunkle RE. Assessing capacity for self-care among the aged. *J Aging Health.* 1989;1(4):430–450.
8. Kart CS, Engler CA. Predisposition to self-health care: who does what for themselves and why? *J Gerontol.* 1994;49(6):S301–S308.
9. Quill TE, Brody H. Physician recommendations and patient autonomy: finding a balance between physician power and patient choice. *Ann Intern Med.* 1996;125(9):763–769.
10. Wagner EH, Austin BT, Von Korff M. Organizing care for patients with chronic illness. *Milbank Q.* 1996;74(4):511–544.
11. Von Korff M, Gruman J, Schafefer J, Curry SJ. Collaborative management of chronic illness. *Ann Intern Med.* 1997;127(12):1097–1102.
12. Emanuel EJ, Emanuel LL. Four models of the physician–patient relationship. *JAMA.* 1992;267(16):2221–2226.
13. Bartlett EE. Reducing the malpractice threat through patient communications. *Health Prog.* May 1988:63–66.
14. Kemper DW, Lorig K, Mettler M. The effectiveness of medical self-care interventions: a focus on self-initiated responses to symptoms. *Patient Educ Counseling.* 1993;21:29–39.
15. Lorig K, Kraines RG, Brown BW Jr, Richardson N. A

workplace health education program that reduces outpatient visits. *Med Care.* 1985;23(9):1044–1054.
16. Kemper DW. Self-care education: impact on HMO costs. *Med Care.* 1982;20(7):710–718.
17. Fleming GV, Giachello AL, Andersen RM, Andrade P. Self-care: Substitute, supplement, or stimulus for formal medical care services? *Med Care.* 1984;22(10):950–966.
18. DeFriese GH, Konrad TR. The self-care movement and the gerontological healthcare professional. *Generations.* Fall 1993:37–40.
19. Boston Woman's Health Book Collective. *Our Bodies, Ourselves.* New York: Simon & Schuster; 1971.
20. Kemper DW. *Healthwise Handbook: A Self-Care Manual for You.* Boise, ID: A Healthwise Publication; 1976.
21. Vickery DM, Fries JF. *Take Care of Yourself.* Reading, MA: Addison-Wesley Publishing Co; 1976.
22. Vickery DM, Kalmer H, Lowry D, Constantine M, Wright E, Loren W. Effect of a self-care education program on medical visits. *JAMA.* 1983;250(21):2952–2956.
23. Vickery DM, Golaszewski T, Wright EC, Kalmer H. The effect of self-care interventions on the use of medical service within a Medicare population. *Med Care.* 1988;26(6):580–588.
24. Clark NM, Becker MH, Janz NK, Lorig K, Rakowski W, Anderson L. Self-management of chronic disease by older adults. *J Aging Health.* 1991;3(1):3–27.
25. Lorig K, Mazonson PD, Holman H. Evidence suggesting that health education for self-management in patients with chronic arthritis has sustained health benefits while reducing health care costs. *Arthritis Rheum.* 1993;36(4):439–446.
26. Levine PH, Britten AFH. Supervised patient-management of hemophilia: a study of 45 patients with hemophilia A and B. *Ann Intern Med.* 1973;78(1):195–201.
27. Berg J, Dunbar-Jacob J, Sereika SM. An evaluation of a self-management program for adults with asthma. *Clin Nurs Res.* 1997;6(3):225–238.
28. Vickery DM. Demand management, self-care, and the new media. In: Harris LM, ed. *Health and the New Media: Technologies Transforming Personal and Public Health.* Mahwah, NJ: Lawrence Erlbaum Associates; 1995:45–63.
29. Riley K. Medical advice close as the phone. *Washington Times.* February 4, 1996:A10.
30. Borfitz D. Medical call centers serve multiple functions: for now, health plans taking the lead. *Strat Health Care Marketing.* 1996;13(3):4–8.
31. Gilbert S. Companies say hotline triage reduces emergencies, comforts patients. *Dallas Morning News.* November 26, 1995:12A.
32. Borzo G. Phone counseling services are booming, as physicians and health plans seek new ways to manage patient use of medical care. *Am Med News.* October 16, 1995:3,35.
33. Wechsler H, Leveine S, Idelson RK, Rothman M, Taylor JO. The physician's role in health promotion: surveys of primary care practitioners. *N Engl J Med.* 1983;308:97–100.
34. Valente C, Sobal J, Muncie H, Levine D, Antlitz A. Health promotion: physician's beliefs, attitudes and practices. *Am J Prev Med.* 1986;2:82–88.
35. Levinson W. Physician–patient communication: a key to malpractice prevention. *JAMA.* 1994;272(20):1619–1620.
36. Sommers PA. Minimizing malpractice risk: a patient approach. *Group Pract J.* September–October 1987:86–90.
37. Eriksen MP, Green LW, Fultz FG. Principles of changing health behavior. *Cancer.* 1988;62:1768–1775.
38. Wilson D. Assessment of an intervention in primary care: counseling patients of smoking cessation. In: Tudiver F et al, eds. *Assessing Interventions: Traditional and Innovative Methods.* Newbury Park, CA: Sage Publications; 1990.
39. Prochaska JO. Disease management needs new paradigms. *J Gen Intern Med.* 1995;10:472–473.
40. Prochaska JO, DiClemente CC, Velicer WF, Rossi JS. Standardized, individualized, interactive, and personalized self-help programs for smoking cessation. *Health Psychol.* 1993;12(5):399–405.
41. Strull WM, Lo B, Charles G. Do patients want to participate in medical decision making? *JAMA.* 1984;252(21):2990–2994.
42. Eraker SA, Politser P. How decisions are reached: physician and patient. *Ann Intern Med.* 1982;97:262–268.
43. Kaplan SH, Gandek B, Greenfield S, Rogers W, Ware JE. Patient and visit characteristics related to physicians participatory decision-making style: results from the Medical Outcomes Study. *Med Care.* 1995;33(12):1176–1187.
44. How is your doctor treating you? *Consumer Reports Health.* February 1995:81–88.
45. Sitza J, Wood N. Patient satisfaction: a review of issues and concepts. *Soc Sci Med.* 1997;45(12):1829–1843.
46. Moorey S. The psychological impact of cancer. In: Tiffany R, Webb P, eds. *Oncology for Nurses and Health Care Professionals.* 2nd ed. Vol 2. London: Harper & Row; 1988.
47. Kendon A. Some functions of gaze direction in social interaction. *Acta Psychol.* 1970;26:22–63.
48. Lacross MB. Nonverbal behavior and perceived counselor attractiveness and persuasiveness. *J Counseling Psych.* 1975;22:563–566.

49. Lochman JE. Factors related to patients' satisfaction with their medical care. *J Community Health.* 1983; 9(2):91–109.
50. Cegala DJ, McNeilis KS, McGee DS, Jona AP. A study of doctors' and patients' perceptions of information processing and communication competence during the medical interview. *Health Commun.* 1995;7:179–203.
51. Thompson J. Communicating with patients. In: Fitzpatrick R, ed. *The Experience of Illness.* London: Tavistock; 1984:87–108.
52. Glaskow RE. A practical model of diabetes management and education. *Diabetes Care.* 1995;18(1): 117–126.
53. Piette JD, Mah CA. The feasibility of automated voice messaging as an adjunct to diabetes outpatient care. *Diabetes Care.* 1997;20(1):15–21.
54. Arnold MS, Stephen C, Hiss RG. Guidelines vs. practice delivery of diabetes nutrition care. *J Am Diet Assoc.* 1993;93:34–39.
55. McPhee SJ, Schroeder SA. General approaches to the patient: health maintenance and disease prevention. In: Tierney LN, McPhee SJ, Papadakis MA, eds. *Current Medical Diagnoses and Treatment.* Norwalk, CA: Appleton & Lange; 1995.
56. Anderson RM, Fitzgerald JT, Oh MS. The relationship between diabetes-related attitudes and patients' reported adherence. *Diabetes Educ.* 1993;19:287–292.
57. Lewis BS, Lynch WD. The effects of physician advice on exercise behavior. *Prev Med.* 1993;22:110–121.
58. Bandura A. Self-efficacy mechanism in physiological activation and health-promoting behavior. In: Madden, J IV, ed. *Neurobiology of Learning, Emotion, and Affect.* New York: Raven Press; 1991:229–269.
59. Prochaska JO, Velicer WF, Rossi JS, et al. Stages of change and decisional balance for 12 problem behaviors. *Health Psychol.* 1994;13(1):39–46.
60. Bandura A. The anatomy of stages of change. *Am J Health Promotion.* 1997;12(1):8–10.
61. Alemi F, Stephens RC. Computer services to patients' homes through telephones. *Med Care.* 1996;34(suppl 10):1–55.
62. MacStravic S, Montrose G. *Managing Health Care Demand.* Gaithersburg, MD: Aspen Publishers, Inc; 1998.

GARY MONTROSE leads the consulting practice of Ashby * Montrose & Co located in Denver, Colorado. Over the past 20 years he has provided strategic, business, and program planning services for provider organizations, health plans, and Fortune 100 technology and pharmaceutical companies in the areas of ambulatory care, disease, demand, and decision management. Mr. Montrose has served on several editorial boards and has taught health care strategic planning as adjunct faculty at the University of Denver. He is coauthor of the recently released book *Managing Health Care Demand.*

CHAPTER 11

Nurse Advice Services

Barry W. Wolcott

Chapter Outline

- Introduction
- Historical Incentives and Services
- Incentives in Today's Marketplace—the Changing Face of Nurse Advice Services
- Importance of Clinical Knowledge Systems
- Technology Factor
- Process Engineering—the Hidden Motor
- Toward an Integrated Future—Redefining Medical Management Services

INTRODUCTION

After accidentally spilling acid on his thigh while working in his laboratory, Alexander Graham Bell yelled into his experimental instrument, "Mr. Watson, come here; I need you." Thus, the first telephone call was, in fact, a call for assistance with a medical problem.

As the telephone has moved from wall-mounted rarity to its current hip-mounted omnipresence, its medical uses have similarly expanded. Today, telephone-based, nurse-assisted symptom assessment is but one aspect of a panoply of telephone-based medical services. In 1998, over 60 million Americans have easy access to such services. How did this evolve?

As telephones became commonplace in individual homes and physicians' offices in the late 1950s, patients enjoyed the new convenience of simply "calling the office nurse" to see what to do about new symptoms; calling the doctor at his home, after hours, regarding acute symptoms became common.

However, unlike lawyers, physicians never viewed telephone encounters as constituting an ongoing professional interaction with their patients—as a professional medical service for which they were entitled to fee-for-service reimbursement. Consequently, the telephone remained a nonmedical instrument. In the minds of most physicians, the telephone was an impediment, rather than an adjunct, to their practice. This perception, and the distortions it introduces into clinical practice, continue today.

HISTORICAL INCENTIVES AND SERVICES

By the 1960s, physicians' incomes had risen significantly, and physicians could afford to indulge in what would have been a luxury just years before: increasing their discretionary personal time uninterrupted by patient demands. At the same time, increasing personal incomes created a demand among the general public for medical services to be provided at times convenient to the patient—outside "normal" physician office hours. Naturally, conflict ensued.

- Increasing demand for after-hours physician services led to more after-hours calls to physicians.

- Physicians began to employ commercial answering services to "screen" the burgeoning number of after-hours calls from their patients and identify patients actually needing to speak with the doctor. Physicians grouped together in ever-larger "call groups" to further decrease exposure to after-hours care requests.
- Patients, perceiving the answering services and unknown (to them) physicians of such groups as barriers to their goal of obtaining medical care at a time of their choosing, sought alternatives to directly speaking with their doctors.

By the early 1970s, increasing numbers of patients wanting care "now" (and with comprehensive insurance) turned to hospital-based emergency departments (EDs) for after-hours services. As a result, emergency rooms serving the small group of critically ill and injured became EDs offering on-demand acute medical services to everyone 24 hours a day; free-standing urgent care centers (UCCs) also arose to meet this demand. The fee-for-service nature of both EDs and UCCs (and a fear of malpractice exposure) made it unlikely that these facilities would offer telephone-based advice (for which they could not be reimbursed) other than "just come in and be evaluated" to callers seeking advice. While patients had on-demand access to acute care services, markedly increased demand meant long waits at most EDs (and many UCCs), not to mention high costs of care for many nonemergency medical conditions.

In the early 1980s, nonmedical entrepreneurs realized that they could prosper by providing a new service matching two perceived marketplace needs: the general public's "need" (more accurately, desire) for on-demand medical advice, and hospitals' need for increased local market share. They created a licensable product (Ask-A-Nurse) through which individual hospitals in a given market could offer the public in their geographic region free telephone-based access to registered nurses able to provide advice and information about medical topics of interest to callers. If a nurse in a sponsoring hospital-operated call center established that a caller needed an office evaluation or a walk-in evaluation at a UCC, the nurse would preferentially direct that caller to offices of physicians on the staff of (or UCCs operated by) the sponsoring hospital. These referrals would directly (or indirectly) increase the sponsoring hospital's market share.

Public acceptance of telephone-based nurse advice was immediate and dramatic. Rapidly successful, the Ask-A-Nurse model drew local and national competitors offering similar products with similar goals. However, by the early 1990s reaction to the magnitude of medical care costs forced extensive modifications to traditional fee-for-service reimbursement—most commonly, limitations on "at-will" use of medical services without scheduled appointments. At the same time, rising numbers of people seeking acute care medical services in hospital-based EDs and UCCs were uninsured. In some markets, hospitals sponsoring nurse advice lines found that programs intended to increase market share in the general public of their affiliated physicians, UCCs, and EDs were counterproductive. Such programs either conflicted with the new "gatekeeping" rules of payers or brought increased numbers of uninsured patients to hospital-operated facilities.

In the same period, managed care plans seeking to expand their membership noted the high popularity of nurse advice services in the fee-for-service market. Plans decided to offer these services as a value-added benefit of membership, and they funded extensive marketing efforts showcasing their nurse advice services.

Unlike local hospitals, these usually geographically diffuse health plans did not operate their own call centers; rather, they contracted with outside vendors to provide nurse advice services to beneficiaries. Entrepreneurs, recognizing the increased margin of providing the services rather than just licensing software and marketing programs, rushed to open large regional call centers capable of serving the vastly increased market created by the almost universal provision of such services by managed care companies. While some hospitals (usually in regions of low managed care penetration) continue to operate local nurse advice services, the predominant players are those who must deliver medical services in an at-risk environment: managed care organizations (MCOs), large physician groups, integrated delivery systems, and so forth.

By the mid-1990s, several national vendors were operating telephone-based nurse advice systems from large regional call centers that served beneficiaries of most large plans. Competition among vendors rapidly moved nurse advice services from a value-added benefit, distinguishing an individual plan in a local market, to a commodity offered by all plans in a market.

As pressures mounted on profit margins, plans began to insist that all aspects of their business produce reductions in the aggregate costs of care provided to populations. Plans moved to eliminate value-added services that could not contribute to cost reductions.

Naturally, vendors of nurse advice services began to emphasize their ability to help managed care plans lower aggregate care costs. Vendors called attention to their ability to appropriately redirect many callers with acute symptoms from EDs and UCCs (where they would have sought care had the nurse advice service not been available) to self-care or care in primary care physician offices.

INCENTIVES IN TODAY'S MARKETPLACE—THE CHANGING FACE OF NURSE ADVICE SERVICES

By the final years of the 1990s, those at risk for the costs of care are contracting with vendors of telephone-based nurse advice services to provide their beneficiaries experiencing new (or newly worsened) symptoms with recommendations regarding the medically appropriate timing and provider of care for their problems. The underlying expectations are that

- giving the right advice by telephone to each case actually lowers aggregate costs (in other words, the savings resulting from correctly redirecting many callers to far less intense care than they would have sought on their own more than offset the added costs of correctly redirecting a few callers to more intense levels of care than they would have sought on their own)
- beneficiaries will value and follow the recommendations made by the nurses of the telephone advice service
- physicians, regulators, and opinion setters will accept these services as reflecting an acceptable standard of care for their patients
- insuring against potential liability remains feasible

As MCOs seek significant return on investment from telephone-based nurse advice services, controlling the costs of delivering these services becomes a critical element in call center management. Efforts to control costs while maintaining quality service necessarily focus on the following:

- controlling call center size
- maximizing call center efficiency
- defining those roles requiring nursing participation

Call Center Size

Callers and service purchasers commonly judge the quality of call center operations by the busy signal rate, the average waiting period before a call is answered, and the abandonment rate (how often callers hang up before completing a call). Each group wants these rates to be very low.

As the absolute number of nurses on duty in a call center increases, these rates become smaller. However, a call center employing a large number of nurses requires high volumes of calls in order to economically employ the nurses on duty. Vendors can most easily create these large call volumes by either routing calls from many clients to a single call center or by operating geographically separate, computer-linked call centers that function as a single, integrated center. This latter model has the additional advantage of decreasing the absolute number of nurses individual call center managers must hire.

Therefore, persistent pressure for high quality as indicated by these measures favors creation of large, regional call centers linked by sophisticated, computer-controlled telecommunications. This quality quest threatens small, local vendors of such services.

Call Center Efficiency

Many nonmedical call center–based services have average contact times of less than 1 minute. In such settings, decreases of but a few seconds in the average length of each call result in major changes in aggregate center costs. Thus, efforts to increase efficiency in such settings usually focus on shortening average call length.

However, a telephone-based nursing evaluation of acute symptoms takes longer—10 to 15 minutes on average. Thus, because aggregate costs in this setting are far less sensitive to average call length, managers direct less effort at this aspect of center process. Rather, they focus mainly on better matching of the numbers of nurses on duty to actual call arrival rates. (It is important to note that achieving these average call lengths requires sophisticated telecommunication switches and computer systems; without them, average call lengths rise prohibitively. Amortizing the overhead costs of these capital-intense technologies continues to favor large regional call centers over smaller local centers.) While linking call centers as discussed above does assist in this matching, an ability to schedule nursing work shifts of less than 8 hours would allow a major improvement in efficiency.

Defining Roles Requiring Nursing Participation

Service efficiency would improve if non-nurses could perform some of the tasks involved in providing telephone nurse advice. For this reason, some call centers already employ clerical personnel to assist in directing callers to pre-recorded or interactive voice technology messages, answering nonmedical (eg, customer service) questions, arranging appointments, etc.

Telecommuting would be the easiest way to enlist nurses to work less than 8-hour shifts. Unfortunately, current residential telephone systems rarely have sufficient bandwidth to allow call center nurses to work part time from home in a manner fully integrated into the call center process. Technologic improvements will likely soon close this gap and allow telecommuting for nurses.

IMPORTANCE OF CLINICAL KNOWLEDGE SYSTEMS

The most common "expert medical system" in use today is the personal judgment of individual medical professionals—physicians, nurses, therapists. Such individual judgments by nurses—based upon their individual education, training, and experience as modified by their individual memory—was (and remains) the most common basis for telephone-based medical advice for newly symptomatic callers by members of physician office staffs.

Not surprisingly, such a system, which was based upon the knowledge of individual nurses, exhibited persistent and large inter-nurse and intranurse variance in the advice provided in a given clinical setting. To minimize this variance, leaders of centralized nurse call centers of the 1970s and 1980s developed symptom-specific written guidelines for the telephone-based evaluation of callers with new symptoms. Clinical guidelines indicated which associated subjective findings a nurse should always consider during these telephone evaluations.

Nursing experts created these clinical guidelines, and physicians then reviewed and modified them. They provided a consistent basis for call center nurses' telephone interviews of callers, a uniform standard for training of newly hired call center nurses, and a basis for quality assurance reviews of individual nursing performance. Additionally, modification of these written guidelines during regular expert review would allow continual improvement in overall process quality.

A paucity of research limited the development of such guidelines. While the questions asked during telephone-based nursing assessments were a type of clinical test, no valid data documented their sensitivity or specificity, and no accurate data existed regarding the "pretest probability" of the possible causes of individual symptoms. Therefore, while guidelines represented the collective wisdom of their authors, they also represented their authors' collective biases.

The weakest guidelines were either a list of etiologies a nurse should exclude when speaking to a caller with a specific new symptom, or a symptom-specific list of questions a nurse should ask (with no accompanying explanation of why the questions were appropriate). The best symptom-specific guidelines were constructed using classic Baysean analysis techniques. Their authors

- accepted that while telephone-based evaluation of newly symptomatic callers could effectively exclude specific etiologies for those symptoms, it could not effectively diagnose the presence of a specific etiology (telephone-based evaluation could frequently *rule out*, but could not *rule in*)
- explicitly stated the possible etiologies the nurses' telephone-based evaluation was to consider
- explicitly estimated the pretest probability for each such etiologic possibility
- explicitly estimated the consequences of erroneously excluding at the initial telephone contact ("missing the presence of") each possible etiology
- explicitly stated the action to be recommended if a specific etiology could not be excluded
- linked the answers to specific questions the nurse should ask each caller with a specific new symptom to excluding (or failing to exclude) specific possible etiologies for the symptoms
- had undergone sufficient, explicit peer review that helped them conclude that their methods represented a reasonable national standard of practice while also reflecting any medically appropriate plan-specific variations from such national standards

TECHNOLOGY FACTOR

Pen and paper generally represent the outer limits of the technology used in office-based telephone nurse evaluations; sophisticated computer systems are essential to larger scale operations. Effective computer systems allow

- efficient distribution of incoming calls among linked call centers and among nurses within individual call centers
- rapid confirmation of callers' plan membership (eligibility to receive services)
- utilization of medical guidelines conforming to the medical standards of the physicians in the sponsoring health plan for each caller
- incorporation of prompts to remind the nurses of the components of the appropriate guideline as they are speaking to an individual caller
- creation of a medical record during each call that can be provided to the caller's physician for inclusion in the individual medical record and can serve as medicolegal documentation of the call process
- retention of information regarding specific calls in a relational database, allowing later data aggregation across a population and creation of (and analysis of) specific population subgroups

PROCESS ENGINEERING—THE HIDDEN MOTOR

People calling a telephone-based nurse call center for evaluation of a new symptom are entitled to expect a clinically appropriate recommendation. Additionally, most would agree that these callers are entitled to expect to receive the same recommendation were they to call many times to different nurses with the same story or to call the same nurse many times with the same story. Nurse-staffed call centers are just beginning to incorporate the process engineering essential to measuring and minimizing process variance; very soon, this level of consistency will be a core competency for successful centers.

Soon, call center operators will be expected to document how they

- clearly link the medical knowledge system underlying the recommendations callers receive to (and routinely modify these recommendations based upon measurement of) medical outcome
- routinely measure internurse and intranurse variation
- routinely identify sources of nursing variance
- use these measurements and identifications to make appropriate process modifications
- measure the effect of all implemented process changes

To do this, tomorrow's successful call center operator will require

- significant expertise in
  - the science of telephone-based symptom assessment
  - the operation and management of a technologically sophisticated call center
  - the operation and management of a medically sophisticated evaluation center
  - the process engineering of medical activities
  - the human engineering required for effective interactions of multiple medical professionals
- the support of a technologically sophisticated computer support system as described above

TOWARD AN INTEGRATED FUTURE—REDEFINING MEDICAL MANAGEMENT SERVICES

As noted earlier, a historical anomaly effectively excluded telephone contact with patients from the physician's practice of medicine and relegated telephone contact to the nonphysicians' business aspects of medicine. Because physicians initially did not charge for (and, therefore, eventually could not charge for) telephone contacts with their patients, physicians had no imperative to develop their expertise in the clinical use of the telephone; until very recently, nurses alone have developed and evaluated such clinical expertise.

For some time, there has been clear evidence that far less costly (and more pleasing to patients) telephone-based nurse–patient encounters could replace face-to-face doctor–patient encounters in a variety of clinical situations, including initial evaluations of new symptoms by nurses. However, the resistance of fee-for-service physicians to such techniques has precluded their widespread use.

That is now rapidly changing. Effective telephone-based programs (employing nurses supported by computer-based expert systems) that assist patients nationwide to manage some aspects of various medical conditions (eg, pregnancy) and chronic diseases (eg, asthma, heart failure, low back pain) already exist.

Pressures to reduce aggregate medical costs while maintaining medical quality are forcing physicians either to include these methods within their practice or to risk being replaced by other, less costly providers who will include them. Non–value-added office visits to physicians will go the way of non–value-added hospitalizations attended by physicians.

In the near future, patients with a variety of new and chronic health problems will regularly visit their medical providers in a variety of "virtual offices." During these "virtual visits," expert systems will assist patients as they interact with individual personal monitors (eg, peak flow meters, glucometers, sphygmometers, pulse oximeters, and so forth), telephone-based nurses and physicians, personal home computer programs and CD-ROM presentations, Internet applications, interactive voice response units, pagers, and personal digital assistants. Practice guidelines underlying the virtual office expert systems will recommend effective interventions individuals can carry out themselves. Face-to-face visits with physicians will be reserved for evaluation and management of individual clinical outliers not responding to management appropriate for the majority.

Additionally, other expert systems operating through similar technologies will expedite various medical quasi-administrative processes.

- New plan members will provide detailed medical histories and risk assessments and select providers whose known skills match their projected medical needs (eg, "Mrs Jacobs, since you have insulin-requiring diabetes and hypothyroidism, would you like to select a personal physician from among those in our network with special expertise in the outpatient management of these conditions?").
- Computer systems will compare physician chart entries and physician orders for a patient in an ED with accepted practice guidelines. The expert system will then preauthorize all requested services that are within the guideline's standards and automatically request specific further information of the physician when care requests seem at variance from the guideline's standard (eg, "Dr Johnson, could you please record whether or not the patient has T-waves elevations, as that information is required to preauthorize thrombolytic therapy?").
- A patient normally living in Denver but experiencing a lacerated forearm one evening while traveling in Boston can be directed to a highly appropriate level of care (eg, "Mr James, four blocks north of your hotel, Dr Swanson's office at 324 Broad Street is open now. Dr Swanson has the ability to evaluate and treat the type of cut you describe in her office. Additionally, since she is an affiliate of our health plan and you have our Gold Coverage, there will be no copayment required. She will also send a copy of her findings to your regular doctor, Dr Highfield, in Denver. Is that satisfactory?").

Historically, medicine has been rather Darwinian: successful physicians have been those who adopt new methods to improve the outcomes of their patients, and physicians rejecting these tools have disappeared. Examples include the ascendancy of scientific-based physicians at the onset of the 20th century, adoption of general anesthesia for surgery and incorporation of asepsis during the middle and end of the 19th century, introduction of antibiotics and imaging in the middle 20th century, and understanding of medical genetics as the 20th century closed. Adoption of techniques of the "virtual medical office" will likely characterize yet another generation of physician "survivors."

SUGGESTED READINGS

DaSilva V, Steinberg B. A force field evaluation tool for telephone service in ambulatory health care. *J Ambulatory Care Manage.* 1991;14(4):68–76.

Daugird A, Spencer D. Characteristics of patients who utilize telephone medical care in a private practice. *J Fam Pract.* 1989;29(1):59–64.

Moreland H, Grier M. Telephone consultations in the care of older adults. *Geriatr Nurs.* January/February 1986:28–30.

Morrison R, Arheart K, Rimner W. Telephone medicine in a Southern University private practice. *Am J Med Sci.* 1993;306(3):157–159.

Nash DB. *The Managed Care Manual.* Philadelpha: Total Learning Concepts; 1997.

Poole SR, Schmitt BD, Carruth T, Peterson-Smith A, Slusarski M. After-hours telephone coverage: the application of an area-wide telephone triage and advice system for pediatric practices. *Pediatr.* 1993;92(5):670–679.

Rao JN. Follow-up by telephone. *Br Med J.* 1994;309:1527–1528.

Sorum PC. Commentary: compensating physicians for telephone calls. *J Am Med Assoc.* 1992;272(24):1949.

Wasson J, Gaudette C, Whaley F, Sauvigne A, Baribeau P, Welch D. Telephone care as a substitute for routine clinic follow-up. *J Am Med Assoc.* 1992;267(13):1788–1793.

Wolcott B. Editorial: for whom the (phone) bell tolls. *Ann Emerg Med.* 1989;18:323.

BARRY W. WOLCOTT, MD, is chief medical officer at Access Health. He focuses on the development of clinically sound medical delivery support systems and their successful incorporation into both health care delivery systems and the practices of individual physicians. He was a founding partner of Informed Access Systems prior to its 1996 merger with Access Health. He is a graduate of Johns Hopkins University School of Medicine, has served in a variety of senior roles in the Army Medical Department, and is a member of the affiliate faculties of the schools of medicine of the Uniformed Services University and of George Washington University.

PART V

Emergency Department Services

The best efforts to provide preventive services and to manage disease states still do not reduce the use of the emergency department to zero. The least desirable method of managing costs in this arena is for a health plan to simply deny payment of a claim for anything that is deemed "not an emergency." This results in frustration all around, especially with the physicians and hospitals, as well as with the member. On the other hand, a health plan is not in a position of paying any claim that comes its way. Contracting terms may provide some relief, and new legislative initiatives surrounding "prudent layperson" interpretations of medical emergency will diminish complaints a bit; these brute force approaches are no match for good management of emergency services in the first place.

In major hospitals, the emergency department is no longer the emergency "room," but is now a sophisticated medical service. It is an important goal in managed care that emergency services be used appropriately—not only to manage costs—but to yield improved clinical outcomes. The chapters in Part V discuss efficient use of emergency services as well as two focused techniques that have been successfully applied in this setting.

CHAPTER 12

Efficient Use of Emergency Medicine Services

Casey J. Jason

Chapter Outline

- Introduction
- Prehospital Triage
- Emergency Department Triage
- Site and Staff Selection for Immediate Care
- Site and Staff Selection for Continuing Care
- Conclusion

INTRODUCTION

This chapter looks at the areas of emergency department operation that could be targets for controlling excessive cost. Two important areas—prehospital and emergency department triage—can be controlled and correlated with expected emergency department expenses. Once an emergency department visit occurs, the appropriate caretakers for ongoing care must be carefully chosen to avoid needless inefficiencies and expense.

Because the field of emergency medicine is evolving, it is becoming more difficult to define and efficiently utilize emergency medicine resources. We must continue to identify deficiencies and develop improvements in the delivery of acute patient care.

Emergency medicine began in the 1960s in Alexandria, Virginia, with Jim Mills as a leader and advocate of the Alexandria Plan. Mills and his colleagues formulated the Alexandria Concept of Emergency Medicine to address several issues.

- Acutely ill patients were often being denied adequate medical care.
- Staffing was performed by physicians with inconsistent interest in the care of the acutely ill.
- No medical specialty addressing emergency care had been created.
- No committed physicians trained in emergency medicine were staffing the hospital 24 hours per day.

The Alexandria Plan involved using committed full-time emergency department physicians to take care of acute and emergency illness. This Plan later developed into the American College of Emergency Physicians. Jim Mills was its first president.

Since the 1960s, emergency medicine has grown considerably. Within the specialty of emergency medicine, other services are now being offered, including chest pain centers (see Chapter 14), observation units (short stay units, see Chapter 13), workers' compensation clinics, and urgicenters. What began as an effort to eliminate an important deficit in health care delivery has been expanded to address other perceived inadequacies in the health care system. Experts are now asking, How can this emergency department resource be used more efficiently, and, from a payer's viewpoint, what should its role be?

Appropriate interventions can improve the quality and efficiency of care provided by an emergency department. These interventions focus on four aspects of emergency department visits: prehospital triage, emergency department triage sorting, site and staff selection for immediate care, and site and staff selection for continuing care.

PREHOSPITAL TRIAGE

A 45-year-old man with back pain considers whether to go to the emergency department or to his physician's office. He cannot decide. His health care plan has an after-hours nurse advice line (or "triage" service; see Chapter 11). He calls the advice line. A recorded voice explains that callers with life-threatening emergencies should call 911; otherwise, the voice explains, callers should wait for a nurse or state their telephone number so that a nurse can return their call. After the caller waits for 3 minutes, a nurse asks him to explain his chief complaint. Then the nurse asks a series of "pathway" questions that lead to a given recommendation for the caller's care (eg, home health care).

The above is an example of an *algorithm-based telephone triage* system, which sorts acuity and diseases with a series of questions. An automated group of proprietary algorithms guide nurses as they eliminate clinical problems one by one, from the most severe to the least, until the appropriate endpoint recommendation occurs, which may be a visit to the emergency department, urgicenter, or physician's office—or home care.

The goal is to recommend the proper treatment location based on the severity of the illness. Because nurses are sharing decision making with the patient, the word *advice* is avoided (despite the rather ubiquitous use of the term "nurse advice line"). Rather, *recommendations* are made. A second component is to differentiate the possible providers available so that the appropriate referral is made. Patient satisfaction with these triage systems is usually high.

In *protocol-based telephone triage*, a patient states a chief complaint, which prompts a threshold number of questions and leads to a recommendation of either an emergency department visit, an office visit, or home care. This approach can best be thought of as a scorecard where a critical number of positive answers triggers either emergency department, urgicenter, or other care. These questions first address life-threatening symptoms to avoid catastrophes and prompt an immediate emergency department referral, while positive answers to questions such as "Did you feel the pain while stretching or lifting?" result in an alternative setting being recommended. Patient satisfaction with protocol-based telephone triage tends to be high.

A *protocol-based, electronic patient-driven instrument* is an example of an attempt at pre-sorting calls in order to optimize registered nurse (RN) time for only those callers seriously considering emergency department care. After a recorded sorting procedure that may be bypassed, the patient is interviewed by a nurse using a protocol-based system. The most expensive parts of the system (RN and clerical) are bypassed unless the patient opts to speak with an RN. Satisfaction with this model has not yet been fully determined but is expected to grow as patients become accustomed to the system.

With any of these methods, several goals must receive high priority.

- efficient triage of patients into the appropriate setting
- high utilization of services by appropriate patients
- uniform delivery of service, whether by company or by licensee (eg, hospital, physician group, etc)
- cost of service reasonable relative to savings it yields

With changes occurring simultaneously in preventive health care, including chronic disease prevention programs, the decrease in emergency department visits will be multifactoral. Preliminary results from a study of commercial health plans suggest that the effect of telephone triage on the number of visits to physician offices and the effect of telephone triage on the number of visits to emergency departments cannot be measured separately. To truly measure the effect of telephone triage, one must look at how it affects both the number of office visits and the number of emergency department visits. Those groups having the most restricted access to preventive health care (individuals using Medicaid, low-income individuals) would be expected to show the largest decrease in emergency department visits because of telephone triage programs. Unfortunately, low-income individuals do not always have access to telephone triage programs. For Medicare and commercial patients, telephone triage programs would have the greatest effect on physician office visits, a savings that would not be reflected in emergency department statistics. The three triage systems are summarized in Table 12–1.

Not all patients using these services are considering emergency department care; therefore, using only saved emergency department visits to justify implementing a telephone triage program is misleading. Though difficult to document, saved office visits and lost time from work for patients using the service can also be used to demonstrate the service's value.

EMERGENCY DEPARTMENT TRIAGE

Given that prehospital triage may or may not decrease the number of emergency department visits, what happens after patients enter the emergency department certainly affects the department's clinical and economic success. Punitive, retroactive denial of emergency department care based upon perceived "inappropriate" use has become, rightly, such a sensitive issue that better ways must be found to assess illness severity after a patient presents to the emergency department. The practice of transferring patients from one treatment center to another for care has inspired intense medical and legal interest. Although there is a burgeoning amount of legal opinion on the issue, the following sections can be used as a primer.

Transfer

The emergency department has become the staging area for defining both emergency department and payer responsibilities for patients. Three major pieces of legislation have included provisions affecting emergency department responsibilities and reimbursement (Table 12–2): the Emergency Medical Treatment and Labor Act of 1986 (EMTALA), the Consolidated Omnibus Budget Reconciliation Act of 1986 (COBRA), and the Balanced Budget Act (BBA) of 1997.

EMTALA was created in 1986 to protect low-income patients and establish emergency department responsibilities to safeguard patient care. The burden was placed on the emergency department to provide this care and be responsible for any repercussions.

Since the passage and revision of COBRA in 1986, Section 1867 of the Social Security Act[1] (amended 1989 and 1990[2]), emergency departments have gone from concern over "antidumping" penalties to problems as diverse as

Table 12–1 Summary of Triage Systems

Service Type	Likelihood of False Positives	Likelihood of False Negatives	Patient Satisfaction
Algorithm-based telephone triage	Low	Low	High
Protocol-based telephone triage	Moderate	Low	High
Protocol-based, electronic patient-driven instrument	Moderate	Low	To be determined

Table 12–2 Legislation Affecting Emergency Department Responsibilities and Reimbursement

Act	Purpose	Who Is Affected
EMTALA	Requires Medicare participating hospitals to evaluate whether patient has an emergency medical condition, and if so, to stabilize the patient.	Emergency department
COBRA	Restricts transport of unstable patients for financial reasons.	Emergency department payers (potentially)
BBA 1997 (concerning emergency department care of Medicare/Medicaid patients)	Requires health plans participating in Medicare/Medicaid to reimburse based upon a "prudent patient standard."*	Payers
	• Prohibits prior authorization requirements.	
	• Creates guidelines for coordinator of poststabilization care.	

*Consumers have the right to access emergency health care services when and where the need arises. Health plans should provide payment when a consumer presents to an emergency department with acute symptoms of sufficient severity—including severe pain—such that a "prudent layperson" could reasonably expect the absence of medical attention to result in placing health in serious jeopardy, serious impairment to bodily functions, or serious dysfunction of any bodily organ or part.

- the nature and type of screening exams
- appropriate stabilization of a patient prior to transfer (or discharge)
- delay or referral of care based upon financial considerations

For managed care groups having specific hospitals "in plan" for care, the safe and appropriate transport of patients from one hospital to another is important in avoiding litigation.

To put the problem into perspective, in the 10-plus years that COBRA has been in force, relatively few violations have been noted or penalties levied. More than 900 million emergency department visits occurred between 1986 and 1996, yet they produced only 1,757 complaints and 1,729 investigations.[3]

- Only 0.5% of hospitals with emergency departments were fined (27 fines).
- Five incidents involved physicians.
- Less than 25% of allegations were confirmed.
- Termination of services occurred in 1.2% of hospitals investigated.
- Inappropriate transfers were involved in 23 cases.

The possibility that unrecognized or unreported violations have occurred always exists; however, the lessons in the more than 10 years since COBRA enactment have been important. An appropriate screening exam, attention to detail, and documentation help to prevent what is a very small but important risk to the emergency department and potential cause of litigation involving managed care.

A new dimension has been added with the pending "Prudent Patient" legislation (HR 815 and S 356 in the House of Representatives and Senate, respectively). This legislation considers a patient's perspective on whether he or she should be seen in the emergency department. This federal legislation is similar to existing Prudent Patient legislation in Maryland,[4] amended 1996,[5] and approximately 12 other states. The question of access to health care represented by Prudent Patient and other pending national and state legislation revolves around a patient's ability to know the severity if not the nature of his or her illness.

BBA 1997, which deals with emergency department treatment of Medicare and Medicaid patients, represents the legislative reaction to patient resentment over preauthorization and retroactive denials. The bill contains a number of provisions potentially affecting managed care.

- Prior authorization would not be required for emergency medical care.
- Services would be covered whether or not a contract was in place.
- Authorization access for care (nonemergent) would be required 24 hours a day.
- All costs related to transfer under COBRA Section 1867 would be covered by the care plan.

BBA 1997 does not have the same effect as the proposed national Prudent Patient legislation. Specifically, BBA 1997

- affects Medicare and Medicaid patients, including those in managed care
- prohibits prior authorization requirements
- establishes guidelines (written by the Secretary of the Department of Health and Human Services) for coordination of poststabilization care for emergency departments and managed care
- does *not* compel self-insured Employee Retirement Income Security Act (ERISA) plans to follow guidelines
- does *not* compel compliance for health plans not having Medicare or Medicaid patients in states without Prudent Patient legislation

This represents a process change for authorization of emergency department care that has gathered momentum and popular public support. The issue is not safe transport of the patient or appropriate emergency department use, but rather that all patients who feel that they need emergent care should receive it as defined by a prudent patient standard.

In Maryland and other states, discussions do not center on whether the emergency department visit is appropriate but rather on the limits to which it is appropriate. This is an important issue for managed care, because the users of the emergency department for minor illness in many cases are commercial, Medicare, or Medicaid patients desiring convenience,[6,7] or those without a primary care physician. Estimates of visits that could have been handled in sites other than the emergency department vary from less than 20% to about 80%.[8-11]

It is generally accepted that most emergency department visits are inappropriate for the level of care needed. This raises two issues: Does it make financial sense to see these people in the emergency department? Is it logical to treat nonemergency cases in an emergency setting?

Estimates of marginal emergency department costs[12,13] and the assumption that the cost shifting from the uninsured does not materially affect the cost for insured patients are questionable. Marginal costs—which include the facility, the staff, and care for low-income people—materially affect the cost of seeing the ambulatory nonemergent insured patient, estimated at over $5 billion in "excess" per year.[14] Given the overcrowding at many emergency departments and the adverse medical and financial effect that the crowding has on having truly emergent patients moved efficiently,[15] the ambulatory patients qualifying for care would be better served elsewhere.

The efficient use of the emergency department can occur only if several important steps occur. First, uniform, scientifically defensible triage capable of comparison among institutions must precede the patient's physician evaluation and treatment. Second, prompt evaluation and continuing care in the proper setting must take place. Third, the appropriate personnel, including physician staff, must be present to care for the patient.

Triage

Triage involves the classification of patients into severity categories that should directly correlate with the speed and intensity of care in the emergency department, as well as the likelihood of admission and death. What would seemingly be a critical first step in patient evaluation is not presently done in a disciplined, consistent, or reproducible fashion. In any system, the goals should be to direct patients to the proper level of care while minimizing the risk of false negatives (ie, the patient is more acutely ill than the health care provider realized).

The triage program should be capable of comparison from institution to institution. This issue is of such concern to patients, physicians, and hospitals that bills HR 815/S 356, Access to Emergency Medical Services Act, and HR 1415, Patient Access to Responsible Care Act, mandate consideration of presenting illness intensity as a guide for access. A compromise between detail and simplicity must be struck so that the system is reproducible with a high yield of valuable information. This information must include intensity of illness rather than outcome as the dichotomous endpoint (ie, treat in the emergency department or refuse care),[16,17] probability of selected outcomes based upon the current standard of care, and adjustments for changes in medical practice.

The problems of the current methods of triage have been cited.[18,19] These problems include[8,18–20]

- interviewer bias both in managed care and emergency department
- variability in interviewer skills and adequacy of interviewer technique
- endpoint validation (eg, return rate for those triaged out, emergency department versus other site, admissions)
- admission rate for those triaged out and its appropriateness
- the use of chief complaint for either inclusion or exclusion from treatment

As a recent journal editorial stated, "The time to evaluate these approaches to patient triage is now."[21] Development of statistical tools to assess acuity and the probability for important clinical endpoints such as admission, discharge, or death in the emergency department is occurring at two leading research institutions (Robert Lowe, University of Pennsylvania; Michael Samuhel, Research Triangle Institute, Research Triangle Park, personal communication, November 1997). This effort is expected to offer a dynamic analytical tool reflecting current and evolving standards of care, as well as correlating with the expected cost for this care.

SITE AND STAFF SELECTION FOR IMMEDIATE CARE

With the appropriate sorting system, responsible choice of alternative treatment sites will be possible. These will include urgent care centers or even committed physician offices. As overflow because of unavailable office appointment times during the day, as well as after-hours illness, remains an ongoing problem, alternative treatment locations become important. For the reasons mentioned previously, the emergency department should not usually be a first choice of care center. Urgicenters represent a well-recognized and appreciated source of low overhead care,[22] although cost is better contained by a physician's office that offers extended hours.[23] With regard to urgicenter or office alternatives, a number of important issues must be considered:

1. location
   - They must be convenient and easily accessible from the patient's home.
   - Reasonable access to a higher level of care must be available.
2. personnel/equipment
   - Proper personnel and equipment should be present, with particular attention being given for those who might deteriorate during their stay.
   - A pleasant, well-lit environment should greet the patient.
   - Proper computer/electronic systems should be available to transmit clinical and billing information.
   - Minimum standards of care should be established for physicians and staff.
3. quality assurance
   - Documentation should be equal to the standard of emergency medicine.
   - Adverse outcomes should be reported to the health care plan and the primary care physician.

- Clinical summaries including 24- and 72-hour return rates should be reported.
- Primary care physician notification of clinical condition and disposition should occur.
- Regular quality assurance reports for both health care plan patients and summary total should be reported to the plan on a regular basis.
- Standard operating procedures should be established.

In summary, the same high standard of care should be present whether the location is an emergency department, an urgent care center, or a physician's office. Board certification in the appropriate primary care field, such as internal medicine or family practice, should be required, although emergency medicine would be an appropriate alternative. The best use of the emergency department for these nonurgent cases would be avoiding it altogether if the appropriate acuity were present and facility available. Alternative treatment facilities fitting the above standards must be made available. Please refer to Chapter 13 for a description of the fast track alternative.

SITE AND STAFF SELECTION FOR CONTINUING CARE

In many cases, an admission may not be necessary.[24] It is critical to have an internist or primary care physician (the hospitalist; see Chapter 16) on site who is familiar with how a managed care system should work. Having the best in clinical knowledge is a prerequisite but is inadequate in the total picture. The physician serving this patient must have familiarity with or access to information about the following:

- present medical problem and its relationship to prior medical history
- treatment course in progress with primary care physician or subspecialist
- plan preferences for
  - subspecialists
  - procedures/special diagnostics
  - hospitals
  - tertiary-level care
  - subacute, skilled nursing services
  - recordkeeping
  - quality assurance procedures

The hospitalist[25] must be clinician, diplomat, and team leader in the truest sense. He or she should be regarded as an ally, not an adversary, of the primary care physician. This person should be capable of integrating the non–office-based care, including, but not limited to, hospital care (special studies, consultants, medical problems and subacute care [including medical follow-up]), and skilled nursing facility care.

CONCLUSION

Efficient use of the emergency department must be viewed as a continuum. The choice is not merely between admission or discharge, but rather among many options. The choice must be guided by a skilled practitioner familiar with how managed care works. The emergency department represents an exciting area for appropriate, acuity-driven intervention, as well as alternative care decisions. The challenge should be welcomed and dealt with appropriately by both emergency medicine departments and payers.

REFERENCES

1. 42 USC § 1395dd.
2. 42 USC § 1395a,b,d.
3. Lewis RJ, Guisto JA, Meislin HW, Spaite DW. Analysis of federally imposed penalties for violations of the Consolidated Omnibus Budget Reconciliation Act. *Ann Emerg Med.* 1996;28:45–50.
4. MD Health-Gen Code Ann § 19.701 (1993).
5. MD Health-Gen 61r0109 (1996).
6. Shesser R, Kirsch T, Smith J, Hirsch R. An analysis of emergency department use by patients with minor illness. *Ann Emerg Med.* 1991;20:743–748.
7. Rubin MA, Bonnin MJ. Utilization of emergency department by patients with minor complaints. *J Emerg Med.* 1995;13:839–842.

8. Young GP, Wagner MB, Kellerman AL, Ellis J, Bonley D. Ambulatory visits to hospital emergency departments. *JAMA.* 1996;276:460–465.
9. Buesching DP, Jablokowski A, Vesta E, et al. Inappropriate emergency department visits. *Ann Emerg Med.* 1985;14:672–676.
10. Guterman JJ, Frakaszek JB, Murdy D, et al. The 1980 patient urgency study: further analysis of the data. *Ann Emerg Med.* 1985;14:1191–1198.
11. Haddy RI, Schmaler ME, Epting RJ. Nonemergency emergency room use in patients with and without primary care physicians. *J Fam Pract.* 1987;24:389–392.
12. Williams RM. The cost of visits to emergency departments. *N Engl J Med.* 1996;334:642–646.
13. Steinbrook R, ed. The role of the emergency department. *N Engl J Med.* 1996;334:657–658.
14. Baker LC, Baker LS. Excess cost of emergency department visits for nonurgent care. *Health Aff.* 1994;13:162–171.
15. Krochmal P, Tamrah R. Increased health care costs associated with ED overcrowding. *Am J Emerg Med.* 1994;12:265–266.
16. Derlet RW, Nishio D, Cole LM, et al. Triage of patients out of the emergency department: three-year experience. *Am J Emerg Med.* 1992;10:195–199.
17. Derlet RW, Kinser D, Ray L, et al. Prospective identification and triage of nonemergency patients out of an emergency department: a 5-year study. *Ann Emerg Med.* 1995;25:215–223.
18. Lowe RA, Bindman AB, Ulrich SK, et al. Refusing care to emergency department patients: evaluation of published triage guidelines. *Ann Emerg Med.* 1994;23:286–293.
19. Brillman JC, Doezema D, Tandberg D, et al. Triage: limitations in predicting need for emergent care and hospital admission. *Ann Emerg Med.* 1996;27:493–500.
20. O'Brien GM, Shapiro MJ, Woolord RW, et al. "Inappropriate" emergency department use: a comparison of three methodologies for identification. *Acad Emerg Med.* 1996;3:252–257.
21. Adams SL, Fontanarosa PB. Triage of ambulatory patients. *JAMA.* 1996;276:493–494.
22. Wong JC. Efficiency and effectiveness in the urgent care clinic. *Postgrad Med.* 1996;99:161–166.
23. Forrest CB, Starfield BS. The effect of first contact care with primary care clinician on ambulatory health care expenses. *J Fam Prac.* 1996;43:40–47.
24. McCormick B. Managed care M*A*S*H. *AMA News.* 1995;3:22–23.
25. Wachter RM, Goldman L. The emerging role of "hospitalists" in the American health care system. *N Engl J Med.* 1996;335:514–517.

CASEY J. JASON, MD, FACEP, FAAP, is the midatlantic vice president and medical director for the hospitalist and skilled nursing facility program for Cove Healthcare. He is also assistant clinical faculty in the department of medicine at Georgetown University. He actively collaborates with metropolitan District of Columbia managed care organizations to improve coordination and efficiency of both hospital emergency departments and inpatient medical services. Dr. Jason has extensive experience in directing proper utilization of emergency medical services, including 14 years as a practicing emergency department physician and 3 years as associate director of the Washington Hospital Center emergency medicine department.

CHAPTER 13

The Fast Track Emergency Department

Angela Zotos

Chapter Outline

- Introduction
- Observation Unit
- Staffing the Fast Track
- Best Practices
- Key Considerations when Designing a Fast Track Program in the ED
- Results Achieved

INTRODUCTION

Emergency departments (EDs) have been the front door of the hospital for many patients who lack health insurance. Health care providers have responded to the increasing demand for emergency services by developing new systems that reduce waiting times, improve accuracy of diagnosis, move the patient to the appropriate level of care quickly, and decrease the overall time spent in the emergency department. "Fast tracks" have developed over the last 6 to 7 years because of the growing numbers of patients using EDs for primary care. The ED's fast track sections are clinics staffed by advanced practice or midlevel providers (physician assistants, nurse practitioners) and, occasionally, primary care physicians. Instead of waiting with the more acutely ill patients, these patients (with complaints such as sore throats, jammed fingers, simple puncture wounds, congestion, etc) are triaged into a separate area, often resembling an office setting. In this area, they can be evaluated, treated, and discharged expeditiously.

In a well-functioning fast track, the cost of the ED visit can be reduced to nearly that of an office visit. The fast track approach allows the patient to be seen within 15 minutes of arrival to the department and treated and released within 30 minutes. Since patients often rate their satisfaction based upon their length of stay (LOS), reducing LOS in a fast track can have tremendous effect on a hospital's patient satisfaction indicators.

Fundamental success in this area requires the commitment of staff, clearly defined policies and procedures, and a thorough understanding of the population to be served. Fast tracks treat non–acute care patients with easy access, high quality, and low cost. They require a paradigm shift from acutely ill (trauma) care to primary care.

OBSERVATION UNIT

Another variation on the fast track concept is an observation unit. Patients who are not sick enough to be admitted and not well enough to go home can be monitored more closely so that an informed decision can be made by the health care provider. Emergency physicians do not want to mistakenly tell people that they are not acutely ill. There is growing concern that managed care systems may have a higher likelihood of missed diagnoses. Therefore, the observation unit can serve a dual purpose; it frees up acute care ED beds while providing appropriate care to patients needing additional testing and treatment, yet it also prevents unnecessary inpatient admissions. Observation areas are typically adjacent to the ED and are managed by ED physicians. Intensive evaluation, management, and stabilization occur over several hours to, for example, rule out a myocardial infarction, congestive heart failure, manage an arrhythmia, or normalize a blood glucose level.

STAFFING THE FAST TRACK

Hospitals and EDs across the country are looking for ways to streamline care delivery and provide an extra pair of hands at the most economical cost. Multiskilled workers and alternatives to physicians, such as physician assistants, are growing in popularity, especially in areas such as the fast track ED. Several training programs for physician assistants are now offering an emphasis in emergency medicine. Fast tracks may also use nurse practitioners, professionals extensively trained in assessment and diagnosis that have served several specialties over the last 20 years, including critical care and obstetrics. Nurse practitioners enjoy the "education" portion of their jobs and are often thought to be better patient educators than physicians. Traditionally, physicians have not had a great deal of training in educating patients. Overall, nurse practitioners' interpersonal skills are usually better than those of physicians, their technical skills are equivalent for the types of care they render, the patient outcomes are equivalent, and access to care is improved.[1]

The American College of Emergency Physicians has guidelines and sample job descriptions for physician assistants and nurse practitioners in EDs. Typical staffing ratios (traditional nursing formulas that allow specific numbers of full-time equivalents per department visit, or physician formulas that allow three visits per hour) cannot be adopted universally because the midlevel practitioners' responsibilities can extend beyond those of a nurse or a physician. Therefore, staffing should be based on the ED's LOS and volume targets. Initially, staffing with two midlevel providers working an overlapping shift each day with ancillary support as needed will be sufficient for a six-bed fast track unit.

BEST PRACTICES

There are four core processes to be considered for optimizing the fast track. *Access in* refers to the rapid and appropriate triage of patients. Rapid triage can be accomplished by developing protocol-based triage, utilizing three to five key questions based upon the patient's presenting complaint. This process replaces a long assessment and therefore can move the patient immediately into a treatment area, eliminating patient waiting time. Registration is next to the triage area. There, essential information required to initiate a patient record is collected. Triage should occur within 5 minutes of arrival to the ED.

Level of care results in the rapid, effective differentiation of urgent from nonurgent patients. The fast track provides access to health care alternatives to ED treatment for nonurgent patients. Therefore, access is improved, ED use is appropriate, and costs are controlled. The ED can focus on truly critical patients. When a triaging system is developed, the lower severity classifications can fluctuate between the ED and fast track. For examples, levels one and two in the ED could also be the two levels seen in the fast track, depending upon the episodic complaints. All areas within the ED are flexible and redirect patients if initial triage proves to be incorrect. Triage in the fast track is not based on acuity of complaint but on the potential for quickly making a diagnosis and completing a management plan. Limiting costly, time-consuming lab and X-ray testing is essential. Although patients may not be acutely ill, patients with problems that require extensive diagnostic testing or a long observation period should not be seen in the fast track area.

Diagnostics/treatment/interventions should be minimal in the fast track area. The initial history and physical assessment can be initiated by the nurse and verified and expanded if necessary by the nurse practitioner or physician assistant. Testing should be minimal and can be completed with rapid-response lab technology. Core processes can be streamlined using documentation systems such as preprinted templates based on the patient's initial complaint. This focuses documentation on essential assessment data and diagnostic testing if needed.

Discharge and disposition should focus on teaching patients how to recognize signs and symptoms of an illness earlier so that a visit to a physician's office may be planned. During this time, patients who utilize the fast track setting as an alternative to a primary care physician can be informed about local physicians who are accepting new patients, and referrals can be made. The entire discharge and disposition should be completed within 5 minutes, with the patient acknowledging understanding. Preprinted discharge instructions for common illnesses (eg, sore throat, sprain) seen in the fast track ED improve adherence to time constraints.

KEY CONSIDERATIONS WHEN DESIGNING A FAST TRACK PROGRAM IN THE ED

Location, Location, Location

It is preferable to establish separate entrances for patients who walk in and those who come by ambulance. Triage should be the first interaction that patients have with the system, and nonacute patients should be triaged to a fast track that has a separate waiting room and clinical area. This will avoid the confusion when patients are seen out of their order of arrival to the ED. Having the fast track area located next to the ED allows for sharing of staff and materials and prevents costly duplication of registration, ancillary, and support services. If the fast track area and ED are separate, the fast track nurse may have to perform many or even all of the clerical duties, thereby eliminating the overhead costs for administrative assistants. Nurse workload and ability to carry out clinical responsibilities in a timely way must be considered before making such a change.

A Schedule That Complements the ED

The fast track should be opened initially during peak hours for the ED. Data on patient arrival patterns, LOS, and ED workload by hour and day can be helpful in deciding when a fast track should be open. Most fast tracks are open from 8 AM until 10 PM daily. As the community becomes more aware of the fast track, the hours can be expanded. Reimbursement can be affected by operating hours, because in order to utilize the billing codes for the ED, the fast track must be available 24 hours per day.

Streamlined Processes

Established patient care protocols that allow the nurse to initiate the care plan before the patient is seen by a physician, physician assistant, or nurse practitioner will reduce waiting times. Clearly defined policies and procedures are integral to the successful design of a fast track. The most common diagnoses for patients seen in fast tracks are viral illnesses, isolated extremity injuries, minor lacerations, and rechecks.

RESULTS ACHIEVED

In emergency medicine, there are two critical—and related—success factors that contribute to maintaining a competitive advantage: time and patient satisfaction. A key determinant of patient satisfaction is wait times. Patient average LOSs in EDs have dropped dramatically since fast tracks were developed.[2] Fast track admissions can be triaged, evaluated, and discharged within 30 minutes, instead of the typical 4- and 5-hour waits that ED patients sometimes experience. Another indicator is the percentage of "walk-outs" experienced by EDs. This phenomenon has nearly disappeared in some instances, with very few patients leaving without being seen. In teaching hospitals, this walk-out number can be higher.

Denial of payment for non-emergent treatment is another measure of hospital success. Denials can be reduced when care is delivered in the appropriate setting. Nearly half of all ED patients can be seen in less expensive settings. While charges probably cannot be lowered to that of a physician's office visit for the same condition, charges overall in the fast track can be substantially lower than charges in the ED. As legislation affecting how a managed care organization reviews claims from the ED or for urgent services comes into play (see Chapter 12 regarding "prudent layperson" definitions of coverage mandates), the fast track ED, with its lower costs, becomes an important tool in managing these services. In fact, there have been some managed care plans that have negotiated a flat rate with a hospital that has a fast track ED; the flat rate covers all urgent and emergent services, and in turn, the health plan does not reject the claims for medical review. This agreement creates a winning situation for both organizations, but it can be undertaken only if both sides can accurately estimate the expected volume and acuity of cases.

Collaboration between ED physicians and midlevel providers in planning and guideline development is key to the success of fast tracks. This collaboration enhances quality and increases the satisfaction of all the providers involved. Staff satisfaction can also improve through the implementation of a fast track. A less congested work area is healthier; it reduces the number and magnitude of patient and family complaints, the number of patients forgotten in the system, and overall stress levels. The ED staff can focus on the critically ill patients without worrying that they are ignoring the nonacutely ill patients.

Implementing a fast track should not be considered a quick fix to ease ED congestion. Bottlenecks in EDs can be caused by a variety of factors (eg, too few treatment areas, extended waits for ancillary services such as laboratory tests and X-rays, and scarcity of physicians). While a fast track can improve wait times overall, it does not necessarily eliminate these problems. As mentioned above, coordination of workload, LOS, and triage criteria can help optimize a fast track operation. Additionally, a clear, concise vision for care; committed staff; and clearly defined protocols and policies will help ensure a fast track's success.

REFERENCES

1. Wright SW, Erwin T, Blanton DM, Covington CM. Fast track in the emergency department: a one-year experience with nurse practitioners. *J Emerg Med.* 1993;10(3): 367–373.

2. Nollman J, Colbert K. Successful fast tracks: data and advice. *J Emerg Nurs.* 1994;20:483–486.

ANGELA ZOTOS, RN, MS, is a senior manager in the Health Care Consulting Practice at Ernst & Young. She earned a BSN from Oakland University and an MS in health care administration from Simmons College. She has extensive clinical and consulting experience. Her clinical experience is focused on emergency and surgical services. Her consulting experience includes postmerger integration, transformation management, and work redesign.

CHAPTER 14

Chest Pain Centers

Suzanne K. White

Chapter Outline

- Introduction
- Traditional Approaches to Managing Chest Pain
- Drivers for Change in the Management of Chest Pain
- The Chest Pain Center Approach
- Clinical and Economic Benefits of a Chest Pain Center Approach
- Chest Pain Center Development
- Conclusion

INTRODUCTION

Acute myocardial infarction (AMI) remains the leading cause of death in the adult population in the United States. Each year, there are 600,000 deaths due to AMI in the United States. Chest pain accounts for 5% of emergency department (ED) visits, or 4.4 million people annually. In fact, chest pain is one of the most common complaints in EDs. Of those visiting EDs, 10% to 15% experience an AMI. Recent advances in the treatment of AMI have greatly reduced its morbidity and mortality, yet these treatments are time dependent and necessitate rapid initiation.

Good outcomes of treatment require quick recognition of signs and symptoms of an AMI by the patient, quick diagnosis of AMI by the physician, and identification of atypical signs and symptoms in patients with an AMI by the physician. This is one of the tenets of a good managed care program: to improve quality and outcomes (as discussed in Part XI) and to do so expeditiously. Conversely, the rapid identification of chest pain for which a cardiac origin has been clearly ruled out allows for an appropriate response in a more cost-effective manner. This chapter will discuss the development of chest pain centers and their clinical and economic impact.

TRADITIONAL APPROACHES TO MANAGING CHEST PAIN

Outcomes have historically not been ideal for most patients who experience chest pain. Patients often wait too long after the onset of symptoms of AMI before seeking medical care. Median delay from chest pain onset until the patient arrives in the ED is greater than 2 hours. But 26% to 44% of patients delay longer than 4 hours. If a patient with an AMI is treated within 60 to 70 minutes, left ventricular damage can be minimized by aborting the infarct, and mortality is decreased.[1] With delay, substantial myocardial necrosis can occur, minimizing the effect of medical intervention.

After the patient arrives in the ED, significant delays may occur before the physician makes the diagnosis of AMI and implements definitive care such as thrombolysis. Delays can occur in obtaining electrocardiograms (ECGs), instituting thrombolytics, preparing and administering medication, and seeking consultation in patients with clear evidence of AMI. Many factors influence these delays. Delays may be due to gender bias, staff's perception of pain as noncardiac, and lack of rapidly available serum markers for AMI. Delays in administering thrombolytics lead to larger infarct size, increase the number of complications, and increase mortality.[2]

Physician's failure to correctly diagnose AMI in patients with atypical signs and symptoms has been another long-standing problem. From 4% to 13% of patients with an AMI are released from the ED with false assurance that they do not have coronary artery disease. Many of these patients have complications from their AMI, and 11% to 25% die. Given the difficulty in diagnosing AMI, combined with the complications from this serious disease process, AMI is the most expensive cause of malpractice litigation against emergency physicians, constituting 20% of all dollars paid.[3]

A fear of malpractice will prompt emergency physicians to admit, often to the coronary care unit (CCU), almost all patients with chest pain. Traditionally, routine care of patients with any probability of AMI was placement in the CCU. Admission to the CCU was acceptable in prior years because the economics of American medicine rewarded providers for doing more without regard to the level of cost incurred or even outcome achieved. Under this system, physicians and hospitals were financially motivated to admit patients, even just to rule out AMI. The cost associated with this traditional AMI rule-out approach is about $8 billion a year.[4]

DRIVERS FOR CHANGE IN THE MANAGEMENT OF CHEST PAIN

Today, changes in the U.S. health care system demand increased attention to cost-effectiveness in the treatment modalities chosen for evaluation of chest pain. A commitment to new clinical knowledge and state-of-the-art care has been supported by the creation of the National Heart Attack Alert Program (NHAAP) of the National Heart, Lung and Blood Institute. This program was established to promote the rapid identification and treatment of AMI with the goal of reducing AMI morbidity and mortality. In 1991, when the NHAAP began, the average door-to-needle time was 60 to 70 minutes. Now it is typically 39 minutes.[5]

Another driver includes changing reimbursement and managed care. As hospital per diems and case-rate payments undergo downward pressure, inpatient reimbursement beyond a single day is unlikely to be profitable. More important, prepaid reimbursement will make controlled access to inpatient beds an imperative for financial survival. Under this reimbursement, chest pain centers will serve as disciplined gatekeepers to inpatient cardiac beds.

Lastly, an increased demand for outcome data is a driving force. The government, managed care plans, accrediting organizations, and consumers are demanding data about quality and cost. If institutions do not review data internally, external entities will do it for them, and the data may not be accurate. This will be discussed in more detail later in the chapter.

THE CHEST PAIN CENTER APPROACH

Because of the failure of traditional approaches and faced with the current drivers described, many hospitals have established chest pain centers (CPCs). Many CPCs have designated resources of personnel, protocols, space, and equipment for patients presenting with chest pain.

What Is a Chest Pain Center?

In 1992 a survey of the American College of Emergency Physicians leadership (319 participants) revealed that 9% of EDs had CPCs.[6] In 1994, a study by Bahr reported that there were 500 CPCs in the United States,[7] and in 1996, he reported that there were between 700 and 1,000 CPCs in the United States.[8] The literature reveals that there are various names for CPCs: chest pain units, chest pain EDs, chest pain evaluation units, short-stay ED CCUs, and ED monitored observation beds. Sometimes CPCs are not in the ED but in the hospital and near the CCU. They come in all shapes and sizes. Some have been developed as marketing ploys to attract incremental revenues while others are impressive displays of organizational efficiency and clinical expertise.

A national study by Zalenski was conducted to determine the prevalence of CPCs in the United States, describe the chest pain diagnosis protocols and techniques, and compare hospitals with and without CPCs. The initial findings reveal that 22.5% of hospitals have CPCs, and most CPCs are in EDs. In hospitals with CPCs, there was increased community education and decreased door-to-needle time. He also found that greater market competition in the area made a hospital more likely to have a CPC.[9]

The National Congress of Chest Pain Centers has defined a CPC as a grass-roots, community-based unit focused on early recognition and treatment of patients with acute myocardial infarction or underlying occult coronary artery disease and prevention in future generations.[10] A CPC should not be a marketing ploy but a way to evaluate chest pain in a cost-effective manner to gain the best outcome for the patient. A tightly controlled managed care environment requires this type of approach.

The components of a CPC include the following[6]:

- attack program (reducing time to treatment, NHAAP)
- chest pain unit (with appropriate design and staffing)
- observation program
- outreach program
- quality management program (to monitor outcomes)

Attack Program

Sixty percent of patients with AMI have clinical presentation suggesting a high or moderate probability of AMI based on history, physical, and ECG. Mortality is decreased 1.6% if thrombolytics are administered in 1 hour.[1] The overall goal of an attack program is to decrease delays in the initiation of therapy for an AMI. Many factors contribute to delay in initiating therapy: delays in obtaining an ECG, delays in decision making on instituting thrombolytics, delays in preparing and obtaining the medication, and asking for consultation in patients with clear evidence of AMI.[6] Many hospitals have developed protocols and pathways to minimize delays in instituting therapy to patients with chest pain. An example of an algorithm for patients with chest pain developed by the NHAAP is shown in Figure 14–1. A successful program depends on improvement in the efficiency and time of delivery of quality care.[11]

Chest Pain Unit

A chest pain unit (CPU) is a geographically designated area typically within the ED that is operated under guidelines (a clinical pathway) for the emergency evaluation and treatment of patients who complain of chest pain. The design and location of a CPU will vary among hospitals. Most units are adjacent to the ED if space is available. Some hospitals have placed CPUs close to CCUs. An ED with a smaller volume of chest pain patients may treat these patients in a usual ED bed with a special cart of appropriate equipment. No matter where these patients are treated, the area must be designed to expedite administration of acute therapy to the patient with AMI.[6]

Cardiovascular monitors are necessary for all patients. Monitor technicians or continuous human surveillance are not necessary if the monitors are equipped with advanced features like arrhythmia detection alarms and memory, and ST segment trend monitoring. Several sources are available on design of ED CPUs. The American Institute of Architects guidelines on health care

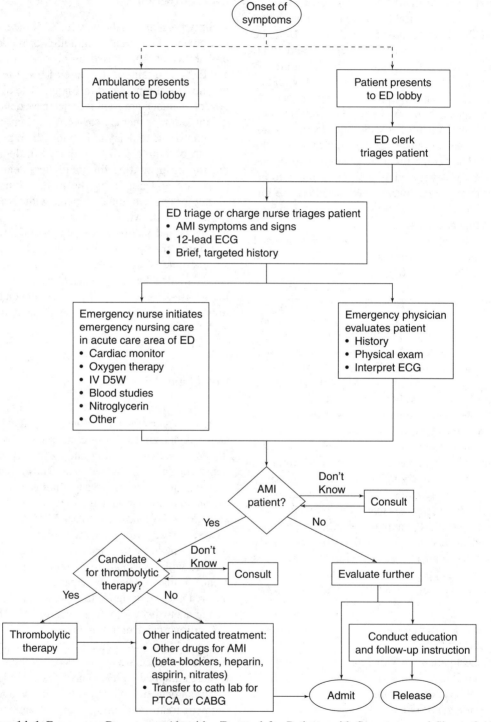

Figure 14-1 Emergency Department Algorithm/Protocol for Patients with Symptoms and Signs of AMI. *Source:* Reprinted from National Heart Attack Alert Program, National Institutes of Health.

facilities include a section describing ED observation units.[12] The American College of Emergency Physicians textbook on ED design has a chapter on the design of ED observation units and a chapter on the design of "Chest Pain EDs."[13] The American College of Emergency Physician Observation Section has published information on the management of ED observation beds.[14]

CPUs must be able to provide services to selected patients over a 9- to 12-hour time period. A single nurse for each patient is not required, but because of the need for continuous surveillance, additional ED staff are necessary if the CPU is adjacent to the ED. Time studies have shown that these patients require about twice the amount of physician time that traditional ED patients require.

Observation Program

Many patients with AMI have an initial clinical presentation that suggests low probability of AMI. The history, physical exam, ECG, and initial serum markers may not suggest an AMI. Despite this clinical presentation atypical of AMI, physicians may be afraid to send the patient home. A report from the Multicenter Chest Pain Study Group of the American College of Emergency Physicians has shown that 50% to 60% of patients who present to the ED with chest pain require extended evaluation if virtually all patients with AMI are to be identified. All patients with atypical chest pain cannot be admitted; therefore, an observation bed is a more feasible site to evaluate the patients with a low probability of AMI. These units are described as a geographically designated area (preferably within or contiguous to the ED) that is operated under guidelines (a clinical pathway) for the ongoing evaluation and treatment of patients who complain of chest pain after their emergency evaluation in the CPU is complete and are found not to have an AMI. These programs minimize unintentional ED release of patients who may be developing an AMI.[6]

Outreach Program

Another component of a CPC approach is an outreach program to minimize delays in seeking medical care. The median delay in seeking medical care is greater than 2 hours.[1] An outreach program serves as a community education tool regarding heart disease and positions the organization within the community as a source of care for those needs. The ultimate goal is to educate and change the community's behavior so that chest pain patients having a heart attack and patients with stuttering chest discomfort symptoms that indicate the potential of a heart attack will seek treatment more quickly.

Multiple initiatives have been implemented in hospitals. Some of these include Early Heart Attack Care community education programs, advertising campaigns, and comprehensive school health programs.[15]

A working group of the NHAAP recently published a paper to assist in the prevention of prehospital delay in patients at high risk for AMI. Patients with previously diagnosed coronary heart disease (CHD), including a previous AMI, have the same or greater delay times as those without prior AMI or CHD. The working group recommended that primary care clinicians in the office and in inpatient settings provide these patients and their family members or significant others contingency counseling about actions to take in response to symptoms of an AMI or acute cardiac ischemia. The content of the recommended educational message includes three components: information, emotional issues, and social factors. A sample form for presenting patient information is presented in Exhibit 14–1. It can be individualized by physicians and others to include instructions for any special medications such as nitrates, aspirin, or other medications that the patient may need; the emergency medical service (EMS) phone number in the community; and the location of the hospital with 24-hour ED service closest to the patient's home and work. Physicians and other health care providers can suggest that patients keep this form on their refrigerators or with their other emergency numbers and that they also keep a copy at work.[16]

Quality Management Program

The structure and function of a chest pain program must be continuously reviewed. This review should be based on continuous quality improvement principles to ensure quality patient care and proper utilization of resources. This improvement process is used to identify problems

---

Exhibit 14–1 Patient Advisory Form

What To Do If You Think You Are Having a Heart Attack

Patient's Name: _____

Physicians now have treatments that can stop heart attacks and lessen damage to the heart. To make sure you can benefit from these treatments, you need to act promptly if you begin to experience symptoms that might signal a heart attack.

1. This is what you may feel:
   - chest pain, discomfort, or pressure
   - left arm pain or discomfort
   - pain radiating to your neck or jaw
   - shortness of breath
   - sweating
   - upset stomach
   - discomfort in the area between your breastbone and navel
   - a sense of dread
   - other: _____

2. Medication instructions:
   - Chew one 325 mg tablet of uncoated adult aspirin.
   - Place one tablet of nitroglycerin under your tongue as soon as you feel discomfort. Take a second tablet if the discomfort does not go away in 5 minutes. Take a third tablet after 5 more minutes if the discomfort does not go away.
   - Other: _____

3. If the symptoms stop, call your physician at _____

4. If symptoms continue for more than 15 minutes, call the emergency medical services phone number below immediately. (Often this is 9-1-1, but you should check to make sure.) Never wait longer than 15 minutes.
   At home, the emergency phone number is _____
   At work, the emergency phone number is _____
   At _____, the emergency phone number is _____

5. Know the location of the nearest 24-hour emergency department.
   At home, the closest emergency department is _____
   At work, the closest emergency department is _____
   At _____, the closest emergency department is _____

Place this form next to the phone near your other emergency numbers!

Signed: _____ MD/RN

Source: Reprinted from National Heart Attack Alert Program, National Institutes of Health.

in patient care, analyze the patient care system, and devise changes in the patient care system to address any problems. The NHAAP recommends examination of the stages through which the AMI patient passes before and during treatment in the ED. These time points and intervals, shown in Figure 14–2, are:

- Time 0: Onset of symptoms
- ED Time 1: Door (arrival at the ED)
- ED Time 2: Data (initial ECG)
- ED Time 3: Decision (to administer thrombolytic treatment, signified by ordering thrombolytic agent)
- ED Time 4: Drug (infusion of thrombolytic agent started)

With each interval, various barriers and impediments to timely care can occur in the ED. Identifying the causes for delays in ED evaluation and treatment, and adopting interventions to minimize these delays, will improve overall care of the heart attack patient. Reducing delay times is applicable to all time points in the ED.[11]

The Myocardial Infarction Project II,[17] a collaborative project in Connecticut, developed a data collection instrument. This instrument was used to collect data on the following:

- patient characteristics (demographics, co-morbidities, Killip class, degree of congestive heart failure in patients with AMI, etc)
- processes of care (usage of thrombolytics, aspirin, beta-blockers, ejection fraction, angiotensin converting enzyme [ACE] inhibitors, calcium channel blockers, percutaneous transluminal coronary angioplasty

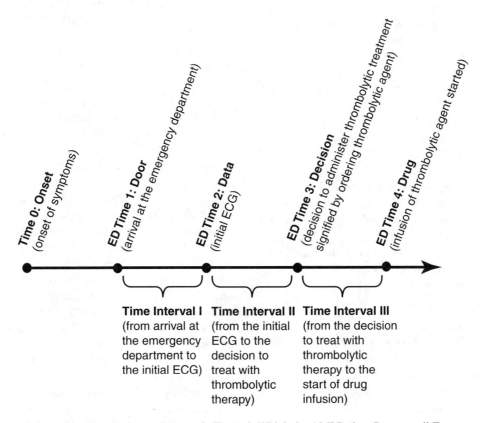

Figure 14–2 Process Time Points and Intervals Through Which the AMI Patient Passes until Treatment in the Emergency Department. *Source:* Reprinted from National Heart Attack Alert Program, National Institutes of Health.

[PTCA], coronary artery bypass graft [CABG], etc)
- outcomes (in-hospital mortality and length of stay)

The Health Care Financing Administration has also begun to perform a nationwide quality assessment of the Medicare population and AMI through the Cooperative Cardiovascular Project.[18] Patient care is being assessed through institutional compliance with 13 indicators judged representative of quality AMI care. The indicators are

1. confirmed diagnosis of AMI
2. in-hospital timing and use of aspirin
3. prescription for aspirin at discharge
4. thrombolytic treatment in patients with ST segment elevation
5. time from arrival to treatment with thrombolytic therapy
6. use of intravenous nitroglycerin for persistent chest pain
7. prescription for beta-blockers at discharge
8. prescription for ACE inhibitors for patients with low left ventricular ejection fraction (LVEF)
9. documented smoking cessation advice
10. administration of low- or full-dose heparin
11. avoidance of calcium channel blockers in patients with low LVEF
12. catheterization or transfer of patient for recurrent angina
13. performance of exercise stress test in patients not undergoing cardiac catheterization

There is a great deal of overlap in the examples of criteria to evaluate AMI care. In fact, there are dozens of other processes that could be examined in the care of patients with chest pain. A focus on critical processes is important and has good prospects of improving patient care. Health care organizations must develop the ability to internally measure their success, or someone else will measure it for them.

CLINICAL AND ECONOMIC BENEFITS OF A CHEST PAIN CENTER APPROACH

Patients who present to the ED with obvious AMI and ST segment elevation should be treated within 30 minutes of hospital arrival because thrombolytic therapy is substantially more effective when given early in the course of treatment. In the Myocardial Infarction Triage and Intervention Trial, mortality was reduced from 8.7% to 1.2% if patients were treated within 70 minutes of chest pain onset.[1]

A CPC approach can provide for more focused evaluation and treatment of patients with suspected AMI. Protocols and pathways are guidelines within which the technical, nursing, and medical staff operate while caring for patients within the CPU or observation area and assist in organizing and streamlining care of the patient. With appropriate guidelines, patients at high risk can be admitted directly to the CCU. Low-risk patients can be evaluated and appropriately released from the ED. Patients at moderate risk can be managed in the CPU or observation unit in the ED or even in a monitored bed in accordance with the predetermined protocol for evaluation. Through using consistent guidelines, patients in this category can be separated into high- and low-risk categories on the basis of cardiac serum markers.

Patients with moderate risk of AMI and nondiagnostic ECG may require about 9 hours of comprehensive evaluation with subsequent provocative stress testing before going home. It's been said that the true value of a CPC may be the reduction in the number of hospital admissions for patients with noncardiac chest pain. Such admissions are estimated to cost $1.5 billion to $3.5 billion annually. The rapid and safe evaluation and release from a CPU for these patients costs 20% to 50% of the typical 1- to 3-day inpatient workup.[19–21]

Gaspoz et al looked at the outcomes of patients who were admitted to a short-stay unit to rule out AMI. Out of 512 consecutive admissions, 425 were discharged home without evidence of AMI or serious complications. The mean length of stay (LOS) was 1 to 2 days with a median LOS of 1 day. Eighty-seven patients, or 17% of all admissions, were transferred to other hospital beds. The rate of AMI was 3%. No deaths occurred and at 6 months, the cardiac survival rate was 99% for patients sent home directly from the observation unit. The cost was half of what CCU care would have cost; the study reported a cost of $415 per day for the observation unit, $1,040 per day for the CCU, and $625 per day for the step-down unit.[20]

In another study, DeLeon and colleagues compared a cardiac profile test with standard creatine kinase and lactate dehydrogenase electrophoresis in 798 cases of possible AMI. In 495 patients, the enzyme screen was suggestive of AMI but without diagnostic ECG changes. Instead of being placed in the CCU, the patients were kept in an observation unit for up to 20 hours, with an average of 11.1 hours. Using the profile, 327 patients were able to go home, and 168 patients were admitted. Only 30 (18%) of these admitted patients had subsequent enzyme evidence of myocardial necrosis. Use of this unit resulted in an 80% reduction in the cost of ruling out AMI for the 327 patients not admitted. The average cost of patients seen in the CPU and sent home with a diagnosis of noncardiac chest pain was $598 after an average LOS of 11.1 hours. Patients previously admitted to the CCU to have AMI ruled out, then discharged with a diagnosis of noncardiac chest pain, spent an average of 3 days in the hospital at an average cost of $3,103.[21]

Roberts et al compared the costs of hospitalizing patients to those of treating patients in an ED-based accelerated diagnostic protocol and observation unit. The mean costs and LOS of all patients randomized to the observation unit, including those subsequently hospitalized, were lower than mean costs and LOS for those randomized to the hospital. They concluded that the observation unit patients cost $1,528, compared with $2,095 for the admitted patients. Use of the observation unit saved $567 in total hospital costs per patient treated, and no deaths or complications occurred among these patients. Observation unit patients spent fewer hours in the hospital, 33.1 versus 44.8, and the hospital gained in efficiency because it did not have to admit and discharge the patients.[22]

The Rapidly Ruling Out Myocardial Ischemia (ROMIO) study concluded that a rapid protocol in an observation unit was more cost-effective than routine hospital care. The average LOS was 12 hours in the observation unit as compared with 24 in the hospital. The initial cost was $893 for the ED and $1,349 for the hospital, and 30-day charges were $898 for the ED and $1,522 for the hospital. No diagnoses were missed.[23]

According to the Cardiology Preeminence Roundtable, data from case study hospitals reveal that ED-based rule-out programs under the current reimbursement system generate a per case profit equal to that resulting from a one-day inpatient rule-out. The economic advantage of observation unit rule-out programs is important in the light of the future of reimbursement. The financial survival of providers will be contingent on aggressive cost reduction without compromise in quality.[24]

The Roundtable found that ED-based rule-out programs cost about $500 less per patient than those for inpatient rule outs. A 300- to 400-bed hospital could see annual variable cost savings of about $200,000 from the combination of 30% fewer chest pain admissions yielded by ED-based rule-out programs and a $500 variable cost savings per case. If the hospital has prepaid reimbursement, then a direct profit is realized. This mechanism also gives hospitals the ability to enable 50% more patients to be definitively diagnosed while still achieving a lower net cost.[24]

A CPU also reduces patient anxiety and stress and provides an opportunity for trained personnel to educate patients about behavior and lifestyle modifications. A significant number of patients admitted to CCUs and found not to have an AMI have been shown to have a higher incidence of subsequent cardiovascular events. While patients are awaiting enzyme results, education can be initiated.[15]

CHEST PAIN CENTER DEVELOPMENT

Many factors should be considered when developing a CPC.

1. Get the right players involved. Appropriate team members are critical to the success of CPC development. These members should include an emergency physician and nurse, a cardiologist, a hospital administrator, and laboratory and cardiology department leaders.
2. A physician champion is critical.
3. A vision is necessary. If the purpose is for marketing alone, the program will eventually fail. Successful programs are the result of clinical expertise and efficiency.
4. Baseline data must be collected, including
   - number of chest pain patients presenting to the ED and number admitted
   - number of AMI and rule-out AMIs discharged
   - LOS for rule-out patients
   - cost per visit to the ED for chest pain patients
   - cost per admission of rule-out AMI and AMI
   - time to treatment (door, data, decision, drug)
   - availability of beds (ED, CCU, step-down, telemetry)
5. Benchmark data should be considered when the data are appropriate and available.
6. Space and facilities should be evaluated.
7. Protocols and pathways should be reviewed to make sure they are current. If there are no protocols or pathways, develop them.
8. Review current reimbursement per visit and per admission for rule-out AMIs. Does admission of rule-out AMI patients remain economically attractive?
9. Study the managed care market. With managed care and provider reimbursement decreasing, economic viability of providers is directly contingent upon appropriate utilization and minimization of incurred costs. With the emerging payment mechanisms, inpatient admissions, additional tests, daily bedside visits, and prolonged LOS contribute to financial liabilities for "at-risk" providers. As aggressive managed care and capitation spread to provider markets, innovations in clinical systems and practice that reduce total costs and maintain or improve quality will become highly valued assets central to financial viability.
10. Commitment to developing the unit once the decision is made requires administrative support and resources.
11. A mechanism for continued quality improvement must be in place.

Predictions

Looking toward the next decade, several predictions can be made about the future of managing chest pain.

- There will be improved strategies for administration of thrombolytic agents and new and better agents. A new thrombolytic, Reteplase, is the only thrombolytic approved by the Food and Drug Administration that can be administered in a simple double-bolus dose. This new drug requires less than 1 hour for delivery and is easier to administer during an AMI emergency situation. The faster thrombolytics can be administered, the less damage to the heart muscle, which results in reduced costs, fewer hospital days, fewer recurrent problems, and reduced mortality rate because of decreased tissue damage to the heart.[25]
- Protocols and pathways will be developed that break down the rule-out population into at least four categories.
  - discharge to home
  - brief 3- to 6-hour rule outs
  - 12-hour rule outs
  - 24-hour rule outs[26–28]
- There will be increased use of more specific and prognostically helpful assays such as

creatine kinase-MB (CK-MB) subforms and troponins I and T. CK-MB subforms have been shown in recent trials to reflect AMI earlier than CK-MB does, and, therefore, may be useful for identifying patients who should receive thrombolytic therapy. It is not known yet whether serial myoglobin results can provide similar information.
- Troponins I and T are believed to be specific to the heart and could be used to exclude AMI in patients with ambiguous CK-MB data. They appear to rise to abnormal levels in patients with myocardial ischemia but not infarction by CK-MB standards. Troponins may be used for risk stratification of the population of patients that rules out for AMI.[26,27]
- There will be CPCs in urgent care facilities. With the increased focus on rapid identification and treatment of AMI, urgent care centers have begun to establish protocols for management of these patients. The establishment of full centers will be a future strategy for quality and marketing.

As mentioned earlier, the increasing demand for data (clinical and financial) by external entities and the increasing prevalence of managed care and prepaid reimbursement systems will continue to influence the establishment of comprehensive CPCs.

CONCLUSION

As described in this chapter, a CPC is a cost-effective approach to provide care to patients experiencing chest pain. A center assists in recognizing and accommodating an ED physician's reluctance to discharge a patient with suggestive but nondiagnostic chest pain, reduces the patient's anxiety and stress, and provides an opportunity for staff to educate patients about behavior and lifestyle modifications. The care of patients experiencing an AMI is changing rapidly. Consumers will continue to expect new therapies, technologies, and a better understanding of their health problems. This care will continue to be provided in hospitals as well as other settings. Wherever the location, a comprehensive CPC can provide a systematic method of care.

REFERENCES

1. Weaver MD, Cerquerira M, Halstrom AP, et al. Prehospital-initiated vs. hospital-initiated thrombolytic therapy: the myocardial infarction triage and intervention trial. *JAMA*. 1993;270;1211–1216.
2. Dracup K, Moser DK, Eisenberg M, et al. Causes of delay in seeking treatment for heart attack symptoms. *Soc Sci Med*. 1995;40:379–392.
3. Karcz A, Holbrook J, Burks MC, et al. Massachusetts emergency medicine closed malpractice claims: 1988–1990. *Ann Emerg Med*. 1993;22:553–559.
4. Barish RA, Doherty RJ. Establishing a chest pain center in an academic medical center: The University of Maryland Experience. *Clinician*. 1995;13:39–43.
5. American Health Consultants. Timing is all: therapy within 30 minutes ideal. *Cost Manage Cardiac Care*. 1997;2:100–103.
6. Graff L, Joseph T, Andelman R, et al. American College of Emergency Physicians information paper: chest pain units in emergency departments—a report from the short-term observation services section. *Am J Cardiol*. 1995;76:1036–1039.
7. Bahr R. Introduction: the shifting paradigm to earlier heart attack care. *Clinician*. 1995;13:4–6.
8. Bahr R. Concept of community chest pain centers in emergency departments. *Clinician*. 1996;14:5–6.
9. Zalenski R. National Survey of Chest Pain Centers: rationale and potential results. *Clinician*. 1996;14:21.
10. National Congress of Chest Pain Centers. New data build the case for chest pain centers. *Cardiovasc Dis Manage*. 1996;2:2.
11. National Heart Attack Alert Program Coordinating Committee, 60 Minutes to Treatment Working Group. Emergency department: rapid identification and treatment of patients with acute myocardial infarction. *Ann Emerg Med*. 1994;23:311–329.
12. American Institute of Architects Committee on Architecture for Health. *1992–1993 Guidelines for Construction and Equipment of Hospitals and Medical Facilities*. Washington, DC: American Institute of Architects Press; 1993.
13. Riggs L Jr, ed. *Emergency Department Design*. Dallas, TX: American College of Emergency Physicians; 1993.

14. Brillman J, Mathers-Dunbar L, Graff L, et al. for the Short-Term Observation Services Section of the American College of Emergency Physicians. Management of observation units. *Ann Emerg Med.* 1995;25:823–830.
15. Bahr R. Wiping out heart disease before the year 2000: an obtainable goal, a prediction for the future. *J Cardiovasc Manage.* May/June 1993:77–80.
16. National Heart Attack Alert Program. *Educational Strategies To Prevent Prehospital Delay in Patients at High Risk for Acute Myocardial Infarction.* NIH publication no. 97-3787. Bethesda, MD: National Institutes of Health, National Heart, Lung and Blood Institute; 1997.
17. Meehan TP, Radford MJ, Vaccarino LV, et al. A collaborative project in Connecticut to improve the care of patients with acute myocardial infarction. *J Qual Improvement.* 1996;22:751–761.
18. Vogel RA. A nationwide quality assessment of acute myocardial infarction through the Cooperative Cardiovascular Project. *Clinician.* 1995;13:52–55.
19. Hoekstra JW, Gibler WB, Levy RC, et al. Emergency department diagnosis of acute myocardial infarction and ischemia: a cost analysis. *Acad Emerg Med.* 1994; 1:103–110.
20. Gaspoz JM, Lee TH, Cook EF, et al. Outcome of patients who were admitted to a new short-stay unit to "rule out" myocardial infarction. *Am J Cardiol.* 1991; 68:145–149.
21. DeLeon AC, Farmer CA, King G, et al. Chest pain evaluation unit: a cost-effective approach for ruling out acute myocardial infarction. *South Med J.* 1989;82: 1083–1089.
22. Roberts RR, Zalenski RJ, Mensah EK, et al. Costs of an emergency department-based accelerated diagnostic protocol vs. hospitalization in patients with chest pain. *JAMA.* 1997;278(1):671–676.
23. Gomez MA, Anderson JL, Karagouniet LA, et al. An emergency department-based protocol for rapidly ruling out myocardial ischemia reduces hospital time and expense (ROMIO). *J Am Coll Cardiol.* 1996;28:25–28.
24. Cardiology Preeminence Roundtable. *Perfecting MI Rule Out: Best Practices for Emergency Evaluation of Chest Pain.* Washington, DC: The Advisory Board Co; 1994.
25. Bode C, Smalling RW, Berg G, et al. Randomized comparison of coronary thrombolysis achieved with double-bolus reteplase and front-loaded, accelerated alteplase in patients with acute myocardial infarction: the RAPID II (reteplase and alteplase patency investigation during myocardial infarction). *Circ.* 1996;94: 891–898.
26. Lee TH. Coronary care, year 2000: historic trends and future directions. *Clinician.* 1995;13:30–33.
27. Hamm CW, Ravkilde J, Gerhardt W, et al. The prognostic value of serum troponin T in unstable angina. *N Engl J Med.* 1992;327:146–150.
28. Adams JE, Bodor GS, Davila-Romain BG, et al. Cardiac troponin I: a marker with high specificity for cardiac injury. *Circ.* 1993;88:101–106.

SUZANNE K. WHITE, MN, RN, FAAN, FCCM, CNAA, is senior vice president, patient services, and chief nursing officer at Saint Thomas Health Services in Nashville, Tennessee. She received her BSN from Barry University in Miami, Florida, and a Master's in nursing from Emory University in Atlanta, Georgia. Her prior experience includes executive positions at Saint Joseph's Health System in Atlanta, Emory University Hospital, and Duke University Medical Center. Prior to joining Saint Thomas, Ms. White was a senior manager in health care consulting with Ernst & Young LLP.

PART VI

Acute Inpatient Care

Acute inpatient care was once the primary focus of managed care (when managed care was called an alternative delivery system). It indeed remains so, but is now complemented by all of the other approaches discussed in this book. Although inpatient utilization has fallen to low levels in the 1990s, acute inpatient costs remain high. Inpatient cases have a higher degree of acuity, they are more procedure centered, and, perhaps most important, significant advances have been made in acute care, accompanied by higher costs. Thus, acute inpatient care remains highly important to any form of managed health care.

Part VI begins with a chapter that reviews basic medical/surgical acute inpatient care. This is the basic blocking and tackling of managed care, and the basics must be done well for the other forms of medical management to be optimized. The remaining three chapters in this part each discuss a particularly powerful approach to adding to these basics.

Chapter 15

Managing Basic Medical-Surgical Utilization

Peter R. Kongstvedt

Chapter Outline

- Introduction
- Administrative Costs Versus Medical Costs
- Demand Management
- Specialty Physician Utilization Management
- Institutional Utilization Management
- Conclusion

INTRODUCTION

There are many facets to the management of utilization, and this book examines them. As managed care has become more prevalent, the divisions between the management of specialty physician care, inpatient care, outpatient care, case and disease management, and indeed all aspects of health care delivery have blurred. However, there remains a core set of activities that may be considered fundamental to managing utilization of medical and surgical services. This chapter provides an overview of that core set. In doing so, the chapter covers information presented in greater detail in other chapters, underscoring the close relationships among many aspects of medical services management.

ADMINISTRATIVE COSTS VERSUS MEDICAL COSTS

Experienced health maintenance organization (HMO) managers know well that investment in utilization management (UM) is well leveraged in the classic sense of the word *leverage*. In other words, there is a high rate of return for money spent in this activity—it results in lower health care costs. The degree of leverage in the past has been high (ie, costs for medical management have resulted in savings that far exceeded those costs). It is now more difficult to measure that economic return, because there are very few surviving models of *un*managed care left. It is challenging to separate the management activities and assign each one an economic value. Therefore, it is hard to know which medical management activities provide the greatest return on a plan-to-plan basis. As is pointed out in several chapters in this book, the return is generally positive, and the reader can only speculate on what costs would be if management were no longer present. It is, however, a fair statement that the cost invested in medical management is more than paid for in lowered medical costs.

This chapter is adapted from PR Kongstvedt, Managing Basic Medical-Surgical Utilization, in *The Managed Health Care Handbook*, 3rd ed, PR Kongstvedt, ed, pp 249–273, © 1996, Aspen Publishers, Inc.

DEMAND MANAGEMENT

Demand management refers to activities of a health plan designed to reduce the overall requirement for health care services by members. In addition to helping to lower health care costs, these services may also provide a competitive advantage to a plan by enhancing its reputation for service and by giving members additional value for their premium dollar. Demand management services fall into five broad categories, which are briefly discussed below to place them in context to basic medical-surgical UM functions. For an in-depth discussion of self-help and nurse advice line services, see Part IV.

Nurse Advice Lines

Nurse advice lines provide members with access to advice regarding medical conditions; the need for medical care, health promotion, and preventive care; and numerous other advice-related activities. Such advice lines have been in use in closed panel HMOs for many years, where they are occasionally referred to as "triage" nurse lines. (The term "triage nurse" is not recommended because of its military connotations. Triage is a term used in battlefield medicine that refers to the separation of casualties into three categories: immediate attention required, attention can be delayed, and casualty is beyond hope and will be given only palliative care.) Plans may staff these lines with their own nurses or may purchase the service from a number of companies. Hours of operation are almost always extended; 24-hour service may even be provided (especially if a plan uses a commercial service). A geographically large plan or a commercial service is likely to use a toll-free line to make it easier for members to access the service.

Special market segments such as Medicare and Medicaid populations may benefit from dedicated programs. Attention to the special problems and concerns of seniors will go a long way to improving health status and can be a major contributor to the overall management of care in this population. Easy access to medical advice in the Medicaid population may allow these members to avoid a trip to the emergency department.

A fever health education program at Kaiser decreased pediatric clinic utilization by 35% for fever visits and 25% for all acute visits.[1] In another study, the combination of a 24-hour nurse advice service and a self-care program (see below) resulted in a savings of $4.75 per dollar invested, while the self-care program alone resulted in a savings of $2.40 per dollar invested.[2]

Self-Care and Medical Consumerism Programs

Self-care and medical consumerism programs provide information to members to allow them to care for themselves or to better evaluate when they need to seek care from a professional. Member newsletters with medical advice are used extensively by HMOs. The most common example of a more proactive approach is a self-care guide provided by the plan. These books are generally written in an easy-to-understand manner and provide step-by-step advice for common medical conditions, as well as preventive care. Information about the wise use of medical services, or how to be an informed consumer, would also fall into this category. Self-care programs have been evaluated since the early 1980s, with typical results around $2.50 to $3.50 saved for every dollar invested.[3] In one structured study in a staff-model HMO, the targeted use of such self-care manuals resulted in decreased outpatient visits and a 2-to-1 return on the cost of the program.[4] Other studies have reported savings of $2.40 to $2.77 per dollar invested.[2]

Shared Decision-Making Programs

Shared decision-making programs encourage the member to be an active participant in choosing a course of care. While this general cooperative philosophy may be prevalent in the routine interactions between patients and physicians, shared decision-making programs are more focused, providing highly detailed information to patients regarding specific procedures. By providing this information, the programs give patients a deeper understanding not only of the disease process, but of the treatment alternatives. Some HMOs that use these programs will not finalize authorization for certain elective procedures—transurethral resection of the prostate, for example—until the member has completed the shared decision-making program.

A number of commercial services have appeared in the past few years to produce these programs. Many use interactive CD-ROM, videotape, and computer programs to provide the information. Supplemental access to a nurse advice line, as well as the ability to discuss the alternatives with the physician after the patient has reviewed the material, is also routine.

Medical Informatics

Medical informatics is a very broad term that applies to the use of information technology in the management of health care delivery. The broader topics surrounding the use of data in medical management are discussed in Chapter 37. For purposes of this chapter, medical informatics refers to the use of information technology in helping to manage demand for services. There are two broad categories to be mentioned: the use of informatics by the member, and the use of informatics by the plan.

Use of informatics by the member might include accessing an on-line service, such as one that provides health-related information to members. Business-related information may also be available, as well as electronic mail and communications with the plan. The plan may do this through a dedicated direct dial-in service, or it may do so through a more public arena; several plans have developed Web sites on the Internet. Many plans have placed kiosks in easily accessible locations. These locations might include a large employer's place of business, the lobby of the health plan, a large medical facility, or a public area such as a shopping mall. The kiosk provides information regarding prevention and certain common medical conditions. It may also provide access to business information such as the types of benefits available.

The Internet has also become a source of this type of information. While in some cases this information is provided by the plan, far more numerous are Internet sites that provide health-related information that is neither regulated nor monitored for quality. The constitutional right to free speech allows for the publication of misinformation, even potentially dangerous misinformation. Therefore, medical managers may want to become familiar with and inform plan members about high-quality Web sites (along with a note explaining that advice can vary from one source to another and still be of good quality).

The plan may use information systems to anticipate demand for services, or to analyze how demand for services can be better managed. For example, an analysis of the use of urgent care or emergency services may be related to hours of operation, location of primary care, work patterns at a large employer, and so forth. By looking for patterns, the plan may be able to develop strategies for lowering demand for one type of service by substituting another type of service.

Preventive Services and Health Risk Appraisals

Preventive services, a hallmark of the HMO industry, are discussed in detail in Parts II and III. Common preventive services include immunizations, mammograms, routine physical exams and health assessments, and counseling regarding behaviors that members can change to lower their risk of ill health (smoking cessation, dietary counseling, stress reduction, and so forth). Counseling and education may also be applied to specific clinical conditions; for example, in one study of a managed indemnity plan, an employer held prenatal education programs at its work site and found that participants in the educational programs had an average cost per delivery that was $3,200 less than the cost for nonparticipants.[5]

The health risk appraisal is a tool designed to elicit information from a member regarding certain activities and behaviors that can influence health status. These appraisals obtain information about behaviors that are generally known to be harmful or that indicate a predisposition for a serious illness. This information is used by the plan and is provided to the member's primary care physician (PCP), who will then be in a better position to counsel the member.

In plans that have a large Medicare enrollment, the plan may take extra steps in performing an initial assessment. The most common of these extra activities is an in-home assessment of the new Medicare member. A trained nurse or medical social worker may determine, for example, that if the plan gives the new Medicare enrollee a bathmat or shower chair, it will significantly reduce the risk of a hip fracture from falling in the bathtub. An inventory of the member's diet may also yield valuable information that will enable the new member's provider to improve health status by lowering sodium intake or lowering saturated fats in the diet.

SPECIALTY PHYSICIAN UTILIZATION MANAGEMENT

Management of medical services requiring authorization is discussed in detail in Chapters 20 and 21. This chapter offers a subset of that discussion. Therefore, the reader needs to review all three chapters to gain a reasonably broad understanding of this category of medical management.

Managing the utilization of referral physicians and consultants (both physicians and nonphysicians) is an area of great importance. In most managed health care plans, the costs associated with non–primary care professional services will be substantially greater than the costs of primary care services—often between 1.5 and 2.0 times as high. This is due to the increased fees associated with consultant services and the hospital-intensive nature of those services; in other words, more than half the costs of consultant services may be associated with hospital cases.

Often overlooked are the associated utilization costs generated by consultants. It is not only the fees of the consultants themselves that add to the cost of care but also the cost of services ordered by consultants, such as diagnostic studies, facility charges for procedures, and so forth. One 1987 study in a non–managed care environment found that each referral from a PCP generated nearly $3,000 in combined hospital charges and professional fees within a 6-month period after the referral.[6] It may be safely assumed that the value of a referral has increased considerably since 1987. These costs are not routinely added to the cost of consultant services when data are compiled, but control of consultant services will often lead to control of these outside services as well.

Definitions

The definition of referral or consultant services includes physicians' fees that are not considered primary care, in other words, all physicians' fees that are not from general internists, family physicians, and general pediatricians. If you have chosen to include obstetrics and gynecology (OB/GYN) as primary care, then you will need to decide which of the services provided by OB/GYN (eg, surgery, routine Pap smears and pelvic examinations, colposcopy, and so forth) are included as primary care and which are consultant care.

In general, most managed care plans count consultant physicians and nonphysician professionals (eg, psychologists) in the consultant cost category, and ancillary services (eg, laboratory, radiology, pharmacy, and the like) are dealt with separately. In keeping with that division, control of ancillary and pharmaceutical services utilization is addressed separately in Part IX.

Data

To manage consultant services, you must first be able to capture utilization and cost data in an accurate and timely manner. If you do not have that ability, your efforts to control utilization in this category will be severely hampered. The issue of data capture and reporting is discussed further in Chapter 37. There is no standard for reporting data on referral utilization as there is for reporting data on hospital utilization. Nevertheless, certain measures are used frequently, and managers find them helpful.

In HMOs that do not have any benefits for services provided without an authorization from a PCP, a useful measure is referrals per 100 encounters per PCP. In this measure, one counts the total number of referrals made by a PCP for every 100 primary care encounters. This correlates to a referral percentage. For example, 11 referrals per 100 encounters per PCP equals a referral rate of 11%. More commonly used is the referral rate per 1,000 members per year. Like the measurement of hospitalization rate, this looks at an annualized referral rate for every 1,000 members. Although this is less directly related to a PCP encounter than referrals per 100 primary care encounters, the nomenclature is standard across many types of plans.

It is important to know whether you are counting initial referrals or total visits to a referral consultant. In other words, if you are counting only the initial referral or authorization, you may be missing a large portion of the actual utilization. It is not uncommon, especially in loosely controlled systems, for a single referral to generate multiple visits to a consultant. For example, if a PCP refers a member with the request to evaluate and treat, this is carte blanche for the consultant to take over the care of the patient, and succeeding visits will be to the consultant and not to the PCP.

It is therefore far more useful to track actual visits. Better yet is to track both initial referrals and actual visits, because that will give you a clearer idea of how the consultants are handling the cases. In a tightly controlled system, such as an HMO with a strict policy granting authorization for one visit only for any referral, the numbers may be almost the same. In a system with loose controls, the number of actual visits may be two to three times greater than the initial referral rate. Specialty visit rates in commercial HMOs averages 1.2 encounters per member per year (PMPY), with a range of 0.8 to 1.3 encounters PMPY; visits to medical specialists were slightly higher than for surgical specialists.[7] Figure 15–1 illustrates specialty visit rates in HMOs.

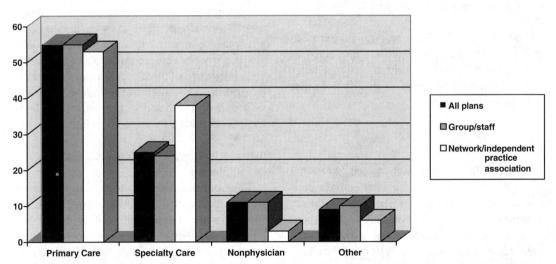

Figure 15–1 Specialty Physician Visit Rates in HMOs (as a Percent of Total Ambulatory Encounters). *Source:* American Association of Health Plans (formerly GHAA/AMCRA), 1992 Utilization Data Supplement to the Eighth Annual HMO Industry Survey (Washington, DC).

Selection of Referral and Consulting Providers

The ability to select providers on the basis of a demonstrated pattern of practice can have a considerable impact on referral expenses. There are large differences in the efficiency of practice among providers within each specialty, and if patients are preferentially sent to those consultants and referral specialists who demonstrate cost-effective practice, the plan can achieve considerable savings.

This is especially important in plans that allow self-referral to consultants by members, such as preferred provider organizations, point-of-service (POS) plans, and "open access HMOs." If you have a loose system that allows open access to any consultant at any time other than through selection of providers, you can exert little control except perhaps by making fee adjustments after enough documentation of overutilization. The problem with using fee adjustments to control utilization (ie, lowering a consultant's, or the entire provider panel's, fees as utilization goes up) is that it can lead to an "I'd better get mine first" mentality. In that situation, providers may begin churning visits and increasing utilization to increase revenues, worried that next month the fees may drop even farther.

The ability to evaluate referral practice behavior is no easy task; evaluations must consider a long period of time and a significant number of events. Please see Chapters 38 and 39 for further discussion on this topic.

Authorization System

Without an authorization system, there is a markedly diminished chance of effectively controlling referral utilization. Through education, you may be able to decrease consultant utilization somewhat, but unless there is a primary care gatekeeper or case manager system in place, it is not likely that you will achieve optimal results. If you have been able to carefully select consultants through practice pattern analysis, you may get improvement in referral expenses, but not to the same degree that a PCP authorization system will allow.

The corollary to this is the possibility that a PCP can deliver many of the same services as a consultant, but at considerable savings and in a more appropriate setting. Even in non–managed care systems, PCPs manage a substantial proportion of their patients' care.[8] Therefore, the reason for using a PCP authorization system to manage consultant costs is twofold: to reduce consultant utilization through services delivered by the PCP and to manage those referrals that are made.

The remainder of this chapter will assume that there is some type of authorization system in place. That system can be rigid or loose. Further discussion of medical services requiring authorization, and authorization systems themselves, is found in Chapter 20.

Methods To Achieve Tight Control of Specialty Physician Services

Single Visit Authorizations Only

An authorization system that allows only one visit per authorization is one that provides optimal control, even if it is not ultimately the type of system a plan chooses to use (as noted below as well as in Chapter 20). In essence, every time a member is referred to a consultant, the PCP gatekeepers (or care coordinators, or whatever you choose to call them) must issue a unique authorization. That authorization is good for one visit and will be used to pay only one claim. Claims submitted by the consultant with multiple charges will be compared to what was authorized, and only the authorized services will be reimbursed.

This sounds strong in theory, and it is strong. Unfortunately, it is sometimes difficult to enforce and may not always be desirable from a member relations standpoint. A mechanism for review of claims that do not exactly match the authorization must be put in place to avoid penalizing members and consultants if the PCP fails to document the authorization correctly. It is also sometimes difficult in practice to pull out overcharges or add-ons to a claim, particularly when the claims adjudicators get overworked. Nonetheless, this system is both workable and necessary for optimal control.

It is vital to inform people—through full and fair disclosure—of such a system before they enroll in your plan. The usual methods of informing members include enrollment literature, new member kits, the identification card issued by your plan, the evidence of coverage certificate that you issue to a member, the referral form itself, the plan newsletter, and even signs in your consultants' offices. Consultants will usually agree to allow signs in their offices when they understand that improving compliance with authorization procedures will enhance their revenue both by speeding up claims processing and by decreasing their bad debt load.

After you have informed members, you must periodically reinform them. Most people will not remember everything they hear, even after hearing it multiple times. There will always be some who deny ever knowing about the need for authorization, but you can only do the best you can.

There are common exceptions to the rule of one authorization per visit. These include chemotherapy and radiation therapy for cancer, obstetrics, mental health and chemical dependency therapy, physical therapy, and rehabilitation therapy. Other plans may choose additional exceptions. For example, they may automatically allow one or two home health visits after short-stay obstetrics.

Even for these exceptions, however, plans should not have open-ended authorizations. There should be an absolute limit on the number of visits that can be authorized at once. For example, plans may wish to limit initial mental health referrals to two or three visits and then require the therapist to discuss the case with the PCP or mental health case manager before any further authorizations are allowed (see Chapter 32). Physical therapy should likewise be limited to an initial number of visits, and then the therapist must discuss the case with the PCP before any further authorizations are issued. For chemotherapy cases, the oncologist should discuss the case with the PCP and outline the exact course of treatment, which could then be authorized all at once. The overriding principle is that open-ended authorizations are simply blank checks. Plans that allow them will pay the price.

Prohibition of Secondary Referrals and Authorizations

Another facet of controlling referral utilization is the prohibition of secondary referrals by consultants. This means that a consultant cannot authorize anything for a member. In other words, if a consultant feels that a patient needs to see another consultant, that must be communicated back to the PCP, who is the only one able to issue an authorization for services.

This extends to subsequent visits to the consultant and to testing and procedures as well. For example, if a consultant has an expensive piece of diagnostic equipment in the office, there may be a subtle pressure to use it to make it pay for itself. One widely noted study looking at physician ownership of radiology equipment documented a fourfold increase in imaging examinations as well as significant increases in charges among physicians who used their own equipment compared to physicians who referred such studies to radiologists.[9] Similar results have been reported for laboratory services[10] and a wide variety of ancillary services.[11]

The issue of physician-owned diagnostic and therapeutic equipment or services, a difficult one to address, is receiving increasing attention in government regulations, at least for Medicare.[12] Perhaps the best method for dealing with this issue is simply to prohibit or markedly restrict the use of such services. Most managed care plans contract with a limited number of vendors for such ancillary services and may limit referral to only those vendors. Ancillary services are discussed in Chapter 25.

Even in the absence of these pressures, secondary referrals may simply be unnecessary. For example, an endocrinologist may be concerned about a referred patient's chest pain and may refer the patient to a cardiologist when in fact the patient's PCP had worked up the problem and was tracking it carefully. This happens more often than one might think because patients may not always communicate or even understand what previous care they have received, and the PCP may not have considered it necessary to put that information into the referral letter or form.

Last, the prohibition on secondary authorizations extends to procedures, including hospitalizations. A consultant must obtain the authorization from the PCP or the plan (depending on the plan's policy about precertification) before any procedures (eg, colonoscopy) or admission to the hospital. This is not to be punitive but to ensure that such decisions are handled in the most cost-effective manner. For example, a referral surgeon may not be aware of the preadmission testing program, may use a noncontracting hospital, or may be used to admitting the patient the day before surgery simply as a convenience (though this practice is pretty rare these days). When authorization is required, such problems can be detected and dealt with easily.

Review of Reasons for Referral

It is the responsibility of the medical director to review the reasons for referral by the PCPs. In the tightest of all systems, this review takes place before the referral is made. In other words, the medical director or associate medical director (or in some instances a utilization committee) must approve any authorization prospectively. This system is obviously cumbersome and may be seen as demeaning to the PCPs, but it is definitely tight, even if prohibitively expensive. It is perhaps best suited to a tightly controlled closed panel or a training program where interns and residents are involved.

More acceptable is retrospective review of referrals. In this case, the medical director, associate medical director, or UM committee reviews referral forms after the fact, although preferably not long after. Reviews may be of all referrals, which potentially achieves tight control but is unrealistic, or of randomly selected referrals, which will be less tight but still quite useful.

More useful is to evaluate PCP referral rates and patterns as well as utilization patterns of referral physicians to determine where retrospective review will have the greatest potential.

The preferred vehicle for review is the referral form (or authorization form), which contains the reasons for referral. If the referral form does not contain clinical information, or if referral authorizations are captured electronically, then periodic chart review, similar to a quality assurance audit, needs to be used.

In this review, the medical director is looking at reasons for referral that are inappropriate or poorly thought out. It is surprising how often one encounters reasons for referral such as "Please evaluate and treat." This is potentially a blank check. Another commonly encountered referral is one in which the patient's complaints are simply echoed (eg, "Patient complains of pain in foot"). In these cases, one is not sure what the referring physician is thinking.

A referral should be made after adequate thought and actions have already been taken. The referring PCP should indicate why the patient is being referred, what the PCP thinks the diagnosis is or what he or she is concerned about, what has already been done, and what exactly the PCP wants the consultant to do. By failing to indicate the results of their own work-up or significant findings on the patient's history and physical examination, PCPs make themselves look lazy and make the job of the consultant that much less efficient.

When the medical director encounters sloppy reasons for referral, he or she need not reprimand or embarrass the PCP. It is more appropriate to discuss the case clinically, suggesting options that the PCP may have tried before referring or ways in which the referral could have been more effective. The goal of these discussions is to foster that type of internal questioning behavior in the PCP so that the medical director will not have to do it. You want each PCP to consider all the options before making a referral and to make referrals count. This often means breaking old habits, but then that is what medical management is about.

Large Case Management by Specialty Physicians

Even in HMO or POS plans, there may be times when the plan may wish to have a referral specialist function as a PCP. This would occur when a member has a chronic and high-cost problem that is clearly outside the scope of a PCP's training and practice. In those events, the plan's large case management (LCM) or disease management function becomes proactive in managing the case (see Chapter 17 and Part X). As part of the case management, a standard PCP may no longer be responsible for the patient's care; instead, a specialist may function as the PCP for that case only. For example, a member with active and aggressive acquired immune deficiency syndrome (AIDS) may be better cared for by an infectious disease specialist rather than a PCP. Although that assumption may not hold in every case, this alternative will sometimes be preferable to forcing a PCP to manage catastrophic cases.

Self-Referrals by Members

Members referring themselves to consultants for care is a chronic problem in managed care plans with authorization systems. In POS plans that have benefits for self-referral, as well as open access HMOs, plan design allows self-referral. But in a traditional HMO or POS plan, new members who are not used to the system and signed up because of the benefits offered may not recall or note the requirements for authorization and are more apt to self-refer and later be surprised that there is reduced or no coverage for the service. This is a particularly common problem for new Medicare enrollees.

In these situations, plans need to consider their policy on first offenders. Many HMOs will pay for the first self-referral if it is a new member, if the plan recently changed to an authorization system, or if plan managers want to be nice. In such cases the plan documents a warning so that benefits for self-referral may be denied on subsequent occurrences. Most POS plans do not cover any self-referrals at the higher level of benefits, but some will remind the member via their explanation of benefits statement that the benefits would have been higher if the member had obtained authorization.

Compensation and Financial Incentives for Specialty Physicians

Financial arrangements are not the topic of this book, so only two pertinent issues are raised at this time. Capitation is a powerful and effective tool for controlling consultant utilization but can be a trap if not used wisely. (Readers who are unfamiliar with capitation are urged to review the topic in *The Managed Health Care Handbook,* 3rd Edition, before using capitation.) Simple capitation arrangements without proper controls on utilization, such as an authorization system and review of reasons for referral, can lead to serious overutilization unless the referral physician is able to exert strong controls on utilization without managerial controls.

Financial incentives or risk/bonus arrangements for PCPs and contracting consultants can be quite useful, especially incentives for PCPs. These incentives are not an attempt to bribe physicians but to share the savings of cost-effective practice. Incentives should not be so great as to raise the danger of inappropriate underutilization but should be enough to have an effect.

INSTITUTIONAL UTILIZATION MANAGEMENT

Utilization of hospital (or, more accurately, institutional) services usually accounts for up to 40% or more of the total expenses in a managed health care plan. That amount can be even greater when utilization is excessive. Control of these expenses is therefore prominent among most managers' priorities.

The expense of any medical service is a product of the price of that service times the volume of services delivered. Pricing for institutional services is beyond the scope of this book; this chapter focuses on managing the volume of institutional services. Simple reduction of bed days may be of value but can lull the inexperienced manager into a sense of complacency. Control of institutional utilization is therefore to be understood in context with control of other areas of utilization as well.

Measurements

Definition of the Numbers

First you must choose exactly what you will measure and how you will define that measurement. It is common for most plans to measure bed days per 1,000 plan members per year (a formula to calculate this is given below). Deciding what to count as a bed day is not always straightforward, however.

In some plans, outpatient surgery will be counted as a single day in the hospital. This is done on the assumption that an outpatient procedure will cost the plan nearly the same as or sometimes more than a single inpatient day would cost. Some plans count skilled nursing home days in the total, and some add commercial, Medicare, Medicaid, and fee for service into the total calculation. In some plans the day of discharge is counted; in most it is not (unless it is charged for by the hospital). Plans must also decide whether to count nursery days when the mother is still in the hospital or only if the newborn is boarding over or in intensive care.

Most plans count commercial days separately from other days, especially Medicare days. Plans with a significant Medicaid population may wish to track it both separately and together with commercial. Most plans do not count outpatient surgery as an inpatient day but report that number separately; likewise, most plans report skilled nursing days separately.

How to count nursery days is a difficult decision. The argument that skilled nursing days are not counted as hospital days because the cost is so much less may also be used for nursery days while the mother is in the hospital. In most hospitals, the nursery charges for a normal newborn are relatively low. If the newborn requires a stay beyond the mother's discharge, the charges usually are higher. If the neonate is in the intensive care unit, charges will obviously be quite high. If you have negotiated an all-inclusive per diem rate or a case rate that takes normal nursery days into account while the mother is in the hospital, you may have no need to count them separately. If you must pay a high rate for nursery days, you will probably want them counted in the total.

Further discussion about utilization reports may be found in Chapter 37.

Formulas To Calculate Institutional Utilization

The standard formula to calculate bed days per 1,000 members per year is relatively straightforward. You may use it to calculate the annualized bed days per 1,000 members for any time period you choose (eg, for the day, the month to date, the year to date, and so forth).

When calculating bed days per 1,000, use the assumption of a 365-day year as opposed to a 12-month year to prevent variations that are due solely to the length of the month. The formula is as follows:

$$[A \div (B \div 365)] \div (C \div 1,000)$$

where A is gross bed days per time unit, B is days per time unit, and C is plan membership.

This may be broken into steps. Exhibit 15–1 illustrates the calculation for bed days per 1,000 on a single day; Exhibit 15–2 illustrates the calculation for bed days per 1,000 for the month to date.

Expected Utilization and Variations

Inpatient utilization is almost always lower in HMOs than in any other types of health plans. Table 15–1 provides examples of utilization data under a variety of different options. Note that the data in Table 15–1 is for 1993, the most recent data available for analysis at the time this book was written. By 1995, even utilization figures in some parts of the country were at least 20% or more lower than those shown in Table 15–1.

There are two common reasons for variations in hospital utilization rates across the country. One reason is easily understood; the other is not. Easily understood is the relationship between

Exhibit 15–1 Example of Bed Days for a Single Day

Assume: Current hospital census = 10
Plan membership = 12,000

Step 1: Gross days = 10 ÷ (1 ÷ 365)
= 10 ÷ 0.00274
= 3,649.635

Step 2: Days per 1,000 = 3,649.635 ÷ (12,000 ÷ 1,000)
= 3,649.635 ÷ 12
= 304 (rounded)

Therefore, the days per 1,000 for that single day equal 304.

---

how tight the UM program you have is and its results. The tighter you make the program, and the more actual medical management is going on, the lower your utilization numbers will be. Conversely, if you choose for various reasons not to enforce a UM program stringently (eg, you may not be marketing a tight system), you will have proportionate increases in the hospitalization rate.

Less easily understood are the profound geographic variations in inpatient utilization. Rates of utilization on the East Coast are consistently and significantly higher than those on the West Coast.[13] In fact, there are geographic variations in utilization in cities of similar size that are not terribly far apart[14–18] and even significant geographic variations in a single metropolitan service area (Blue Cross and Blue Shield of National Capital Area, unpublished data, 1993). There is no rational explanation for this from the standpoint of the patients. The answer must lie with the practice habits of physicians in different areas. At the very least, this perplexing disparity based on geography points out that significant improvement in utilization may be achieved, especially in the eastern United States.

Despite low utilization in HMOs and other forms of managed care plans, there are researchers who strongly believe that there remains a significant amount of unnecessary utilization even now. The most aggressive of these is found in a report by Milliman & Robertson in which the authors state that almost 60% of inpatient utilization is unnecessary.[19]

Exhibit 15–2 Example of Bed Days for the Month to Date (MTD)

Assume: Total gross hospital bed days in MTD = 300
Plan membership = 12,000
Days in MTD = 21

Step 1: Gross days MTD = 300 ÷ (21 ÷ 365)
= 300 ÷ 0.0575
= 5,217.4

Step 2: Days per 1,000 in MTD = 5,217.4 ÷ (12,000 ÷ 1,000)
= 5,217.4 ÷ 12
= 435 (rounded)

Therefore, the days per 1,000 for the MTD equal 435.

Table 15–1 Hospital Utilization Rates, 1993

	Commercial			Medicare			Medicaid		
	BD/K	Disch/K	ALOS	BD/K	Disch/K	ALOS	BD/K	Disch/K	ALOS
Indemnity and HMO	273.1	61.2	4.46	2,474	309	8.0	930.1	165.4	5.62
HMO (all plan types)	242.2	66.3	3.8	1,526	224.5	7.0	568	132.1	3.8
Staff	251.5	71.1	3.7	1,501	209.6	7.0	439	124.9	3.5
Group	242.0	67.0	3.6				N/A	N/A	N/A
Network	197.5	58.9	3.6	1,565	228.3	N/A	480	122.0	3.6
Independent practice association (IPA)	262.9	68.6	4.0				603	142.7	3.7

Note: Indemnity and HMO data combined in first row—unable to accurately break out. Indemnity and HMO data combined excludes Medicare, Medicaid, workers' compensation, government pay, uninsured, nonpay, and no charge. Indemnity-only utilization estimated to be approximately 20% higher than noted in table for commercial. For Medicare, staff and group figures are combined and network and IPA numbers are combined. BD/K = bed days per thousand; Disch/K = discharges per thousand; ALOS = average length of stay; N/A = not applicable.

Courtesy of Ernst & Young LLP.

Common Methods for Managing Utilization

Management of institutional utilization may be best presented by discussing the key categories for managing the process: prospective, concurrent, and retrospective review and LCM. Prospective review occurs before a case happens, concurrent review occurs while the case is active, and retrospective review occurs after the case is finished. LCM refers to managing cases that are expected to result in very large costs, so as to provide coordination of care that results in both proper care and cost savings.

Prospective Review

Precertification. Precertification refers to a requirement on the part of the admitting physician (and often the hospital) to notify the plan before a member is admitted for inpatient care or an outpatient procedure. There is a widespread and rather erroneous belief that the primary role of precertification is to prevent unnecessary cases from occurring. Although that may occasionally happen (particularly in workers' compensation cases), it is not the chief reason for precertification.

There are three primary reasons for precertification. The first is to notify the concurrent review system that a case will be occurring. In that way, the UM system will be able to prepare discharge planning (discussed below) ahead of time as well as to look for the case during concurrent review rounds. In some instances, the LCM function (see below) may be notified if the admission diagnosis raises the possibility that it will be a highly expensive case (eg, a bone marrow transplant).

The second major reason for precertification is to ensure that care takes place in the most appropriate setting. Perhaps an inpatient case is diverted to the outpatient department, or a case is diverted from a nonparticipating hospital to a participating one or to a facility that has been designated as a center of excellence for a selected procedure.

The third reason is to capture data for financial accruals. Although it is unlikely that a plan can capture every case before or while it is taking place, a mature plan that is running well can capture the vast majority of cases, perhaps 90% to 95%. By knowing the number and nature of hospital cases as well as potential catastrophic cases, the plan may more accurately accrue for expenses rather than having to wait for claims to come in. This allows management to take action early and to avoid nasty financial surprises.

In any case, for inpatient cases the plan usually assigns a length of stay guideline at the time the admission is certified. (Length of stay is discussed below.) The plan may also use the precertification process to verify eligibility of coverage for the member, although most plans have a disclaimer stating that ultimate eligibility for coverage will be determined at the time the claim is processed.

In the case of an emergency or urgent admission, it is obviously not possible to obtain precertification. In that event, there is usually a contractual requirement to notify the plan by the next business day or within 24 hours if the plan has 24-hour-per-day UM staffing. Most plans have contractual language with both the physicians and the hospitals imposing financial penalties (eg, a percentage of their fee or a flat penalty) for failure to obtain precertification. For plans that allow members to seek care from noncontracted providers (eg, POS plans), the responsibility to contact the plan rests with the members if they choose not to see a network physician; in such cases, most plans impose benefits penalties (eg, a higher coinsurance or a flat penalty rate) on a member who fails to obtain proper precertification.

Preadmission Testing and Same-Day Surgery. One of the easiest and also the most common methods for cost control is preadmission testing and same-day surgery. A member who is going to be hospitalized on an elective basis has routine preoperative tests done as an outpatient and is admitted on the day of the surgery. Both these policies are confirmed at the time of precertification.

For example, imagine that a member has elective gallbladder surgery scheduled for 10:00 AM on Thursday. On Tuesday the member goes to the hospital for the preoperative tests. The results are made available to the admitting physician, who performs the admission history and physical while the patient is still an outpatient and either delivers the results to the hospital or calls them in on an outside line to the hospital's transcription department. The member arrives at the hospital at 6:00 AM on Thursday, is admitted, and has surgery as scheduled.

Many health plans make arrangements for laboratory work to be done with a contracted laboratory at reduced rates or have in-house capabilities to perform the laboratory work. Occasionally, a hospital will refuse to accept the results of these laboratories. If the laboratory is accredited and licensed, the hospital has little grounds to require a plan to use its laboratory, electrocardiography, and radiology services for preoperative admission testing. In these cases the plan's management team must discuss this issue with the hospital administrator and negotiate an agreement for the hospital to accept the plan's laboratory work or to agree to perform the work at equivalent costs to the plan. If the hospital refuses to cooperate, the plan needs to decide whether to direct the elective cases to another, more cooperative hospital.

Mandatory Outpatient Surgery. It has become popular for health plans to produce mandatory outpatient surgery lists, lists of procedures that may be performed on only an outpatient basis unless prior approval is obtained from the plan medical director. In developing its own mandatory outpatient surgery list, a plan can build from lists used by similar plans or even Medicare. No two lists are identical, which causes some confusion with physicians and hospitals. Although there is consensus on many common procedures (eg, a carpal tunnel release), there are always procedures that are migrating from inpatient to outpatient (eg, at the time this book was written, outpatient cardiac catheterization had only become popular in the last few years). That confusion probably tends to encourage physicians to use outpatient surgery when in doubt.

As mentioned earlier in this chapter and elsewhere, a plan should be sure that it will actually achieve the desired savings before instituting mandatory outpatient surgery requirements. In some cases, hospitals or free-standing outpatient surgery facilities have charges that are equal to or greater than those for an inpatient day. In other cases, the facility charge may be lower, but the unbundled charges for anesthesia, recovery, supplies, and so on can drive the cost higher than anticipated.

Concurrent Review

Concurrent review means managing utilization during the course of a hospitalization (as opposed to an outpatient procedure). Common techniques for concurrent review involve assignment and tracking of length of stay, review and rounding by UM nurses, and discharge planning. The roles of the medical director, the PCP, and the attending or consulting physicians are discussed later in this chapter, as is the relationship between concurrent review and LCM.

Assignment of Length of Stay. A common approach to hospital utilization control is the assignment of a maximum allowable length of stay (MaxLOS), which sometimes appears in the guise of an estimated length of stay, but with teeth. With the MaxLOS, the plan assigns a length of stay on the basis of the admission diagnosis, and that is all the plan will authorize for payment. For example, an admission for gallbladder surgery may be assigned 3 days. It is assumed that the patient will be admitted on the day of surgery and go home 3 days later. Any stay beyond that day is not covered. In those plans that cannot or will not restrict payment, the MaxLOS is used only to trigger greater involvement by the medical director.

The MaxLOS is determined by International Classification of Diseases, Ninth Edition, Clinical Modification (ICD-9-CM) code, or diagnostic code, although diagnosis-related groups (DRGs) are similar in concept. Selecting a norm for the MaxLOS is not always easy given the regional variations. Looking at the local fee-for-service experience may or may not be helpful, depending on a plan area's history of achieving good control of utilization. Also, a number of organizations and companies sell such data.

The advantage of using MaxLOS designations is threefold. First, they allow plans to cover a relatively large geographic area with few personnel, which may be necessary in a start-up open panel plan. Second, these designations have a certain legitimacy and keep a plan from having to negotiate every time. Third, MaxLOSs are relatively clear-cut, so plan personnel need less training. Even though MaxLOSs are clear-cut, it is still important to verify, usually through the UM nurse, that diagnoses are accurate.

But there are three problems with using MaxLOS designations. First, it is easy to get complacent. If a plan chooses certain values for MaxLOS designations, it may never reevaluate those values. Second, designated time becomes free time. In other words, there is less incentive to evaluate critically every day in the hospital for appropriateness and alternatives if plan personnel and the physician feel that there is still time on the meter. Third, using such a mechanical system often achieves less than optimal results. Intensive medical management by qualified personnel should produce better control of utilization, but such personnel are not always available. The topic of concurrent review against criteria is discussed below.

A plan must also know what the consequences of exceeding the MaxLOS will be. In many plans, exceeding the MaxLOS results in either a denial of payment for services rendered after the MaxLOS has been reached or a reduction in payment, usually by a percentage amount. If a plan has failed to inform its membership of a MaxLOS program and the plan does not have sole source of payment clauses with its providers and hospitals, the plan may not be able to enforce a MaxLOS designation easily.

Role of the Utilization Management Nurse. The one individual who is crucial to the success of a managed care program is the UM nurse. It is the UM nurse who will be the eyes and ears of the medical management department, who will generally coordinate the discharge planning, and who will facilitate all the activities of utilization control.

Staffing levels for UM nurses will vary depending on the size of the geographic area, the number of hospitals, the size of the plan, and the intensity with which UM will be performed (eg, by on-site hospital rounding). It is common for plans to staff one UM nurse for every 6,000 to

8,000 members, assuming that the UM nurses will be making rounds on all hospitalized patients and that utilization is reasonably tightly controlled, but not on a 24-hour-per-day basis. Staffing ratios have considerable variation, however, with one study reporting the average number of full-time nurse reviewers at 0.16 per 1,000 enrollees, with a range of 0.01 to 0.8 per 1,000.[20] Plans that perform telephone review only may staff at ratios that are half the average. It is also necessary to provide clerical support to do intake, to follow up on discharge planning needs, to take care of filing, and so forth.

The scope of responsibilities of the UM nurse will vary depending on the plan and the personalities and skills of the other members of the medical management team. In some plans, the role simply involves telephone information gathering. In other plans, there will be a more proactive role, including frequent communication with attending physicians, the medical director, the hospitals, and the hospitalized members and their families; discharge planning and facilitation; and a host of other activities, including active hospital rounding.

The one fundamental function of the UM nurse is information gathering. Information about hospital cases must be obtained in an accurate and timely fashion. It falls to the UM nurse to be the focal point of this information and to ensure that it is obtained and communicated to the necessary individuals in medical management and the claims department.

Necessary information includes admission date and diagnosis, the type of hospital service to which the patient was admitted (eg, medical, surgical, maternity, and so forth), the admitting physician, consultants, planned procedures (type and timing), expected discharge date, needed discharge planning, and any other pertinent information the plan managers may need.

In some plans, information gathering is done strictly by telephone; in other plans, hospital rounding is done in person by the UM nurse. When the telephone is used, it is used first to check with the admitting office to determine whether any plan members were admitted and then to check with the hospital's own UM department to obtain any further information.

Telephone rounding is usually done in cases where there is too much geographic area to cover and the plan cannot yet justify adding more UM nurses (eg, in a start-up individual provider association or preferred provider organization [PPO] covering five counties). It may also be done in those rare instances where a hospital refuses to give the UM nurse rounding privileges on hospitalized plan members. There are certainly situations where a plan may in fact delegate rounding and review to the hospital's UM department, but those are not common; examples include arrangements where the hospital is at significant financial risk (eg, through capitation or DRGs). Telephone rounding may also be used when there are not tight controls on utilization; then, the UM nurse is looking for clear outliers rather than trying to achieve optimal utilization control.

Hospital rounding in person is far superior to telephone rounding. When rounds are conducted daily by a UM nurse on every hospitalized member, plans obtain the most accurate and timely information, sometimes even information that they might not get otherwise.

For example, in a good quality management program (see Part XI), the rounding UM nurse will be able to watch for quality problems or significant events that would trigger a quality assurance audit. A rounding nurse will also be able to pick up information about a patient's condition that may affect discharge planning—information that the attending physician may have failed to communicate (eg, the need for home durable equipment that must be ordered).

The UM nurse may also be able to detect practice behavior that increases utilization simply for the convenience of the physician or hospital. For example, a patient may be ready for discharge but the physician missed making rounds that morning and will not be back until the next day, or the hospital may have rescheduled surgery for its own reasons and the patient will have to spend an extra and unnecessary day. In these types of situations, the UM nurse must not be put into an adversarial position but should refer such cases to the medical director.

Personal rounding by a plan's UM nurse has the added advantage of increasing member satisfaction. Many people feel uncomfortable talking to physicians and welcome the chance to express their fears or feelings to the UM nurse. In other cases, inquiring about how members are feeling can let them know that plans care about them as people and that plans are not simply trying to get them out as fast as possible.

When hospitals refuse to grant rounding privileges to the UM nurse, they often explain that they already have a UM department. These departments are usually not adequate for a plan's needs because they do not address that plan's specific member satisfaction and quality assurance needs. Another frequent excuse is that the hospitals want to protect their patients' confidentiality. But no patient confidentiality will be violated if the plan's UM nurse is rounding on only plan members (who have agreed in their application to allow access to records). If a hospital refuses to allow a plan's UM nurse to round, a plan must seriously question doing business with that hospital. In most cases, a hospital will cooperate fully and willingly.

The heart of concurrent review is the evaluation of each hospital case against established criteria—review against criteria. Many plans, especially open panel plans and PPOs, use published or commercially available criteria for such reviews[21–24] to facilitate evaluation by UM nurses. Experienced nurses use such criteria as an aid in managing utilization, but they do not blindly depend on it. It is possible to keep a patient in the hospital for less than adequate reasons but still meet criteria; the seasoned UM nurse is able to evaluate each case on its merits.

Most plans have now automated this function to improve the efficiency of UM nurses. Software allows the MaxLOS to be generated automatically from the admission diagnosis or procedure. Member and benefit eligibility is checked, diagnostic and procedure codes are generated from entered text, review criteria are automatically displayed for both admission and concurrent review, unlimited text may be entered to allow tracking, census reports are produced, statistics are generated, and so forth. UM software also links to the claims system so that claims are properly processed, including special instructions from the nurses.

Discharge Planning and Follow-Up. Good discharge planning starts as soon as a patient is admitted into the hospital, or even before. The physician and the UM nurse should be considering discharge planning as part of the overall treatment plan from the outset. This planning includes an estimate of how long the patient will be in the hospital, what the expected outcome will be, whether there will be any special requirements on discharge, and what needs to be facilitated early on.

For example, if a patient is admitted with a fractured hip and it is known from the outset that many weeks of rehabilitation will be necessary, it is helpful to contact the facility where the rehabilitation will take place to ensure that a bed will be available at the time of transfer. If it is known that a patient will need durable medical equipment, the equipment should be ordered early so that the patient does not spend extra days in the hospital waiting for it to arrive.

An often overlooked aspect of discharge planning is informing the patient and family. If the patient and family do not know what to expect, they may be surprised when the physician tells them that the patient is being discharged. This is especially true if the patient has received hospital care in the past and has certain expectations. Informing the patient and family from the start about when they can expect discharge, how the patient will be feeling, what they might need to prepare for at home, and how follow-up will occur will all help smooth things considerably.

In the case of short-stay obstetrics, the government has now decided to regulate that the minimum length of stay is 2 days. However, 1-day stays for obstetrics are still acceptable if the patient, the physician, and the plan all agree. In the case of short-stay obstetrics, the patient and family must be prepared for the homecoming. Active discharge planning for short-stay obstetrics is crucial, and the plan must offer home health visits to mothers who have had a short-stay delivery.

Discharge planning is an ongoing effort beginning with admission or preadmission screening. The UM nurse is in the ideal position to coordinate discharge planning. In addition to making sure that all goes smoothly to effect a smooth and proper discharge from the hospital, the UM nurse can follow up with the member by telephone after discharge to ensure that all is well.

Primary Care Physician Responsibilities. There are two basic models for managing hospital cases: the PCP model and the attending physician or "hospitalist" model. In the PCP model, the PCPs are expected to manage the care of their patients in the hospital even when patients are hospitalized for care delivered primarily by consultants or specialists; most commonly this occurs when the patient is hospitalized for surgery or for a severe medical condition (eg, a myocardial infarction), or when the patient has a drawn-out course of treatment (eg, recovery from a stroke). In the PCP model, the most important functions of the member's PCP are also the most obvious: to make rounds every day and to coordinate the patient's care.

When a patient is receiving care from a consultant, it is very important for the PCP to round daily. This serves a number of purposes. First, it helps ensure continuity of care while the patient is in the hospital (eg, the PCP may be able to add pertinent clinical information as needed). Second, it provides a comforting, emotionally supportive presence for the patient, which results in better bonding between physician and patient. Third, it allows for continuity after discharge because the PCP is aware of the clinical course and discharge planning.

UM by the PCP is highly effective when a member is receiving hospital care from a consultant. The PCP is able to discuss the case with the consultant and suggest ways to decrease the length of stay (eg, home nursing care) that the consultant may not be used to considering. The PCP will presumably know the patient well enough to determine the patient's ability to do well in alternative situations.

The PCP will also be able to communicate effectively with a consultant if the consultant fails to see the patient on rounds. For example, if a busy surgeon misses a patient on rounds because the patient was in the bathroom, the surgeon, because of a heavy operating room schedule, may not make it back to see that patient until late at night. If the patient is actually ready for discharge, the PCP can communicate with the surgeon that morning and arrange for discharge.

There will be situations where the PCP is unable to make rounds in person. This happens most frequently when a member is admitted to a tertiary hospital where the PCP does not have privileges. For example, cardiac bypass surgery may be done at a teaching hospital with a closed medical staff. In these situations, it is important for the PCP to be in frequent telephone contact with the attending physician on the case to keep up with developments and to aid in the discharge planning process. For example, the PCP may be comfortable with accepting the patient back in transfer during the recovery period or may be able to suggest home nursing care. In addition to controlling utilization, this helps ensure continuity of care, and the attending physician will almost always remark to the patient about how attentive the PCP has been.

Equally important to good medical management is for the PCP to avoid the trap of "That's the way it's always been done, and it's good enough for me!" The PCP and the specialist must be open to evaluating new methods of treatment and considering high-quality but cost-effective ways of caring for people.

As a corollary, PCPs must be confident and assertive about their own abilities. Unfortunately, because of the highly specialized nature of medicine, there are times when a PCP is looked down upon by a consultant. Certainly a consultant who depends on the PCP for referrals will not knowingly exhibit behavior that the PCP will find offensive, but there often remains an unspoken agreement that the consultant will call the shots once the patient is admitted.

PCPs may raise objections about getting involved with the care of patients admitted to a consultant's service. First, the PCP may feel intimidated by the consultant's knowledge about the medical problem. When this happens, there is no reason why the PCP cannot read up on the subject, at least in a major medical text, and ask questions. Also, the individual is the PCP's patient, and the consultant is a consultant. It is the PCP's responsibility to follow the care of the patient and to be aware of the medical issues involved. Simply asking the consultant questions about that care is appropriate and necessary and will frequently result in improved understanding by all parties as well as improved utilization control.

A PCP may consider such questioning confrontational and may not want to question the competence of the consultant. But the PCP is not questioning the consultant's competence (assuming that the consultant is indeed competent); rather, he or she is discussing the case and asking the consultant for an opinion about alternatives. The fear of such confrontations is far greater than it should be. The PCP has nothing to be shy about; PCPs are trained physicians specializing in primary care, and the consultant is helping care for the PCP's patient, not vice versa.

Specialist Physician Responsibilities in the Primary Care Physician Model. Even in a PCP model, the consultant has responsibilities. The interaction between consultant and PCP is highly important to good medical management and utilization control. Beyond that, it is reasonable for the plan, through the medical director, to communicate certain expectations of all consultants. It has been clearly shown that even in intensive care units where little discretion would be expected in treatment decisions, HMOs have 30% to 40% lower utilization (measured by length of stay, charges, and use of ventilators) when compared to fee-for-service environments, even when the figures are adjusted for case mix.[25] Clearly, consultants and specialists in a managed care environment have considerable effect on resource use.

First, plans expect all consultants to be aware of and to cooperate with policies on testing, procedures, and primary care case management. Second, plans that use PCPs as gatekeepers or managing physicians should expect consultants to be in communication with PCPs about their patients and to provide written reports on consultations (some plans go as far as refusing payment to a consultant until the PCP receives a written report). Third, care should be directed back to the PCP as soon as it is practical to do so, and the consultant will reinforce the plan's philosophy of primary care. Last, the consultant will not subauthorize further nonurgent care for the member without first discussing the case with the PCP. The PCP may already have worked up a problem that the consultant is seeing for the first time, or the PCP may be able to perform the medical duties that the consultant is requesting.

In a loosely controlled plan there will be fewer expectations of the consultant than in a tightly controlled plan. As has been mentioned numerous times, the better the control of utilization you hope to achieve, the more you have to deal with practice patterns and physician behavior. Consultants are able to add significantly to the cost of care not only from their own fees but through additional fees generated by extra days in the hospital and through testing, procedures, and secondary referrals to other consultants.

Rounding Physician or Hospitalist Model. In the rounding physician model, sometimes called the *designated admitting physician* or *hospitalist* model, one physician is designated to care for all admissions of a group or health plan to a given hospital or hospital service (eg, to a medical service). This model is sometimes found in group and staff model HMOs, but is also beginning to appear in some open panel HMOs as well. The PCP relinquishes responsibility for the admission, and the rounding physician assumes responsibility.

The rounding or designated physician may be on site full-time or may simply carry a lighter outpatient load, devoting greater time to rounding on hospitalized patients. In the large closed panels, as well as the open panel plans that are adopting this system, it is more common for the designated physician to be full-time on site at the hospital. In some cases, the hospitalist is a full-time specialty physician who practices only in the hospital; in other cases, this duty is shared by members of the medical group in rotation. The rounding physician is usually an internist but may belong to another qualified specialty.

The reasoning behind this approach is that a dedicated on-site physician will be closer to the care that the patient is receiving and in a better position to coordinate needed services as well as closely monitor care for quality and appropriateness. A dedicated hospitalist is better able to obtain diagnostic study reports, consultations, and so forth in a timely manner. Some large organized medical groups have gone so far as to create entire hospital care groups that include not only a hospitalist physician, but a physician's assistant or clinical nurse practitioner, a dedicated rounding nurse, and other clinical team members (eg, a clinical pharmacist or a social worker). Of course, there will be many clinical conditions where the hospitalist is not at all in a primary caregiver situation—in the early stages of an acute myocardial infarction, during chemotherapy, for obstetrics, for surgical procedures, and so forth. Even in these cases, however, the hospitalist follows the case as a PCP would (see above).

The hospitalist model works best in a capitated environment in which the medical group and the hospitalist share in the same capitation payment. Alternately, if a hospital system is receiving global capitation for services, it may wish to employ the hospitalist to manage and monitor cases, even when the outside medical group has no direct financial stake in the cost of institutional services. Even in situations where a hospital system is capitated for services, there is commonly some level of savings sharing between the hospital and the plan physicians.

Large groups also find that the hospitalist model increases their overall efficiency by keeping physicians from going into a hospital for just one or two patient visits. In all cases, it lowers the administrative burden, since the medical director is working with 1 physician in the hospital rather than with 20.

In some plans, it is not practical for a PCP to follow all cases in the hospital even though the plan may not have a formal rounding physician program. The reasons for this may include high use of teaching hospitals with closed medical staffs, communities where PCPs simply do not hospitalize cases (which can occur in both urban and rural areas), or plans that do not use a PCP gatekeeper system. In any case, the attending physician in this situation is usually a specialist or consultant and has responsibility to manage the case and to interact with the plan. The responsibilities of the attending physician in this model are very similar to the PCP's. Interaction with the plan is necessary, and the consultant needs to cooperate with plan policies and procedures. The main difference in this model is the person with whom the UM nurse and medical director interact. The hospitalist model is further discussed in Chapter 16.

Medical Director's Responsibilities. In addition to monitoring all the elements discussed in this chapter, there are a few specific functions that the medical director should be performing.

Communications. The medical director will have to become involved in the most difficult cases from a management standpoint. There may be difficulty with the PCP, a consultant, a hospital, or the member or member's family. There are times when the medical director must deal with uncooperative individuals, and this can certainly be difficult. The medical director must take a compassionate, caring, but firm stance. It often seems easiest simply to give in to a difficult person, but that can only be done so many times before it becomes a habit that damages the plan's effectiveness. Medical directors should empathize and sympathize with, not submit to, someone else's perspective. Although the medical director will occasionally want to loosen the reins, it is important for the medical director to remain firm when the situation is clear and to back up his or her subordinates and the PCPs when they are right.

If the medical director is heard from only when there is a problem, his or her effectiveness will be diminished. The medical director should have reasonably frequent contact with PCPs and important consultants even when all is well. This can be especially useful when discussing cases. If the medical director discusses cases, suggesting appropriate alternatives even when there is no pressing need to make a change, the participating plan physicians will be much more accepting of the medical director's opinions when change is definitely needed (assuming that the medical director has helpful opinions in the first place, of course).

The usefulness of frequent contact cannot be underestimated. By asking thoughtful questions in a nonthreatening manner, and by constantly stimulating thought regarding cost-effective clinical management, the medical director may slowly reinforce appropriate patterns of care. Physicians may begin asking themselves the questions the medical director would ask and begin improving their practice patterns on that basis.

Daily Review of Utilization. A task that the medical director should perform for optimal utilization control is reviewing the hospital log daily. This may seem an onerous task, and it can be, but it is the only way the medical director will consistently spot problems in time to do something about them. For example, finding that surgery was not done on the same day as admission may prompt a call to the PCP or surgeon to prevent recurrence of that type of problem. If possible, it is even better for the medical director to review the hospital log with the UM nurse early enough each day for meaningful action to be taken—usually before noon, when many hospitals automatically charge for another day. Large plans with highly competent UM nurses and UM departments may get to a point where the medical director need not review every case every day but simply will review any problem cases or outliers. Even in these situations,

the medical director should periodically review every case to be certain that the UM department is performing as well as expected.

Retrospective Review

Retrospective review occurs after the case is finished and the patient is discharged. Retrospective review takes on two primary forms: claims review and pattern review.

Claims Review. Claims review refers to examining claims for improprieties or mistakes. For example, it is common for plans to review large claims to verify whether services were actually delivered or whether mistakes were made in collating the claims data. In such large cases, the plan may actually send a representative on site to the hospital to review the medical record against the claims record.

Pattern Review. This refers to examining patterns of utilization to determine where action must be taken. For example, if three hospitals in the area perform coronary artery bypass surgery, the plan may look to see which one has the best clinical outcomes, the shortest length of stay, and the lowest charges. The plan may then preferentially send all such cases to that hospital. Pattern review also allows the plan to focus UM efforts primarily on those areas needing greater attention (ie, Sutton's Law: Go where the money is!).

One other use of pattern review is to provide feedback to providers. Although not as powerful as active UM by the plan's own department, feedback sometimes can have an effect.[26] When combined with other management functions and financial incentives, feedback is a useful management tool (see Chapter 39 for an in-depth discussion of the use of feedback in modification of physician behavior).

Alternatives to Acute Care Hospitalization

There are many instances where patients are ill or disabled but do not need to be in an acute care hospital. Despite that, these patients often stay in acute care hospitals. The reasons for this are many. In some cases, the patient started out needing the services of an acute care hospital (eg, a patient had surgery but the recovery phase requires far fewer resources than are available in the hospital). In other cases, there is simply no place for the patient to go (eg, a patient is recovering from a broken femur but lives alone). In a few cases, a patient is kept in the hospital for the convenience of a physician who does not want to make house calls or rounds at another institution. Last, there are times when a patient is kept in the hospital simply because "That's the way it's always been done!" The role of post–acute care in managed care is discussed in detail in Part VIII.

Subacute Care, Skilled or Intermediate Nursing Facilities. A useful alternative to consider is the skilled or intermediate nursing facility or subacute facility. These facilities are best suited to prolonged convalescence or recovery cases. For example, if a patient with a broken femur requires more traction than can be provided safely at home and needs many months to recover, the cost for a bed day in a nursing facility will be much less than the cost for a bed day in the acute care hospital. The principle also applies in rehabilitation cases such as stroke or trauma to the brain when the damage is too extensive for the patient to go home immediately. Although there are few (if any) reasons anymore to admit someone for uncomplicated back pain, if a plan's physician does so, a nursing facility is the most appropriate place for the bed rest to take place.

Recently, the subacute care industry has begun to focus on making its facilities a practical alternative to an acute care hospital for a larger variety of medical cases. For example, some subacute care facilities provide a cost-effective location for the administration of chemotherapy that requires close supervision. The treatment of many medical conditions such as acute pneumonia or osteomyelitis when the patient is too sick to be cared for at home may be done in a subacute facility. In some cases, the patient may be able to be cared for at home, but it is still more cost-effective to deliver the therapy in the subacute facility due to more favorable pricing achievable through economies of scale. In order for a subacute facility to effectively vie for this type of business, it must transform itself into something other than a nursing home.

The main problem with the use of subacute facilities or nursing homes is objection from the patient or the family, particularly in the case of young patients. There is a stigma attached to nursing homes that makes some people consider them warehouses for older people. To overcome this, a plan needs to take a proactive approach.

First, the plan should contract with only those nursing or subacute care facilities that meet its (and implicitly, its members') notions of pleasant surroundings. Plans should not simply choose the least costly facility. A good nursing facility will be interested in working with plans to ensure that their patients will be given a private room (a private room in a nursing facility is still less costly than a semiprivate bed in an acute care hospital) or at least will be placed in a room with another patient who has a similar functional status.

Second, plans should discuss the alternative with the patient and the family well in advance of the actual move. Nothing is as distressing for patients as suddenly finding out that they will be shipped out in the morning to a nursing home. If possible, plans should have the family visit the nursing facility to meet the staff and see the environment before the patient is transferred.

Last, plans should not abandon the patient. In other words, plans should have someone, preferably the physician and the UM nurse, regularly visit patients in a nursing home. It is easy to reason that, because the patient is in the nursing facility for long-term care, visits are unnecessary; after all, the nurse would call if there was a problem. That may be true from a medical standpoint, but it is not true from a human relations standpoint.

How a plan handles a nursing facility will have an impact on its marketing. Plans that coldly shunt people into a nursing facility simply to save money will rapidly get a reputation for placing their needs over those of their members. Members will complain to their benefits managers or to other potential members, and plans will develop enrollment problems. If, however, plans demonstrate caring and compassion, taking the time to alleviate the emotional distress that may be caused, they will find that most people are quite understanding and accepting of this alternative.

The other issue to consider in the use of nursing facilities is monitoring the case with regard to a plan's benefit structure. It is easy for a case to go from prolonged recovery to permanent placement or custodial care. It can be emotionally wrenching both for the member's family and a plan to face up to the end of benefits. The problem of who will pay for long-term custodial care is a national dilemma, and it becomes personal when a family is faced with high costs because the benefits offered by a plan do not continue indefinitely.

If it is possible or likely that benefits will end, it is wise early on to make the benefits structure clear to the family. This does not have to be done in a cold and calculating manner but rather by laying out all the possibilities so that the family may begin early planning themselves.

Step-Down Units. As an alternative to free-standing nursing facilities, many hospitals with excess capacity have developed step-down units. Even if they have not, many hospital administrators are willing to consider them in negotiations.

In essence, a step-down unit is a hospital ward or section of a ward that is used in much the same way as a skilled nursing or subacute care facility. A patient who requires less care and monitoring, such as someone recovering from a hip replacement (after all the drains have been removed), may need only bed rest, traction, and minimal nursing care. In recognition of the lesser resource needs, the charge per day is less.

The step-down unit has the advantage of being convenient for the physician and UM nurse and is more acceptable to the patient and family. It also does not require transfer outside the facility. Although the cost per day is sometimes slightly higher than that of a nursing facility, the difference may be worth it in terms of member acceptability.

Outpatient Procedure Units. In many instances, performing a procedure in an outpatient unit is less expensive than admitting a patient for a 1-day stay. This is not always true because, with the increased popularity of outpatient surgery, some hospitals have raised their outpatient unit charges to make up the lost revenue and increasing complexity of outpatient procedures. Plans should pay careful attention to outpatient charges when negotiating with hospitals.

Free-standing outpatient facilities are also an alternative. These may be affiliated with a hospital or may be independent. As they do with hospitals, plans can and should negotiate the charge structure so that they indeed receive the cost savings that outpatient surgery should allow.

Hospice Care. Hospice care is care given to terminally ill patients. It tends to be supportive care and is used most often when such care cannot be given in the home. It is not always covered by health plans, but it does sometimes take the place of acute care hospitalization and should be considered when appropriate.

Home Health Care. Home health agencies are proliferating, and home care is becoming increasingly accepted. Services that are particularly amenable to home health care include nursing care for routine reasons (eg, checking weights, changing dressings, and the like), home intravenous treatment (eg, for osteomyelitis, certain forms of chemotherapy, or home intravenous nutrition), home physical therapy, respiratory therapy, and rehabilitation care.

Plans should have little trouble negotiating and contracting with home health agencies for services. It is becoming popular for hospitals to have home health care services to aid with caring for patients discharged from their facility, and plans may be able to negotiate for those services with your overall contract. Furthermore, as Medicare continues to tighten payments for home care, many agencies are looking for alternative sources of revenue. As with hospitals or any other providers of care, home health and high-technology home care agencies need to be evaluated in terms beyond simple pricing breaks. An active quality management program, the presence of a medical director, and evidence of attention to the changes that are constantly occurring in the field are all requisites for contracting.

A warning about home health services is in order. Because the physician and UM nurse seldom visit the patient receiving home health care, the home health nurse often must determine how frequently and how long the patient should receive services, and this can lead to some surprising bills. It is highly advisable to have a firm policy regarding how many home health visits may be covered under a single authorization and that continued authorization requires physician review.

Large Case Management

LCM, also referred to as catastrophic case management, refers to specialized techniques for identifying and managing cases that are disproportionately high in cost. For example, active AIDS can be an expensive disease process, as can a high cervical spinal cord injury, a bone marrow transplant, and many other events. This highly important subject is discussed in detail in Chapter 17 as well as Part X, so only a brief discussion will occur here in the context of overall management of medical-surgical utilization.

Identification of large cases may be straightforward because the patients are in the hospital the first time plans identify them, as is the case for trauma. Other cases may be identified before they are ever hospitalized. For example, examining the claims system for use of dialysis services may identify an end-stage renal disease patient. Proactively contacting patients with potentially catastrophic illnesses not only can save the plan considerable expense by managing the care cost-effectively but can also result in better medical care because the services are coordinated.

Prenatal care is a specialized form of LCM because active coordination occurs before the newborn is delivered. Prenatal LCM involves identification of high-risk pregnancies early enough to intervene to improve the chances of a good outcome. With the staggering costs of neonatal intensive care, it takes only a few improved outcomes to yield dramatic savings. Methods for identifying cases include sending out information about pregnancy to all members, reviewing the claims system for pregnancy-related claims, asking (or requiring) the PCPs and obstetricians to notify the plan when a delivery is expected, and so forth. After the UM department is informed of the case, the member may be proactively contacted, and a questionnaire may be given to assess for risk factors (eg, very young maternal age, diabetes, medical problems, and so forth). If risk factors are noted, then the plan coordinates prenatal care in a very proactive manner. Although it is impossible to force a member to seek care and to follow up on problems, it is possible to increase the amount and quality of prenatal care that is delivered. A special problem exists when the pregnant patient is also abusing drugs; close coordination with the substance abuse program must then occur.

The degree to which the plan can become involved in LCM is in part a function of the benefits structure. In a tightly run managed health care plan, it is common for the UM department to be proactive in LCM; in simple PPOs, LCM is often voluntary on the part of the member (in other words, if the member chooses not to cooperate, there is little impact on benefits). Even in situations requiring strictly voluntary cooperation by the members and physicians, it is surprising how often LCM can be highly effective.

In addition to the standard methods of managing utilization, LCM often involves two other techniques. First is the use of community resources. Some catastrophic cases require support structures to help the member function or even return home. Examples of such support include family members, social service agencies, churches, special foundations, and so forth.

The other common technique is to go beyond the contractual benefits to manage the case. For example, if the benefits structure of the group has only limited coverage for durable medical equipment, it may still be in the plan's interest to cover such expenses to get the patient home and out of the hospital. In self-funded groups, the group administrator may actually be willing to fund benefits outside the contract simply as a benefit for an employee or dependent who is experiencing a terrible medical problem.

In all events, the hallmark of LCM is longitudinal management of the case by a single UM nurse or department. Management spans hospital care, rehabilitation, outpatient care, professional services, home care, ancillary services, and so forth. It is in the active coordination of care that both quality and cost-effectiveness are maintained.

CONCLUSION

The provision of basic medical-surgical services involves a broad continuum of care. Managing utilization of these services must focus on managing basic demand, managing referral and specialty services, and managing institutional services.

The management of referral and specialty services affects not only professional expenses but costs associated with testing and procedures, including hospitalization, that may be generated by the consultant. The ability to select only those consultants and referral specialists who practice cost-effectively can yield cost savings, but optimal control depends on an authorization system, and lack of such a system will hamper your abilities to meaningfully decrease utilization over the long term.

The control of hospital or institutional utilization is one of the most important aspects of controlling overall health care costs. The methods used to control hospital utilization vary from relatively weak and mechanical to tightly controlled, longitudinally integrated, and highly labor intensive. The control of hospital utilization is a function that must be attended to every day to achieve optimal results, and special attention must be paid to LCM to produce the greatest savings.

REFERENCES

1. Robinson JS, Schwartz ML, Magwene KS, Krengel SA, Tamburello D. The impact of fever health education on clinical utilization. *Am J Dis Child.* 1989;143:698–704.
2. Goldstein MA. *Modern Healthcare.* August 21, 1995: 126–130.
3. Vickery DM, Kalmer H, Lowry D, et al. Effect of a self-care education program on medical visits. *JAMA.* 1983;250:2952–2956.
4. Elsenhans VD. Use of self-care manual shifts utilization pattern. *HMO Practice.* June 1995.
5. Burton WN, Hoy DA. First Chicago's integrated health data management computer system. *Managed Care Q.* 1993;1(3):18–23.
6. Glenn JK, Lawler FH, Hoerl MS. Physician referrals in a competitive environment: an estimate of the economic impact of a referral. *JAMA.* 1987;258:1920–1923.
7. American Association of Health Plans. *1995 Sourcebook on HMO Utilization Data.* Washington, DC: American Association of Health Plans; 1995.
8. Dietrich AJ, Nelson EC, Kirk JW, et al. Do primary physicians actually manage their patients' fee-for-service care? *JAMA.* 1988;259:3145–3149.
9. Hillman BJ, Joseph CA, Mabry MR, et al. Frequency and costs of diagnostic imaging in office practice—a comparison of self-referring and radiologist-referring physicians. *N Engl J Med.* 1990;323:1604–1608.
10. Office of the Inspector General. *Financial Arrangements between Physicians and Health Care Businesses: Report to Congress.* Dept of Health and Human Services Publication no. OAI-12-88-01410. Washington, DC: Department of Health and Human Services; 1989.
11. State of Florida Health Care Cost Containment Board. *Joint Ventures among Health Care Providers in Florida.* Tallahassee, FL: State of Florida; 1991.
12. The Ethics in Patient Referrals Act—Omnibus Budget Reconciliation Act of 1989.
13. Health Care Knowledge Resources. *Length of Stay by Diagnosis and Operation.* Ann Arbor, MI: Health Care Knowledge Resources; 1991.
14. Chassin MR, Brook RH, Park RE, et al. Variations in the use of medical and surgical services by the Medicare population. *N Engl J Med.* 1986;314:285–290.
15. Smits HL. Medical practice variations revisited. *Health Aff.* Fall 1986:91–96.

16. Wennberg J, Gittelsohn A. Variations in medical care among small areas. *Sci Am*. April 1982:120–135.
17. Wennberg JE, Freeman JL, Culp WJ. Are hospital services rationed in New Haven or overutilized in Boston? *Lancet*. 1987;1:1185–1189.
18. Chassin MR, Kosecoff J, Park RE, et al. Does inappropriate use explain geographic variations in the use of health care services? A study of three procedures. *JAMA*. 1987;258:2533–2537.
19. Axene DV, Doyle RL. *Research Report: Analysis of Medically Unnecessary Inpatient Services*. Milliman & Robertson; 1994.
20. Kelley SK, Trutlein JJ. A survey of human resources in managed care organizations. *Physician Executive*. 1992;18(6):49–51.
21. Doyle RL. *Healthcare Management Guidelines, Vol 1: Inpatient and Surgical Care*. Milliman & Robertson; 1990.
22. InterQual. *The ISD-A Review System with Adult Criteria*. Chicago: InterQual; 1991.
23. InterQual. *Surgical Indications Monitoring SIM III*. Chicago: InterQual; 1991.
24. Utilization Mangement Associates. *Managed Care Appropriateness Protocol (MCAP)*. Wellesley, MA: Utilization Management Associates; 1991.
25. Rapoport J, Gehlbach S, Lemeshow S, Teres D. Resource utilization among intensive care patients: managed care vs. traditional insurance. *Arch Intern Med*. 1992;152:2207–2212.
26. Billi JE, Hejna GF, Wolf FM, et al. The effects of a cost-education program on hospital charges. *J Gen Intern Med*. 1987;2:306–311.

CHAPTER 16

The Hospitalist Model: A Method for Managing Inpatient Care

David W. Plocher, Jean Stanford, and Bruce Meltzer

Chapter Outline

- Introduction
- The Hospitalist Model
- The Hospitalist Model and Clinical Outcomes
- The Hospitalist Model and Community Physicians
- Hospitalists and the Continuum of Care for Patients and Families
- Some Potential Pitfalls
- Recruiting and Managing Hospitalists
- Conclusion

> We're really popular with local physicians around the holidays.
>
> —*A hospitalist, commenting on local physician acceptance of a hospitalist program*

INTRODUCTION

The "hospitalist" model of inpatient care is gaining considerable popularity across the country (see Chapter 15 for a description of the traditional models of inpatient care in a managed care setting, as well as a brief description of where this model of inpatient care fits into the overall scheme of advanced care management). Many hospitals are considering hiring hospitalists, many multispecialty groups are assigning some of their own members to full-time hospital duties, and several payers are even providing their own hospitalists in high-volume inpatient settings.

Some movements, such as the ones involving creation of physician–hospital organizations (PHOs) or the purchase of physician practices, gain rapid momentum for competitive reasons—rather like a prairie fire sweeping through hospital board rooms (for further discussion of these types of organizational models, see *The Managed Health Care Handbook,* 3rd Edition, Aspen Publishers, 1996). In this chapter, we intend to provide physicians and health care executives with insight into the hospitalist model so that its best features can be adopted, if appropriate, and some of its already-apparent pitfalls can be avoided.

THE HOSPITALIST MODEL

"Hospitalist" is a relatively new term; it was coined by Wachter and Goldman in 1996 in the *New England Journal of Medicine.*[1] They describe "a new breed of physicians we call 'hospitalists'—specialists in inpatient medicine—who will be responsible for managing the care of hospitalized patients in the same way that primary care physicians are responsible for managing the care of outpatients."

As Bruce Meltzer observes, there is little difference between what a hospitalist does and what a third-year resident does (personal communication, January 1998). Indeed that is correct, agrees John Nelson, a hospitalist since 1988 and cofounder of the National Association of Inpatient Physicians, except that hospitalists are paid more than third-year residents (personal communication, January 1998). This raises an obvious potential barrier for transfer of this model into an academic medical center, though creative management can potentially overcome this barrier and capitalize on an already-built structure.

According to Christine Wiebe, "Most hospitalists were trained as general internists, while others are specialists, such as pulmonologists or critical care physicians. Some work for hospitalist groups who contract with primary care physicians to cover their patients in the hospital, while others work for hospitals or managed care groups. Some multispecialty groups have rotating hospitalist duty, where an internist from the group is always on duty at the hospital to handle the group's inpatients. Some hospitalists rotate between inpatient and outpatient settings, while others work exclusively in the hospital. Hours vary, too, with some hospitalists working from 9 AM to 5 PM, while others work long blocks of time with similar periods off."[2]

Managed care payers are looking closely at the hospitalist program. Many of them, in fact, pioneered the concept in the United States. Kaiser (which refers to hospitalists with the colorful term of "rounders"),[3–5] Family Health Plan (FHP; since acquired by PacifiCare), Humana Health Plans,[4] and a number of others use hospitalists for inpatient care.

There is a distinction between the term "hospitalist" and the term "intensivist," which is also widely used. An intensivist specializes in the management of critically ill patients, usually in an intensive care setting.[6–9] A hospitalist primarily deals with patients with internal medicine problems (chest pain, pneumonia, abdominal pain), whether critical or not, that require inpatient hospitalization. Very few hospitalists handle obstetric, pediatric, or oncology cases, according to Nelson (personal communication, January 1998).

Health economist Uwe Reinhardt of Princeton University notes that physicians used to make a significant portion of their incomes by taking care of inpatients but that managed care is reversing economic incentives in favor of outpatient care.[3] Thus, as ambulatory care becomes a much more important part of a physician's revenue base, it makes less economic sense for each physician to manage inpatients as well as outpatients. Reinhardt believes that the hospitalist model is cost-effective and will be adopted widely across the United States.

Indeed, the model is being used in a number of communities, urban and rural. Mahendr S. Kochar, professor of medicine and dean of graduate medical education at the Medical College of Wisconsin, said the number of hospitalists, now estimated at about 2,000 in the United States, eventually will grow to 20,000 or more.[10] Hospitals from Muskegon, Michigan,[3] to San Diego have adopted the model. Wachter predicts that

> the hospitalist model will become the predominant form of hospital care throughout the country, as it already has become in San Francisco, San Diego, and Minneapolis. This is an example of the newly competitive health care market forcing the system to reexamine traditional ways of providing medical care. The model it has produced appears to reduce costs without compromising quality of care, patient satisfaction, doctors' satisfaction, or medical teaching.[11]

As Wachter and Goldman point out, the hospitalist model has been in wide use in Europe and Canada for many years. W. Rubenstein commented in the *New England Journal of Medicine*[12] that he had been practicing under the hospitalist model in Canada for 20 years. However, his hospital had recently converted a 30-bed ward, he reported, *from* a hospitalist care model *to* a community physician model and found that patient satisfaction increased, length of stay decreased, and continuity of care improved due to the community physicians' knowledge of the patients, families, and care resources in their neighborhoods.

As with most fads and other popular ideas, some institutions may adopt the hospitalist model too hastily, overlooking the model's limitations. Rather than rapidly converting to a hospitalist model without considering the ramifications, institutions must carefully examine the hospitalist model and tune the model to make it most useful for them.

THE HOSPITALIST MODEL AND CLINICAL OUTCOMES

Wachter and Goldman argue that use of hospitalists should result in better quality of care. Wachter states

> While a typical primary care doctor may supervise the care of one or two hospitalized patients as part of their day, a hospitalist generally cares for about 20 hospitalized patients on a full-time basis. The primary care doctor, as a result, may see fewer than five patients annually suffering from any one condition requiring hospitalization. The hospitalist may care for as many as 50 patients annually who suffer from the same condition. The increased expertise born of the greater experience of hospitalists coupled with their greater availability makes a compelling argument for the new model.[11]

For example, Elizabeth Tucker-Sanfelippo, member of a hospitalist team in Milwaukee, was quoted in the *Milwaukee Journal Sentinel* as saying: "We are here 24 hours a day, so we know where things are. The more you do hospital skills, the better you get. It's easy to realize the efficiencies."[10] As recounted by Ken Terry,[3] the advent of managed care revealed the lack of knowledge that some primary care physicians had about management of the acutely ill. Some capitated providers felt that primary care physicians were too quick to call specialists to manage inpatient episodes. Terry describes an independent practice association (IPA; or perhaps more accurately, an open panel plan [see the glossary]) that established a hospitalist program to get better control of inpatient costs.[3]

Payers appreciate the availability of hospitalists in the inpatient care setting because they believe that hospitalists can streamline the delivery of care so that patients can be discharged sooner, simply because they will not be waiting for orders to be written or test results examined. Every day spent waiting for physician input costs the payers a great deal of money.[4]

One important advantage of hospitalists is that full-time inpatient physicians become very familiar with care pathways and can implement them more efficiently than community practitioners who encounter them infrequently. However, this very familiarity may lead to some conflict with the patient's community physician, especially if the hospitalist is following a pathway that recommends care at home that the community physician would have treated as inpatient care.[3] If the community physician is accustomed to hospitalizing a patient with pneumonia and the hospitalist is following a care path that does not call for hospitalization, there may be conflicts between the two physicians.

No peer-reviewed comparative studies of hospitalists' cost/quality of care have been done to our knowledge. However, many institutions that employ hospitalists are measuring their effectiveness for their own purposes. Scripps Health Corporation found that hospitalists made a significant difference in length of stay.[3] Since they formed their hospitalist program in 1992, emergency department (ED) admissions have declined and bed days have dropped by about 35% for commercial patients.[3] Patient satisfaction ratings have remained about the same for hospitalist-managed versus community-physician-managed patients. Long Island Jewish Medical Center found that its hospitalist program decreased its patients' hospital stays by 17% and dropped costs per hospital stay by 15% without affecting satisfaction and quality.[13] Park Nicollet Clinic in Minneapolis has been using hospitalists for 3 years and has found that average stays dropped a half day and costs per stay plunged 20%, with no change in patient satisfaction rates.[14] Since the hospitalist program was instituted, "Park Nicollet's average length of stay for the 17 most common DRGs [diagnosis-related groups] has decreased from 4.8 to 4 days. For the 12 most expensive DRGs, the average hospital bill per patient has dropped from $7,100 to $5,300. Specialist referrals also dropped by 12 percent in the program's first year."[3(p66)]

THE HOSPITALIST MODEL AND COMMUNITY PHYSICIANS

There may be vehement objections to hospitalist programs when they are first proposed in a community. Some physicians strongly resist changes to their practice patterns and do not believe that the same quality of care can be maintained if the patient's regular physician does not manage the case.[5]

While some organizations are hiring hospitalists in order to improve the efficiency of inpatient care, others are doing it to help strengthen their relationships with community physicians by relieving them of the burden of dashing across town to make rounds at lunch or taking night calls for ED admissions.[3] "The hospitalist is my other arm," said Harry Jacob, a Long Island internist for 22 years. "While I am sitting in my office, the hospitalist, who is efficient at expediting medical care, can tell me what is going on with my patients in the hospital."[13(p1)] Tibbett Speer reports that primary care physicians in groups using hospitalists gain 4 hours of office time per week to see patients because they no longer must do rounds.[14] Anecdotally, some community physicians also comment that they are now freed of hospital committee meeting obligations, which they see as a benefit.

Primary care physicians have more responsibilities under managed care than they did under indemnity systems because they have acquired so-called gatekeeper (or perhaps more appropriately, care management) responsibilities. As gatekeepers, primary care physicians are responsible for closely monitoring their ambulatory patients (eg, managing referrals to specialists). Adding intensive cost management of inpatients to this load is perhaps going to be the straw that breaks the camel's back. Since hospitalized patients now are usually sicker and often have multisystem disease, and since close management can dramatically reduce length of stay and inpatient costs, it is a real burden for primary care providers to remain in close contact with a few inpatients as well as their full office load.[14,15] It appears to be more efficient to pay a full-time hospitalist to manage 20 inpatients than to have 10 primary care providers going back and forth to the hospital to manage two patients each.

Specialists often find the hospitalist programs to be threatening, at least initially. The major concerns seem to be potential loss of referrals (which is not as big an issue in capitated environments) and disruption of existing referral relationships with primary care physicians. The former may well be a real concern, because hospitalists do become more adept at managing patients with fewer specialty referrals as they become more skilled at intense inpatient care. The latter can be managed by paying close attention to the primary care providers' wishes on referrals and retaining those patterns as much as possible. A hospitalist program that does not respect the community physicians' referral patterns will have more acceptance problems than one that does not disrupt them.

An alternative perspective on the generalist hospitalist is offered by Morris Jutcovich, proponent of the specialist hospitalist (personal communication). Dr. Jutcovich, President of MEDEXCEL, maintains that the advantages over the generalist include the following:

- Primary care physicians can still have their preferred specialty care physicians see their patients. Specialty care physicians do not have to face a workload reduction, because each specialty care physician hospitalist is still allowed access to primary care physi-

cians who have previously been referral sources.
- Specialty care physicians are assigned the case types specifically matching their specialty.
- Specialty care physicians use fewer consultants than generalist hospitalists.
- At least in Dr. Jutcovich's organization, specialty care physicians can conduct office follow-up on the same patients after discharge because they maintain an office practice for MEDEXCEL.

HOSPITALISTS AND THE CONTINUUM OF CARE FOR PATIENTS AND FAMILIES

One concern that is often voiced about the hospitalist movement is whether hospitalists will have the opportunity to know their patients if they see them only during inpatient episodes. As some physicians point out, families and patients are stressed when someone is sick enough to be admitted. It may be asking a lot to expect them to start building a relationship with a new physician. "There is life before and life after a hospitalization," agreed John Eisenberg, administrator of the federal Agency for Health Care Policy and Research. "It's pretty tough to get to know people in 4.9 days," he said, referring to the average length of a hospital stay. "I think it's a very serious concern that the continuity of care could suffer from these hand-offs."[2] "We view it with concern for what it means for the patient," said Robert Graham, executive vice president of the American Academy of Family Physicians. "Hospitalization can be a time when the patient feels most vulnerable. That can be a terrible time to lose contact with the physician that you've come to trust."[2]

Yet the patient satisfaction results discussed above show that patients have quickly become accustomed to hospitalists and do not seem to bear out the concerns—at least at those hospitals reporting results. Perhaps the key ingredient in promoting patient satisfaction is focusing on service as an important ingredient in the hospitalist program—perhaps as important as or even more important than the focus on cutting the length of stay.

SOME POTENTIAL PITFALLS

There are some potential downsides to the hospitalist model. Val Dean, executive vice president and chief operating officer of Colorado's largest health plan, FHP of Colorado, Inc, was quoted in the *Denver Business Journal* as saying that "primary care physicians actually enjoy an informal 'continuing education' program by visiting their patients in the hospitals and learning from the specialists and other physicians at the facility. What are we going to do to substitute for that kind of education? I think we can come up with it, but we must make sure we are smart about it."[5]

Other physicians are not so sure that this is a real issue. They point out that few community physicians are in solo practices any more, so they interact with other members of their practice group. In addition, there are many opportunities for community physicians to interact with specialists and other physicians in the course of managing ambulatory care.

Some wonder whether the hospitalist movement will provide only temporary efficiencies. Eisenberg believes that the efficacy of hospitalists is probably situational.[2] His assessment is that in the long run the most promising model will be the large multispecialty group rotation model. This would allow the group physicians to maintain patient relationships, and the inpatient physicians would be communicating closely with the physicians in their own group. The efficiency of the hospitalist would be combined with the close collaboration of group practice.

Other pitfalls concern the selection of physicians for hospitalist positions. If these physicians are not well respected in the physician community, it will be hard to get community physicians to entrust their patients to them. If there is no emphasis on service to the community physicians, if the hospitalists rupture long-standing specialty referral patterns that the community physicians have established, if patients feel depersonalized or brushed off, then the hospitalist model will indeed fail.

Financial arrangements may be a pitfall, though the literature offers few examples where financial arrangements have proven difficult. Kaiser, a capitated system, uses hospitalists, but so do hospitals that are still primarily in a fee-for-service environment. Anyone considering implementing a hospitalist program would be well advised to investigate payment issues, but most payers are in favor of hospitalist programs and have an incentive to help make the project work.

RECRUITING AND MANAGING HOSPITALISTS

The physicians who opt for a hospitalist position seem to be motivated by the chance to deal with complex patient situations and challenging cases.[2,10,14,16] They appear not only to want the challenges of caring for acutely ill patients but also to prefer a practice style of intense work for a period of time followed by complete freedom while other hospitalists take all calls. They also seem to appreciate the sense of closure that acute inpatient care provides. There is a very limited, though intense, period of patient contact, then the patient either is discharged or has deceased. The patients do not usually keep returning to manage chronic problems. ED physicians have similar experiences.

It is possible that hospitalists will not be able to maintain their positions for their entire careers. "I just burned out," Denver physician Lawrence Repsher, a pulmonologist and former hospitalist, told the *Denver Business Journal*. "It's a pretty tough life. I enjoyed it, especially the challenges, but it got to be old. I wanted my nights and weekends. It's a young man's game."[5]

Employed hospitalists' compensation seems to run between $100,000 and $200,000, according to published reports.[2,17] Compensation slightly in excess of the office-based physician might be warranted in light of the higher technology demands, as well as the round-the-clock working hours.

There is some variation in hospitalist scheduling. Some hospitalists work shifts; others work intensively for long periods (as long as several weeks) and then get a large block of time off.[2,18] There can be a major disadvantage to using the shift approach. If the hospitalist works a 12-hour shift, for example, patients may see several hospitalists in one inpatient episode. Combine this physician rotation with the discontinuity of care from the patient's primary care physician and there is real potential for care management problems, as well as patient dissatisfaction.[19] There may be equal disadvantages in block scheduling due to exhaustion, so there may be no one right answer to the scheduling problem. Santiago[18] reports that one physician is totally exhausted on the last day of a 1-week block. The pace may not be sustainable. Furthermore, it is unclear whether the hospitalist can be viewed by the family as the appropriate counselor and confidant when the patient is facing end-of-life care decisions.

CONCLUSION

The hospitalist model has the potential of transforming and streamlining the care of acutely ill inpatients. Further, by working only in hospitals, hospitalists have the opportunity to identify and implement useful innovations in patient care that would be difficult for community-based physicians to deploy. As with any new movement, there is a possibility of going overboard. When considering a hospitalist program, it is important to consider the following issues:

- what the hospitalist skill mix (intensivists, specialists, generalists) will be
- whether the hospitalists will rotate (as some multispecialty groups are doing) or will be dedicated entirely to inpatient work (if they rotate, there will be discontinuity with their outpatient panel; if they are dedicated to inpatient work only, there is a real danger of burnout)
- how the program will be reimbursed for hospitalists' services (fee for service, capitation, etc)
- how to recruit and retain hospitalists who

are respected by their peers and able to communicate well with patients and families who are under stress
- how to maintain excellent communication with community physicians to preserve the quality of care and ensure that the patient is discharged back to a service that fully understands the patient's condition and care plan
- how to ensure continuity of care for patients during their inpatient stay as hospitalists go on and off duty and how to rapidly build a trusting relationship with patients as they are admitted to the hospitalists' care
- how to keep the ambulatory physicians from losing their acute care skills entirely and how to prevent isolation from peers that may result from office-only practices
- how to manage relationships with specialty physicians to ease their concerns about displacement and maintain their relationships with their community physicians

This model of care management for hospitalized patients in a managed care setting has much to offer, but care must be taken not to embrace it without exploring the advantages and disadvantages of the model.

REFERENCES

1. Wachter RM, Goldman L. The emerging role of "hospitalists" in the American health care system. *N Engl J Med.* 1996;335(7):514–517.
2. Wiebe C. Physicians turn to hospital practice in new 'specialty' (hospitalists merge general medicine with inpatient care). *Am Med News.* 1997;40(33).
3. Terry K. Discharging primary care doctors from hospital rounds. *Med Econ.* 1996;73(22).
4. Balaban D. HMOs spawn new specialists. *Kans City Business J.* 1997:1.
5. Smith B. "Hospitalists" challenge traditional care: new specialty of doctors spreads in metro area. *Denver Business J.* 1997;48(26):2B(3).
6. Carlson RW, Weiland DE, Srivathsan K. Does a full-time, 24-hour intensivist improve care and efficiency? *Crit Care Clin.* 1996;12(3):525–551.
7. Teener JW, Raps EC, Galetta SL. Intensive care neurology. *Curr Opin Neurol.* 1994;7(6):525–529.
8. Scheinkestel CD. The evolution of the intensivist: from health care provider to economic rationalist and ethicist. *Med J Aust.* 1996;164(5):310–312.
9. Cunnion RE, Masur H. Physician staffing in intensive-care units (commentary). *Lancet.* 1996;348(9040):1464–1465.
10. Manning J. Doctor in the house: hospitalists save time for other doctors, patients. *Milwaukee J Sentinel.* September 7, 1997:1.
11. Wachter RM. Press release, University of California at San Francisco via DowVision. November 19, 1997.
12. Rubenstein W. The role of "hospitalists" in the health care system. *N Engl J Med.* 1997;336(6):445.
13. Nahas DK. A new breed in medicine: "hospitalist." *NY Times.* January 11, 1998.
14. Speer TL. The balancing breed: hospitals use specialist physicians instead of primary care doctors to control costs. *Hosp Health Networks.* 1997;71(3):44(3).
15. Reiff A. Doctors speak out on area health care trends. *Cent Penn Business J.* 1997;13(13):21.
16. Benmour E. Caritas to hire "hospitalist" who will oversee patient care. *Business First—Louisville.* 1997;13(52):12.
17. Jeffrey NA. Hospitalists let internists, family doctors skip rounds. *Wall Street J.* May 20, 1997:A1.
18. Santiago R. The doctors are in. *Crain's Cleve Business.* 1997;18(31):17.
19. Erikson J. Turmoil in Tucson: physicians at Thomas-Davis Medical Centers P.C. battle owners FPA Medical Management Inc. *Am Med News.* 1997;40(34):1.

JEAN STANFORD is the associate director of health care consulting at Ernst & Young in Washington, DC. She is a specialist in health care delivery markets and how they are evolving across the United States. She was the technical lead for the development of the spider model for the analysis of health care markets, for internal IDS analysis, for governance, and for physician integration. Previously, Ms. Stanford worked for IBM and a number of health care organizations, including the George Washington University Medical Center.

BRUCE MELTZER, MD, works for the Center for Health Care Emerging Technology for Ernst & Young in Boston, Massachusetts.

Chapter 17

Case Management and Managed Care

Catherine M. Mullahy

Chapter Outline

- The Case Manager's Role
- Patient Profile: Not Every Case Needs a Case Manager
- On-Site Versus Telephone-Based Case Management
- Case Managers in Managed Care
- The Case Management Work Format and Process
- Utilization Review: Preadmission and Concurrent Review and Case Management
- Preadmission and Concurrent Review Case Management Reports
- Red Flags: Indicators for Case Management
- Timing Case Management Intervention
- Beyond the Case Management Basics
- A Long-Term Solution to a Long-Term Problem

THE CASE MANAGER'S ROLE

Managed care and *case management* are not interchangeable concepts. Managed care is a system of cost containment programs; case management is a process. It is one component in the managed care strategy.

The following definition of case management has been adopted by the developers of the leading credentialing process for case managers, the Commission for Case Manager Certification (CCMC), previously the Certification of Insurance Rehabilitation Specialists Commission (CIRSC): "Case management is a collaborative process which assesses, plans, implements, coordinates, monitors, and evaluates the options and services required to meet an individual's health needs, using communication and available resources to promote quality, cost-effective outcomes." The credentialing group went on to clarify the role by stating that case management is not episodic but "occurs across a continuum of care, addressing ongoing individual needs" rather than being restricted to a single practice setting.[1(p1)]

Case managers work in the provider sector in hospitals, rehabilitation facilities, managed care organizations, home health agencies, infusion care companies, and other practice settings, as well as in the payer sector, representing employers through third-party administrators (TPAs) or self-administered programs, employed within health maintenance programs or by major insurance carriers. Independent case managers, professionals working outside the medical care provider and claims payer systems, can be found

---

This chapter is adapted from CM Mullahy, Case Management and Managed Care, in *The Managed Health Care Handbook*, 3rd ed, PR Kongstvedt, ed, pp 274–300, © 1996, Aspen Publishers, Inc.

in any of the practice settings mentioned and may also be working directly for a patient or other family member.

Case managers are not the claims police. Though they work to ensure cost-effective treatment, case managers are not overrated number crunchers who review treatment simply to find the cheapest scenario. Case managers are coordinators of care, catalysts, problem solvers, facilitators, impartial advocates, and educators.[2] They are professional collaborators with physicians and negotiators with durable medical equipment providers, home health care agencies, therapists, and many other providers. They make certain that the patient is following the treatment plan prescribed by the physician and that the equipment delivered to the home is the equipment that was ordered, not the same bed's super-deluxe version, which just happens to cost $400 more per week. As a liaison with insurance claims staff, case managers clarify claims information. With benefits personnel, and in the best interests of the patient and the payer, they sometimes pursue alternatives to the plan package.

PATIENT PROFILE: NOT EVERY CASE NEEDS A CASE MANAGER

For years, it has been known that most health care costs are generated by the 3% to 5% of patients that are at high risk, critically injured, or suffering from a chronic disease. As an example, in one 10-month period, one firm spent over $1.8 million in health care benefits for its employees and their dependents (2,520 covered lives). Fully half of that cost was distributed to 30 individuals (4% of the employees). This means that one half of the benefit dollars spent, over $900,000, was focused on 1.1% of the total covered population. Twenty-two employees spent $588,702; expressed differently, 3% of the employees accounted for 33% of the group's total in paid claims—or, 0.9% or *less* than 1% of those covered spent 33% of the dollars.[2]

In an insurer's review of its plan year covering 11,000 employees, a report showed health benefits expenditures of $36 million. A program designed to flag each case totaling more than $50,000 produced 35 cases responsible for $5 million in benefits. Those 35 cases represent 0.3% of the employees; less than one half of 1% of the group spent 14% of the group's dollars.[2] This is the central message of this chapter: you don't have to manage all of the patients all of the time. You do have to track those complex cases, those patients who are most likely to fall through the cracks in our health care delivery system because of the layers of care they require.

By developing systems to identify and manage the high-risk, high-cost cases (cancer, acquired immune deficiency syndrome [AIDS], stroke, transplant, head injury, severe burns, high-risk pregnancy, neonates, spinal cord injuries, neuromuscular diseases, etc) from day one, case management promotes quality care and contains costs. By wrapping the case management approach around all lines of medical coverage, case managers can be appropriately attentive to potentially problematic cases, more creative in problem solving, and better able to address spiraling expenses before they take off. The cost-to-savings ratio will vary depending on the case. (If a case manager is not saving any money, he or she is doing something wrong.) At the low end, savings might be 1:3; at the high end, for a well-managed traumatic brain injury or premature baby case, savings of 1:30 to 1:50 can be expected. As a bonus, case management also tackles other problem areas that push up health care costs and concerns: patient compliance, prevention of complications, patient satisfaction with medical services, and timely return to work. According to the National Pharmaceutical Council's Task Force on Noncompliance, the annual cost of noncompliance alone exceeds $100 billion every year.[3] A case manager's professional intervention and guidance improves patient outcomes and morale by providing direct communication and personal attention, helps make the best use of limited benefit dollars, and helps eliminate repeated occurrences of the same afflictions.

Throughout the course of care, the case manager will work in four major areas of activity:

medical, financial, behavioral/motivational, and vocational.

Medical Activities

This area encompasses all those activities a case manager performs to ensure that the patient receives the most effective medical and nursing care, including the following:

- contacting the patient in the hospital, in the rehabilitation unit, or at home to assess the patient's condition, understanding of his or her injury and its ramifications, and ability or predisposition to follow the treatment plan
- contacting the members of the medical treatment team (the physician, nursing staff, clinical practitioners, rehabilitation therapists, etc) to discuss the patient's course of progress and needs, and utilizing the information in discharge planning and the initial needs assessment
- arranging for all services required for discharge or relocation (equipment, home nursing care, therapy, transportation, transfer to another facility, home utilities, etc); coordinating efforts with the primary registered nurse (RN), discharge planner, or social services administrator to eliminate duplication of service and conserve benefit dollars
- visiting with the family
- checking the home for safety factors and architectural barriers and arranging for any needed safety aids and modifications
- on follow-up, reevaluating equipment, ensuring supplies are replenished, monitoring home nursing services, and arranging for equipment repair; evaluating activities of daily living, home programs, and modifications to treatment
- identifying problems, anticipating complications and acting to avoid them, providing health instruction to the patient and family, and referring the patient back to the physician or other health team member when appropriate
- identifying plateaus, improvements, regressions, and depressions; counseling accordingly or recommending help
- making personal visits or contacting the physician or other appropriate practitioner to clarify the diagnosis, prognosis, therapy, activities of daily living, expected permanent disability, and so on
- assisting in obtaining payer authorizations for any modalities of treatment recommended, and investigating and suggesting alternative treatments when appropriate
- assisting in obtaining information and forms regarding a living will, health care proxy, do-not-resuscitate order, etc
- acting as a liaison between the physician and the insurance company when necessary
- sharing pertinent information about the patient with the physician and working together with the physician to achieve the best outcome

Financial Activities

Some of the specific services a case manager might contribute on behalf of a patient include

- assessing the patient's benefit plan (indemnity, group medical, managed care, workers' compensation, disability, auto, dental, disease-specific, etc) for coverage and limitations; negotiating with the plan for out-of-plan coverage as appropriate to make best use of the plan's financial resources
- negotiating for more cost-effective rates for provider services
- suggesting medically appropriate alternatives (a timely move from an acute care facility to a skilled nursing facility or home care, for example) to accomplish treatment plan goals more cost-effectively
- counseling the patient or family on budgeting and notifying creditors
- identifying financial distress and referring the patient or family to appropriate community resources

- helping the patient or family sort and prioritize unpaid bills
- acting as a liaison among the insurance company, referral source, employer, patient, and family to alleviate financial and other problems or misunderstandings
- educating the payer regarding the risk (financial exposure) of noncompliant, untreated, or unmanaged cases, and the documented success rates medical case management achieves, protecting payer funds

Behavioral/Motivational Activities

- exploring the patient's feelings about him- or herself and his or her injury or illness and helping the patient with the associated trauma and frustration
- monitoring the family's feelings regarding the patient's illness and observing the family's ability or inability to manage under new emotional stress
- offering reassurance and information about the patient's condition
- if qualified, counseling in the areas of marital discord, role reversal, dependency, and sexual problems arising from the injury or illness

Vocational Activities

- obtaining a history of past education, employment, hobbies, and job skills and uncovering vocational interests and future goals
- if appropriate, overseeing psychovocational testing, work evaluations, schooling, on-the-job situations, transportation, and anything else needed to assist the patient in becoming or remaining gainfully employed
- assisting the patient in using the recuperative period in a constructive fashion (studying, upgrading skills, preparing for job interviews, etc)
- visiting the patient's place of employment and talking with the personnel director or immediate supervisor about the employer's expectations and the patient's needs
- completing a job analysis and discussing the possibility of the patient's return to work in the same job, perhaps after job modification or lightening of duties
- sharing the above information with physician at appropriate times[2]

ON-SITE VERSUS TELEPHONE-BASED CASE MANAGEMENT

Case management is not a hands-on role. Case managers are not actively practicing nurses, clinicians, or caregivers. They do not diagnose an ailment, prescribe a medication, or set the course of treatment. They do offer their expertise and observations to suggest alternative care options. Using on-site visits and information-gathering conversations, a case manager can make sure a noncompliant patient is following the treatment plan outlined by the physician or note the possible complications from the medications recommended by the patient's ear, nose, and throat specialist but never mentioned to his or her cardiologist.

Although case managers do not offer hands-on care, they cannot be truly effective if every case is addressed in a totally hands-off manner. Telephone work is necessary for maintaining lines of communication without driving up costs. Case management over the telephone is particularly effective for preventive and case screening measures, and for tracking low-intensity patients or patients who have improved to the point where in-person case management is no longer needed. However, when all communication among the case manager, patient, family, physician, and payer occurs over the telephone, oversights in care can result, especially in cases where the patient is noncompliant, undereducated, or poor. The vulnerability of the patient coupled with the legal and monetary exposure of the provider and payer may call for, at the least, a minimum of on-site interaction.[2]

Case management by telephone is almost always less expensive than on-site case management, and its use has grown in our current managed care environment. The increasing practice of telephone-based case management is not in itself alarming; however, the increasing prevalence of poor-quality telephone-based case management is a problem. Much information can be lost over the telephone unless the individual is very skilled and devoted to the particulars of the job. Callers are encouraged to get beyond the "no" by asking questions that demand more than a "yes" or "no" answer, and to explore answers by asking leading questions. The question is not, Are you taking your medication? but rather, What medications are you taking and when?

Many case managers are hard pressed to convince payers that on-site assessment is necessary. But if it can be established that care decisions were based only on lowering costs, employers, providers, payer groups, and case managers could be held liable in a wrongful action suit. To protect their interests and liabilities, it behooves each party to be fully aware of how care decisions are made. It is the case manager's responsibility to say "No, I must be on site to review this case" or "No, I'm unable to put that plan into action" if she or he feels the level of care being provided is substandard or places the patient at too great a risk. Further, providers need to maintain accurate outcomes data and can use case managers as their eyes and ears.

CASE MANAGERS IN MANAGED CARE

An integral part of the managed care process, case managers are introduced to patients and cases in a variety of ways. They may be a member of the discharge planning team employed on site at a hospital; part of a major insurer's in-house case management team; an independent case manager working on contract for an employer or TPA; a community-based social worker/case manager; or on staff at a rehabilitation facility, infusion therapy company, home health agency, or other provider location. The referral source might be an insurance company with clients covered under workers' compensation, auto, or group medical plans; a TPA that is paying claims for a client company; or a corporate human resources manager. It might be a state Medicaid office with case management services within a line of insurance or a population segment, such as high-risk newborns or children who are dependent on technological medical assistance. Case managers are also contacted directly by families seeking to monitor the care of an out-of-state relative or friend, for example. There are individuals and firms providing a broad range of case management services, and those specializing in specific diseases or patient groups, such as premature babies, individuals with diabetes, or those suffering from Alzheimer's disease, AIDS, or breast cancer.

For optimum outcomes, a case manager will be called in on the case as early as possible. If case management services are strategically coordinated with preadmission review and concurrent review services, early intervention and its benefits often occur. However, there are times when a case manager is not notified until a case has reached a threshold of $30,000—a little late in the game, but not past the point of no return.

Although many managed care organizations (MCOs) employ case managers as part of their utilization management departments, in other situations, case management services are outsourced to an independent case management service. Services are customarily billed on an hourly basis, or on a flat-fee basis, where a set fee is established for each review conducted. More frequently, with the increased use of managed care strategies, case management services are being purchased at a capitated rate, similar to preadmission and concurrent review services. In a capitated rate structure, a per case, per month fee is established, and it is up to managers of a case management department to accurately predict the case load and needs of the covered lives.

Case management services may be covered by language in the benefit plan or requested as an alternative to policy benefits. Sometimes part of a comprehensive managed care program, case management services are offered in conjunction with preadmission review and concurrent review. In these cases, all three services might be offered at a capitated rate, or on a stand-alone (per service, per case) basis.

THE CASE MANAGEMENT WORK FORMAT AND PROCESS

Money is pouring into our health care system. But improved treatment and services are not flowing out at the same rate. Case management is a catalyst that pushes performance to more cost-effective levels, promoting better outcomes and the maintenance of quality care.

(See the case management flowchart presented in Figure 17–1.)

Gathering and Assessing Information

A case manager's approach to a new case is influenced by the referral source (generally the payer) and the line of insurance; her or his latitude in creatively and effectively managing a

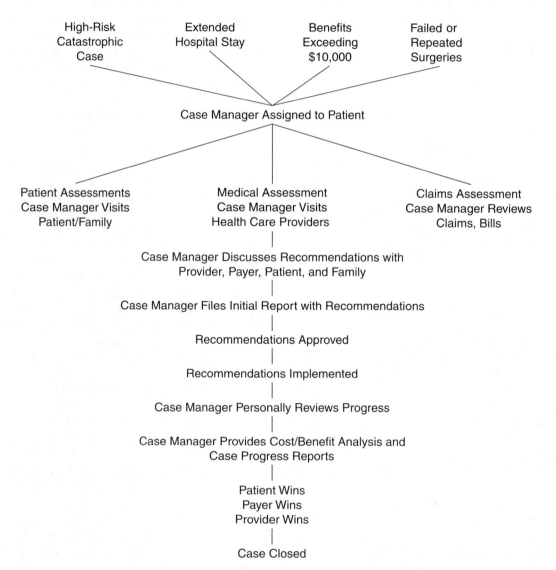

Figure 17–1 Case Management Work Format Flowchart. Courtesy of Options Unlimited, Case Management Services Division, Huntington, New York.

case will vary with the amount the payer has at risk. Generally, the self-insured employer, paying dollar-for-dollar for benefits, is more interested in and involved in the case management process and more readily approves out-of-plan benefits to make the most of benefit dollars. On the other hand, a large employer paying a capitated, one-rate-fits-all fee to a major insurer for its employees' health benefit coverage is often less inclined to work with a case manager on an individual case.

Appropriate and effective case management is possible only when the information gathered is accurate and thoughtfully analyzed. This gathering process will include conversations with the major players—the referral source or payer, patient, family, physicians, and other key members of the medical treatment team. The case manager will introduce him- or herself and explain the role of case management, making certain that each person understands what the case manager will bring to the table. Medical records must be consulted, and employers and attorneys must be contacted as needed. The right questions must be asked. Does the wheelchair fit through the doorjambs in the patient's home? Does the cardiac patient think hypertension occurs only when he has a headache, and does he take his medication accordingly? Is the wife of the man who had a massive cardiovascular accident (CVA) expecting him to be up and back in the office in a month?

Furthermore, all data must be carefully considered. Too often, case managers fall into the habit of transferring information from their notes to a report without asking themselves the same direct questions they should be asking their patients, payers, and providers: What is hindering better progress here? What can I do to encourage the patient's family to help with her care? Should I aggressively pursue this seemingly necessary service on an out-of-plan basis?

Initial Assessment

The words "initial needs assessment" carry a variety of meanings depending on the listener. An initial needs assessment is the case manager's first activity, undertaken to prepare a report to the referral source (payer) that will include a description of the patient; the patient's condition, diagnosis, and prognosis; and the case manager's recommendations. Some organizations think of an initial needs assessment as a four-page document prepared by the case manager following on-site visits with the claimant, family, physician, and employer. Others feel a thorough telephone conversation will cover their needs (and their liability), or request that the case manager visit with the patient but not with other participants in the care plan when conducting an initial needs assessment.

Talking with the Referral Source

Before beginning an initial needs assessment, the case manager should know if the patient is covered under the specific line of insurance paying for case management. To determine the client's responsibility on this case, for this individual, under this policy, it is not too rudimentary to start with the basics: What is the line of insurance? Is this patient covered under this policy? Suppose the case manager works in the preadmission and concurrent review department of a health care provider group and receives a call that James Jones has just been admitted to the hospital with which the provider group is affiliated. Upon checking, the case manager determines that James' father, John, is covered by a plan in which the group's practitioners are participating physicians (or member physicians) and that James is listed as a dependent on his father's plan. However, the case manager discovers that James' injury occurred at work, making it a workers' compensation case. James is not eligible for benefits under his father's group medical plan but may be covered under workers' compensation. (This topic is discussed in detail in *The Managed Health Care Handbook,* 3rd Edition.)

To assess the case for possible high-risk or long-term cost factors, the case manager will ask how long the patient has been ill. Even with minimum description—"The car accident occurred 2 years ago," "It's a spinal cord injury," "This is his third hospitalization in 18 months"—the case manager begins to get a clear picture of short- and long-term needs, and can begin considering any required adjustment to the treatment plan, the potential requirement for long-term case management, or a closer case review. The person in a coma rarely jumps up during week two to return to his or her normal lifestyle; hence, a long-term case management plan would be in order. If an individual citing lower back pain has been in physical therapy for 3 years, a wake-up call to the treating physician might be in order. Other questions for a case manager to put to a payer include, What dollars are available for how long? Are there any limits or restrictions on the type of care provided? Type of care facility? Length of stay? Is there coverage for a skilled nursing facility versus an acute care center? Does the provision for home nursing services include 24-hour care, or is it limited to one 4-hour shift each day?

The line of insurance itself indicates certain questions to a case manager. In workers' compensation cases, one such question is, How did the injury happen? This might be one in a series of injuries at the same workstation, causing the case manager to urge the employer's risk manager to investigate that job procedure and workstation before another employee is disabled and before the employer is facing a wrongful injury lawsuit.

More details about the case manager's conversation with the referral source follow in Exhibit 17–1.

Exhibit 17–1 Communicating with Referral Sources

1. A referral is made to the case manager by the payer, employer, hospital discharge planner, attending nurse, or the MCO's pre-certification department.
2. The case manager gets the appropriate details and confirms the needs of the referral source (eg, expectations, fees, format and time frame for reports, etc).
3. The case manager requests case background (eg, the status of the patient, the diagnosis and the prognosis, the type of insurance coverage, the patient's eligibility under the policy, the policy benefit limits, the plan's flexibility, the restrictions on care, etc).
4. The case manager confirms the initial needs assessment and report parameters in writing to the referral source and/or payer.
5. The case manager makes a follow-up call to review the confirmation letter.
6. The case manager documents all conversations.

Source: Reprinted from CM Mullahy, *The Case Manager's Handbook,* 2nd ed, p 160, © 1998, Aspen Publishers, Inc.

Talking with the Patient

When interviewing the patient, the case manager is trying to obtain an overview of the patient's current medical history, the particular individual, and the situation, as well as to encourage the patient to be participatory in his or her own care program. Initial questions will center on the patient's understanding of his or her medical diagnosis and prognosis. How does the patient view the situation? The individual might answer, "My doctor told me I have lupus." The case manager must then ask, "What do you think that means? Will it affect your lifestyle?" By listening carefully to patient responses, a case manager will be able to determine the individual's level of understanding and acceptance (or denial) of the problem.

The case manager should never assume that a patient has the ability to understand the diagnosis; the ability to accept the diagnosis; or enough information and understanding of that information to be a cooperative, compliant participant in the health care plan. Perhaps the family is withholding information from the patient in a misguided effort to protect the patient. Perhaps the referral source, the physicians, and the case manager all have a clear understanding of the patient's condition—a malignant tumor that has already metastasized to other organs—but the patient and family have no concept of how this will affect their future. They might have heard the information but chosen to edit it to a version more easy or convenient to accept. "I had a growth, but it was removed and I'm fine now." "Dad can go back to his job in 2 weeks, and my college tuition will be no problem."

A case manager also needs to be able to spot those who want to be lifelong members of the health care delivery process. Turning a chronic headache pattern into an undetectable brain tumor allows one some respite from life's greater responsibilities.

A crucial line of questioning, often overlooked by all members of the medical system, including case managers, centers on medications. There is a gap, the distance between life and death, between what a patient perceives as a problem and what the medical profession knows is a problem. Whether the patient takes an interest in his or her medications or not, the case manager should ask to see all pills and medications being taken, including over-the-counter capsules and herbal vitamins. The case manager should also ask related questions: Which of these are you taking? How often are you taking them? What do you think they are for? Sometimes patients halve their doses, stop taking medications midway through the course of treatment, or take medications only on the days when the presenting problem is noticeable. In some cases, this medical manipulation has no significant consequences. In other cases, the ill effects are harrowing.

Also important are questions regarding the patient's vocation and avocations. Is this person actively involved in a church? Other church members might provide the family with care respite. Is he or she an avid golfer, fisher, or skeet shooter? Does he or she enjoy working? An optimistic person, fully experiencing life, is more likely to be a cooperative patient than the individual who is not participatory by nature. Someone seeking to get back to all of life's business will follow a treatment plan; someone who was recently laid off may choose a "disability mentality," where the illness becomes his or her job and social life.

At the end of the interview, the case manager should obtain a signed consent form (Exhibit 17–2) from the patient or the patient's guardian. This will enable the case manager to review the patient's medical records and to share information regarding the patient with his or her physician(s) and attorney, if the case is in litigation.

Exhibit 17–2 Patient Consent Form

> **CONSENT**
>
> Date:_____
>
> To ensure appropriate medical case management services, I, _____, authorize any physician, hospital, or other professional involved in my treatment to disclose medical, hospital, vocational, or related information. I authorize that the information may be shared with other professionals, agencies, or insurance companies that may be involved in the provision or payment of necessary services.
>
> A copy of this authorization may be accepted, if necessary.
>
> Signed_____
> Guardian_____
> Witness_____
>
> *Source:* Reprinted from CM Mullahy, *The Case Manager's Handbook,* 2nd ed, p 68, © 1998, Aspen Publishers, Inc.

Talking with the Family

Families affected by an injury or illness often will experience role changes, dependency shifts, anxiety, anger, and an inability to make decisions, particularly in long-term cases. Because of this, it is helpful for a case manager to interview the family early on to determine family dynamics. Is the family taking an overprotective stance with the patient? Is the family spokesperson speaking for the patient unnecessarily? "He needs to eat more." "She isn't sleeping well." Is there so much fear associated with this illness that other members of the family are developing symptoms, having emotional outbursts, or consulting the bottle in an effort to regain a feeling of balance or control in their lives?

In many ways, the patient's health will be supported by the emotional and physical health of the family. The case manager will want to not only gauge the strength of the family structure but also compile a medical family tree. Do certain illnesses run in the family? Does the 42-year-old man recuperating after a heart attack have a family with a history of cardiac disease and middle-age deaths?

The case manager needs answers to the following questions: What was the prime caretaker's role in the family prior to this illness? Did he or she run the household? Hold down a job? Does the caretaker still have those responsibilities in addition to caring for the patient? How is the caretaker reacting to the illness? Is the caretaker physically and emotionally capable of supporting and caring for the patient?[2]

All these elements will influence the case management plan and sometimes even dictate what the case manager can hope to accomplish. For example, the family with three active, inquisitive, dial-turning children under age 7, plus an infant who requires oxygen, is going to need part-time home nursing assistance following discharge; also helpful will be an oxygen system with outdoor tanks, removing the siblings' temptation to tamper.

Talking with the Treating Physician

When a case manager works as a collaborative partner with a physician, as well as all other members of the medical team, there is greater opportunity to track a patient's progress, ensure that the patient is and remains participatory and compliant, and check that each element of the treatment plan is carried out appropriately. To build such partnerships, a case manager should schedule a personal meeting with the physician at his or her convenience when the case is complex. In less medically complex or physically distant cases, a telephone conversation with the treating physician is effective.

The case manager will ask questions such as, What is the diagnosis? What is the treatment plan and prognosis? What do you think will be the outcome for this person, both short term and long term? Do you anticipate any complications? What have you told the patient? What do you think he or she understands?[2] This last question is important because the patient, the physician, and the case manager all need to be speaking the same language. Patients often choose to forget the components of conditions that they have difficulty accepting. This impacts the treatment plan. It is the case manager's job to make certain the patient has all the information necessary to cooperate and follow the treatment plan.

If the case manager knows up front that there is a limit on care dollars, he or she has the responsibility to make the physician aware of the limit and share in the goal of using the money in the best way possible. Although some care options may be ideal, the expenses connected with them make them poor first choices. A good alternative may not be perfect, but it will not pose any risk to the patient and may cover care and services over a longer period of time.[2]

Independent Medical and Second Opinion Exams

In some cases, an independent medical exam or a second opinion exam will be requested. A case manager's involvement depends on the type of exam performed. An independent medical exam is generally used by insurance carriers to determine the diagnosis, the need for continued treatment, the degree of disability (partial or total), the duration of a disability (temporary, long-term, or permanent), and the patient's ability to return to work. Independent medical exams are requested when treatment appears excessive, when the recovery time appears overly extended, or when there is a delay in the patient's return-to-work schedule. They are also employed upon request to authorize surgery, expensive equipment, or unusual diagnostic testing, or when there is an increase in the number of treating professionals. The physician conducting the exam most often remains in a nontreating role. A case manager may assist in setting up the exam and may accompany the patient, but in most instances will not be present at the exam.

Also used to determine a diagnosis, a second opinion exam is often performed to help clarify a complex medical outlook or to prepare alternatives to the current or proposed treatment. In group medical plans, a second opinion exam is sometimes required prior to certain surgical procedures that the carrier or the latest utilization review statistics show to have a high usage rate (such as hysterectomies, hip replacements, cardiac bypass, magnetic resonance imaging scans, disc surgery, etc). Such exams are also called for when there is a conflict between potential treatment plans, when a questionable treatment is in place, or when the existing treatment plan is not achieving the expected outcome. The case manager who arranged for the second opinion exam is usually in attendance, and the physician conducting the exam often will become a treating physician.

To get greater benefit from independent medical exams and second opinion exams, a case manager should thoroughly understand the purpose of any exam ordered and be specific about what the physician's report should address. The examining physician should be given as much information as possible (operative reports, diagnostic test reports, X-rays, computed tomography [CT] scans, etc) and be given enough time to review all the data prior to the actual exam. After reviewing the physician's report to confirm that it is responsive to the initial request for information, the case manager should speak to the physician to discuss findings and clarify any unanswered issues.[2]

Talking with Service and Equipment Providers

Many case managers find it helpful to work with one representative at a durable medical equipment, home medical equipment, or home health care agency. In this way, equipment, services, contracts, and billing can all be reviewed in one phone call. In addition, it helps case managers get answers when they need them, and very often, answers are needed immediately (especially on Friday afternoons, when it seems every patient in the country is simultaneously declared ready for discharge).

Prior to selecting providers or arranging for services, a case manager should review the benefit plan contract to make certain that its language supports the use of home nursing visits, durable medical equipment, and so on. It is the case manager's responsibility to verify that the contract she or he arranges agrees with plan language and will be approved when the bill for the services/equipment finally arrives in a claims department.

There are many questions case managers should ask: What are the options included with this piece of equipment? What specifically is it designed to do? What are the terms—lease, rent, rent with option to buy, outright purchase? This patient will be using this equipment for at least 6 months; what discount will you offer for a long-term rental? Is repair service available 24 hours a day? What are the costs for various levels of service? What services do your homemakers provide, and how do they differ in price and services from the home health aides?

Talking with Community Resources

The case manager need not spend benefit plan money just because it exists. There are numerous local, state, and national agencies—as well as disease-specific organizations, foundations, and philanthropic groups—that may provide services, guidance, and equipment free of charge. The United Way, Meals on Wheels, and "I Can Cope" programs and loaner wheelchairs from the American Cancer Society are examples of available assistance. Easter Seals offers support on a sliding scale for children and adults with crippling diseases. Some local volunteer fire departments provide ambulance services at no charge.[2]

Planning

Case management is a process of identifying and solving problems. The first and key issue is whether the treatment is appropriate and being provided in the best possible setting. If the patient is not being well served, the case manager can help create a better system of care. The case manager's evaluation of the patient's current status will be the foundation for the case management plan. The case manager must look at what the patient's needs are and how they can best be met in terms of quality and cost. One factor should never drive the others; there must be equilibrium among needs, quality, and cost. Given the patient's diagnosis, current medical status, and prior medical history, is the treatment plan attaining the most desirable results? Does it appear that it will lead to an eventual recovery, or have there already been too many complications? Is the treatment plan sound? Is it appropriate, reasonable, and really necessary for this patient? Is it forcing the patient into any undue hardship or discomfort?

Is the patient in the most appropriate and most cost-effective setting for his or her problem? Imagine that John is in the hospital, his surgery has been completed, and now he is being observed and given medication, physical therapy, or pain or infusion care services. Does he have to remain in the hospital? Once patients can be effectively managed without all the expensive support services of an acute care facility, they should be moved to a more appropriate and less costly arena for care—the home or another setting.

During assessment and planning, the case manager will also be evaluating the money available and the exposure faced. Whose pocket is it, and how large is the pocket? If unlimited dollars are available, should they be spent whatever way the providers want, regardless of necessity? Sometimes this attitude does prevail. Case managers need to look for the "value-locked dollar" for a demonstration that the treatment is necessary, reasonable, and will achieve good results and that the treatment plan is the most cost-effective way to provide the requisite care.[2]

Reporting

A case manager's report back to the referral source, payer, or internal department head should reflect those issues that most concern the payer or facility. If the case manager is on staff at a health maintenance organization (HMO) and the lines of insurance are predominantly group medical, reports will address medical issues for the most part. In a disability case where the client is the employer, the case manager needs to focus on return-to-work issues. A case manager in a rehabilitation facility will detail patient progress and outcomes information, and relate it to cost. In a workers' compensation case, carriers are responsible for both medical costs and lost earnings. This payer will want to know the extent of medical involvement, the severity of injury, and the likelihood of some permanent incapacitation. When reporting to a claims supervisor, the case manager will want to include specific medical information and parenthetical explanations to help the reader interpret the medical terms (and to help educate him or her about information likely to appear in other reports regarding the diagnosis or prognosis). The desired frequency and length of case management reports should be confirmed with the referral source.

Reports should be written at least once a month. All pertinent case activity should be recorded in a specific, regular format. Readers should not be punished with months' worth of casework, and payers should not be put off with the attached large invoice. By reporting in manageable increments of 3 to 4 weeks, case managers gain better control of client files, outcomes tracking, and invoicing and keep the payer up to date on the case. Significant activities or events requiring clarification should be reported in a timely fashion, first by phone and subsequently through written documentation (within a few days).

How extensive should reports be? Some payer organizations have very specific guidelines, limiting initial report writing time to 2 hours or even a half an hour. Others request a verbal report, asking that the case manager not even take the time to send a document, even a fax. In this type of situation, the case manager needs to educate the referral source. Case management reports have practical and legal value as documents chronicling case management activity.

Suppose the case manager, during a phone conversation, reports to the payer a previously undocumented call to the patient or the physician. Will either of them remember this exchange of information? What if the case moves into litigation? What if the patient takes a turn for the worse? Especially when planning services, negotiating services, or putting alternative plans in place, case managers need to document—in writing—decisions and their implementation. This is just good case management administration.

Case management reports should follow a certain format and contain the name of the referral source, the mailing address and phone number for reporting, the line of insurance, the date of occurrence of the accident or injury, a code for the name of the insured, and the name of the claimant or patient. In addition, the report should include any pertinent information obtained from the payer, patient, family, employer, medical records, physician(s), and other medical professionals; a review of the policy coverage and limits; any suggested alternative treatment program; and a discussion of relevant community resources.[2] In their own best interests, case managers should also use these reports to educate readers on the positive impact of case management on outcomes and costs.

Obtaining Approval from the Payer

Once the case management plan has been devised and the report has been sent to the client, the case manager must then obtain approval to proceed with the recommendations in the report. There are always going to be times when case managers have to use their own judgment and consider whom they are representing. An employer or referral source might say directly, "I want John out of that facility; it's too expensive." If case managers feel that patients are in the most appropriate center and that there is no less costly setting, they cannot allow the client to override their professional judgment. The case manager cannot service the client first and the patient last; the interests of the patient must always predominate. Case managers are not in the business of slashing away at the federal or corporate health budget while sacrificing patients' well-being and safety.[2]

Coordinating and Monitoring: Putting the Plan into Action

Plans are sometimes put in motion as early as the initial evaluation stage. Case managers may not have completed gathering all the information or submitted a report when they get the go-ahead to put services in place. When an involved case has been referred from a company the case manager has worked with before, the company might request a verbal report from on-site. During that phone conversation, the case manager might obtain approval to begin the recommended intervention.

The case manager not only has the responsibility to put appropriate services in place, but also should make certain that the services and treatments put in place remain cost-effective, of good quality, and necessary—the case manager should monitor the case. Sometimes a client company will want a case manager to make a one-time visit, arrange for services, and be done with the case. Then who is watching for changes in the patient's needs or tracking and assisting with increases or decreases in services—the home infusion company or home care agency that obviously has a stake in the case's progression? Who is tracking the continued adherence to the physician's treatment plan?

The monitoring process varies from case to case. It may include semimonthly home visits by the case manager or periodic phone calls made by the patient to the case manager. In active cases where multiple services are in place, the case manager must make monthly on-site visits. If there are no services in place, but the patient has been discharged and asked to take specific medications or dress a wound a certain way, the case manager will make check-in calls to see how the patient is coping. When a patient sounds poorly or acknowledges problems, the case manager should call the treating physicians and assess the situation. Perhaps the treatment plan needs to be reevaluated.[2]

Evaluating the Plan

Along with monitoring the medical treatment plan and its effectiveness, the case manager will evaluate and reevaluate the case management plan over the course of intervention. Is the treatment working? Have any complications developed? How is the family coping? Does the caregiver need a respite? Each case will go through modification and redevelopment. Changes in patient status will require new measures of care.

The case manager should review the treatment plan and the patient's progress at least once every 30 days. Short-term referrals, which generally run less than 3 months and are characterized by intense activity at the outset that tapers off as the patient improves, are always reassessed prior to the patient's discharge from a facility or program. Long-term programs, such as geriatric care, are evaluated at intervals of 3, 6, or 9 months. In a brain or spinal cord injury case, care may be evaluated at 1-year intervals. Long-term care evaluations can become challenging because the goal of case management is stability; in some cases, things can go smoothly for long periods of time and there will seemingly be nothing to report.

Further, quality of life is less easily measured than the quantity of money spent on care. Is a continuation of the program warranted? Are the dollars spent on John's care every day worth it? Treatment might be necessary for a 6- to 9-month period, but the patient may not require facility services for that entire time. Although making great strides in the first 2 months, the patient may show no further improvement after 3 months. Perhaps the patient has hit a plateau and needs a break from the rigorous therapies. The next step might be to place the patient in a less expensive day program, then perhaps return him or her to the inpatient facility for another round of intensive therapy if improvement again becomes noticeable.

Over the course of care, as a treatment facilitator, the case manager maintains communication with the treating physicians to share concerns and observations regarding developing conditions, and with physical therapists, social workers, community center personnel, employers, and anyone else who may contribute to the patient's care and welfare. The case manager may need to reestablish ties to a specialist to request assistance.[2]

UTILIZATION REVIEW: PREADMISSION AND CONCURRENT REVIEW AND CASE MANAGEMENT

Generally speaking, utilization reviews fall into three categories: prospective (before the event, called preadmission or precertification), concurrent (during the event), or retrospective (after the event). Each type of review uses certain criteria to determine whether there is a need for further action, decision, or intervention, and to evaluate the necessity and efficiency of the medical services. In addition to tracking the appropriateness of medical care and expenses, the review process itself can also be used to identify cases for case management if the organization or reviewer is aware of the red flags that indicate a need for case management intervention, such as multiple hospital admissions, certain International Classification of Diseases, Ninth Edition, Clinical Modification (ICD-9-CM) diagnostic codes, claims for apnea alarms, electric hospital beds, infusion care services, and so on. These indicators are discussed further below. From a case management perspective, the opportunity to explore alternatives, assist the patient, and preserve benefit dollars is already missed when the case manager is confronted with a claim for $42,000 resulting from a hospital stay of 28 days. Could the patient have gone to a skilled facility for 2 of those weeks? Were nursing and other services in the home a possibility? With alternatives, would there have been opportunities for fee negotiations? Would fee negotiations have been possible with the hospital itself? The lack of early intervention in this case carried a $42,000 price tag.

It is amazing that carriers, TPAs, employer groups, and even some MCOs often set up preadmission review without linking it to some kind of case management program. Reviews are performed in a management vacuum; it is assumed there are no savings to be gained. And, except for those savings possibly realized through the denial of a few days in the hospital or avoidance of an inpatient stay, there will not be any savings to record. Without a connection to case management, preadmission review accomplishes nothing more than maintaining a census of inpatient admissions. And preadmission review alone, without concurrent review, is incapable of reducing lengths of stay or allowing alternative care plans to be considered.

The maximum opportunity for success exists when one organization provides preadmission and concurrent review along with case management services. Too often, particularly in organizations other than large HMOs, one company does the reviewing and another provides the case management. The delays that inevitably occur between identifying a high-cost case, referring it for case management, assigning the case, and actually managing the case make the system ineffective instead of the ongoing process of evaluation, identification, assessment, planning, and implementation that would be ideal. The key in case management is how the case manager gets involved and how soon. For example, one has missed an opportunity if a case manager starts working with a patient with an injured spinal cord 20 or 30 days after the initial hospitalization. Earlier involvement could have resulted in a transfer of this patient to a spinal cord injury treatment center and the prevention of some complications that would, after 20 or 30 days, have already occurred; that will be more costly to treat; and that prolong the period of rehabilitation.[2]

Case managers are facilitators who have the expertise to understand complex cases and the ability to effect change. They assist patients by getting information and expediting the delivery of services. To perform effectively, case managers need to work within a system that allows involvement to occur at an optimum time. Because a seemingly simple procedure can unexpectedly become complex and expensive, each admission needs to be reviewed as it occurs. This does not mean that each case will require case management intervention. Most will not. But the strategy of reviewing each will promote better outcomes for patients and payers.

The sample case presented in Exhibit 17–3 was created to illustrate what would probably occur with and without an integrated system in place. Exhibit 17–4 is a letter designed to be sent to plan participants to explain the advocacy role of the case manager and the nature of the case management process.

For example, the author once received a referral from a claims department after it was notified by a provider who had conducted a preadmission review 7 weeks prior and noted a diagnosis of cancer of the stomach. A claims examiner now had the end-of-month printout and

Exhibit 17–3 Case Samples Without and with Preadmission Review, Concurrent Review, and Case Management

Case A

Scenario—Mr. Jones sustains an injury to his right knee following a fall from a ladder and reports the injury. He is out of work for 1 week, and his supervisor hasn't heard from him or when he's coming back. The worker's family physician is treating the injury conservatively with rest and minimal activity. It's 3 weeks later and the supervisor now hears from the worker's coworkers that there is now an infection in the knee and the worker is scheduled for a surgical procedure. No date for return to work is known. Another week passes. The worker is out of the hospital but still having problems. The supervisor doesn't know what the problems are but the worker's prolonged absence is increasing the workload on the department, and the supervisor also is behind on his work. It's now 6 weeks since this "little fall" (in the words of the supervisor) and it has gone on "too long." The treating physician has told the worker that he can go back to "light duty" and maybe his old job in another month. The supervisor tells the claims examiner there is no "light duty" and the worker continues to remain home. Someone sees the worker mowing his lawn, word reaches the employer, who notifies the claims examiner and requests surveillance. It is clear where this is going, isn't it?

Case B

Scenario—Mr. Jones sustains an injury to his right knee following a fall from a ladder. As is required, he reports the injury to his supervisor. The supervisor advises him that a case manager will be contacting him to help him get appropriate care, answer questions he may have, and assist him in returning to work. The case manager contacts the injured worker and learns that he has sustained a 4-inch laceration to the knee, which required several stitches in the emergency department. She also learned during her phone assessment with the employee that he is unsure about how to care for the wound, or what dressing is needed and how often it should be changed. He also does not know the signs of infection to check for and has not yet scheduled a follow-up visit with his family physician. Because the case manager asked about prior medical history, she discovered that the worker had a "little bit of diabetes" (in the words of the worker) and was lacking knowledge about this disease and, in fact, was told he had cataracts and that his vision is a little "blurry."

The case manager assessed the following as problems:
- a large laceration requiring daily dressing changes and inspection of the wound
- cataracts, which resulted in blurred vision and the inability to detect subtle changes in the wound
- unmanaged diabetes, which prolongs and complicates the wound healing process

The case manager implemented the following:
- skilled nursing visits daily to inspect the wound, change the dressing, and assess diabetic care needs
- referral to physician the following day (after explaining risk factors for infection to office nurse)
- call to supervisor apprising him of status of employee (during this call, obtained description of employee's job [physical demands, etc], discussed some possible modifications to be considered, and suggested a call to the worker by the supervisor to "touch base"—express concern and good wishes).

continues

Exhibit 17–3 continued

Within a week, healing was progressing well and following calls to employee and the treating physician, it was determined that the worker could return to work as long as he did not have to use a ladder or work in a crouched position.

The supervisor was able to modify the worker's position (climbing the ladder was needed only occasionally and another worker could do this; crouching position was done rarely and this, too, could be done by another). Employee could also be checked daily by the company nurse, who would also monitor his diabetes.

Eleven days after the injury, the employee returned to a modified form of his job. The case manager maintained contact with all parties, ensured that the wound was completely healed in 3 weeks and that the worker could then return to all of his duties.

Costs:

Medical: Hospital admission for wound infection and intravenous (IV) antibiotics, wound incisions, and drainage

Hospital @ $1,500 × 7 days = $10,500

Surgery: $2,500

Physical therapy, 3 times a week × 4 weeks (and continuing) = $900

IV antibiotics at home following hospital stay @ $550/day plus nursing visit @ $140/visit × 7 = $4,830

Physician fees: $2,000

Replacement of earnings @ $450/week × 6 = $2,700

Total medical: $20,730 (and continuing)

Total lost earnings: $2,700 (and continuing)

Total costs: $23,430

Indirect costs: decreased productivity, litigation, employee morale

AND IT'S NOT OVER!

Costs:

Medical: Nursing visits for wound care/dressing changes @ negotiated rate of $75 × 10 days = $750

Physician fees: 2 visits for wound care/diabetic management = $200

Replacement of earnings @ $450/week × 2 = $900

Total costs: $1,650*

*Case management is another cost consideration. In this kind of case, case management started early would cost less than $1,000.

Results from Case A:

Increased costs

An employee with continuing medical complications

Adversarial relationship between employer and employee

Pending litigation

Decreased productivity

Decreased morale

Results from Case B:

Savings (net): $20,780. Actual costs and case management fees were deducted from costs of case that would have occurred as in Case A.

A productive employee with a better outcome and the recipient of a true advocacy program

A business that can return to its *own* business needs and goals

Courtesy of Options Unlimited, Case Management Services Division, Huntington, New York.

Exhibit 17–4 Letter Explaining Case Management to Plan Participants

---

January 15, _____

Dear _____:

  Please allow this letter to serve as an introduction and explanation of services that have been requested on your behalf by _____ of Third-Party Administrator (TPA), which is the company administering the health care benefits on behalf of your employer, _____.

  _____ is a private consulting firm utilized by TPA on behalf of its insured to assist TPA with the problems resulting from a variety of medical conditions. This service is at no cost to you and is a benefit provided by the company.

  Our nurse consultants work with you, your family, and treating physicians in coordinating whatever care and services are necessary in order that you may receive the best results possible. This intervention is not intended to interrupt or interfere with any care you are currently receiving, nor is this a "hands-on" service.

  In order to determine just how we may be of assistance, one of our consultants, _____, would like to meet with you at your home. Because our consultants are frequently out of the office, would you please call us COLLECT at (999) 999-9999 in order that we can put _____ in touch with you.

  Enclosed please find a brochure that further describes our services. Should you have any questions or concerns, please feel free to contact me directly. Please accept my personal assurance that every effort will be extended on your behalf.

Very truly yours,

Case Manager

cc: Claims Department

  Courtesy of Options Unlimited, Case Management Services Division, Huntington, New York.

---

had also just received a claim for 1 week of total parenteral nutrition (TPN) and other services totaling $10,000. The examiner thought a case management referral was in order. And it was, but it came a little too late. The services continued a second week as arranged; the provider refused to negotiate retrospectively to lower costs because he knew his services were payable at 100%. (He knew that the patient's benefit plan would pay full price for his services because he called the claims department and learned this from a customer service representative.) The patient died after a second admission to the hospital. Perhaps the TPN services could have been negotiated more cost-effectively. Perhaps a hospice program could have been arranged, allowing the patient to die at home with his family around him. Perhaps money could have been saved. In this instance, there were preadmission and concurrent review and case management and a benefit plan that would have permitted alternatives, yet because each system functioned independently of the others, realizing an alternative was impossible.

When preadmission and concurrent review and case management functions are integrated, the coordination can avoid duplication of involvement, help a claims department manage its workload, assist in the development of prevention and wellness programs, support the evaluation of benefit use, and expose the need to redesign plans.[2]

PREADMISSION AND CONCURRENT REVIEW CASE MANAGEMENT REPORTS

Preadmission and concurrent review summary reports (Exhibit 17–5) and other documentation of case events constitute an ongoing profile of a case. Case-specific reports (Exhibit 17–6) help establish a case history and can be used to track the details of a case, which can be extremely helpful if the patient moves from low- to high-risk status. Produced for all hospital admissions, all scheduled pregnancies, and all emergency cases, case-specific reports incorporate notes made by nurse reviewers. They are valuable for internal use in a preadmission and concurrent review department, provide the rationale for case management referral, contain important background information for the case manager assigned to the case, and are forwarded to the claims examiner.

The review summary report shows that only 1 patient out of 10 was referred for case management. One review summary prepared by the author showed a surprisingly high incidence of admission for pregnancy complications for one employer group, and it led to the formation of a maternity screening and management program and the prevention of two premature births. The savings to the group far outweighed the costs of the managed care program.[2]

RED FLAGS: INDICATORS FOR CASE MANAGEMENT

Cases that benefit most from case management commonly involve the most expensive services. Use of these services is thus a red flag. Other indicators include a high frequency of admissions in a short period and an unusually lengthy hospital stay. A stay of 10 days or longer for a surgical hospitalization indicates multiple problems or complications now and points to problems down the road as well. This is where a case manager needs clinical knowledge—a feel for what constitutes a big case. Exhibit 17–7 is a tip sheet that includes red flags for case management intervention as well as indicators for claims review.

Different red flags should be used for different lines of insurance. Looking for case management indicators, a case manager will not apply the same dollar limit per claim in a workers' compensation case as he or she applies in a group medical case. In workers' compensation, for each lost-time injury there is an established guideline, and if the injured person is still out of work a month beyond the date calculated using the guidelines, then that fact becomes a red flag. Many physicians use the reference *The Medical Disability Advisor: Workplace Guidelines for Disability Duration*, written by Presley Reed and published by Reed Group. A six-volume set of care guidelines for hospital admissions and stays, physician's office treatments, home health care, dentistry, recovery times before returning to work, and medicines has been developed by Milliman & Robertson Inc. These guidelines are followed by the health plans—among them Prudential, CIGNA, US Healthcare, Kaiser Permanente, and many Blues—of more than 50 million Americans.

Other indicators of a problem: extension of treatment, treatment recommended by a physician at his or her physician-owned facility, a patient receiving physical therapy and chiropractic manipulation at the same time, a variety of practitioners consulting on a seemingly straightforward case, a case that continually bypasses its return-to-work date, and a patient taking large numbers of pain medications or antidepressant medications.

In group medical coverage the concerns will be different. Group plans cover employees and

Exhibit 17–5 Preadmission and Concurrent Review Summary Report

Group #001   Third-Party Administrator   1/1/97–1/31/97

Date Reported	Employee SSN	Patient Name	Diagnosis	Type	Date of Admission	Date of Discharge	Status
1/2/97	000000000	J Smith	Fracture	Emergency	1/1/97	1/2/97	Closed
1/3/97	000000000	C Jones	Normal Delivery	Emergency	1/25/97		Open
1/5/97	000000000	K Williams	Lump in Breast	Scheduled	1/8/97		Open
1/7/97	000000000	S Allen	Myocardial Infarction	Emergency	1/11/97	1/18/97	Refer CM
1/12/97	000000000	T Hans	Herniated Disc	Scheduled	1/21/97	1/25/97	Closed
1/14/97	000000000	L Mooney	Miscarriage	Emergency	1/13/97	1/14/97	Closed
1/16/97	000000000	J Bono	Appendicitis	Emergency	1/15/97	1/18/97	Closed
1/18/97	000000000	N Strong	Derangement Knee	Scheduled	1/25/97		Open
1/25/97	000000000	P Duffy	Depression	Scheduled	1/28/97		Psych
1/28/97	000000000	I Grello	Pregnancy	Scheduled	3/25/97		Open

Total Admissions for Period = 9   Total Discharged = 5   Total Referred for Case Management = 1

TOTAL CASES FOR PERIOD = 10

Courtesy of Options Unlimited, Case Management Services Division, Huntington, New York.

Exhibit 17–6 Preadmission and Concurrent Review Case-Specific Report

CareWatch ID #: 00676
Date Reported: 08/31/97
Reported by: RENY

Group/Carrier:

Employee Information:
Name: G. Jones SSN: 123-45-6789
Address: 12 Amhurst Street, Mid-Island, NY
Hire Date: 03/01/91 Effective Date of Coverage: 06/01/91
Telephone:

Patient Information:
Name: G. Jones DOB: 01/25/67 Age: 30
Relation: Employee Sex: Male
Confinement Type: Emergency
Admission Date: 08/28/97 Length of Stay: 2 days
Discharge Date: 08/30/97
Procedure: initial hosp. care/eval. and management
Hospital: COMM. HOSPITAL
Address: ROUTE 111
SMITHTOWN, NY 11787
Telephone: (516) 979-9800 Fax:

Admitting Physician Information:
Doctor: Dr. J. Kahn
Telephone: 555-1212 Fax:
Diagnosis: hemorrhage—cerebral

CASE REMARKS
9/3/97: t/c to hospital, claimant was discharged on 8/30/97 but could not give me any other info. CTR t/c to MD, spoke Evelyn Spencer, who said that the claimant has an app't. with the MD today and she will call me back after he has been seen by the MD. CTR
t/c to claimant, who said he felt dizzy and went to the ER, he was admitted to ICU and had a CAT scan, was told he had an elevated BP and is on medication. He continues to feel dizzy sometimes and gets tingling in his tongue. Has an appt. today at 12:30 PM, will f/u on 9/8. CTR
9/8/97: t/c to claimant—per family member he is having some type of outpt. test today. f/u with claimant 9/9. IK
9/9/97: t/c to MD—told me that claimant was readmitted to hosp. for one day 9/8 to have arteriogram done. Diagnosis is seizure disorder and AV malformation and he was started on Dilantin. Will be referring him to neurologist. Will f/u with claimant. MF
9/10/97: t/c to claimant—still feels dizzy, has appt. with his MD today. Will f/u with claimant 9/14 for outcome and neuro. appt. IK
9/14/97: T/C to claimant—per his father, he has an appt. with neurologist Dr. Kahn (didn't have no.) tomorrow at 1 PM; he still has dizziness and numbness of tongue. f/u with claimant/MD 9/16. IK
9/16/97: t/c to claimant—told me that he had appt. with neurologist yesterday and that he referred him to another MD (neurosurgeon?) and that appt. is for next week 9/22 (claimant did not know name of MD offhand). Continues to take Dilantin and continues to feel dizzy, even though he stopped smoking. Claimant mentioned that MD might have to operate on his brain because "there is something wrong with blood vessel in his brain." Obtained Dr. Kahn's phone number 516-555-1212. Will f/u with MD. MF

continues

Exhibit 17–6 continued

9/16/97: t/c to MD—not in because of holidays. Will be back in office on 9/21 after 1 PM. MF
9/21/97: t/c to Dr. Kahn—per Sue pt. has AVM, will not be seen again in MD's office until sometime around 10/12, not aware of ref. to another MD, not aware of potential for surg. at this time. f/u with claimant to obtain name and no. of referral MD. IK
9/21/97: t/c to claimant—no answer × 2. IK
9/24/97: t/c to claimant—left message on answering machine. MF
9/30/97: t/c to claimant—no answer. Will try one more time tomorrow if no answer or return call, then will close case. MF
10/01/97: t/c to claimant—no answer × 2. IK. MULTIPLE attempts made to contact claimant; per MD office no further therapy scheduled at this time. Case closed. IK
MONITOR FILES FOR FUTURE CLAIMS******************

CareWatch ID #: 00954
Date Reported: 11/08/97
Reported by: BARBARA

Group/Carrier:

Employee Information:
    Name: G. Jones   SSN: 123-45-6789
    Address: 12 Amhurst Street, Mid-Island, NY
    Hire Date: 03/01/91   Effective Date of Coverage: 06/01/91
    Telephone:

Patient Information:
    Name: G. Jones   DOB: 01/25/67   Age: 30
    Relation: Employee   Sex: Male
    Confinement Type: Emergency
    Admission Date: 10/30/97   Length of Stay: 4 Days
    Discharge Date: 11/03/97
    Procedure: initial hosp. care/eval. and management
    Hospital: COLUMBIA PRESBYTERIAN MED CTR.
    Address: 207 ST & BROADWAY
             NEW YORK, NY 10032
    Telephone: (212) 305-2500   Fax:

Admitting Physician Information:
    Doctor: Dr. Z. Binder
    Telephone: (212) 555-1212   Fax:
    Diagnosis: hemorrhage—cerebral

CASE REMARKS
CASE KNOWN TO OPTIONS FROM PREVIOUS ADMISSION—VERY DIFFICULT TO FOLLOW—CLAIMANT DID NOT RETURN PHONE CALLS.
11/8/97: t/c Dr. Binder office. MD not available. will have secretary (Aline) call me back. vc
11/8/97: t/c to hospital pt info. patient discharged 11/3/97. vc
11/8/97: t/c claimant. no answer. vc
11/8/97: t/c hospital medical records. dept closed (hrs. 9–12, 2–3:45) direct #212-555-1212

continues

Exhibit 17–6 continued

> 11/9/97: t/c to MD—MD is away, per Aline, residents are following claimant. She will get info. from them and return call. MF
> 11/9/97: t/c from Aline at Dr. Binder's office—told me that claimant is being followed by Dr. Sachs and that I should speak to Pat his secretary for further info. Number is 212-555-1212. Transferred me to that number—according to Pat, MD is away and she could not tell me about hosp. stay. Claimant does not have a follow-up appt. yet, she has to call him this week and set something up. Told me that claimant did not have surgery and during hosp. stay claimant was under the care of Dr. Frank 212-555-1212. MF
> 11/9/97: t/c to Dr. Frank—not in yet, left message with secretary, Lisa. MF
> 11/10/97: t/c to Dr. Frank—not in yet; left message with secretary, Lisa, for MD to call back. BR
> 11/11/97: t/c to claimant—spoke to man who rents a room from claimant's father. Told me that claimant does not live here anymore. Claimant's father is out right now, he will give him my phone number for him to call me back with number where claimant can be reached. MF
> 11/11/97: t/c to claims. Renee will pull most recent claims and check on address and call me back. MF
> 11/11/97: t/c to MD office—spoke to Lisette who told me that she gave the MD the messages. She will speak to him again and try to get info and call me back. Asked if she had claimant's address and phone number and she transferred me to billing to speak to Terry. Per Terry, claimant does not appear to be in computer system at office or with hosp. Check system several times. Told me to call back after 1 PM and speak to Carmen and perhaps she could help. MF
> 11/12/97: t/c to Dr. Frank. Claimant had a minor cerebral hemorrhage. Dx. is arterial malformation of the brain; Dr. Sachs is performing surgery at a later date; (212)555-1212; individual not in any danger; need to contact Dr. Sachs for more detailed info. JG/br
> 11/15/97: t/c to Dr. Sachs office/Pat: they have been unable to contact claimant; he needs to see Dr. Sachs & then surgery can be scheduled. BR
> 11/15/97: t/c to claims. Renee says claimant admitted to Community Hosp. of W. Suffolk on 11/13.
> 11/15/97: t/c to C.H.O.W.S./UR Dept./Mrs. King—claimant adm. 11/13 via ER with seizures; was in ICU—now on telemetry; under the care of Dr. Zeller, (516)555-1212 has no additional info @ this time. BR
> 11/15/97: t/c to Dr. Sachs/Pat—given above info; she will inform MD to f/u with Dr. Z; BR
> 11/15/97: t/c to Dr. Zeller's office—informed of pending consult with Dr. S # given; Dr. Zeller in with patient; will call with claimant when finished. BR
> 11/15/97: t/c from Dr. Zeller, claimant c/o numbness of tongue which MD feels is seizure activity; Dilantin increased—c/o of dizziness; CAT scan WNL; EEG pending; will be disch. tonight or tomorrow; f/u with Dr. S. BR
> 11/15/97: t/c to claimant; spoke with father; corrected birthdate obtained (12-06-34): will f/u with claimant tomorrow to schedule CM assessment; in rm 254, father & son
> work for the same company. BR
> CASE REFERRED FOR CASE MANAGEMENT.
>
> Courtesy of Options Unlimited, Case Management Services Division, Huntington, New York.

their dependents, and a case manager might target catastrophic illnesses, premature deliveries, cancer cases, plus other chronic and devastating long-term diseases, such as AIDS or multiple sclerosis. Other things to watch for include multiple hospitalizations, multiple physicians, expenses beyond a certain threshold (eg, $10,000), and particular kinds of services, such as chemotherapy, radiation therapy, and infusion care.[2]

Exhibit 17–7 CareSolutions and AccuClaim Red Flags

CareSolutions Red Flags

Diagnosis:	Cancer	Neuromuscular diseases	Head injury	Psychiatric
	AIDS	Spinal cord injuries	Severe burns	Multiple trauma
	Stroke	Alcohol and substance abuse	High-risk pregnancy	High-risk infant
	Transplant	Cardiovascular	Chronic respiratory illness	
Potential treatment:	Ventilator dependent	TPN/enteral	Home care	
	IV antibiotics	Extended ICU	Chemo	
Frequent hospitalizations:	3 admits same year/same or related problem			
Cost of claim:	Same illness over $10,000 so far this year			
Location of claim:	Complex care delivered in rural setting, small hospital, or facility with poor outcome history/diagnosis			
Patterns of care:	Failed or repeated surgeries, hospital-acquired infections, malpractice concerns			

Diagnostic codes: ICD-9-CM Case Management Referral Indicators

042–044	HIV infection	358	Myasthenia gravis (repeat hosps.)	800	Fx vault of skull
140–239	Neoplasms (cancer)	359	Muscular dystrophy (repeat hosps.)	806	Fx of vertebral column w/SCI
250	Diabetes with complications			850–854	Intracranial injury excluding those w/skull Fx
252	(Possible mult. hosps., coma, renal, eye, neuro)	430–438	Cerebral vascular disease, car. hemorrhage	860–869	Internal injury of chest, abdomen, and pelvis
277	Cystic fibrosis, porphyria, metabolic disorders (mult. hosps.)	496	COPD	870–879	Open wound of head, neck, and trunk
		501–503	Asbestosis and Silicosis		
279	Immunity deficiency disorders (repeat hosps.)	584–586	Renal failure	925–929	Crushing injury (may involve extensive trauma)
286–287	Coagulation defects (repeat hosps.)	644	Early or threatened labor	948	Burns over 25% of body
290–299	Psychoses	655–656	Fetal abnormality	952	SCI without spinal bone injury
300–316	Neurotic, personality and other nonpsychotic mental disorders	710	All collagen (SLE+)	994	Effects of external causes—lightning, drowning, strangulation
		714	Rheumatoid arthritis w/inflammatory polyarthropathies		
330–337	Hereditary and degenerative diseases of CNS (Alzheimer's, Huntington's chorea)	740–759	Congenital anomalies, spina bifida, cardiac septal defect	996–999	Complications of surgical and medical care
		760–763	Maternal causes of perinatal morbidity and mortality		
340–349	CNS disorders, MS, CP, quadriplegic, paraplegic, anoxic brain damage	765.1	Premature birth		

continues

Exhibit 17–7 continued

AccuClaim Red Flags

Surgical and anesthesia claims: All surgery claims over $1,000 and all cases with more than two line items should be referred for a medical review. Alert for GYN, orthopaedic, plastic surgery. If the surgical claim is referred, corresponding anesthesia claims should be referred also to verify complexity of claimed procedure.
Information to obtain: 1) operative report; 2) anesthesia time; 3) R&C charges for EACH CPT code.

Podiatrists: All claims that exceed $800 should be referred.
Information to obtain: 1) operative report if a surgical procedure is being billed; 2) R&C charges for EACH CPT code.

Physical therapy and occupational therapy: Claims that exceed 6 weeks of treatment should be referred.
Information to obtain: 1) PT evaluation; 2) therapy progress notes that include long- and short-term goals and the range of motion results; 3) letter of medical need from treating MD with diagnosis, frequency of treatment, and estimated duration.

Chiropractic care: Claims that exceed $300 should be referred.
Information to obtain: 1) complete copy of the medical records—NO summaries. Include diagnosis, treatment plan, frequency of treatment, estimated duration.

Durable medical equipment: This is an area of extreme abuse and overutilization of services and fees. The following claims should be referred: oxygen concentrators and related equipment, hospital beds, wheelchairs, ANY monitors, respirators/ventilators, requests for home modifications (ramps, etc).

Home health services: All claims for nursing, aides, or related services should be referred.
Information to obtain: 1) itemized bills; 2) nursing notes.

Infusion care services: All claims for the following infusion services should be referred: IV antibiotics and other medications, TPN (total parenteral nutrition), chemotherapy, analgesia (pain medications).
Information to obtain: 1) MD's prescription; 2) itemized billing for medications, nursing, and related services and supplies.

Any of the following should be referred: 1) appeals; 2) difficult providers; 3) ambulatory surgical centers; 4) large hospital bills: over 7 days LOS—to review for LOS, medical needs vs. custodial needs.

continues

Exhibit 17-7 continued

Procedure Codes: CPT AccuClaim Referral Indicators

Integumentary system
11000–11044 For cosmetic vs. medical
15780–15791 For cosmetic vs. medical
15810–15840 For cosmetic vs. medical
17304–17310 For cosmetic vs. medical
19318–19500 For cosmetic vs. medical

Musculoskeletal
27290–27295 Amputation
27590–27598 Amputation

Pulmonary system
30400–30630 For cosmetic
31300–31660 Laryngectomy—tracheotomy, etc
32310–32545 Lung surgery

Cardiovascular
33200–33220 Pacemaker surgery
35450–35458 Vascular vs. cosmetic
37799 Unlisted procedure
38999 Unlisted procedure
39599 Unlisted procedure

Digestive
41100–41155 Mouth, tongue (for cancer)
43600–43640 Stomach (biopsy, etc)
44100–44340 Intestinal
47100–47135 Liver

Urinary system
50200–50380 Kidney, incl. transplant
51550–51597 Bladder (especially for cancer)

Maternity
59000–59100 High-risk procedures
59120–59140 High-risk procedures

Nervous system
61304–61576 Craniectomy
62180–62258 Spine
64999 Unlisted procedure

Eye and ear
65771 Radial keretotomy
68899 Unlisted procedure
69300 Cosmetic
69399 Unlisted procedure

Courtesy of Options Unlimited, Case Management Services Division, Huntington, New York.

TIMING CASE MANAGEMENT INTERVENTION

At what point in the review process should a referral be made for case management intervention? As discussed earlier, there are some basic indicators or red flags to look for and there are other, more individualized considerations. Some indicators may actually be evident during the very first call from a hospital admissions department, treating physician, or patient's family to a preadmission review department or company. A preterm delivery, a high-risk pregnancy, a cerebral vascular accident suffered by a teenager, a spinal cord injury, or a traumatic brain injury with coma are all conditions for which there is a high probability of a lengthy hospital stay, a need for additional care and services upon discharge, high costs, and benefits to be gained through case management.

Other conditions would also merit an early referral, not necessarily because of a particular diagnosis but because of surrounding circumstances. For instance, diabetes is not by itself a condition that would necessarily promote a case management referral, but the fourth hospital admission in 2 months of a patient with diabetes might. Why are these readmissions occurring? Is the patient noncompliant or noneducated? Is the treating physician a retiring family practitioner? Perhaps an endocrinologist is needed?

Consider a patient with an admitting diagnosis of cellulitis. At first glance, this is not a situation appropriate for case management. However, perhaps as the patient's stay in the hospital continues, more is revealed about this 46-year-old woman: she is also hypertensive, had a coronary bypass 2 years earlier, is diabetic, and weighs 250 pounds, clearly morbidly obese for her height of 5 feet, 4 inches. This woman might eventually require a below-knee amputation secondary to her multiple conditions. The potential for this occurrence warrants an assessment by a case management professional. Patients like this woman would likely be overlooked by a system for case management referral that was driven solely by one ICD-9-CM code or one set dollar limit. Each similar case presents such substantial opportunities for improved outcomes, prevention of complications, and reduction of expenses that not referring becomes a costly risk.[2]

BEYOND THE CASE MANAGEMENT BASICS

Case Management's Contribution to Claims Management

By helping identify the small percentage of claimants responsible for generating the majority of claims and the bulk of benefit payouts (those in need of case management intervention) and educating claims administrators regarding medical issues, case managers serve a vital function in claims departments. They help providers, MCOs, insurers, and TPAs look good to employers and payers by better managing benefit dollars; help patients get care approval in a timely fashion; and help speed the claims administration process without losing patients through the cracks in the system.

Nothing speaks more loudly to a client than a report taken from its own group experience. With a claims run, the case manager can show that out of a group of 500, with total claims paid of $200,000, fewer than 20 individuals (4%) filed claims totaling 80% ($160,000) of that sum. With this information in hand, a case manager can work with the claims administrator and the employer/payer to improve that claims experience. When the few cases are properly managed, the whole group benefits from lower claims costs.[2] (It must be emphasized that a case manager's work is accomplished without compromising the patient/employee's right to privacy. A case manager can save a company big bucks; the chief executive officer has no need to know and will never know the name of the individual in each case.)

Using a computer program, a case manager can conduct a group run, a profile that may include all hospital admissions, all workers' compensation cases, all short-term disability cases, all cases lasting over a year, and so on. The purpose is to begin examining the claims experience of the group to answer the question, Where have the dollars gone?

For one client, the author prepared a group claims run to find those patients in need of case management intervention. For the first check, a wide net was cast—all hospital admissions. (This field could be narrowed later by setting specific length-of-stay parameters.) The first month's claims run showed that 1% of the group generated 34% of the claims; the next month, 2% generated 67% of the total. In the third month, 2% of the group was responsible for 73% of the benefit dollars paid, and 0.3% (three employees) accounted for 44% of the total. This 3-month run also showed us those cases requiring costly care from month to month, a clear indicator for case management intervention.[2]

Case managers also work with individual reports. The specific limit for this hypothetical report is $15,000. The first patient that the computer identifies has claims for one hospitalization and one major surgical procedure, a colostomy. The surgery was successful, the postoperative problems minor; there was no real opportunity here for case management to have a major impact. The next individual who has reached the $15,000 limit has a series of claims for an unresolved ulcer of the foot, diabetes, hypertension, and vascular disease. This patient is a health care time bomb. What's the real problem here? Why isn't the ulcer healing? Is this person receiving appropriate care? When reports break out claims history by ICD-9-CM or current procedural terminology (CPT) codes, the case manager can ascertain the presenting problems and procedures taken to alleviate problems; actual claims files will indicate potential difficulties such as complications from the interaction of various medications. Case managers can use the tools of the claims department to help resolve health issues, while claims departments can use the skills of case managers to better their service.[2]

Cost Benefit Analysis Reports

Cost benefit analysis reports are one form of case management documentation; they illustrate in financial terms that the costs spent on case management services (and the services that are put in place as part of an alternate care plan) translate into dollar savings, or dollars spent versus dollars saved. The report format can be customized or modified to meet departmental or client company needs, and report citations may change as a case management program develops. Generally, a cost benefit analysis report should include an overview of the case management intervention (a brief narrative), a summary of the intervention, case management fees, savings (avoided charges, potential charges, discounted and negotiated reductions, and reductions in services, products, and equipment), actual charges, gross savings (potential charges minus actual charges), net savings (gross savings minus case management fees), and the status of the case (open or closed).

There are many opportunities for case managers to improve treatment quality, outcome, and lifestyle for patients. Arranging for home care can increase patient morale and save money; additional savings are realized when a case manager asks providers for prompt-pay discounts or reduces the level of care or hours of care through continual assessment of the patient's progress. Reductions, discounts, negotiated rates, all-inclusive per diem rates, and "freebies" (the free ambulance service provided by some community fire departments, for instance) are examples of savings reported in a cost benefit analysis report.

Savings achieved by avoiding potential charges are more difficult to quantify but should be reported as well. Consider this scenario: A case manager is referred a patient who, in prior months, had an admission every 1 to 2 months for diabetic complications and an emergency hospital stay of 5 to 7 days. The case manager discovers that Julie does not understand her diagnosis, is minimally compliant, and frequently ignores dietary restrictions and blood and urine testing. During the case management intervention of 3 months, the case manager spoke to Julie's physician regarding these problems, referred Julie for formal education and a diet counseling program, and involved Julie in daily monitoring of her own progress. The pattern of admissions and complications was halted. Over 6 months of case management intervention, there were no further hospital admissions. The dollars in acute care that could have been spent, but were not, are savings achieved via avoided or potential charges.[2]

Combined with outcomes data (and including outcomes data as part of the summary of case management intervention), cost benefit analysis reports chart the success of alternative treatment plans and serve as strong arguments for the effectiveness of case management and managed care.

Wellness Programs

A good case management program should come full circle, with outcomes data providing the rationale for wellness programs designed to address the problems before they arise so employers and payers spend even less money treating them, and patients are relieved of having to live through the treatments. If a preadmission and concurrent review program or a claims report sequence is pointing out patients whose illnesses are protracted and all of them are smokers, perhaps a "smoke out" wellness program is needed. If every third worker in the warehouse has been out on disability for lower back pain, a case manager might design a wellness program incorporating exercise, review of and instruction on improved lifting patterns, and a facility review to make site modifications as needed to reduce the lifting injuries. As mentioned earlier in the chapter, effective pregnancy counseling and case management intervention can prevent premature labor and the problems arising from low-birthweight babies.

Once a company puts a case management program in place, the next step is to begin using the case management outcomes data wisely to reduce the company's exposure and liabilities by addressing those areas where it is most vulnerable.

24-Hour Coverage Programs

Like wellness programs, 24-hour coverage programs take the best facets of case management and managed care programs and put them to broader use. Combining total health care and disability management, 24-hour coverage is a program that coordinates all aspects of health care management. This eliminates the oversight, duplication of services, and paper chase that results when care and management of care are split into categories based on whether or not the slip on the ice occurred on the job (workers' compensation) or at home (group medical coverage), includes a jaw injury (dental coverage), or removes the patient from the work force for 3 months (short-term disability). Rather than pass this individual from management system to management system, 24-hour programs coordinate the entire care program as it moves from site to site, and coverage plan to coverage plan. This puts the focus back on the patient and the care, better managing his or her needs and therefore better managing the costs.

Disease Management

As it was defined in early 1995, disease management bore a striking similarity to case management. An article in the *Journal of Subacute Care* called disease management a coordinated care strategy, citing a Blue's National Coordinated Care Management program as an example and calling it "a new strategic direction for managing customer healthcare experience. The program presents an opportunity to enhance patient care and decrease benefit costs by identifying and selecting chronically ill individuals who represent high-cost users of medical care and linking those individuals with appropriate providers and outpatient interventions. The program involves three separate but integrative components: 1) Identification; 2) Intervention; and 3) Monitoring and Evaluation, that are designed to provide a comprehensive approach to the management of an individual patient's care."[4(p17)]

Sound familiar? Look again at the description of case management at the beginning of this chapter and the section on the case management work format and process to see just how familiar. The reader is also referred to Part X for further discussion of disease state management.

In *Medical Marketing & Media*, there was less consensus about what disease management covered. However, it was summarized as "a system of viewing healthcare disease by disease and examining the interrelated elements in the treatment process with outcomes research to improve quality and lower costs."[5(p48)] The article further defined disease management as "An integrated system of customized interventions, measurements, and refinements to current processes of care designed to optimize clinical and economic outcomes within a specific disease state by facilitating proper diagnoses, maximizing clinical effectiveness, eliminating ineffective or unnecessary care, using only cost-effective diagnosis and therapeutics, maximizing the efficiency of care delivery and improving continuously."[5(p53)]

While the majority of case management programs have focused on the management of the sickest and costliest individuals in a group, most experts would agree that earlier, more creative, nonepisodic management presents far greater opportunities to prevent these health care disasters. Health care organizations and payers have been striving to improve the quality of care, to control costs, and to actively involve plan members in this process. Whereas case management focuses efforts on an individual patient, disease management targets groups of individuals with diagnostic conditions that have historical and financial evidence of being costly and that will be significantly improved with more integrated and systematic management. Several diseases have already been identified as having the greatest potential for change: asthma, diabetes, high-risk pregnancy, and cardiac disease.[2]

The major thrust of effective disease management programs is in the prevention of acute episodes. The Diabetes Treatment Centers of America in Nashville, Tennessee, successfully reduced hospital admission rates for patients enrolled in its program to 67.3% below the national average for persons with diabetes nationwide. Another successful program at the Denver-based National Jewish Center for Immunology and Respiratory Medicine reports outcomes that show asthma hospitalizations decreased 83%, emergency department visits decreased 45%, and hospital days decreased 82% for this high-cost patient group.[2]

A LONG-TERM SOLUTION TO A LONG-TERM PROBLEM

Case management was improving outcomes and preserving benefit dollars long before "health reform" became a catch phrase bandied about in political circles, and case management will continue to help maintain quality care while making the most of the dollars available. As an integral part of effective managed care programs, case management is a long-term solution to a long-term problem—the attempt to find a balance in our health care delivery system—for patients, families, physicians, employers, and payers confronted by diverse health care challenges, new medical technologies, broad ethical questions, and cost concerns. As a managed care tool, case management works. As a health care discipline, it is here to stay.

REFERENCES

1. McCollom P. Position statement by the Interim Commission for Certification of Case Managers (CCM). Presented at the meeting of the CCM Interim Commission Committee; January 27, 1995; Orlando, FL.
2. Mullahy C. *The Case Manager's Handbook*. 2nd ed. Gaithersburg, MD: Aspen Publishers, Inc; 1998.
3. Dearing G. Improving patient compliance in the best interests of all. *Managed Healthcare News*. 1996;12(12):1, 15–16.
4. Falcon SP, Berg SS, Kosel KC. National coordinated care management: focused disease management strategies for the 21st century. *J Subacute Care*. 1995;3(2):16–19.
5. Castagnoli WG. Is disease management good therapy for an ailing industry? *Med Marketing Media*. 1995;30(1):46–53.

SUGGESTED READINGS

Books

Benefits Source Book. Marietta, GA: Employee Benefit News, Enterprise Communications; updated annually.

Blancett S, Flarey D. *Handbook of Nursing Care Management.* Gaithersburg, MD: Aspen Publishers, Inc; 1996.

Center for Healthcare Information. *Case Management Resource Guide* (updated annually). Irvine, CA: Center for Healthcare Information.

Cohen EL, Cesta T. *Nursing Case Management: From Concept to Evaluation.* 2nd ed. St. Louis, MO: Mosby–Year Book; 1997.

Kemether NA, ed. *Crisis Management and Catastrophic Care: A Guide for Rehabilitation Specialists.* Richmond, VA: Vocational Placement Services; 1985.

St. Coeur M, ed. *Case Management Practice Guidelines.* St. Louis, MO: Mosby–Year Book; 1996.

Schwartz GE, Watson SD, Galvin DE, Lipoff E. *The Disability Management Sourcebook.* Washington, DC: Washington Business Group on Health and Institute for Rehabilitation and Disability Management; 1989.

Thorn K. *Applying Medical Case Management: AIDS.* Canoga Park, CA: Thorn Publishing; 1990.

Periodicals

Business & Health
5 Paragon Drive
Montvale, NJ 07645
(201) 358-7200

Business Insurance
740 North Rush Street
Chicago, IL 60611-2590
(800) 678-9595

Case Management Advisor
3525 Piedmont Road NE
Building 6, Suite 400
Atlanta, GA 30305
(800) 688-2421

The Case Manager
10801 Executive Center Drive, Suite 509
Little Rock, AR 72211
(501) 223-5165

Case Review
4676 Admiralty Way, Suite 202
Marina del Rey, CA 90292
(310) 306-2206

Group Practice Managed Healthcare News
201 Littleton Road, Suite 100
Morris Plain, NJ 07950-2932
(201) 285-0755

The Journal of Care Management
PO Box 210
Green Farms, CT 06436-0210
(203) 259-9333

Managed Healthcare News
105 Raider Boulevard
Belle Mead, NJ 08502
(201) 285-0855

The Remington Report
30100 Town Center Drive, Suite 421
Laguna Niguel, CA 92677-2064
(800) 247-4781

Risk & Insurance
747 Dresher Road, Suite 500
Horsham, PA 19044-0980
(215) 784-0860

Risk Management
205 East 42nd Street
New York, NY 10017
(212) 286-9364

The Self-Insurer
17300 Redhill Avenue, Suite 100
Irvine, CA 92714
(714) 261-2553

CATHERINE M. MULLAHY, RN, CRRN, CCM, is a case management consultant and a spokesperson for the case management industry. She is founder and president of Options Unlimited, a medical case management and benefits consulting firm in Huntington, New York. Ms. Mullahy is a commissioner, secretary, and chair-elect for the executive committee of the Commission for Case Manager Certification (CCMC) and chair for CCM Certification Compliance Review, and she has served on ongoing expert panels in connection with the development of the CCM credential since its inception. She is editor of *The Case Manager* magazine, and the second edition of her book *The Case Manager's Handbook* was published by Aspen Publishers, Inc, in 1998.

Chapter 18

Critical Paths: Linking Care and Outcomes for Patients, Clinicians, and Payers

Richard J. Coffey, Janet S. Richards, Susan A. Wintermeyer-Pingel, and Sarah S. LeRoy

Chapter Outline

- Background and Terminology
- Scope and Uses of Critical Paths
- Environment for Critical Paths
- Approach to Developing Critical Paths
- Use of Critical Paths
- Alternative Formats and Sample Uses
- Resource Formats
- Calculate and Use Float/Slack Time Information
- Results
- Conclusion

Critical paths are important tools to link patients and clinicians to managed care organizations (MCOs), other payers, and integrated delivery systems (all of which will be collectively referred to as MCOs in this chapter) to achieve high-quality and cost-effective care. Critical paths have proven to be effective tools to improve the planning, coordination, communication, and evaluation of care. This chapter provides an overview of the concepts, approach, and uses of critical paths, and provides guidance for developing and implementing critical paths, based upon the knowledge gained at the University of Michigan Health System (UMHS) and other organizations (UMHS includes the University of Michigan Hospital and Health Centers and the University of Michigan Medical School). In a managed care environment, there is greater emphasis on coordination of services and efficient use of resources across multiple settings, such as inpatient, outpatient, and home.

Critical paths foster collaborative goal setting among multiple care providers, for specific case types. Outcomes that have been discussed and agreed upon by a whole team are more likely to be achieved because they have a team focus. Changes or variations in outcome trends are more likely to be explored and acted upon. There is less chance of confusion for the patient, the family, the care provider, or the payer concerning the intent of care and expected outcomes.

Outcomes related to processes for their achievement (the path) are more likely to assist payers and health care providers to agree upon resources for care provision. Data support the process, particularly when benchmarking has been incorporated into the pathway development. Critical paths assist health care providers to have input into the payers' guidelines for "reasonable" care.

This chapter is adapted from RJ Coffey et al, Critical Paths: Linking Outcomes for Patients, Clinicians, and Payers, in *The Managed Health Care Handbook*, 3rd ed, PR Kongstvedt, ed, pp 301–317, © 1996, Aspen Publishers, Inc.

BACKGROUND AND TERMINOLOGY

Critical path method (CPM), program evaluation and review technique (PERT), project management, and related approaches have their roots in construction and industrial applications, where there is a need to coordinate multiple contractors and activities to complete a project on time and within limited resources. Within the health care industry, several different terms are used, including critical paths, CareMaps, clinical pathways, clinical guidelines, clinical protocols, CPM, and algorithms. There are no universally accepted definitions of these terms, although the underlying concepts and tools are very similar. Once the concepts are understood, an organization can choose its preferred terminology.

Coffey et al describe the basics of critical paths as they have been applied in health care: "A critical path is an optimal sequencing and timing of interventions by physicians, nurses, and other disciplines for a particular diagnosis or procedure, designed to minimize delays and resource utilization and to maximize the quality of care."[1(p45)] "A critical path is the sequence of activities that takes the most time to complete."[2(p15)]

When first introduced, the term *critical path* may cause some confusion in health care organizations due to multiple interpretations of the term *critical*. Clinically, "critical" refers to the urgency of a patient's clinical condition, such as a patient in critical condition within the critical care unit. In CPM, however, "critical" refers to the sequence of activities that take the most time. Most clinicians are comfortable using this meaning of critical path. If, however, clinicians object to the term, there are other alternatives.

- clinical path, which emphasizes coordination of all clinical activities
- time-limiting path, which clarifies that the goal is to coordinate resources and care to minimize the duration of care[2,3]
- CareMaps, which clarifies that the planned activities describe the care provided (CareMaps also include outcome information)[4,5]

Schriefer offers a useful distinction between the general terms associated with pathways, and those associated with algorithms or guidelines. "The pathway provides an overview of the entire production process from start to finish, not only pieces in the process, and can be used to reduce variation in the production process."[6(p485)] "Conversely, algorithms often guide clinicians through the 'if, then' decision-making process, such as a variation from a pathway. Algorithms, which were initially developed for handling complex mathematical equations, usually address patient responses to a particular treatment or condition."[6(p485–486)]

SCOPE AND USES OF CRITICAL PATHS

Using critical paths is like looking through a microscope. Just as microscopes have different levels of magnification, critical paths have different scopes—each used for a different purpose.[1] The contrasts of these scopes is particularly important for managed health care organizations. Scopes include the following:

- *Inpatient care.* These critical paths are initiated at the time of either admission or a surgical procedure and typically end when the patient is discharged. As length of stay is shortened, some critical paths now include selected pre- and posthospitalization care as well.
- *Complete episode of care.* These critical paths begin at the time the patient presents at the physician's office requiring diagnosis and end when the patient has completed all therapeutic care related to that episode of illness. This scope of critical path application addresses care across multiple geographic settings, including inpatient care in a hospital, outpatient care at a clinic or physician's office, and home care.
- *Specialized applications.* Critical path methods can also be used for specialized applications, such as for ambulatory surgery

patients, renal dialysis patients, or patients in an intensive care unit. As an example, UMHS is currently developing a model for managing the care of outpatients in a new cough and dyspnea clinic.
- *Life and health management.* These critical paths are developed for management of chronic conditions. These might be used to coordinate the care of patients with hypertension, asthma, cancer, or other illnesses, to achieve the best-quality and most cost-effective care practices. Coffey, Fenner, and Stogis describe a taxonomy of health care, health, and social services that might be included in a critical path addressing life and health management.[7] This taxonomy includes many services not considered part of the traditional health care system.

The scope of the critical path affects the geographic settings of care and the resources involved. The scope for critical paths will be addressed again later.

Critical paths have many important uses. The key uses include the following:

- *Clarifying the "big picture" of planned care.* Traditionally, physicians write orders each day, but often other members of the care team are unaware of the overall plan for care. Lacking knowledge of an overall plan, nurses, pharmacists, therapists, ancillary departments, and others carry out each day's orders but cannot plan ahead. Hence, breakdowns in communication and delays are common. Critical paths direct care toward agreed-upon endpoints that are expected outcomes.
- *Planning and coordinating care.* During critical path development, the teams of physicians, nurses, pharmacists, therapists, and others discuss the coordination of appropriate care based upon data, published research, expert opinion, and consensus. Thus, the different specialties and disciplines are acting in a coordinated, rather than independent, manner.
- *Establishing expectations.* Critical paths developed by a multispecialty, multidisciplinary team establish specific expectations of actions, timing, and outcomes for everyone.
- *Reducing variation of care.* An almost guaranteed outcome of using critical paths is more consistent care. During development of the pathways, the team members evaluate alternative approaches to care and select a standardized approach that accomplishes the best outcomes.
- *Educating and orienting.* Critical paths provide an excellent tool to educate staff, students, and others regarding treatment plans and expected outcomes. This represents a substantial deviation from the usual way of educating house officers or residents, medical students, nurses, and others. Instead of allowing all residents and medical students to order whatever they find interesting, pathways guide them to order those tests and therapies that are proven most effective.
- *Benchmarking.* Critical paths provide an excellent mechanism to study how alternative care plans affect patient outcomes. Many hospitals compare critical paths and learn from those with the best outcomes.
- *Communicating among clinicians, patients, families, payers, and others.* Critical pathways help everyone—clinicians, patients, families, payers, and others—to understand the planned care and expected outcomes. MCOs, for example, might approve services based upon the critical path.
- *Improving the working environment.* The process of developing and using critical paths encourages cooperation and mutual understanding of everyone's role in providing high-quality, cost-effective care. This leads to an improved working environment.[1]

ENVIRONMENT FOR CRITICAL PATHS

Successful development and use of critical paths is not just a matter of learning the analytical techniques. Administrative support of this process is crucial to the success of critical paths. To successfully meet pathway outcomes, leaders must dedicate time to critical path development, training, monitoring, and data analysis. Leaders must establish an environment where development, education, and use of critical paths is fostered.

External Environment

The external environment of health care has changed dramatically during the last few years. Businesses, payers, accrediting bodies, government agencies, patients, and others are scrutinizing health care providers much more than in the past. Customers and other external organizations are demanding more information about care provided, clinical outcomes, costs, customer satisfaction, and other measures. For example, the Health Care Financing Administration (HCFA), within the US Department of Health and Human Services, is holding physicians, hospitals, and other providers to much more stringent documentation expectations. Critical paths can be used to help document the care provided.

Urgency To Change

Change occurs only if people believe there is a reason to change. Without this motivation to change, physicians, nurses, other clinicians, payers, and others will continue to practice as they have in the past. Businesses, government agencies, and payers are creating an urgency to control costs without sacrificing quality of care, by working "smarter and better."

Champions

Respected clinicians from all disciplines are necessary for broad acceptance of critical paths. Look for teams of physicians, nurses, pharmacists, therapists, and others that believe critical paths will help them. Working with the champions to demonstrate success with pilot studies will encourage broader participation. Once critical paths are developed, champions are also more likely to comply with them.

Willingness To Challenge Current Practices and Boundaries

It is very important that the environment encourage clinicians and support staff to critically challenge current practices, such as current clinical protocols, the settings where care is provided (eg, inpatient, outpatient, home), the roles of individuals providing services to achieve the desired outcomes (eg, physicians, registered nurses, physician assistants, family members), and the timing of activities. To challenge the boundaries, clinicians and support staff must consider the whole episode of care, not just the inpatient portion. If other care settings are used, a patient may spend little or no time in a hospital, but the patient's care will still be managed for a substantial period.

Standardization Versus Independence

One of the most significant changes facing physicians is increased standardization of clinical practice. The prevalence of completely independent, autonomous clinical practice is decreasing, and many physicians resist that change, calling critical paths, algorithms, and other guidelines "cookbook medicine." For critical paths to succeed, the environment must encourage physicians and other clinicians to standardize care to the extent helpful, then address appropriate exceptions. The idea is to reduce unnecessary variation in care, rather than to replace critical thinking.

Though they sometimes seem to be in conflict, both standardization and innovation are required to develop critical paths. Standardization of practice, using critical paths, guidelines, and algorithms, is the most cost-effective approach to providing high-quality care based upon current best practices. New clinical practices, however, are developed from independent, often innovative, clinical research. Thus, research is required to develop best practices, and then those practices are standardized for broad clinical application using critical paths, guidelines, and algorithms.

Managed Care Covers Same Scope as Critical Path

For broad-scope critical paths to be used, it is important that MCOs cover the same scope of services addressed by the critical paths. For example, a broad-scope critical path addressing the complete episode of care related to a knee replacement might address prehospitalization care in the physician's office, preadmission testing, inpatient care, outpatient physical therapy, durable medical equipment, and home care. However, if a managed care company covers only inpatient care and selected outpatient therapy, clinicians will tend to utilize these more expensive services and minimize services that result in direct costs to the patient. Thus, MCOs should consider extending coverage of services when broad-scope critical paths demonstrate cost-effectiveness and quality.

APPROACH TO DEVELOPING CRITICAL PATHS

The process may vary with the organization and the team, but the following steps provide a useful general approach to developing a critical path[1,2] (see Chapters 35 and 36 for related discussions).

Select Diagnosis, Procedure, or Condition for Path

Although selecting the diagnosis, procedure, or condition for which a critical path will be developed may sound straightforward, there are some important issues to consider. There should be an urgency for change, and a champion for the diagnosis, procedure, or condition selected. In addition, it may be helpful to conduct an initial sensitivity analysis of where costs and problems exist. If, for example, 80% of the costs for a surgical patient are associated with the surgical procedure, spending large amounts of time on a postsurgical critical path may address postsurgical length of stay but may miss the major opportunity to reduce costs.

Define Scope of Critical Path

Will the critical path address inpatient stay only, inpatient plus outpatient follow-up care, the whole episode of care, chronic care management, or another scope? This should be defined before developing the critical path, because it affects the type of care and the clinicians that will develop and use the path.

Select a Multidisciplinary Team

As with quality improvement projects, the team should include all the key clinical and nonclinical staff involved within the critical path's scope of care. Many critical path efforts suffer because they involve only some, not all, of the staff. Incorporating knowledge from several team members will help develop both a useful pathway and support to use the pathway in clinical practice.

Make Flowcharts and Collect Baseline Information

Most critical path efforts begin by making a flowchart of the current process and documenting current practices and outcomes through chart review. This approach helps team members understand the complexities, precedent relationships, and current variations in practices within the process before instituting change. Time estimates for different activities are helpful to clarify understanding.

Question Current Practices and Determine Best Practices

During development and use of a pathway, guideline, or algorithm, it is very important that all current practices be questioned, and literature research be conducted, to determine best practices. The aim is evidence-based pathways, guidelines, and algorithms. Simply replicating current practice in pathways may be an acceptable place to start, but improving practice requires serious questioning of what, when, who, where, how, and why we do things. What criteria are *really* necessary for a patient to be discharged? What care can be provided at home or on an outpatient basis? What intermediate patient care objectives or outcomes are really necessary to accomplish the desired outcomes? What activities contribute? What activities are unnecessary, or not directly related to the key discharge criteria? Why do we do this? Do different practices really result in different outcomes? These questions objectively challenge our current practices, identify activities that are pertinent to attaining and improving outcomes, and eliminate or de-emphasize activities that are less important to outcomes.

Review of clinical and operational literature is helpful to determine evidence-based best practices used at other health care organizations. Benchmarking includes not only documenting results but understanding how those results are achieved. If another organization is found to achieve similar outcomes with substantially shorter length of stay or at substantially lower cost, further information should be gathered about "how" that organization achieves those results. The aim is not necessarily to copy best documented practices, but to use that information to define a minimum acceptable practice. Your clinician group may improve the process to develop a new best practice.

To create more innovative ideas, it may also be helpful to ask questions in a different way. "Why not" questions (eg, Why *can't* we do . . .) invite people to consider whether hard evidence exists to prove that an approach might not work. Asking these types of questions stimulates more creative approaches. If no counterevidence exists, then a new approach may be tested to determine its effectiveness.

Identify Outcomes

When developing a critical path, it is important to begin by defining the specific desired patient outcomes. Ideally, these outcomes should be defined as final goals related to the patient's functional status. When defining outcomes, it is helpful to consider specific outcomes the patient should achieve.

- Define the outcome criteria for discharge from the hospital, to return home, and to return to daily activity. The focus here should be on the most important criteria. All clinical activities should be addressed as part of the critical path, but some are not as important to the overall progress toward these outcomes. It is useful to focus on patient outcomes related to physiological progression or functionality, rather than system outcomes like the patient being transferred or discharged. Focusing on the system-generated boundaries may distract attention from more creative alternatives to achieving the desired patient outcomes. These same outcomes are used to develop the tool for monitoring variance from the pathway and planned outcomes.
- Be specific. Whenever possible, use objective, quantitative terms and measures.
- Be alert to changes in criteria due to new clinical practices, new technology, changing resources available in different settings, and other changes. Research on best practices will be important in this process. For example, UMHS has been able to change the discharge criteria related to stable heart rhythm by using a home care agency with experienced cardiac care nurses to monitor patients at home.[8] The discharge criteria were achieved earlier in the treatment course, and a new critical path emerged.

Define Intermediate Patient Care Objectives

Although not currently done by most teams at UMHS, the next logical step in defining the critical path is to define intermediate patient care objectives necessary to achieve the desired outcomes. Care planning should be based upon the clinical and support activities required to achieve the intermediate patient care objectives leading to the major outcome criteria. To the extent possible, the intermediate objectives should be related to the patient condition rather than system outcomes or constraints.

Determine Activities To Achieve Outcomes

Next, an organization must identify all the activities required to accomplish the outcomes and intermediate objectives. There may be some confusion between activities and events when describing the care plan. Activities are actions that require time and resources to complete, whereas events are milestones that have no time component. Activities are often grouped into categories such as consults, tests, patient activities, treatments, medications, diet, and patient and family education. Including events on the pathway may be helpful for clarifying purposes and milestones.

Determine Precedent Relationships

An activity that must be completed before another activity can begin is called a precedent. Certainly, care providers understand precedent relationships within the scope of their own practice. Although difficult, formalizing the sequence of activities and the precedent relationships is important, particularly for coordination among professionals. In part, this is difficult because care providers have different conceptual frameworks of how care should be organized, different information, and different involvements and priorities for activities. Developing more formalized definitions of precedent relationships and activity times stimulates important discussions that often result in more efficient care. To identify precedents, for each outcome, intermediate objective, and activity you ask, What must be completed before this activity can begin? Using the flowchart/network format helps participants visualize the process and is therefore helpful in encouraging consensus and the discovery of opportunities for improvement.

Determine Activity Times

Some health care organizations discuss the time requirements of activities in general but do not determine times for every activity. They stop short of actually determining the "critical," or time-limiting, path—the path that will take the longest time. Critical paths provide a useful understanding of the process. To calculate the critical path, the times of all activities must be determined. Different approaches can be used to estimate activity times. Initially, most teams develop consensus estimates involving small interdisciplinary efforts. Analyses of medical records can provide frequency data and times of certain events, from which activity times can be estimated. After a pathway is in use, analyses of variations can provide additional data. Formalized time studies are the most accurate but are infrequently done. CPM calculations use average time estimates, whereas PERT calculations use three time estimates: optimistic, most likely, and pessimistic. It should be noted that activity durations can be changed by altering the processes used, productivity of resources, and/or the amount of resources allocated to an activity. For example, after a coronary artery bypass graft (CABG) procedure, an aggressive monitoring of intake, output, and patient weight can shorten the amount of time needed for the patient to "dry out," or reduce to preoperative weight.

Determine the Critical Path

We can find the critical path by summing the times of the respective activities and intermediate outcomes to calculate the total duration of each path through the network or flowchart. As mentioned above, the path with the longest time requirement is called the "critical" path. Because the critical path is intuitive to the clinical team, the team may choose not to formally calculate the critical path or slack times. These calculations are most easily handled by computerized project management software, and many such programs for personal computers are available.

Implement and Monitor Pathways

Once consensus is reached on a pathway, it is implemented and monitored. Pathways should be viewed as guidelines for coordinated care that regularly change based upon changes in practice, new technologies, and resources available in different settings. Consequently, we have found it acceptable to initiate pathways without 100% clinician agreement, particularly during pilot studies to document the effectiveness of alternative care approaches. Clearly, at times, patient condition requires alterations in pathway activities. Outliers are allowed and documented, as are their outcomes. Those data are then used to review and revise the pathway later. By analyzing data comparing variations in practice, costs, and outcomes, the clinicians are able to reduce future variations.

USE OF CRITICAL PATHS

In practice, most clinician effort involves the use of critical paths in daily care of patients, after the pathways are developed. Most health care organizations assign a case manager, pathway coordinator, or another member of the health care team to monitor all patients on critical paths. Richards et al describe a sample process to initiate and use critical paths for an inpatient care episode as follows[9(p36)]:

1. Pathway coordinator is notified of admission.
2. Head nurse/designee assigns appropriate bed on unit.
3. Pathway coordinator initiates patient on pathway by:
   - Documenting in unit log (handwritten or computer database).
   - Entering dates on preprinted orders.
   - Entering dates on pathway.
   - Placing completed pathways in plastic folder on bedside chart and in main chart.
4. Pathway coordinator talks with admitting physician to clarify any questions related to caring for this patient while looking at clinical pathway and preprinted orders.
5. Pathway coordinator talks with the nurse providing care for this patient to clarify any questions.
6. Variance documentation takes place throughout the admission and upon discharge; pathway coordinator completes the variance record and the unit log.
7. Ongoing communication between outpatient and inpatient care providers facilitates smooth transition of patient care through the continuum.

The critical path serves as an important tool for daily communication and coordination about clinical activities, support activities, expected outcomes, and the patient's progress. The critical path is only one tool in the process of caring for the patient, however. Any program that uses pathways must have a method to evaluate the patients' progress while on them, and to evaluate the effectiveness of the pathways.

Variances from patients' expected activity along the critical path or the inability to meet intermediate objectives must be monitored. Because these paths and objectives are constantly monitored, action can be taken immediately when a variance is identified. In some cases, this allows for corrective action before variances occur. For example, if a physician orders a complete blood count and chemistries to be drawn every day, and the pathway specifies that they should be drawn on only days 1, 3, and 5, timely monitoring can help change orders to avoid unnecessary lab tests. While retrospective monitoring does take place, it is less than optimal; variances will already have taken place.

It is also necessary to identify critical events or activities that have a direct impact on pathway outcomes and are schedule dependent. These events and activities include the ordering of needed consults and initiation of discharge planning. While the pathway may describe when you should begin these activities, the variance tool describes the last point at which it can be achieved before it will affect an outcome or resource use. For example, imagine that the pathway describes that the patient should begin ambulation protocol within 6 hours of return from surgery. The outcome is that the patient walks the length of the hallway independently by the time of discharge. The team may decide that an intermediate outcome is that the patient walks at least X feet by 24 hours after surgery. But, if the patient cannot meet the intermediate outcome time frame, a consult may be needed, and the consult time must be built in so the patient can still meet the intended 3-day discharge time.

Another example of critical events or activities that impact pathway outcomes is a 5-day course of continuous chemotherapy where completion of 5 days of chemotherapy is one pathway outcome. A critical event or activity that must occur every day is the initiation of each bag of chemotherapy, on time and infused over the appropriate hours, to meet the final outcome of Y amount of drug given over 5 days or 120 hours. A variance in this process would be the development of patient toxicities, resulting in delay of chemotherapy—a patient variance. On the other hand, if the day 1 bag was hung late due to delay in nursing time to initiate, this would be a clinician variance.

Documentation of variances from the critical path is important to both the care of the patient and the continued improvement of the care processes and critical paths. Richards et al state that

> When a variance occurs between expected and actual treatment plan of care, documentation should identify the variance, its type (patient, clinician, or system), and its effect on outcomes achievement. This should be followed by a review of aggregate data about multiple patients and the long-term outcomes achieved. Only patient variances should be addressed in the patient record. For legal reasons, clinician and system variances are tracked and recorded separately as part of a more confidential quality assurance document. Variance data collection routinely has been labor intensive, especially when the information is collected in narrative form. When variances are collected outside the patient record they should be recorded in a quantitative format that is user friendly and clear, allowing clinicians to use the data to identify trends requiring timely action plans.[9(p35–36)]

ALTERNATIVE FORMATS AND SAMPLE USES

Critical path methods include a number of formats for information displays and associated calculations that can further enhance understanding and provision of health care services. Although some of these formats are not normally used, they offer opportunity for enhancement of critical paths, particularly as the pathways are computerized. In this section, we will briefly summarize four key formats: the activity/precedent table format, the Gantt chart format, the flowchart/network format, and the resource format, and offer an explanation of float/slack time. A more complete description is provided by Coffey et al.[2] Some computer programs include additional formats or views. All of those formats or views are interrelated, so if you change the number of hours or days required for an activity in one view, the other views change to reflect the longer time period. Also, the same information, such as precedent relationships, can be discussed using different formats. In choosing formats, it is best to use those that are most easily understood and used by team members.

Activity/Precedent Table Format

After defining the desired outcomes, the next step in the methodology discussed above is to define all the necessary activities and their relationships. The activity/precedent table is helpful for listing all the activities and reviewing their required precedents, durations, and resource requirements. Calculated start times, finish times, and float/slack times may be displayed in this table also. Use of the activity/precedent table forces a formal consideration of the precedent relationships and duration of all activities, which in turn raises questions about availability of ancillary services and other resources to expedite patient care. The relationships among activities are more difficult to understand in this format than in the flowchart/network format, since there is no indication of which activities are on the critical path. Also, it is difficult to visualize which activities are done on the same day. An activity/precedent table is illustrated in Exhibit 18–1.

Gantt Chart Format

A Gantt chart shows the beginning and ending times for each activity on a bar chart, along a timeline in the units being used. Most health care organizations currently implementing "critical paths" use a form of the Gantt chart, listing the activities to be done each day. This is the most common form of representing a pathway or CareMap. It presents a concise, easy to understand picture of the activities, and in some cases expected outcomes, for each day. The activities are typically organized into groups of consults, tests, patient activities, treatments, medications, diet, and patient and family education. The Gantt chart format is particularly helpful in communicating which activities are being done during each time period. It provides an excellent tool for communications among staff, patients, and family members, and it is very useful for educating clinicians about care requirements. Although it is useful to display activities by day for communication purposes, it may be more useful to use smaller time units, like hours, for planning, coordination, and evaluation.

This format does not work well to illustrate the precedent relationships among activities, nor does it identify which activities are listed on the critical path. Some computer software programs have partially solved this deficiency by including lines linking the information on the Gantt chart to show precedence-related activities. Exhibit 18–2 shows a Gantt chart.

Flowchart/Network Format

The flowchart/network format graphically illustrates the precedent relationships among activities and shows the critical path. This format displays the activities in the care process as a flowchart. The initial flowchart of the current process may be used as a first step, but that flowchart may be refined as precedent relationships and activity durations are revised.

It is helpful to involve direct care providers in creating the flowchart. Using the flowchart may allow creation of the pathway in less time, because it is easier to visualize the relationships of activities than in other formats. Flowcharts are particularly helpful for discussions about existing or changing precedent relationships, clinical practices, and sequences of activities. There may be one or more equal-duration critical paths.

Flowcharts require more space than tables of activities, and they can grow quite large. This format does not work well to communicate what will be done each day. Manually generated networks seldom have supplemental information such as durations of activities or float times, but some computerized project management programs display this additional information in the flowchart/network format. This format is illustrated in Figure 18–1.

RESOURCE FORMATS

There are entry and output forms of the resource table. The data entry table, which is sometimes an extension of the activity table, is used to enter the amounts of different resources required for each activity. If the activity duration is significantly altered, it may alter the resource requirements. Similar to the required activities and precedent relationships, the resource requirements must be carefully challenged. For example, activities that may have been previously done by a physician in an intensive care unit might be done by a nurse in an acute care unit, or even by a visiting nurse in a patient's home. The resource requirements by activity differ from the activity times. The activity time is the amount of chronological time required to complete the activity. The resource requirement is the amount of time or resources required during the activity. For example, it may take 16 hours of pharmaceutical support for a CABG patient, yet the resource requirement during one period may be 1 hour of registered pharmacist time and 1 hour of registered nurse time.

As with activity time estimates, resource requirement estimates may be derived from esti-

Exhibit 18–1 Excerpt from a Sample Activity/Precedent Table for Uncomplicated CABG Patients

ID No.	Activity Name	Duration (Hours)	Precedent Activities
1	Thoracic Surgery Clinic Visit	3	None
2	Anesthesia Clinic Visit	3	1
3	Physical Therapy Visit	1	1
4	Preop Assessment	1	2, 3
5	Preop Identification of Postdischarge Caregiver	1	4
6	Pre- and Postop Patient and Family Teaching	1	5
7	Operative Procedure CABG	6	6
8	Pharmaceutical Support	16	7
9	Hemodynamic Monitoring	16	7
10	Cardiac Monitor	16	7
11	Maintain Ventilator Support	16	7
12	Stabilize Hemodynamics	1	8, 9, 10
13	Discontinue Hardwire Monitoring	1	12
14	Discontinue Hemodynamic Monitoring	1	12
15	Adequate Blood Gases, with Reduced Oxygenation	1	11
16	Extubate	2	15
17	Transfer to Step-Down Unit	1	13, 14, 16
18	Cardiac Monitoring via Telemetry	48	17
19	Discontinue Telemetry	24	18
20	Normal or Preop Cardiac Rhythm	0	19
21	Monitor Intake and Output, Vitals, etc (ongoing)	0	17
22	Diuretic Protocol	36	21
23	Monitor Weight	1	22
24	Weight Approaching Preop Weight	0	23
25	Increasing Activity (plus other related activities)	85	17, 22
26	Bowel Movement	1	25
27	Wean to Nasal Cannula	3	16
28	Discontinue Nasal Cannula	34	27
29	Room Air × 24 Hours	24	28
30	Tolerates Activity on Room Air	0	29
31	Discharge	4	20, 24, 26, 30
32	Positive Life Style Activities		31
33	Postop Appointments Kept		31
34	Weight at Preop Level		31
35	Cardiac Rhythm Stable		31
36	Activity at Least at Preop Level		31

Source: Reprinted from RJ Coffey, JE Othman, and JI Walters, Extending the Application of Critical Path Methods, *Quality Management in Health Care*, Vol 3, No 2, p 24, © 1995, Aspen Publishers, Inc.

Exhibit 18–2 Gantt Chart Showing Excerpt of Activities by Day for Uncomplicated CABG Patients

	Postop Period of Operative Day	*Postop Day 1*	*Postop Day 2*
Treatment	Maintain ventilator support until extubation		
	Wean to nasal cannula	Oxygen by nasal cannula	Room air
	Hardwire monitoring	Telemetry	Monitor intake and output tid
	Vital signs monitored	Vitals every 4 hours	Vitals every 4 hours
	Hemodynamic monitoring		
	Cardiac output every 4 hours		Telemetry
	Pharmaceutical support	Pharmaceutical support	Pharmaceutical support
	Initiate diuretic protocol	Continue diuretic protocol	Continue diuretic protocol
Patient activity	Bed rest until extubated	Ambulate to tolerance qid	Increase ambulation to tolerance qid
	Up in chair at bedside		
Diet	NPO	No added salt, low-cholesterol solid diet	No added salt, low-cholesterol solid diet
	Advance to clear liquids		
Discharge planning		Assess additional home care needs	
		Transfer to step-down unit	
Teaching	Explain intensive care unit procedures	Reinforce incentive spirometer use	
	Explain transfer to step-down unit	Reinforce increasing activity	Reinforce increasing activity
Medications	Potassium as needed		Potassium as needed
	Magnesium as needed		
	Nitroglycerine 1 µg/kg		
	Diltiazem 30 mg tid	Diltiazem CD once a day	Diltiazem CD once a day
Test	Electrolytes (potassium × 3)	Electrolytes	
	Complete blood count		
	Arterial blood gases		
	Chest X-ray		
	Pulse oximetry	Pulse oximetry	

Note: This Gantt chart is for illustration only and should not be used as a standard of care.

Courtesy of University of Michigan Hospitals, Ann Arbor, Michigan.

Critical Paths 231

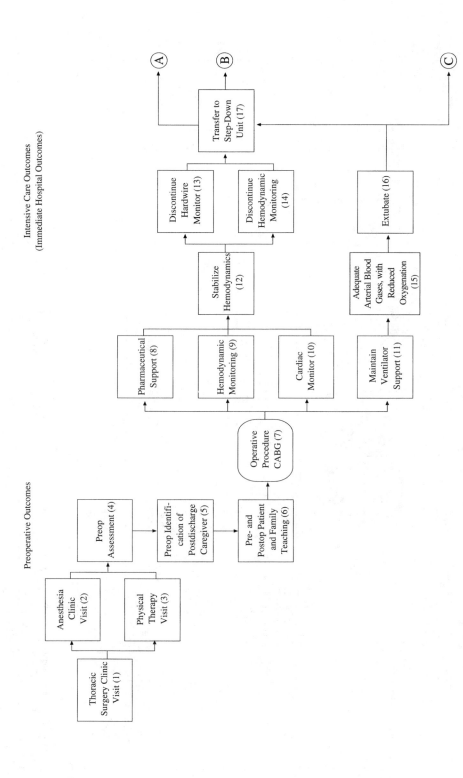

Figure 18–1 Excerpt from a Sample Flowchart of Activities and Outcomes for Uncomplicated CABG Patients. *Note*: This figure is for illustration only and should not be used as a standard of care. *Source*: Reprinted from RJ Coffey, JE Othman, and JI Walters, Extending the Application of Critical Path Methods, *Quality Management in Health Care*, Vol 3, No 2, p 20, © 1995, Aspen Publishers, Inc.

continues

232 Best Practices in Medical Management

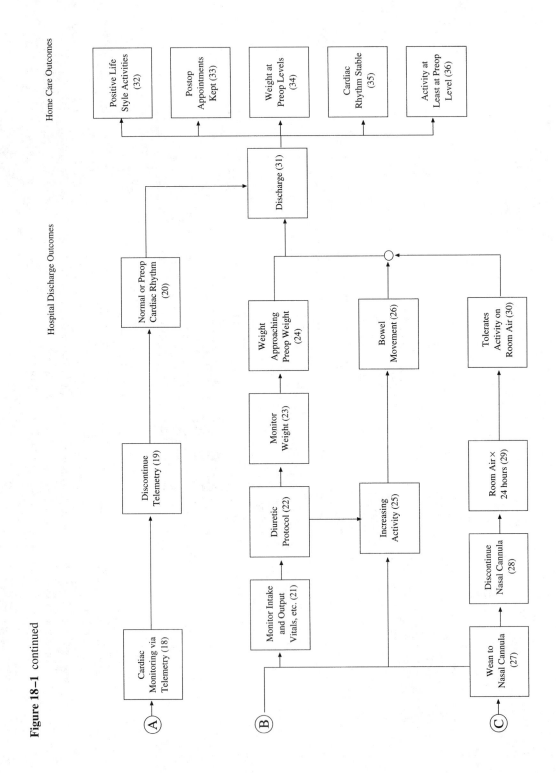

Figure 18–1 continued

mates agreed upon by professionals, estimates derived from times in patient charts, analyses of variances, or time studies. Resource requirements by activity have seldom been included in the critical path work to date in health care. The resource format can be helpful to plan and schedule resource requirements, and evaluate changes in resource use, as more patients are on computerized critical paths. Like the Gantt chart, this format (Exhibit 18–3) does not communicate precedent relationships, nor does it have information about the duration of the activity.

CALCULATE AND USE FLOAT/SLACK TIME INFORMATION

All tasks not on the critical path have "slack" or "float" time. Float time is the amount of time an activity can be delayed without delaying another activity. Although this concept is not currently used in health care, knowing the amount of float time is helpful in prioritizing activities, particularly in clinical situations where the path is very constrained. "Free float" is the amount of time an activity can be delayed without delaying another activity. "Total float" is the amount of time an activity can be delayed without delaying the finish date (though the activity may cut into the float time of successive activities). A path with relatively large float time allows for more tolerance of uncontrollable variation. Clinicians must be extremely vigilant if they have little or no float time for activities; delays of these activities will delay the outcomes or discharge. Although conceptually simple, the calculations related to float time are detailed and best handled by a computer program.

RESULTS

The results associated with implementing critical paths fall into two general categories. First, patients, clinicians, and payers agree that critical paths improve planning, coordination, and communication related to the care of patients. They help expectations to be communicated among clinicians, patients, family members, and payers.

Second, critical paths make available quantitative measures of changes in length of stay, resource use, costs, and so on. These measures are useful to health care administrators and payers. UMHS and other health care organizations have found that critical paths do have a positive impact on these quantitative measures. Some examples follow.

At the CS Mott Children's Hospital of UMHS, data were analyzed for a sample of 300 inpatients admitted to the pediatric cardiology service included on one of the critical pathways for 19 diagnoses/procedures.[9] Charts were analyzed for 130 patients before the critical paths were initiated, and these were compared with results for 170 patients after the critical paths were initiated. Cost and readmission data were obtained from patient accounting and admitting, respectively. "After implementation of case management [with critical paths], 76% (130 of 170) of the patients were discharged within the expected length of stay, which increased from 66% (86 of 130) of patients in the pre–case management group ($x^2 = 3.89$, $p = 0.05$)."[10(p76)] The study also found that the average length of stay decreased by 0.2—to 1.0 day for 11 of 14 diagnoses/procedures for the group that was case managed.[10] However, initiation of case management did not significantly change the incidence of readmissions. After case management, the incidence was 1.2% (2 of 170), whereas before case management, it was 1.5% (2 of 130).[10] In the study, "Discharge readiness was not assessed in patients hospitalized less than 72 hours. At the time of assessment before discharge, 97% (67 of 69 [assessed]) of parents reported readiness for their child's discharge within 24 hours. Follow-up assessment approximately two weeks later revealed that parental perception of discharge readiness was highly reliable with 95% agreement (that is, same or better rating of readiness)."[10(p77)] With respect to charges for the surgical procedures, however, the "data regarding average billed charges for eight cardiac surgical procedures suggested a mean in-

Exhibit 18–3 Sample Resource Table for Uncomplicated CABG Patients

ID No.	Activity Name	Staff Time Requirements				Equipment	
		Physician Time (hours)	Nurse Time (hours)	Tech/Physician Assistant Time (hours)	Other (hours)	Room	Other
1	Thoracic Surgery Clinic Visit	1		0.5	0.75	Exam Room	
2	Anesthesia Clinic Visit	0.5			0.75	Exam Room	
3	Physical Therapy Visit			1		Exam Room	Spirometer
4	Preop Assessment		0.5				
5	Preop Identification of Postdischarge Caregiver		0.5				
6	Pre- and Postop Patient and Family Teaching		0.5				Booklet
7	Operative Procedure CABG	24	12	24	16	OR	

Note: This resource table is for illustration only and should not be used as a standard of care.

Source: Reprinted from RJ Coffey, JE Othman, and JI Walters, Extending the Application of Critical Path Methods, *Quality Management in Health Care,* Vol 3, No 2, p 26, © 1995, Aspen Publishers, Inc.

crease of 13.4%, without adjustment for changes in hospital costs [over a multiyear period]."[10(p76)]

Multiple clinical services have implemented critical paths within the adult hospital of UMHS. Quantitative results include the following:

- For thoracic surgery, average lengths of stay decreased significantly for the four key procedures with pathways, as illustrated in Table 18–1. Some of the procedures have multiple critical paths. The changes in other

Table 18–1 Average Length of Stay for Thoracic Surgery Patients

	Length of Stay (Days)	
Unit and Procedure	Before Critical Path (4/1/1990–1/19/1991)	2 Years after Critical Path (4/1/1992–12/31/1992)
Intensive care unit		
Heart transplant	12.10	8.47
CABG (first time)	4.60	2.53
Esophagectomy	3.60	0.80
CABG (revision)	6.29	2.73
Routine unit		
Heart transplant	14.60	10.44
CABG (first time)	8.50	6.90
Esophagectomy	12.70	11.99
CABG (revision)	6.83	6.58

Source: Reprinted from RJ Coffey et al, Critical Paths: Linking Outcomes for Patients, Clinicians, and Payers, in *The Managed Health Care Handbook,* 3rd ed, PR Kongstvedt, ed, p 315, © 1996, Aspen Publishers, Inc.

Table 18–2 Average Length of Stay for Orthopaedic Surgery Patients

	Length of Stay (Days)	
Procedure	Before Critical Path (1/1/1992–12/31/1992)	After Critical Path (1/1/1993–12/31/1993)
Posterior spinal fusion	10.40	8.39
Total knee arthroplasty	6.39	5.65
Total knee arthroplasty (revision)	8.20	6.33
Total hip arthroplasty	7.24	6.52
Total hip arthroplasty (revision)	10.52	9.26

Source: Reprinted from RJ Coffey et al, Critical Paths: Linking Outcomes for Patients, Clinicians, and Payers, in *The Managed Health Care Handbook,* 3rd ed, PR Kongstvedt, ed, p 316, © 1996, Aspen Publishers, Inc.

resource use, as measured by relative value units (RVUs) to eliminate pricing changes, varied. For 4 of 7 procedures, resource RVUs decreased, and for 3 of 7, resource RVUs increased.

- For orthopaedic surgery, average lengths of stay decreased significantly for the five key procedures with pathways, as illustrated in Table 18–2. And 4 of the 5 procedures also experienced decreases in resource use, as measured by RVUs.
- For urology, Figure 18–2 illustrates a graph of length of stay calculated for many of the diagnoses and procedures with critical paths. Although the length of stay was decreasing before implementing the critical path, the length of stay after implementing the pathway dropped faster.

CONCLUSION

Critical paths are important tools. They help link the patients, clinicians, and MCOs and other payers and increase the quality and cost-effectiveness of care. Critical paths have different scopes of use, including inpatient care, entire

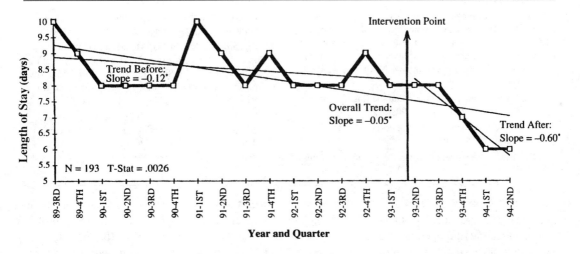

Figure 18–2 Radical Prostatectomy without Complications: Mean Length of Stay and Trend Lines, All Patients, Before and After 6/21/93 Intervention. Total RVU consumption, 881,318. *The slope of the trend line reflects the average increase (or decrease, if negative) in days per quarter (per patient). Courtesy of University of Michigan Medical Center, Ann Arbor, Michigan.

episodes of care, and management of chronic conditions. They are developed collaboratively by teams comprising physicians, nurses, pharmacists, therapists, dietitians, and other clinicians to coordinate the care of a patient with a specific diagnosis or procedure. To be most effective, critical paths must focus on achieving patient care outcomes and intermediate objectives as quickly as possible, while avoiding wasted resources.

The time units used for the critical path should be linked to the scope of care covered by the pathway. For highly specialized and time-sensitive services like surgical procedures or emergency services, the best time unit may be minutes. For intensive care and other services with very short lengths of stay, the best time unit may be hours. For chronic disease management, the best time unit may be months.

Critical paths have improved many aspects of health care organizations. They have effectively helped organizations to plan and coordinate care; establish expectations; reduce variations in care; educate and orient staff; encourage communication among patients, clinicians, payers, and others; benchmark best practices; and reduce length of stay and costs.

Successful development and use of critical paths means doing more than just learning the analytical techniques. Organizations must provide the right environment for critical paths. There must be a sense that change is necessary and a willingness to challenge current practices and boundaries. There must also be champions for critical paths, administrative support, and payers and MCOs that cover the same scope of care as the critical paths.

REFERENCES

1. Coffey RJ, Richards JS, Remmert CS, LeRoy SS, Schoville RR, Baldwin PJ. An introduction to critical paths. *Qual Manage Health Care.* 1992;1(1):45–54.
2. Coffey RJ, Othman JE, Walters JI. Extending the application of critical path methods. *Qual Manage Health Care.* 1995;3(2):14–29.
3. Wintermeyer-Pingel S, Othman E, Althouse B, et al. Coordinated care variance data collection: a "time-limiting pathway" approach. Presented at the National Leadership Conference, Management of Quality: Changing Today for Tomorrow; November 4, 1993; Ann Arbor, MI.
4. Zander K. Estimating and tracking the financial impact of critical paths. *Definition.* 1990;5(4):1–3.
5. Zander K. CareMaps: the core of cost/quality care. *New Definition.* 1991;6(3):1–3.
6. Schriefer J. The synergy of pathways and algorithms: two tools work better than one. *Joint Commission J Qual Improvement.* 1994;20(9):485–499.
7. Coffey RJ, Fenner KM, Stogis SL. *Virtually Integrated Health Systems: A Guide To Assessing Organizational Readiness and Strategic Partners.* San Francisco: Jossey-Bass, Publishers; 1997.
8. Frantz A. Cardiac recovery in home: improving quality while reducing cost. *Remington Rep.* 1993;7:14–15.
9. Richards JS, Kocan MJ, Monaghan H, Wintermeyer-Pingel S, Goldman EB. Clinical paths and patient care documentation. In: Spath PL, ed. *Clinical Paths: Tools for Outcomes Management.* Chicago: American Hospital Association; 1994:33–44.
10. Uzark K, LeRoy S, Callow L, Cameron J, Rosenthal A. The pediatric nurse practitioner as case manager in the delivery of services to children with heart disease. *J Pediatr Health Care.* 1994;8(4):74–78.

RICHARD J. COFFEY, PHD, is director of program and operations analysis at the University of Michigan Hospitals and Health Centers (UMHHC), Ann Arbor, Michigan, and an adjunct associate professor of industrial and operations engineering at the University of Michigan. Dr. Coffey has authored over 45 articles and chapters, coauthored three books (*Transforming Healthcare Organizations, Total Quality in Healthcare,* and *Virtually Integrated Health Systems*), and given over 120 presentations at regional, national, and international conferences.

JANET S. RICHARDS, MS, RN, CNAA, is director of Mercy Health Telemanagement, Mercy Health Services, Ypsilanti, Michigan. She was formerly the programmatic lead for the Coordinated Care Program at the University of Michigan Hospitals and Health Centers. She was coauthor of a chapter titled "Clinical Paths and Patient Care Documentation" in *Clinical Paths: Tools for Outcomes Management.*

SUSAN A. WINTERMEYER-PINGEL, MSN, RN, OCN, is a clinical nurse specialist at the University of Michigan Hospitals and Health Centers and participates in the Coordinated Care Program, working with the adult hematology/oncology population. She coauthored the chapter entitled "Clinical Paths and Patient Care Documentation" in *Clinical Paths: Tools for Outcomes Management* and has presented topics related to management of critical pathways both nationally and locally.

SARAH S. LEROY, MSN, RN, is a clinical nurse specialist in pediatric cardiology at CS Mott Children's Hospital within the University of Michigan Hospitals and Health Centers in Ann Arbor, Michigan.

Part VII

Ambulatory Care

The most common setting of health care, other than the home when one considers self-care for minor conditions, is the ambulatory setting. The focus in Part VII is on clinical care in the office, ambulatory procedures, and the overlaying authorization systems and programs that accompany so much of managed care.

Chapter 19

Management of Clinical Services in the Clinician's Office

Gordon Mosser

Chapter Outline

- Introduction
- Finding the Clinicians' Points of Engagement
- Clinical Practice Guideline Development as an Engagement Strategy
- Planning the Guideline Program
- Guideline Development
- Fostering Improvement of Clinical Care Through Collaboratives
- Holding Practices Accountable
- The Necessity for Trust

INTRODUCTION

Management of clinical services in the clinician's office presents a special challenge. Only clinicians—not health plans—can manage these services. The role of the health plan is to encourage clinicians to manage these services, to provide an attractive pathway for the activity, and to provide support for the tasks involved.

Management of services in the office has three purposes (as does management of care in general).

- to improve the delivery of care and information to patients
- to improve patients' health outcomes
- to eliminate waste from care processes

Office practice management projects must promise to advance at least one of these purposes.

FINDING THE CLINICIANS' POINTS OF ENGAGEMENT

The first task in mounting a health plan program to improve office care is identifying participating physicians' goals, because these goals can be used to motivate physician participation in programs. In other words, the task is to answer the question, What do the physicians want that they might achieve through participation in an office care management program? There are several possibilities, and the relative weight attached to the various answers varies by locale.

The common points of engagement include

- a desire to improve the care and information provided to their patients
- a desire to improve patients' health outcomes
- a desire to eliminate waste to make the physicians more competitive or more profitable in a managed care environment
- a desire to increase fee-for-service billings for legitimate services such as overlooked preventive testing, immunization, or counseling
- a desire to reduce the frustrations and unpredictability of daily office practice by improvements in the processes of care, that is, the flows of hourly events in the office
- a desire to meet contractual requirements commonly included in health plan con-

tracts, that is, requirements to engage in effective quality improvement activities
- a desire to improve their attractiveness to employer-purchasers by gaining experience in quality improvement and waste reduction

Medical directors must explore the wishes of participating physicians so that office practice management programs can be crafted to appeal to physicians. Unless programs meet physician needs, they will have no reason to work with them.

CLINICAL PRACTICE GUIDELINE DEVELOPMENT AS AN ENGAGEMENT STRATEGY

There are essentially two strategies available for engaging physicians to work with the health plan to improve clinical practice in their offices. The first is to measure their performance using administrative data or data from chart reviews. The rationale for this approach is that demonstration of room for improvement will be illuminating and motivating for physicians who want to improve care processes and health outcomes. This approach can succeed in selected settings, but unfortunately, presenting performance data can often engender annoyance and time-wasting debates about the data's validity.

A more attractive and lower risk strategy is to invite physicians to participate in a program to develop clinical practice guidelines.[1] The appeal to them to join in this effort should be linked to the physicians' priorities. For example, if the physicians show special interest in improving outcomes for childhood asthma, the clinical practice guidelines program might address this topic first. If participating physicians want to demonstrate cost-consciousness to influential purchasers, early emphasis should be placed on waste reduction guidelines such as one aimed at decreasing premature computed tomography (CT) or magnetic resonance imaging (MRI) scanning for acute low back pain.

Crafting clinical practice guidelines is an attractive entry point for the management of clinical services in the office. Most physicians enjoy clinical discussions of how best to deal with the diagnosis and management of a given disease or condition. Many appreciate having a structured setting in which to discuss clinical issues with clinicians who practice in otherwise separate settings.

On the other hand, crafting guidelines is only a first step. Guidelines alone do not improve care. They are only plans for care. They must be combined with a management approach in order to achieve any real improvements in the office (see also Part XI), and the best management approach is continual improvement (the approach variously labeled "continuous quality improvement," "total quality management," and the like).[2-4]

The effectiveness of using practice guidelines to improve care is now beyond doubt.[5] Nevertheless, many clinicians continue to be skeptical or to feel threatened, and vigorous promotion of the concept may be necessary.[6]

PLANNING THE GUIDELINE PROGRAM

A health plan seeking to foster management of clinical services in the office should begin by assembling a planning group of participating physicians. This group will establish a guideline development and implementation program for interested physicians. The group should be representative of the participating providers generally and must be accepted by the providers. In some cases, the group can be the health plan's preexisting quality improvement committee.

The group may begin by considering how the guidelines will be developed. In general, they should not be developed anew but should be modified from guidelines obtained from well-respected sources such as the Agency for Health Care Policy and Research or the American College of Physicians. A specific developmental sequence should be agreed upon. (An example sequence is provided below.)

The planning group must also deal with the criteria to be used in selecting topics for guideline development. Commonly, the criteria include the frequency of the condition at issue; the anticipated gain with respect to care, outcome, or waste reduction; and the probability of success. The pace of guideline development should also be set; in particular, the group should decide the number of guidelines to be developed in the first year. A timid start—say, 1 or 2 guidelines—may fail to attract the attention of the participating physicians. An overambitious start—say, 15 guidelines—will overwhelm the practitioners or fail for lack of focus.

The group should choose a standard format for guideline documents. The format may be an annotated algorithm, structured text, or table. Generally, annotated algorithms are the most satisfactory because they are easily understood and because the format encourages logical clarity during the drafting.[7]

Finally, the group should devise a plan for topic-specific collaboratives of various physician practices intent on the improvement of care for the disease or condition in question. It is through these collaboratives that the guidelines will be implemented.

GUIDELINE DEVELOPMENT

At the close of the planning period, a steering committee should be established to choose guideline topics, approve guidelines, and oversee their development and use for the improvement of care. The steering committee may evolve from the planning group or may be appointed by the health plan medical director or the quality improvement committee. As with the planning group, it is important that the steering committee is perceived as representative and legitimate by a broad cross-section of the physicians participating in the health plan. The need is similar to the one for the critical pathway discussed in Chapter 18.

Using the choice criteria developed during the planning period, the committee will choose topics for the first year's work. This task initiates the developmental sequence shown in Figure 19–1.

The next step is to assemble a group of 7 to 12 physicians and other clinicians to draft the guideline for a given topic. The group should be dominated by clinicians who will use the guideline. Thus, if the guideline is to cover primary care treatment of diabetes, most of the physicians should be internists and family practitioners. One or two diabetologists should also be included, as should a nurse and a diabetic educator. The group should normally be led by a physician who is aided by a person skilled in managing small group processes, that is, a facilitator.

The developmental sequence for a guideline document should occur within a well-defined period of time stipulated by the steering committee in advance. Typically, the development of the first draft can be accomplished in four to eight meetings of 2 to 3 hours over 3 or 4 months. A sequence of fewer than four meetings will not allow the group to form properly before it tries to forge consensus; the result is likely to be agreement without commitment. A development period of more than eight meetings is usually unnecessary and runs the risk of decreasing program momentum.

The developmental process should begin with a guideline from a respected source, commonly called a "seed" guideline.[8] It is not necessary to identify all such guidelines since the purpose is not to synthesize them but instead to speed the initiation of the local process. The group should identify its points of doubt or disagreement with the seed guideline and then review the medical literature on these points, revising the seed guideline as it sees fit. The group should be focused on production of a document in the format prescribed by the planning group. Focusing on the document helps to keep the discussions on track and makes the process more efficient.

At the end of the initial drafting period, the document should be subjected to extensive review, comment, and criticism by clinicians who will use the guideline. The purpose of this critique is twofold. First, it will identify omissions and errors in the guideline. Second, and

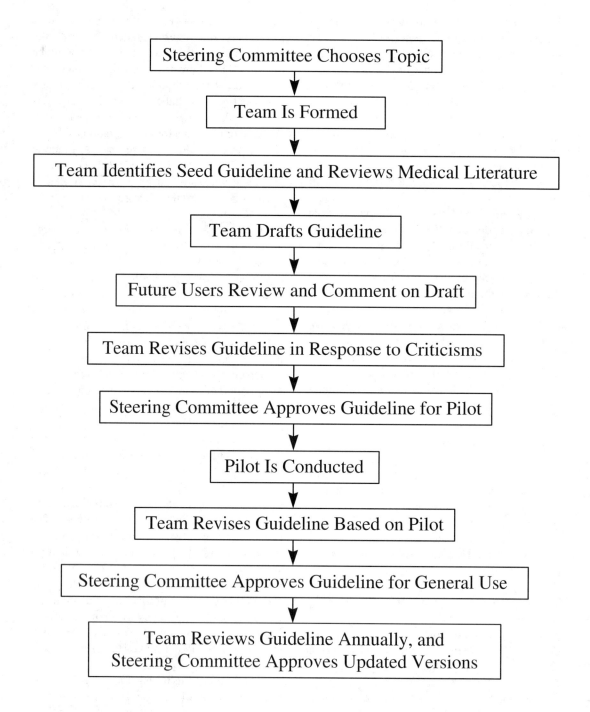

Figure 19–1 Guideline Development. Courtesy of Institute for Clinical Systems Integration, Bloomington, Minnesota.

more important, it will build knowledge of and support for the guideline. It is essential that the drafting group respond substantively to the criticisms and that it modify the guideline when the available evidence supports the criticism. Responding does not mean agreeing in all cases; a suitable response will often be a reasoned defense. However, without responsiveness from the drafting group, the guideline is destined to go unused. The group should be required to answer all criticisms of its draft publicly as part of improving the draft guideline and of gaining support for it through an open, deliberative process.

After revisions are made in response to the critique, the guideline should be presented to the steering committee for approval. The committee should develop clear, brief criteria for guideline approval. The criteria should deal with procedure and not with content. In other words, the guideline should be approved if the work group followed the prescribed process, including, most important, the conduct of the critical review and subsequent revision. The steering committee should avoid redebating the content of the guideline because usurping the authority granted to the drafting group will alienate its members and decrease future support for the effort.

Next, the guidelines should be piloted for 4 to 6 months in a small number of volunteer offices. The experiences of the pilot offices should be conveyed to the drafting group, which should then revise the guideline to take advantage of the knowledge gained.

All guideline documents should be revisited periodically (ordinarily annually) to ensure that they remain current with the literature and with knowledge gained through their use. This review should be performed by the original drafting group once each year. If work group members resign, they should be replaced so that the work group is maintained as long as the guideline is in use. If a guideline is not found useful, it should be explicitly withdrawn and the work group disbanded.

As an example of the sequence of development, imagine the implementation of a guideline for the primary care of asthma in children (discussed in detail in Chapter 30). Asthma would be a natural choice for steering committees in many health plans because the disease is common, undertreatment is frequent in many settings, care is often poorly coordinated, and the prospects for improvement are often good. The drafting team should consist of family practitioners, pediatricians, a pulmonologist, an allergist, a nurse, perhaps a pharmacist, and a facilitator.

A good seed guideline would be the 1997 National Institutes of Health (NIH) guideline.[9] The team would review the NIH guideline, noting any points that seem doubtful or controversial. It would then consult the medical literature on these points and revise the guideline, supporting its position with citations of the literature. It would then circulate the draft to large numbers of family practitioners, pediatricians, and nurses, seeking their criticisms. It might seek out a few highly regarded clinicians not involved in the drafting to provide especially thorough reviews.

Using the criticisms received, the team would revise the guideline, answer each critic in writing, and then submit the guideline to the steering committee for approval to pilot its use. The guideline would then be used for a few months in four or five practices. Using the reports from the piloting practices on the guideline's value and practicality, the team would next revise the guideline again and submit it for approval for general use. After a year, the team would reconvene to review and revise the guideline, taking into account any new evidence in the medical literature as well as reports from practices using the guideline. Revision meetings would continue annually.

FOSTERING IMPROVEMENT OF CLINICAL CARE THROUGH COLLABORATIVES

Once a guideline has been drafted, critiqued, revised, piloted, revised again, and approved, it should be disseminated to all clinicians who would use it. However, this distribution alone will ordinarily have little or no effect.

The key to fostering use of the guideline is the establishment of collaboratives made up of physicians, nurses, and others who are using the guideline in their own offices. These collaboratives provide venues for exchanging information on what works and what does not; for sharing data on success (or failure); for peer challenge and peer pressure; and for teaching provided either by health plan staff, participating physicians, or invited speakers.

As in the initial stage of exploring potential points of engagement, health plan staff should find out what topics appeal to clinicians. Commonly attractive topics are diabetes, asthma, hypertension, coronary artery disease prevention, and preventive services such as cancer screening and immunization. Once a suitable topic or two have been identified, recruitment of interested practices can begin.

The collaborative's meetings should be attended by a physician and one other person, typically a nurse, from each participating practice.

The group should fix its own schedule. A meeting every 2 or 3 months for 2 to 3 hours will ordinarily work well. In between meetings, the participants may choose to meet by conference telephone call.

At the meetings the physicians and nurses should be encouraged to use a disciplined continual improvement approach in their use of the guideline. Typically, this approach will consist of the following steps (Figure 19–2):

- Identify gaps between the guideline and the office's actual practice.
- Set an overall goal for the project, for example, to improve glycemic control among persons with diabetes.
- Set an intermediate goal that will advance the long-term goal, for example, improvement of hemoglobin A1c testing for persons with diabetes.
- Try out some change to achieve the intermediate goal, for example, having nurses add a note to the front of the chart of each person with diabetes, prominently display-

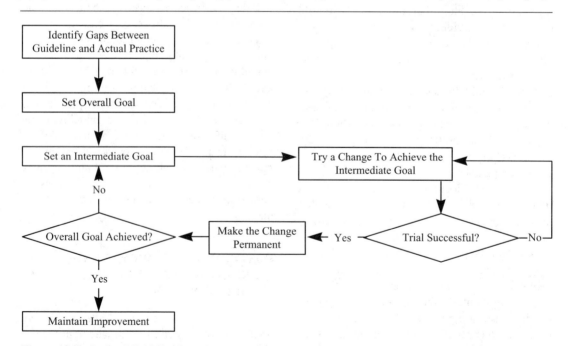

Figure 19–2 Cycle of Guideline Use. Courtesy of Institute for Clinical Systems Integration, Bloomington, Minnesota.

ing to the physician the date of the patient's last hemoglobin A1c testing.
- Determine whether the trial worked and, if so, make the change permanent.
- Choose another intermediate goal and pursue it in a similar fashion until the overall goal is met.

Physicians and their office staff members will commonly benefit from brainstorming and suggestions for achieving improvements. The available action options can be summarized under eight headings.

1. *process redesign*, for example, the addition of the nursing note just mentioned for the care of persons with diabetes
2. *training* of physicians, nurses, and other support staff—usually training of people who were assigned new tasks because a process was redesigned
3. use of *peer influence*, for example, group discussions of a guideline among physicians in the same practice or academic detailing carried out by a respected clinician[10]
4. providing *prompts at the time of care*, for example, use of laminated cards that summarize the guideline and are readily accessible in the examining room
5. providing *performance data feedback*, for example, data sent quarterly to each clinic in a multispecialty group practice to show the clinic what percentage of its hypertensive patients had controlled blood readings at their last visits
6. *patient education*, for example, providing guidelines in nontechnical language directly to patients
7. use of *administrative rules*, for example, requiring that an in-house pharmacy may not fill a prescription for an antibiotic unless a diagnosis is specified on the prescription form
8. obtaining *clinician participation*, for example, bringing together nurses and obstetricians to redesign an office routine for providing prenatal care

These action options have been summarized in various ways in the literature on improving clinical care.[11,12] The health plan medical director and other staff supporting the collaboratives should agree upon one of these available frameworks and use it consistently. It will serve as a source of ideas during brainstorming and as a way of avoiding overuse of weak options, such as distribution of memoranda as reminders.

The role of health plan staff in the collaboratives is critical. At a minimum, they must recruit the participants, organize the meetings, facilitate the group process in the meetings, take minutes, and do the follow-up work (eg, distribution of implementation tools, such as flowsheets for medical records or a journal article of special interest to the group).

The improvement work within the practices should generally be done by the physicians and office practice staff. However, if the practices have fewer than seven physicians, their internal resources may be too meager for this work. In these situations, the health plan will need to consider providing roving staff members to facilitate meetings and to collect and present data within the practices.

Careful records should be kept of the collaborative's activities, and successes should be celebrated as part of building support for the program.

HOLDING PRACTICES ACCOUNTABLE

The practices participating in the collaboratives should be held accountable for their improvement activities. Accountability can be achieved by adopting a system that requires practices to declare annually what they are working on and what they intend to achieve. For each practice, a designated physician should state in writing each year the practice's objectives with respect to the collaborative and the measures to be used in determining whether the objectives have been attained.

At the end of each year, to complete the cycle, each practice should also be required to report on how it fared in working toward its goals. The audience for these reports should be the collective made up of the participating practices as well as the supporting health plan staff. Data on the chosen measures should ordinarily be presented in run charts or control charts. Reports should be made at meetings as well as on paper. Typically, health plan staff will need to assist the practices in preparing their reports.

THE NECESSITY FOR TRUST

A health plan can successfully improve office practices only if trust can be established with participating physicians. Without trust, the physicians will not join in the activity. Without trust, there will be no candor in reporting success or failure.

Establishing trust depends first and foremost on meeting the physicians on their own terms. In other words, establishing trust requires identifying the physicians' points of engagement and selecting topics for collaboratives on the basis of their perceived needs. Beyond these beginnings, developing and maintaining trust depends upon delivering value to the physicians by organizing useful meetings, providing useful training to office staff, providing educational materials for patients in support of guideline implementation, and offering similar assistance.

It will generally be useful for the health plan staff members who support the improvement activities to be different from the health plan staff members who negotiate contracts with the physicians and who inspect them periodically for accreditation purposes.

A medical director contemplating a program for improvement of clinical services in the clinicians' offices should begin by reflecting upon whether trust already exists between the health plan and the physicians or, if not, how it might be engendered. There is no substitute.

REFERENCES

1. Mosser G. Clinical process improvement: engage first, measure later. *Qual Manage Health Care.* 1996;4(4):11–20.
2. Batalden PB, Stoltz PK. A framework for the continual improvement of health care: building and applying professional and improvement knowledge to test changes in daily work. *Joint Commission J Qual Improvement.* 1993;19:425–447.
3. Berwick DM. Continuous improvement as an ideal in health care. *N Engl J Med.* 1989;320:53–56.
4. Langley GJ, Nolan KM, Nolan TW, Norman CL, Provost LP. *The Improvement Guide.* San Francisco: Jossey-Bass, Publishers; 1996.
5. Grimshaw JM, Russell IT. Effect of clinical guidelines on medical practice: a systematic review of rigorous evaluations. *Lancet.* 1993;342:1317–1322.
6. Mosser G. Half a dozen hobbling half-truths about practice guidelines. *Group Pract J.* 1997;46(4):34–40.
7. Hadorn DC, McCormick K, Diokno A. An annotated algorithm approach to clinical guideline development. *JAMA.* 1992;267:3311–3314.
8. Gottlieb LK, Sokol HN, Murrey KO, Schoenbaum SC. Algorithm-based clinical quality improvement: clinical guidelines and continuous quality improvement. *HMO Practice.* 1992;6(1):5–12.
9. National Heart, Lung and Blood Institute. *Guidelines for the Diagnosis and Management of Asthma.* National Institutes of Health publication no. 97-4051. Bethesda, MD: National Institutes of Health; 1997.
10. Soumerai SB, Avorn J. Principles of educational outreach (academic detailing) to improve clinical decision making. *JAMA.* 1990;263:549–555.
11. Handley MR, Stuart ME, Kirz HL. An evidence-based approach to evaluating and improving clinical practice: implementing practice guidelines. *HMO Practice.* 1994;8(2):75–83.
12. Eisenberg JM. *Doctors' Decisions and the Cost of Medical Care.* Ann Arbor, MI: Health Administration Press; 1986.

GORDON MOSSER, MD, is a general internist and the executive director of the Institute for Clinical Systems Integration (ICSI) in Minneapolis. ICSI is a not-for-profit quality improvement organization that bridges 17 medical groups. Its main focus is the development and implementation of health care guidelines. Previously, Dr. Mosser has worked at Share Health Plan, Aspen Medical Group, Rhode Island Group Health Association, and Group Health, Inc.

CHAPTER 20

Clinical Services Requiring Authorization

Peter R. Kongstvedt

Chapter Outline

- Definition of Services Requiring Authorization
- Definition of Who Can Authorize Services
- Claims Payment
- Point of Service
- Categories of Authorization
- Staffing
- Common Data Elements
- Methods of Data Capture and Authorization Issuance
- Authorization System Reports
- Open Access HMOs
- Specialty Physician–Based Authorization Systems
- Non–Physician-Based Authorization Systems
- Conclusion

One of the (relatively) definitive elements in managed health care is the presence of an authorization system. This may be as simple as precertification of elective hospitalizations in an indemnity plan or preferred provider organization (PPO) or as complex as mandatory authorization for all non–primary care services in a health maintenance organization (HMO). It is the authorization system that provides a key element of management in the delivery of medical services. Managed health care organizations without authorization systems are "open access" HMOs, which are discussed later in this chapter.

There are multiple reasons to have an authorization system. One is to allow the medical management function of the plan to review a case for medical necessity. A second reason is to channel care to the most appropriate location (eg, the outpatient setting or a participating specialist rather than a nonparticipating one). Third, the authorization system may be used to provide timely information to the concurrent utilization review system and to large case management. Fourth, the system may help the finance department to estimate the accruals for medical expenditures each month.

It is important to note here that important information on this subject is also found in Chapter 15, which addresses basic medical-surgical utilization. That chapter focuses on specialty physician services, and that information will be only briefly referenced in this chapter, which focuses on the methods for managing authorization systems. Together, the

---

This chapter is adapted from PR Kongstvedt, Authorization Systems, in *The Managed Health Care Handbook*, 3rd ed, PR Kongstvedt, ed, pp 469–478, © 1996, Aspen Publishers, Inc.

chapters offer a relatively broad understanding of this topic.

DEFINITION OF SERVICES REQUIRING AUTHORIZATION

The first requirement in an authorization system is to define what will require authorization and what will not. This is obviously tied to the benefits design and is part of full and fair disclosure marketing requirements in that, if services require authorization, the plan must make that clear in its marketing literature.

There are no managed care systems that require authorization for primary care services. PPOs and HMOs require members to use providers on their panels, and most HMOs require members to choose a single primary care physician (PCP) to coordinate care, but this does not require an authorization. Defining what constitutes primary care services is another issue and is addressed elsewhere in this book as well as more definitively in *The Managed Health Care Handbook,* 3rd Edition.

The real issue is determining what non–primary care services will require authorization. In a tightly controlled system, such as most HMOs (other than open access HMOs, discussed later), all services not rendered by the PCP require authorization. In other words, any service from a referral specialist, any hospitalization, any procedure, and so forth require specific authorization, although there may be certain conventional exceptions such as an optometry visit or a routine Pap smear from a gynecologist. In less tightly controlled systems, such as many PPOs and most indemnity plans, the requirements are less stringent. In those cases, it is common for authorization to be required only for elective hospitalizations and procedures, both inpatient and outpatient.

The tighter the authorization system, the greater the plan's ability to manage utilization. An authorization system per se will not automatically control utilization, although one could expect some sentinel effect. It is the management behind the authorization system that will determine its ultimate effectiveness. If the medical director is unable or unwilling to deal with poor utilization behavior, an authorization system will have only a marginal effect. If the claims department is unable to back up the authorization system, it will quickly be subverted as members and providers learn that it is little more than a burdensome sham.

In any plan there will be times when a member is unable to obtain prior authorization. This is usually due to an emergency or to an urgent problem that occurs out of area. In those cases, the plan must make provision for the retrospective review of the case to determine whether authorization may be granted after the fact. Certain rules may also be defined regarding the member's obligation in those circumstances (eg, notification within 24 hours of the emergency). Such requirements should allow for only automatic review of the case to determine medical necessity—not necessarily automatic authorization—if the plan is notified within 24 hours, even when the plan uses a "reasonable layperson's standard."

DEFINITION OF WHO CAN AUTHORIZE SERVICES

The next requirement of an authorization system is to define who has the ability to authorize services and to what extent. These choices will vary considerably depending on the type of plan and the degree to which it will be medically managed.

In addition to HMOs, there are "gatekeeper" PPOs that are tightly controlled, in which there is a requirement for PCP authorization. In most PPOs and in all managed indemnity plans, there is usually only a requirement for authorization for elective hospitalizations and procedures, but that authorization comes from plan personnel and not from the PCP or any other physician.

For example, if a participating surgeon wishes to admit a patient for surgery, the surgeon first calls a central telephone number and speaks with a plan representative, usually a nurse. That representative then asks a number of questions about the patient's condition, and if predetermined criteria are met, and after the member's eligibility is confirmed (if the plan has that capability), an authorization is issued. In most cases, the surgery must take place on the day of admission, and certain procedures may be done on only an outpatient basis.

It is common practice in HMOs to require that most or all medical services be authorized by the member's PCP. Even then, however, there can be some dispute. For example, if a PCP authorizes a member to see a referral specialist, does that specialist have the ability to authorize tests, surgery, or another referral to himself or herself or to another specialist? Does a PCP require authorization to hospitalize one of his or her own patients?

A relatively common exception to this practice is in the area of mental health and substance abuse (MH/SA). As discussed in detail in Chapter 32, MH/SA services are unique and often lend themselves better to other methods of authorization. Plans or even the accounts themselves may carve out MH/SA from the basic health plan and treat it as a stand-alone function.

Another, less common exception to the PCP-only concept occurs in HMOs that allow specialists to contact the plan directly about hospitalizations. In these cases, the referral to the specialist must have been made by the PCP in the first place, but the specialist may determine that hospitalization is required and obtain authorization directly from the plan's medical management department. Plans that operate this way generally do so because the PCPs have no real involvement in hospital cases anyway and because it is not useful to involve them in that decision.

There is a fundamental split in managed care organizations (MCOs) that require PCP authorization for non–primary care services: whether or not the PCP's authorization needs secondary review by a utilization management committee (UMC). From the mid-1980s until the mid-1990s, it was common for many MCOs to require that the PCP's authorization first go to a UMC for additional review. If the UMC approved the authorization request, then the member and the PCP were so notified (or just the PCP was notified) that the authorization request was valid and the referral went forward; if the UMC decided that the referral was medically unnecessary, investigational, or not a covered benefit, then the authorization would be denied and the PCP so notified. Then the PCP had the much coveted task of explaining that decision to the member.

While this type of secondary review system still exists in some MCOs, most have abandoned it in favor of an older model in which the PCP's authorization is valid immediately. Why the change of procedure? In earlier times (defined as a decade or more ago), MCOs did not have the data systems to properly perform practice profiling (see Chapter 38); in addition, PCPs were generally not used to their role as care coordinator and were more likely to refer cases. As managed care has become more prevalent, information systems have improved and PCPs have become much more experienced with managed care.

Unless secondary review by a UMC is required because utilization is grossly and inappropriately high, the benefits of not requiring the use of a UMC are obvious: administrative costs are much lower, physician satisfaction is higher, member satisfaction is higher, and it is likely that member retention in the MCO will be higher (though that is conjecture). However, without secondary review by a UMC, the organization will need a reasonably sophisticated profiling system that is able to detect patterns, adjust for severity of illness, and provide usable feedback to the plan's medical management and to the PCPs.

In any type of managed care plan, there may be services that will require specific authorization from the plan's medical director. This is usually the case for expensive procedures such as transplants and for controversial procedures that may be considered experimental or of limited value except in particular circumstances. This is even more necessary when the plan has negotiated a special arrangement for high-cost services. The authorization system not only reviews the medical necessity of the service but ensures that the care will be delivered at an institution that has contracted with the plan.

As mentioned above, the tighter the authorization system, the better the plan's ability to manage the care. For optimal control, only the PCP should be able to authorize all services (except those that require the approval of the plan's medical director or MH/SA services [in certain plans]). In other words, even if a member is referred to a specialist, only the PCP can actually authorize any further services such as diagnostic tests, re-referral, or procedures. This is the tightest form of a gatekeeper or case management model. As discussed below, this requires the use of unique authorization numbers that tie to specific bills, and the claims department must be able to properly adjudicate claims based on that medical policy. As a plan reduces the degree of control, utilization will tend to increase.

CLAIMS PAYMENT

A managed care health plan is not a dictator; it cannot issue blindfolds and cigarettes to members who fail to obtain authorization for services. The only recourse a plan has is to deny full payment for services that have not been authorized. This pertains equally to services obtained from nonparticipating providers (professionals or institutions) and to services obtained without required prior authorization.

In an HMO, payment can be completely denied for services that were not authorized. (Point of service [POS] is unique and is discussed below.) In most PPOs and indemnity plans, if a service is not authorized but is considered a covered benefit, payment may not be denied, but the amount paid may be significantly reduced. For example, a plan might pay 80% of charges for authorized services but only 50% of charges for nonauthorized services or might impose a flat-dollar-amount penalty for failure to obtain authorization.

In certain cases, a plan may deny payment for a portion of the bill but will pay the rest. For example, if a patient is admitted the day before surgery even though same-day admission was required, the plan may not pay the charges (both hospital and physician) related to that first day but will pay charges for the remaining days.

In a PPO where a contractual relationship exists between the provider and the plan, the penalty may fall solely on the provider, who may not balance bill the member for the penalty. In the case of an indemnity plan (or a PPO in which the member received services from a nonparticipating provider), the penalty falls on the member, who must then pay more out of pocket.

POINT OF SERVICE

POS is a special challenge for authorization systems and claims management (a thorough discussion of claims management may be found in *The Managed Health Care Handbook,* 3rd Edition). It is necessary to define what is covered as an authorized service and what is not because services that are not authorized will still be paid, albeit at the lower out-of-network level of benefits. Because POS is sold with the intent that members will use out-of-network services, it is not always clear whether a service was or was not authorized.

For example, if a PCP makes a referral to a specialist for one visit and the member returns for a follow-up, was that follow-up authorized? If a PCP authorizes three visits but the member goes four times, does the fourth visit cascade out to an out-of-network level of benefits? If a PCP refers the member to a specialist and the specialist determines that admission is necessary but the member is admitted to a nonparticipating hospital, is that authorized? What if the member is admitted to a participating hospital but is cared for by a mix of participating and nonparticipating physicians? What if a member is referred to a participating specialist who performs laboratory and radiology testing (even though the plan has capitated for such services); is the visit authorized but not the testing? What if the member claims that he or she had no choice in the matter?

The list of "what ifs" is a long one. Most plans strive to identify an episode of care (eg, a hospitalization or a referral) and to remain consistent within that episode. For example, the testing by the specialist referenced above would be denied and the specialist prohibited from balance billing, or an entire hospitalization would be considered either in network or out of network. In any case, the plan must develop policies and procedures for defining when a service is to be considered authorized (and when it is considered in network in the case of hospital services that require precertification in any event) and when it is not.

A special problem occurs in POS plans: sometimes the claim arrives before the authorization. This can easily occur in any plan that has a high rate of electronic claims submission but depends on a paper-based authorization system. In a typical HMO in which only authorized, in-network benefits are available, this situation usually results in the HMO's claims system "pending" (ie, holding) the claim to wait and see if the authorization comes in. But POS is specifically designed to allow for out-of-network care, so a claim that does not have an associated authorization immediately cascades down to be processed as an out-of-network service with lesser benefits; and in some cases, *then* the authorization arrives. The member and provider may complain, and the plan has to rework the claim. This is a suboptimal event; reworking a claim is costly, as is upsetting members and providers.

CATEGORIES OF AUTHORIZATION

Authorizations may be classified into six types:

1. prospective
2. concurrent
3. retrospective
4. pended (for review)
5. denial (no authorization)
6. subauthorization

There is value in categorizing authorization types. By examining how authorizations are actually generated in your plan, you will be able to identify areas of weakness. For example, if a plan's leaders believe that all elective admissions are receiving prospective authorization and discover that in fact most are being authorized either concurrently or, worse yet, retrospectively, the leaders will know that they are not able to intervene effectively in managing hospital cases because they do not know about them in a timely manner. A brief description of the authorization categories follows.

Prospective

Sometimes referred to as precertification, this type of authorization is issued before any service is rendered. This is commonly used in plans that require prior authorization for elective services. The more prospective the authorization, the more time the medical director has to intervene if necessary, the greater the ability to direct care to the most appropriate setting or provider, and the more current the knowledge regarding utilization trends.

Inexperienced plan managers tend to believe that all authorizations are prospective. That naive belief can lead to a real shock when the manager of a troubled plan learns that most claims are actually being paid on the basis of other types of authorizations that were not correctly categorized. This is discussed further below.

Concurrent

A concurrent authorization is generated at the time the service is rendered. For example, imagine that a utilization review nurse discovers that a patient is being admitted to the hospital that day. An authorization is generated, but by the nurse and not by the PCP. Another example is an urgent service that cannot wait for review, such as setting a broken leg. In that case, the PCP may contact the plan, but the referral is made at the same time.

Concurrent authorizations allow for timely data gathering and the potential for affecting the outcome, but they do not allow the plan medical managers to intervene in the initial decision to render services. This may result in care being inappropriately delivered or delivered in a setting that is not cost-effective, but it also may result in the plan's being able to make the course of care more cost-effective even though care has already commenced.

Retrospective

As the term indicates, retrospective authorizations take place after the fact. For example, imagine that a patient is admitted, has surgery, and is discharged, and then the plan finds out. On the surface, it appears that any service rendered without authorization would have payment denied or reduced, but there will be circumstances when the plan will agree to authorize services after they have been rendered. For example, if a member is involved in a serious automobile accident or has a heart attack while traveling in another state, there is a clear need for care and the plan could not deny that need.

Inexperienced managers often believe not only that most authorizations are prospective but that, except for emergency cases, there are few retrospective authorizations. Unfortunately, there are circumstances when there may be a high volume of retrospective authorizations. This commonly occurs when the PCPs or participating providers fail to cooperate with the authorization system. A claim comes in cold (ie, without an authorization), and the plan must create an authorization retrospectively if the service was really meant to be authorized. Because the PCP—not the member—was at fault, the plan cannot punish the member and that claim gets paid.

Most plans have a *no balance billing* clause in their provider contracts and may elect not to pay claims that have not been prospectively author-

ized, forcing the noncompliant providers to write off the expense. That will certainly get their attention, but it may hurt provider–plan relations. Even so, this option sometimes becomes necessary if discussions and education attempts fail.

If the plan's systems allow an authorization to be classified as prospective or concurrent regardless of when it is created relative to the delivery of the service, it is certain that retrospective authorizations will occur but not be labeled retrospective. The PCP or specialist may say "I really meant to authorize that" or "It's in the mail" and call the authorization concurrent. Another possibility is that claims clerks may be creating retrospective authorizations on the basis of the belief that the claim was linked to another authorized claim (see below).

In a tightly managed plan, the ability to create a retrospective authorization is strictly limited to the medical director or utilization management department, the ability to create prospective authorizations does not exist once the service has actually been rendered, and concurrent authorizations cannot be created after 24 hours have passed since the service was rendered.

Pended (for Review)

Pended is a claims term that refers to a state of authorization purgatory. In this situation, it is not known whether an authorization will be issued, and the case has been pended for medical review (for medical necessity such as an emergency department claim, or for medical policy review to determine if the service is covered under the schedule of benefits) or for administrative review. As noted above, if a plan is having problems getting the PCPs or participating providers to cooperate with the authorization system, there will be a significant number of pended claims that ultimately lead to retrospective authorizations.

Denial (No Authorization)

Denial refers to the certainty that there will be no authorization forthcoming. As has been discussed, not every claim without an associated authorization will be denied; there are reasons that an unauthorized claim may be paid.

Subauthorization

This is a special category that allows one authorization to hitch onto another. This is most common for hospital-based professional services. For example, a single authorization may be issued for a hospitalization, and that authorization is used to cover anesthesia, pathology, radiology, or even a surgeon's or consultant's fees.

In some plans, an authorization to a referral specialist may be used to authorize diagnostic and therapeutic services ordered by that specialist. Great care must be taken to control this. If not, linking will occur.

Linking refers to claims clerks linking unauthorized services to authorized ones and creating subauthorizations to do so. For example, imagine that a referral to a specialist is authorized, and a claim is received not only for the specialist's fees but for some expensive procedure or test as well, or a bill is received for 10 visits even though the PCP intended to authorize only 1. The claims clerk (who is probably being judged on how many claims he or she can process per hour) may then inappropriately link all the bills to the originally authorized service through the creation of subauthorizations, thereby increasing the costs to the plan.

STAFFING

Plan personnel required to implement properly an authorization system are the medical director, an authorization system coordinator (whatever that person's actual title), and the utilization review nurses. Various clerks and telephone operators will also be required; the number of these depends on the size of the plan and the scope of the system.

The medical director has three primary roles. The first is to interact with the plan's PCPs and specialty physicians to ensure cooperation with the authorization system. Second, the medical director is responsible for medical review of pended claims. That does not mean that the medical director will have to review every claim personally, but that each claim is ultimately the medical director's responsibility. In some instances the case will be reviewed by the member's PCP; in others it will be more appropriate for a nurse reviewer or even the medical director (or designate) to perform the primary review. Third, the medical director will sometimes have interactions with members when payment of a claim is denied. Although the claims department usually sends the denial letters and responds to inquiries, it is common for members to demand a review of the denied claim on the basis of medical necessity or a belief that the PCP really authorized the service. In those cases, the medical director will often be involved.

The authorization system needs a coordinator to make sure that all the pieces fit together. Whether that responsibility falls to the claims department, the utilization department, the medical director's office, or general management is a local choice. In a small plan, the role of coordinator usually falls to a manager with other duties as well, but as the plan grows it is best to have only one person coordinating the authorization system.

The coordinator's primary purpose is to track the authorization system at all its points. All systems can break down, and the coordinator must keep track of where the system is performing suboptimally and take steps to correct it. In some cases that will require the intervention of others because an authorization system has ramifications in the PCP's office, the hospitals, the utilization review department, the claims department, member services, and finance. If no one is in charge of maintaining the authorization system, people will tend to deny their responsibilities in making it work.

Some thought must be given to the relationship of the authorization system to the utilization review coordinators. Specifically, how much can the utilization review coordinator authorize? It makes sense to allow him or her some ability to create authorizations, especially subauthorizations for hospital services, but a plan must decide whether it will allow the utilization review coordinators to create primary authorizations, particularly for hospital cases. It is common in large HMOs for nurse case managers involved in large case management to have the ability to authorize services without the need to go through a PCP (see Chapter 15 for a discussion of this activity).

COMMON DATA ELEMENTS

The needs of your plan will dictate what data elements you actually capture. In some plans, the management information system will be able automatically to provide some of this information, so you would not have to capture it at the time the authorization is created. The data elements that are commonly captured in authorization systems are illustrated in Exhibit 20–1.

In systems where there are clinical requirements for authorization, the system then must determine what the requirements are on the basis of the diagnosis. For example, if a plan has preset criteria for authorization for cataract surgery, those requirements may be reviewed with the physician calling in for authorization. The same issue applies to mandatory outpatient surgery: if admission is being requested, the procedure may be compared to an outpatient surgery list to determine whether the physician needs to justify an exception. Such reviews should be done only by medically trained personnel, usually nurses. In the case of disagreements with the requesting physician, the medical director must be able to contact the physician at that time or as soon as possible. It becomes less common for a plan to deny authorization based on medical necessity as the plan matures and the participating physicians become more conversant in definitions of medical necessity; however, the other values of the authorization system remain important.

When an authorization is made, the system also must be able to generate and link an authorization number or identifier to the data, so that every authorization will be unique. In tightly controlled plans, any claim must be accompanied by that unique authorization number to be processed.

Exhibit 20–1 Data Elements Commonly Captured in an Authorization System

- Member's name
- Member's birth date
- Member's plan identification (ID) number
- Eligibility status
  - Commercial group number or public sector (ie, Medicare and Medicaid) group identifier
  - Line of business (eg, HMO, POS, Medicare, Medicaid, conversion, private, or self-pay)
  - Benefits code for particular service (eg, noncovered, partial coverage, limited benefit, full coverage)
- PCP
- Referral provider
  - Name
  - Specialty
- Outpatient data elements
  - Referral or service date
  - Diagnosis (International Classification of Disease, Ninth Edition, Clinical Modification [ICD-9-CM], free text)
  - Number of visits authorized
  - Specific procedures authorized (Current Procedural Terminology, 4th Edition [CPT-4], free text)
- Inpatient data elements
  - Name of institution
  - Admitting physician
  - Admission or service date
  - Diagnosis (ICD-9-CM, diagnosis-related group, free text)
  - Discharge date
- Subauthorizations (if allowed or required)
  - Hospital-based professionals
  - Other specialists
  - Other procedures or studies
- Free text to be transmitted to the claims processing department

METHODS OF DATA CAPTURE AND AUTHORIZATION ISSUANCE

There are three main methods of interacting with an authorization system: paper based, telephone based, and electronic.

Paper-Based Authorization Systems

Paper-based systems generally work in plans that allow the PCP to authorize the service without prospective review by the plan. If plan preapproval is necessary before an authorization is issued (except for infrequent services such as transplants), a paper-based system will not be responsive enough. If, however, the PCP has the authority to authorize services, a paper-based system will be adequate, though far from state of the art.

In this type of system, the PCP (or other authorizing provider) must complete an authorization form, which may be used as a referral or admission form as well. A copy of the form is sent to the plan, which enters the authorization data into its system. Claims submitted to the plan may or may not require a copy of the authorization form, depending on plan policy.

Paper-based systems offer some advantages. They are less labor intensive than telephone-based systems and therefore require less overhead. Although electronic systems are even more labor efficient, electronic systems require a higher level of sophistication and support than paper-based systems. Data entry can be done in batch mode because there is little need for real-time interaction. They also tend to be more acceptable to physicians because they are less intrusive regarding clinical decision making, run less risk of violating patient confidentiality, and do not have the problem of busy signals or a physician's being placed on hold during a busy day in the office.

The main disadvantage of paper-based systems is that there is less opportunity to intervene at the time the authorization is made. Once an authorization is issued, it is nearly impossible to reverse it. You may be able to alter future behavior, but neither physician nor member will easily accept an after-the-fact reversal of an authorization. Another disadvantage is that paper-based systems increase the administrative burden on the physician, particularly if he or she is participating in multiple plans, each with its own complicated set of forms. Paper authorizations can get lost in the mail (or mail room) and lend themselves to data entry errors (eg, digit transpositions). Lastly, paper-based authorizations may arrive at the plan well after an electronic claim has been received, resulting in a processing error and a required reissuance of a payment.

Telephone-Based Authorization Systems

Telephone-based systems rely on the PCP or office staff to call a central number and give the information over the telephone. If clinical review is required, it is done at that time. Telephone-based systems can clog up and lead to poor service. If the system is unresponsive, or if PCPs get frequent busy signals or are put on hold, they will stop calling. The investment in a responsive telephone-based system will be paid back in a reduction of pended claims and retrospective authorizations.

Collecting the data and issuing an authorization number may be done either manually or by an automated system. It is extremely rare for a health plan not to use computers for claims payment, although a start-up plan could certainly perform this function manually for a brief period. Because authorization is linked to claims payment, there must be an interface between the two systems.

One approach is to collect all the data on manual logs and then enter them into the claims system through batch processing. Another approach is to automate the entire process. If you have systems capabilities to do so, you may wish to have your authorization clerks or nurses enter the data directly into the computer. Be aware, though, that computer systems can delay you with slow screens, complicated menus and entry screens, down time, training problems, and a host of other difficulties. Some computer systems are made for batch entry, making real-time entry too inefficient. In those situations, you may wish to use a manual log for data capture and authorization issuance until your automated system is well tested. You should also be able to use a manual system as a backup on a moment's notice.

The advantages of telephone-based systems are that they can be more responsive and timely, have greater potential for directing care to the appropriate location and provider, and have the potential of reducing the administrative burden on the PCP's office staff. The disadvantages are that they increase the administrative burden on the plan and, if not run efficiently, can generate great ill will with the PCPs.

Electronic Authorization Systems

Electronic authorization systems are still not as common as paper- or telephone-based systems, but their popularity is rapidly growing. Electronic-based systems require participating physicians and hospitals to interface electronically with the plan, usually through a personal computer or a dumb terminal in the office. Generally, electronic communications with providers focus on claims submission and payment, but they can focus on authorizations just as easily.

Electronic authorizations may be nothing more than an electronic form that the provider completes on line and transmits to the plan. The authorization system may be more complex, involving editing fields to ensure that the referral or admission is to a participating provider and requiring key data elements to be provided. An electronic authorization system may also provide automatic information transfer (eg, member status and demographics). It is also possible for an electronic system to gather clinical information and to compare that information to protocols before processing the authorization, but currently that is not a common feature of such systems.

In electronic systems, the authorization data is generally entered directly (or via electronic batch entry) into the management information system, so that the need for personnel to enter data is reduced. Such systems require a high level of expertise by the plan and a certain level of sophistication by the providers themselves.

AUTHORIZATION SYSTEM REPORTS

The reports needed from an authorization system will depend on the complexity of the system and the management needs. Obviously, the one absolutely necessary report function is linking incoming claims to authorized services.

Hospital logs and reports are discussed in greater detail in Chapter 15. The authorization system should be able to print out a report indicating prospective admissions and procedures, current admissions and procedures, and retrospectively authorized cases. Cases pended for review should also be reported, with data indicating when the claim was received, when it was reviewed, and its current status.

Outpatient reports are also discussed in greater detail in Chapter 37. Reports from the authorization system could include summaries of authorizations by type for each PCP expressed as ratios—for example, total authorizations per 100 encounters per PCP or per 1,000 members per year (annualized). The authorizations could be broken down into prospective, concurrent, retrospective, and so forth. Authorization types may also be expressed as a percentage of the total number of authorizations for that PCP. For example, the total authorization rate may be 8 per 100 encounters per PCP with 50% prospective, 40% concurrent, 6% retrospective, and 4% pended (if it is denied, it is not an authorization, although it is still quite useful to report denial statistics by provider as well).

Another valuable report is an overall comparison of authorization types to paid claims. This report shows the percentage of claims that have been authorized prospectively, concurrently, and so forth. This is valuable in determining your ability to capture the data in a timely fashion. It will be inversely proportional to your plan's rate of incurred but not reported claims (IBNRs).

These reports will allow you to identify noncompliant providers or providers who comply but not in a timely fashion. The medical director will be able to focus on those providers who either do not obtain authorizations or do so in a way that does not allow for active medical management by the medical director (if that is needed). These reports, along with a report on the number and nature of open authorizations (ie, authorizations for services for which a claim has not yet been received), will also allow the finance department to calculate more accurately the accruals and IBNR factor for the plan, reducing the chances of nasty surprises later.

OPEN ACCESS HMOs

As noted early in this chapter, there are some HMOs that do not require a member to go through a PCP in order to access a specialist (thus the name "open access"—access to specialists is open to members). These types of plans were quite popular in the late 1970s and early 1980s, but a string of failures led to their near extinction. However, a few did survive, and as of the time this book was written, open access HMOs have regained a small but noticeable presence in the health care market.

The phoenix-like resurrection of open access HMOs is usually attributed to one or both of the following factors. First, market research indicates that members prefer to access specialists directly without having to go through a PCP. Second, many plans find that they rarely deny a request for a referral to a specialist from a PCP and that the system therefore may be creating unnecessary visits for no good reason.

Although these are the stated reasons for the creation of an open access HMO, the flaws in these two lines of reasoning are pretty clear. First, it did not require too much research to determine that members would prefer direct access to specialists; with direct access to specialists, members can—but do not have to—visit a PCP. This type of model has often been referred to as indemnity insurance or a PPO, and the costs of such systems have usually been higher than the costs of HMOs. The second factor, that of not denying authorization requests, is also not quite right; HMOs have not regularly denied referral requests for some time. The real issue is that the request comes from a physician, not from a member who has no medical training. It is not at all clear whether open access HMOs will now succeed or succumb to the fate of their progenitors.

Even in open access systems, certain services may still require authorization. For example, highly expensive diagnostic studies, inpatient care, surgical procedures, and so forth may still be required, even though it would be the specialist who now requests them. Also, certain services, such as behavioral health and chemical dependency treatment, may be carved out even in open access plans. Lastly, some plans limit the number of self-referrals that a member may make per year (eg, a member may self-refer up to three times per year). This option is rather difficult to track from an information systems standpoint, and issues such as follow-up visits must be clarified (eg, does a follow-up visit count as part of the original self-referral, or is it a second self-referral?). Whether the specialist can initiate diagnostic or institutionally based services should also be made clear.

Having said all of this, it is certainly possible that such systems will have a better chance of succeeding now than they did a decade ago. Physicians and hospitals have changed their practice patterns substantially over the last 10 years, greater abilities to monitor medical resource uses are now available, and performance-based reimbursement models are now more sophisticated. Administrative costs are likely to be lower, and if the system can be monitored and appropriate medical management applied, there is probably more chance of success than existed in prior years.

SPECIALTY PHYSICIAN–BASED AUTHORIZATION SYSTEMS

With all of the attention paid to PCP-based types of MCOs, it is easy to forget that there are a number of advanced MCOs that use specialist physicians in the primary physician role for care coordination and authorization for services. When one encounters this type of care management authorization system, it is usually in a plan that is relatively experienced in overall care management and has a reasonably good management information system.

Not all members of the plan would be under this type of system; in fact, the majority would still use PCPs as their main coordinators of care. However, it is clear that in many cases, specialists are both more efficient and provide higher quality of care for certain clinical decisions. These cases would include patients diagnosed with the human immunodeficiency virus (HIV), certain forms of cancer, certain neurological diseases, certain cardiovascular diseases, brittle diabetes mellitus, and so forth. In these instances, the plan determines that the member falls into the category of one of these disease states and then removes that member from the usual PCP care management system and assigns the member to the appropriate specialist for care coordination. Of course, the member chooses the specialist he or she wants from the plan's participating specialist list. In some cases, however, the plan may have selected a specialty provider to care for all of the members with that diagnosis, in which case the member's choice is limited to physicians in that group. For an in-depth discussion of disease management, see Part X.

NON–PHYSICIAN-BASED AUTHORIZATION SYSTEMS

A few plans have been using a system in which requests for authorization for services come directly from members to the plan; in almost all cases these requests are directed to a registered nurse (RN) who is specially trained in evaluating such requests. In these types of plans, the member calls a central telephone number to request an authorization and speaks with an RN. The member tells the RN the reasons for the request for authorization for non–primary care services, and the RN then accesses computerized algorithms to verify the appropriateness of the request for a referral for specialty services and either authorizes the referral or refers the member back to the PCP. In this type of plan, the PCP has no influence or input into whether or not the plan authorizes the referral and generally may find out only after the event has occurred.

While this type of system looks attractive on its surface, there are some issues that are worthwhile to consider before it is adopted. First, are the clinical algorithms appropriate and adequate? Such algorithms can be purchased, but the plan may find it difficult to put them into place if the PCPs have had little or no input into them. More important, this type of authorization system is always done via telephone, with no information available based on a history or physical examination; therefore, the RN making the evaluation can rely on only information reported by the member. This information is often, but not always, adequate. Therefore, it is likely that authorization for specialty services will occur more often than if PCPs are making the decisions. Counterbalancing that is the improved member satisfaction that the plan enjoys from this more relaxed type of authorization system.

CONCLUSION

An effective authorization system is a requirement of any managed care plan. Whether that system is all encompassing or pertains to only certain types of services is dependent on the type of plan. Key elements to address are what services require authorization, who has the ability to authorize, whether secondary plan approval is required, what data will be captured, how they will be captured, and how they will be used.

CHAPTER 21

Guideline Use for Ambulatory Procedures

Victoria P. Haulcy

Chapter Outline

- Introduction
- Guideline Products in Ambulatory Care
- Guidelines for Managing Financial Risk
- The Future of Guidelines in Ambulatory Care Decisions

INTRODUCTION

Changes in medical technology, health care delivery systems, and spiraling health care costs have created major shifts in the health care marketplace. One noticeable shift is from inpatient care for procedures, with extended lengths of stay, toward outpatient ambulatory procedures. Shifting to more outpatient procedures is believed to help contain costs and facilitate optimal patient outcomes.

Many procedures once believed to require an inpatient hospital stay are now routinely being done in an ambulatory care setting. However, performing these services in this new setting can pose challenges to the physicians and other providers as they seek to provide consistent, high-quality care; keep pace with new techniques and approaches; and prevent postoperative complications. The number of ambulatory care procedures and ambulatory care centers has been growing rapidly. Practitioners, hospitals, and independent centers have had to develop specific organizational and patient care strategies for delivery of ambulatory services: strategies for organizational effectiveness, management, legal matters, job roles, staff training, care delivery, and information management.

Managing information within the ambulatory care setting for clinical and administrative decision making can be an arduous task. Successful information management requires an accurate assessment and understanding of the patient, staff, payer, and regulatory needs. Following this assessment, organizations must select an appropriate information system or platform to support these needs and the corresponding software to assist in decisions, documentation, monitoring, and reporting. The system and its users must also have methods for maintaining confidentiality.

One of the most important elements of information management in the ambulatory care setting is an application to guide and assist in the selection and delivery of appropriate care. Using the right tools to facilitate care delivery will lead to clinical performance improvement, appropriate financial performance, and reduced risk. These tools can also be used to assist in accommodating movement of the patient within the continuum of care from referrals to specialists (Chapter 20), triage to the Emergency Department (Part V), admission or transfer to postacute or skilled nursing facilities (Chapter 23), or even delivery of medical services in a home care environment (Chapter 22).

Various terms—clinical protocols, criteria, boundary guidelines, and others—have been used to describe these types of tools. The methods used to create these tools vary almost as widely as the titles they are given. Guidelines themselves are not a new tool, but they are now more necessary and more widely applied to different clinical settings than ever before. In the past, guidelines were primarily a tool used by utilization management firms to reduce the number of inpatient admissions, as well as the overall lengths of stay per visit. Inpatient admissions and lengths of stay were initially targeted because these areas were thought to offer the greatest potential savings without harm to outcomes.

However, most early decision guideline tools were paper based and cumbersome. Their application was largely dependent on the user, thereby compromising consistency. Without accountability for consistent and appropriate application of best practices, decisions were often based on the judgment of the nurse reviewer, or the insistence of the treating physician, despite the availability of guidelines. Cases were reviewed either prospectively, concurrently, or retrospectively by a nurse care manager who handled utilization management. Having nurses manage risk in this way meant that prospective and concurrent reviews could potentially affect decisions about treatments or procedures before they were done to ensure appropriateness and cost-effectiveness. Retrospective reviews could be used to analyze large volumes of data from multiple sources for establishing baselines and assist in benchmarking outcomes. Chapter 15 provides a discussion of these most basic forms of utilization management.

Although this practice reduced the number of unnecessary admissions and unnecessarily long hospitalizations, and in turn helped employer groups save hundreds of millions of dollars, it also raised some concern. Providers questioned whether medical practice was being second guessed by nurses or by managed care groups that were perhaps more interested in saving money than in quality care. Lack of information on how the guidelines were derived and how they were being implemented by the utilization firm, or on the consequences of practitioner noncompliance to guidelines, further heightened concerns about their use. Critics in the medical community used terms such as "cookbook medicine" to describe guideline usage. Patients also began to question whether the guidelines were medically driven or financially driven at the expense of their health and well-being. Meanwhile, managed care enrollment continued to grow at a rapid pace, making it even more necessary to develop additional solutions for managing cost, reducing risk, and establishing quality outcomes to maintain a competitive advantage.

Looking at moving procedures from inpatient to outpatient settings seemed a natural next step in finding effective ways for organizations and governments to control spiraling health care costs. To cut costs and allay provider and patient concerns about quality care, experts developed guidelines for the delivery of health care in an ambulatory setting. This interest in guidelines is further heightened by the rapid growth and competitiveness of managed care organizations, capitation, and the shift of risk from payers to providers. Better, faster, and smarter guideline tools are required to meet the needs of regulatory bodies that, in addition to cost savings, want specific and documented strategies for showing evidence-based consistency with patient care decisions, quality management, provider profiling, effective outcomes studies, and high patient satisfaction rates. These factors, combined with advancements in hardware and software technology, and the need to access and translate large volumes of data into information, have given rise to a new generation of clinical decision-making tools for this market.

Some studies have emphasized where it may be useful for guidelines to aid in appropriate selection, treatment, and savings (Figure 21–1).

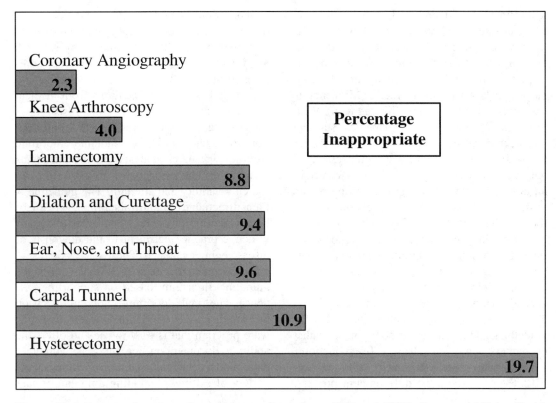

Figure 21–1 Inappropriate Procedures (Common Procedures, 1991 and 1992). Courtesy of Value Health Sciences, Inc, Santa Monica, California.

Additional clinical evaluations have also aided in the identification of and need for guidelines as procedures transition to ambulatory settings. Multiple studies have been done to evaluate the types of procedures and diagnostic tests, ranging from diagnostic hysteroscopy to peripheral angioplasty, that are appropriate for the ambulatory and outpatient setting.[1–6] Likewise, there have been several recent articles highlighting the need for clinical guidelines for many of these ambulatory diagnostics and procedures[7,8] in areas as diverse as treatment of diabetes in older persons (Chapter 29), behavioral health (Chapter 32), and drug utilization (Chapter 26). Clinical decision support is the logical answer to advancements in utilization management; it assures patients and purchasers that consistent best practices are being applied for patient care and managing risk.

GUIDELINE PRODUCTS IN AMBULATORY CARE

There are many guideline products to choose from, including those developed by state and governmental regulating bodies such as the Agency for Health Care Policy and Research, medical associations such as American College of Obstetrics and Gynecology and the American College of Physicians, research groups (eg, the RAND Corporation), private utilization management firms, insurance companies, hospitals, clinics, and a number of private industries. Some products are available to the public at no charge, some are intended for internal use only, and others are licensed or sold to the public. Not all have application to the ambulatory care market or provide a representative list of guidelines to select from. One guideline product that is licensed to organizations and can be applied to the ambulatory care setting is QualityFIRST Guidelines, developed by the Institute for Healthcare Quality, a research and development subsidiary of Health Risk Management, Inc, in Minneapolis (the organization that I am affiliated with). With more than 250 guidelines in its medical-surgical and behavioral health product lines and over 1,900 treatments and diagnostic procedures, of which 27% are recommended to be performed in an outpatient setting, it represents one of the most comprehensive clinical decision support tools on the market today (Figure 21–2).

The product first confirms the diagnosis and then identifies the appropriate treatment, procedure, setting, and duration. An example of the product's impact on ambulatory utilization of specialist services is provided in Table 21–1. This pre-post study suggests that QualityFIRST guidelines had a substantial effect on specialist encounters, achieving at least a 50% reduction.

Paramount to the acceptance of the QualityFIRST guidelines is the development process, which is similar to other guideline development processes. The process begins with an exhaustive international literature search by research analysts with degrees. Information from additional sources, such as medical databases, academic studies, recommendations from medical societies, and results from other research, is used, along with the literature search information, to develop an initial guideline algorithm. Additional research analysts and biostatisticians then review the information to assess the research's validity and strength. The guideline is then directed to a multidisciplinary team of board-certified physicians and other clinicians in active practice pertinent to the diagnosis or disease being evaluated. These panels hold several subsequent meetings to revise and refine the guideline algorithm, based on supporting evidence. The final algorithm, logic, and decision tree are then transferred into an interactive software program that is easy to use and offers the ability to document on-line, integrate with other data, report decisions, and apply within a wide variety of settings, including ambulatory care

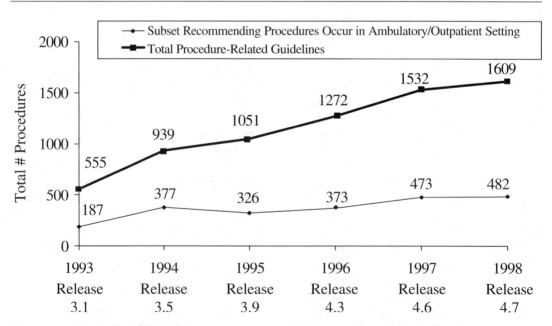

Figure 21–2 QualityFIRST Medical-Surgical Procedures

Table 21–1 One Client's Results from Implementing the QualityFIRST Guidelines (Data Normalized/ 1,000 Members)

	June	July	Aug	Sept	Oct	Nov	Dec
Medicare membership	1,737	1,719	1,680	1,646	1,620	1,625	1,547
Medicare referrals	246	242	242	156	110	78	68
Medicare referrals/1,000 members	142	141	144	96	68	48	44
Commercial membership	755	776	752	712	684	684	652
Commercial referrals	64	69	60	49	32	29	27
Commercial referrals/1,000 members	85	89	80	69	47	42	41

Courtesy of Health Risk Management, Minneapolis, Minnesota.

centers and provider offices. A summary of the research evidence is then made available on-line and can be printed for reference by the user. The program thereby becomes a powerful tool for educating and encouraging behavior change in physicians and nurse care managers.

Each guideline undergoes a similar process for updating annually to ensure information and medical content are up to date, reflect current practices, and incorporate the experience of current clients and guideline users. This evidence-based development process, reporting capability, and continuous quality improvement process assist users in facilitating accreditation. In addition to inpatient and outpatient settings, the guideline also includes directives to alternative settings such as acute rehabilitation care, home health care, hospice, and subacute or skilled nursing facilities, to name a few. By coordinating these into each of their guideline product lines, rather than having a separate ambulatory care guideline, inpatient and outpatient centers using this product can meet patient needs across the entire spectrum of care.

GUIDELINES FOR MANAGING FINANCIAL RISK

In addition to standardizing and reducing the use of inappropriate care and settings, practice guidelines attempt to help manage or reduce the overall health care cost. Milliman & Robertson, Inc, an actuarial and health care consulting firm in Seattle, estimates that the United States could save as much as 25% of its total health care cost if efficient medical practices were adopted. Having reviewed the treatment patterns of more than 25,000 physicians, Milliman & Robertson found that 40% to 50% of hospital days, 10% of office visits, and 35% of ancillary services were unnecessary.[9] This type of information supports the need for sound practice guidelines, not only for ambulatory procedures and treatments, but also for most services.

Outpatient procedures are performed at hospital outpatient facilities, freestanding surgery centers (FOSCs), and physician offices. Surgeries performed in FOSCs are projected to increase dramatically. Physician office–based procedures are also expected to rise. With anticipated growth of total outpatient procedures and of the locations where they are performed, the need for guidelines to assist in quality care is even more apparent.

THE FUTURE OF GUIDELINES IN AMBULATORY CARE DECISIONS

Reduction of treatment variability using evidence-based guidelines will become more important as the shift toward outpatient procedures continues, payers and providers continue to want to manage risk, and consumers continue to demand quality health care. The need to coordinate information will place an emphasis on software integration, such that any guideline system will need to accommodate various hardware platforms and a multitude of systems for long-term success. A good guideline system will also need to facilitate physician acceptance and encourage changes in behavior patterns that help make adherence to guidelines a success for patients, providers, and payers.

REFERENCES

1. Parkin D, Hutchinson A, Phillips P, Coates J. A comparison of diagnosis-related groups and ambulatory visit groups in day-case surgery. *Health Trends*. 1993;25(2):41–44.
2. Nagele F, O'Connor H, Davies A, Badawy A, et al. Outpatient diagnostic hysteroscopies. *Obstet Gynecol*. 1996;88(5):900–901.
3. Wills TE, Burns J. Urethroscopy: an outpatient procedure? *J Urol*. 1994;151(5):1185–1187.
4. Struk DW, Rankin RN, Eliasziw M, Vellet AD. Safety of outpatient peripheral angioplasty. *Radiol*. 1993;189(1):193–196.
5. Powers TW, Goodnow JA, Harris AD. The outpatient vaginal hysterectomy. *Am J Obstet Gynecol*. 1993;186:1875–1878.
6. Macaluso JN, Thomas R. Extracorporeal shock wave lithotripsy: an outpatient procedure. *J Urol*. 1991;146(3):714–717.
7. Weiner JP, Parente ST, Garinick DW, Fowles J, et al. Variation in office-based quality: a claims-based profile of care provided to Medicare patients with diabetes. *JAMA*. 1995;273(19):1503–1508.
8. DeNeef P, Ellsworth A, Schneeweiss R. A system of drug utilization review in ambulatory care. *J Fam Pract*. 1991;32(6):607–612.
9. Burns J, Cordero C, Findlay S, Harris N, McKnight M. Quality costs less. *Business Health*. 1994;12(suppl B):6–11.

VICTORIA P. HAULCY, RN, BSN, MPH, is director of marketing at Health Risk Management, Inc, a provider of products and services for total health plan management. Ms. Haulcy has more than 17 years of experience in health care delivery and medical marketing for medical devices, pharmaceutical, and health plan management. She serves on several advisory boards, including the National Institutes of Health and the American Cancer Society, Hennipen County.

Part VIII

Post–Acute Care Settings

Once considered strictly as skilled nursing, post–acute care has evolved and grown as much as any other segment of health care. Post–acute care may now encompass what is still known as skilled nursing but has expanded. Post–acute care is care that is delivered after an acute hospitalization but in a more cost-effective setting. That care is often in lieu of hospitalization, not after it. Home care has grown dramatically in this decade and is likewise a potentially cost-effective alternative to the acute care facility. Lastly, Part VIII includes a discussion of end-of-life care, or hospice care. Managed medical care must, and does, encompass the entire spectrum of birth to death.

Chapter 22

Home Health Care

Peggy H. Rodebush, Kathleen M. L. Popper, and Barry K. Morrison

Chapter Outline

- Introduction
- What Is Home Care?
- History of Home Care
- Update
- Indicators and Predictors of Home Care Demand
- Home Care Services
- Professional Home Care Disciplines
- Regulations Guiding Home Care
- Financing Home Care Services
- Regulatory Issues Impacting Home Care
- Measuring Quality in Home Care Services
- Examples of Advanced Clinical Practices in Home Care

INTRODUCTION

Home health care has evolved to become a critical component of medical management of illnesses. It serves as a tool used successfully in pre– and post–acute care settings and is vital in the existing environment of cost-efficiency pressures and quality measurement through the continuum of care. There are many different types of home health care, including medical and non-medical care, intermittent and continuous care, custodial and skilled care, and formal and informal care. The limits of each of these categories are usually not driven by the medical needs of the patient but by the financing mechanism available for payment of the services provided. For example, Medicare, as the predominant home care payer, has traditionally consisted of multiple medical disciplines within a highly coordinated plan of treatment. The complete team, if medically necessary, comprises a registered nurse, physical therapist, licensed practical nurse, occupational therapist, speech therapist, social worker, and home health aide.

The limits of care are frequently set in the federal code that authorizes payment for the care and describes the conditions that must be met by providers to participate in the federal programs. The goal of the Medicare program is to improve the health and functional status of patients. Medicare approves payment for this care only as long as progressive improvement can be shown and in some specific chronic cases that require skilled nursing follow-up on a long-term basis (such as monthly urinary catheter change).

Older persons receive most home care because of the age criteria of Medicare and older persons' higher health care needs. There is an increasing number of non-Medicare, younger patients receiving home care services, however. This growing younger market is an extension of the improving clinical capabilities of home care providers and the increasing number of third-party payers that recognize home care as a viable medical alternative or adjunct to more expensive acute and subacute care.

WHAT IS HOME CARE?

Home care encompasses a broad range of medical, social, and support services. It involves the delivery of health care at home typically to persons who are disabled, chronically ill, terminally ill, or recovering.

Care provided may be viewed in terms of intermittent or continuous care. Continuous care is frequently referred to as private duty care, since it is seldom reimbursed by Medicare or third-party payers. This type of care is typically offered by organizations other than those providing intermittent care designed for the capitated Medicare program and for third-party payers who stipulate intermittent care. Continuous and intermittent home care differ in the duration of time for care delivery. Private duty care is usually for service unit increments longer than 1 hour or service units that are billed relative to the number of hours or shifts spent delivering care. A service unit for intermittent home care is described as a patient visit.

Both continuous and intermittent care have complex and supportive care components. Continuous care may range from registered nurse support for ventilator-dependent patients to companions for the older or confined persons. Intermittent care requires highly skilled professionals who can work independently in the home, under a physician's orders, with typically much higher problem solving and technical skills than in many inpatient medical settings. Likewise, home health aides provide intermittent supportive care, such as bathing, assistance in moving about the home, and meal preparation.

HISTORY OF HOME CARE

Care provided to a member of a household by a recognized health care practitioner or member of the household has been in existence for centuries and preceded institutional care. It has been a local phenomenon focused on the neighborhood, village, or town in which the ill person lived. As practitioners' ability to care for the ill improved, the level of the care provided in the home evolved with it.

Health care focused outside the home began to develop as the involvement of religious and academic organizations in health care increased and formal medical education evolved. As these organizations began to serve the ill, the larger, more complex health care organizations began to emerge, providing hospitals where higher levels of care were developed and could be provided.

Home care in the modern sense existed as a cottage industry until the early 1980s, when a lawsuit concerning excessive paperwork and unreliable payment policies led to a revision in the Medicare home health payment policies. The Omnibus Budget Reconciliation Act of 1980 permitted the certification of proprietary home health agencies in states not having licensure laws.[1] Since these revisions, Medicare's annual home health benefit outlays have increased significantly and the number of home health agencies has grown steadily.

UPDATE

Home care agencies have increased from 13,959 in May 1993, to 15,027 as of March 1994 (Figure 22–1). This rate of increase has been fu-

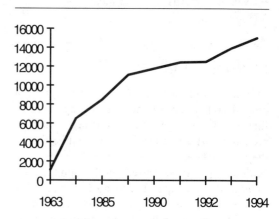

Figure 22–1 Number of Home Care Agencies from 1963 to 1994. *Source:* Data from NAHC Inventory of Home Care Agencies and Office of Survey and Certification, Health Care Financing Administration.

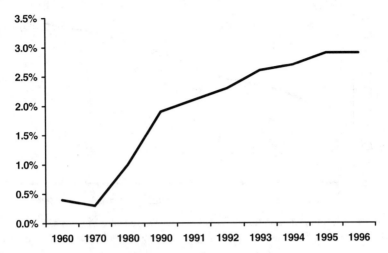

Figure 22–2 Home Care Expenditures as a Percent of National Health Expenditures. *Source:* Reprinted from Office of the Actuary, Health Care Financing Administration.

eled by the increasing demand for care at home. The growth in the number of agencies serving the population has increased home care's share, a small but growing portion, of the total health care dollar (Figures 22–2 and 22–3). The dramatic increase in the number of agencies with the resulting increase in expenditures does not necessarily indicate that the population is overserved. The increase in the number of persons served per thousand indicates an expansion of services to a market with need (Figure 22–4).

INDICATORS AND PREDICTORS OF HOME CARE DEMAND

There are multiple factors contributing to the growth of the home care market, including

- changes in aging demographics
- shrinking hospital system (cost containment pressures) and improved home care technology
- changes in the formal versus informal caregiver mix

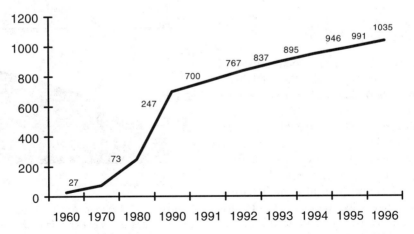

Figure 22–3 National Health Care Expenditure Trends. *Source:* Reprinted from Office of the Actuary, Health Care Financing Administration.

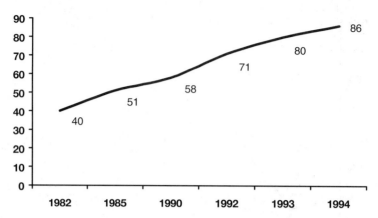

Figure 22–4 Number of Home Health Patients Served per 1,000 Medicare Enrollees. *Source:* Data from Division of Health Care Information Services, Bureaus of Data Management and Strategy, Health Care Financing Administration.

Demographic Shifts

The first major factor contributing to the growth of the home care market is the much-discussed graying of America. The number of persons reaching retirement age and Medicare eligibility age is increasing and is predicted to grow exponentially. Americans' life expectancy has increased from age 63 in 1940 to age 82 today. By 2100, it is projected that the United States will have 20.1 million residents over 85 years old, 50.6 million over 75 years old, and 89.9 million over 65 years old (Figure 22–5).[1] This growing aged population continues to put tremendous pressures on the health care system.

The Shrinking Hospital System

In response to the pressures to control costs and generate positive profit margins, hospitals have begun the process of downsizing. Two methods of measuring these changes are the number of hospital beds and patient days spent in the hospital (Table 22–1 and Figure 22–6). However, as hospital stays shorten, the days that are spent in the hospital are more expensive days. For example, these stays are often spent in the intensive care or cardiac care units. Additionally, after discharge many of the patients still need some reduced level of care. Less costly patient care will facilitate this move from the hospital. Home health care has moved to fill this void.

Formal Versus Informal Caregivers

It is estimated that 9 to 11 million people need home care services. Many of these people will receive care from family members, friends, or others. These "informal caregivers" are noncompensated. An average home health patient received 76 visits in 1996.[2] The demand for these services continues to increase as the population ages. However, there are additional reasons for the growth.

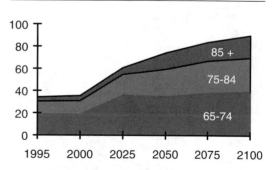

Figure 22–5 Persons Aged 65 and Older in the United States. *Source:* Reprinted from 1996 statistics, Health Care Financing Administration.

Table 22–1 Inpatient Beds Trends

Year	Total Hospitals	Average Beds per Hospital	Beds per 100 Enrollees
1975	6,707	1,132	51.5
1980	6,780	1,152	46.9
1995	6,414	1,074	29.4
1996	6,376	1,056	28.4

Source: Reprinted from 1996 statistics, Health Care Financing Administration.

The population is growing older, and the older the patient, the more home care the patient needs. Informal caregivers are also reaching the age where they will need to receive care. Due to the breakdown of the nuclear family, the dispersion of extended families, and the increased mobility of the American family, there will be fewer informal caregivers. The gap created by the loss of informal caregivers will necessitate a shift to the formal caregiver, and this shift will contribute to the growth in demand for home care services.

HOME CARE SERVICES

The home care market is segmented due to the unique nature of the various services as well as differing reimbursement mechanisms for each service type. A single patient can receive care from one or several service areas. Home care services can generally be divided into the following four groups:

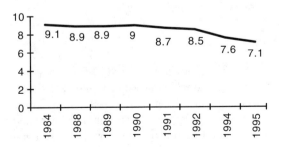

Figure 22–6 Trends in Medicare Average Length of Stay (in Days). *Source:* Data from 1993 and 1996 statistics, Health Care Financing Administration.

1. traditional Medicare-certified and private pay services
2. infusion services
3. medical equipment and supplies
4. respiratory services

Traditional Nursing Services

Traditional nursing services form the largest category of home care services. When they think of home care, most people think of these traditional services, which include services provided by registered nurses (RNs), licensed professional nurses (LPNs), home health aides (HHAs), certified nursing assistants (CNAs), and medical social workers (MSWs). In-home rehabilitation services, frequently grouped with traditional nursing services, are performed by licensed or registered therapists, including physical therapists, occupational therapists, dietitians, and speech language pathologists.

Infusion Services

Infusion services are a higher acuity level of care and often are viewed as a component of traditional care. Infusion services require a higher skill level of nursing and a pharmacy component. These services have experienced rapid and sustained growth, and in the last 10 years their fees and quality of service have been scrutinized. In 1996, infusion services were a $6 billion market.[3]

Medical Equipment and Supplies

Medical equipment and supplies are generally nonclinical items that consist of durable medical equipment (wheelchairs, walkers, hospital beds, and activities of daily living equipment and supplies) and other medical supplies. In 1996, the medical equipment market was $1.5 billion.[3]

Respiratory Services

Respiratory services, often viewed as the clinical component of home medical equipment and supplies, consist of home oxygen and respiratory therapy services. This market was $4.5 billion in 1996.[3]

PROFESSIONAL HOME CARE DISCIPLINES

Formal home care services are offered by a multidisciplinary mix of medical and nonmedical professionals.

Nurses

Nurses include RNs and LPNs. These medical professionals provide skilled services that are required by the complexity of the patient's condition. Nurses may provide assessments, injections, intravenous therapy, psychiatric care, wound care, education, disease management, and case management. Registered nurses have received 2 or more years of formal education and training and are licensed to practice in individual states. LPNs have 1 year of specialized training. They are also licensed in individual states and must operate under the supervision of an RN.

Physical Therapists

Physical therapists (PTs) perform treatment to restore loss of mobility and strength caused by physical impairments. These professionals may use specialized equipment during the conduct of these treatments. An important aspect of therapy is the education of the patient and other health care professionals in proper physical techniques to alleviate pain and prevent initial or future injury.

Occupational Therapists

Occupational therapists (OTs) provide treatments similar to physical therapy but focus on improving the patient's performance of activities of daily living (ADLs). ADLs may include eating, drinking, dressing, bathing, and performing other routine household duties. An OT often must address the physical, social, and emotional needs of the patient.

Speech Language Pathologists

Speech language pathologists (SLPs) provide care to diagnose, restore, and improve the speech function of patients having dysfunction due to stroke or injury. SLPs work to improve the communication function of these patients by using specialized tools and techniques. These therapists also work with patients suffering from problems with breathing and swallowing.

Respiratory Therapists

Respiratory therapists provide care related to the treatment of patients with pulmonary and respiratory dysfunction. This care frequently involves the use of specialized equipment, including ventilators, oxygen concentrators, liquid oxygen dispensing systems, nebulizers, continuous positive air pressure (CPAP), and other respiratory support equipment and supplies.

Medical Social Workers

Medical social workers (MSWs) assess and improve the psychological and social issues of patients. MSWs counsel patients and family in understanding the resources available to patients with illnesses or disabilities. These resources include public and private agencies that may temporarily assist the patient and patient's family, providing food, shelter, funds to pay bills, clothing, and so on. Frequently, the MSW will assist in completing the required documentation and coordinating the supportive needs of more acutely ill patients.

Physicians

Although they are last in this discussion and receive the smallest share of home care funds, physicians are the gatekeepers for most home care services. Both in traditional Medicare and commercial payment scenarios, the physician goes uncompensated for medical supervision of all home care services unless payment is handled indirectly under a full risk arrangement. The physician is responsible for initiating the plan of treatment and all changes, which can be numerous under Medicare, given the progressive rehabilitation requirement and the generally frail condition of the Medicare population. Additionally, physicians may conduct visits to the patient's home, although this is not common. Physicians do work closely with home care service providers to determine patient needs and which mix and frequency of services best meet those needs. Medicare patients under a physician's care require their care plan to be reviewed every 62 days, or more frequently, as the patient's medical needs change. The home care provider usually reviews these Medicare plans of care as part of a multidisciplinary approach to meeting the patient's needs. In many cases, physician time involvement for home care patients approaches (and sometimes exceeds) that for acute hospitalized patients.

Dietitians

Dietitians offer nutritional counseling to those patients needing dietary supportive services as part of their treatment regimen.

Home Health Aides

HHAs frequently provide the majority of services in traditional home care agencies. These caregivers may have specialized training and are not licensed by the state. They assist patients with a large variety of services, including ambulation, bathing, toileting, personal care, and dressing. Under Medicare, these services must be provided under the guidance of an RN.

Nonmedical home caregivers, including HHAs, homemakers, and companions, are also an important component of the service mix. HHA services are reimbursed by Medicare as long as a medical plan of treatment is in effect. Some Medicaid programs have waivers that pay some costs of HHA or homemaker services for the very frail or poor ill under certain conditions. However, these types of home care services, although they improve the quality of life and play a major role in raising health status and safety, are not reimbursable by third-party payers.

Homemakers

Homemakers provide supportive services in the form of general household duties, including meal preparation, laundry, light housekeeping, and shopping. They usually do not participate directly as part of the care for medical needs.

Companions

Companions are frequently called "sitters." These individuals provide a physical presence for those patients who should not be left at home alone. These caregivers do not provide medical care and are generally viewed as custodial.

Volunteers

Volunteers provide a vast number of services to the home care patient. Their involvement is determined by their individual capabilities and the needs of the patient. They are used extensively in hospice programs for bereavement care.

These professionals operate from a variety of organizations, including home care agencies, hospices, staffing (private duty) agencies, registries, medical and supply companies, and pharmaceutical and infusion services companies. These organizations may operate independently, vertically through common ownership with hospitals or skilled nursing homes, or horizontally with other home health agencies through partnerships or common ownership.

REGULATIONS GUIDING HOME CARE

Home care service providers that participate as Medicare providers are subject to Title 42 of the Code of Federal Regulations. This section of the code describes the Conditions of Participation that home health agencies must comply with to become a Medicare-certified agency and to provide care to Medicare and Medicaid recipients. These regulations establish minimum requirements for management and patient care. These regulations, which have undergone numerous changes, were initially based upon the belief that any reasonable and appropriate caregiver could interpret and administer progressive rehabilitative care. Compared to federal hospital and nursing home regulations, home care has endured in a remarkably stable financing structure over the last 30 years.

If providers do not desire to participate in the Medicare and Medicaid programs, then they are subject to any existing state requirements. The majority of states do not have specific requirements for nonparticipating providers. Frequently, private third-party payers require an agency to be Medicare certified in order to care for their beneficiaries and receive reimbursement.

The Medicare program allows both free-standing and hospital-based programs full cost reimbursement up to a regional cap, generally higher for hospital-based agencies, to cover their overhead. State and federal certification and accreditation by the Joint Commission on Accreditation of Health Care Organizations (Joint Commission) and the National Committee for Quality Assurance (NCQA) have traditionally placed higher faculty standards on hospital-based agencies than on freestanding agencies.

For patients to qualify for home health coverage under the Medicare system, the following four conditions must be met:[4]

1. The physician must have determined a medical need for home care and developed a plan of care.
2. The care described in the plan of care must be for intermittent skilled nursing, therapy, or speech services.
3. The patient must be homebound.
4. The home health agency delivering care must be certified to participate in the Medicare program.

Once these four conditions are met, Medicare will pay for[4]

- skilled nursing care either on an intermittent or part-time basis, but not full time
- HHA services on an intermittent or part-time basis, but not full time
- PT, as frequently and as long as it is medically necessary and reasonable
- SLP, as frequently and as long as it is medically necessary and reasonable
- OT, as frequently and as long as it is medically necessary and reasonable (OT can be provided in the absence of any other skilled care)
- medical social services
- medical supplies
- medical equipment (Medicare pays for 80% of the approved amounts, and the patient is responsible for the remaining 20%)

The length of time that care may be delivered is based on the medical reasonableness and necessity of the care to be delivered. Limitations do exist on the number of days and hours of care that may be received.[4]

Part-time care is defined by Medicare as

- 28 hours a week of skilled nursing and HHA care
- services provided 7 days a week if they are provided for fewer than 8 hours per day
- allowable increase to 35 hours if Medicare agrees that patient's condition requires the change

Intermittent care is defined by Medicare as

- 28 hours per week of skilled nursing care and HHA care, with increase to 35 hours a week if the patient's condition requires the change
- services provided for 6 days a week
- in some cases, nursing and HHA services provided for a maximum of 8 hours a day, 7 days a week, for 21 consecutive days, with a defined extension beyond 21 days for extreme cases

These limitations do not apply to therapy services, which may be provided for as long as they are deemed medically responsible and necessary.

The indemnity, health maintenance organization (HMO) and, more recently, large self-insured employer sectors have evolved to a broader understanding of the value of medically necessary home care. Initially, approvals for reimbursement were on a case-by-case exception basis, led by nurse case managers who arranged for complex long-term care, such as intravenous antibiotic therapy, in the home. The main driver was cost, with the added benefit of customer satisfaction. As these sectors became more creative, programmatic handling of home care began, for example, by supporting earlier discharge of new mothers and babies with one or two home visits and follow-up telephone calls. Hospitals initiated these efforts to differentiate themselves and increase margins under case rate contracts.

Commercial HMOs also followed the path of Medicare HMOs in seeking procedure-specific (eg, lumbar laminectomy) or disease-specific carve-outs. Programs focused on specific disease states require highly skilled professionals. Successful implementation of the programs hinges upon close working relationships of the discharge planning teams, which include inpatient and home care program coordinators, payer case managers, and physicians.

Certification of a Medicare agency is the responsibility of the Health Care Financing Administration (HCFA). However, most state health departments have attained "deemed status" to conduct on-site surveys and reviews of agencies in their state. Thus, a single review team applies the higher standards or the combined federal and state standards, making Medicare and Medicaid reimbursement possible. In many states, agencies cannot bill commercial carriers without state (and often, therefore, federal) certification and licensure.

Medicare-certified home care services were loosely regulated in the past. HCFA allowed state regulatory agencies to serve as approval authorities for entry and continued participation in the Medicare system. These approvals came in the form of annual state surveys performed by state employees using a combination of local, regional, and national regulations, more often than not subjective and incorrectly interpreted by providers and regulatory agencies alike. The surveys usually lasted 1 to 3 days and consisted of nonstatistical sampling of medical charts for audits, limited visits to patient homes, and reviews of policies, procedures, and other documents. The results of these surveys were discrepancy lists; the agency had a certain amount of time to develop a correction plan and forward it to the regulators. The agency might or might not then be subject to a reinspection.

These regulations were relatively toothless in the past. However, recent legislation has imposed substantial criminal and other penalties for fraud and abuse of the Medicare system. This new breed of regulations includes the Operation Restore Trust initiatives, surety bond regulations, and the Balanced Budget Act of 1997. Additionally, numerous rulings and mandates from HCFA, the Department of Health and Human Services, fiscal intermediaries, and even the president have substantially altered the way home health agencies currently operate and will operate in the near future.

FINANCING HOME CARE SERVICES

Health care expenditures have significantly increased in the last 30 years. The source of expenditures has undergone a fundamental shift. Private funds were the primary payer source in 1960. In 1996, public, federal, state, and local funds represented almost half of total expenditures (Figure 22–7). Expenditures for home health care services have increased astoundingly since 1980. This growth represents one of the fastest growing expenditures in the Medicare system. It has grown from 2.9% of all Medicare payments in 1980 to nearly 9% in 1996 (Figure 22–8).[2]

Home care services are paid for by a variety of payer sources, both public and private. They may also be paid for directly by the patient or responsible party. The trend in payment sources for home care has also shown a shift in the primary payer for home care services. In 1980, federal funds accounted for 37% of home care pay-

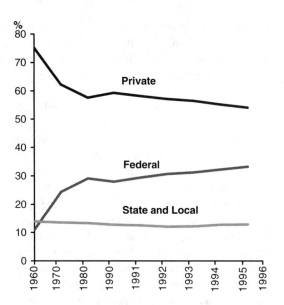

Figure 22–7 National Health Expenditures by Payer Type. *Source:* Reprinted from Office of the Actuary, Health Care Financing Administration.

ments (Figure 22–9). Private funds, including private health insurance and other private sources, contributed 38%. By 1996, federal contributions had risen to 53%, a 16% increase. Medicare represented 86%, $13.6 billion, of those federal funds in 1996. By 1996, private source funds had dropped to 21%, a 17% decrease. During this same period, out-of-pocket reimbursements remained at approximately 20%, and state and local funds contributed 4% in 1980 and 7% in 1996, a 3% increase. Federal programs have emerged as the primary source of funding for home care services.

Public third-party payers constitute the largest sector of funding sources. These payers include Medicare, Medicaid, the Older Americans Act, the Department of Veterans Affairs, Social Services block grant programs, and other community organizations.

REGULATORY ISSUES IMPACTING HOME CARE

There is continuous scrutiny of home health care related to fraud and abuse of the reimbursement system. Operation Restore Trust (ORT) has been successful in detecting this fraud and abuse. The ORT program is being expanded to include 12 states and is projected to eventually be nationwide. The Department of Health and Human Services has identified $1.2 billion for recovery collections, fines, settlements, and restitution in fiscal year (FY) 1997.[2] This FY 1997 total was six times higher than that of FY 1996. Criminal and civil prosecution cases totaled 1,340 in FY 1997, and over 2,700 providers were excluded from participation in federal and state programs.[2] The pressures on home care agencies will continue to grow as home care becomes a central target in these activities. The Balanced Budget Act of 1997 contains additional proposals to fight fraud and abuse in home care, including

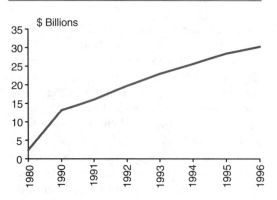

Figure 22–8 Home Health Care Expenditure Trends. *Source:* Reprinted from Office of the Actuary, National Health Statistics Group, Health Care Financing Administration.

- new penalties of $50,000 per violation for providers paying kickbacks for referrals
- requirements that providers disclose Social Security numbers and employer identification numbers to screen out past offenders
- requirements for surety bonds from home health agencies
- a more clear definition of what constitutes skilled services to prevent medically unnecessary visits

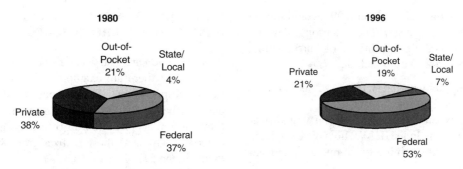

Figure 22–9 Home Health Care Payer Types. *Source:* Reprinted from Office of the Actuary, National Health Statistics Group, Health Care Financing Administration.

- authority to deny payment to providers that bill in excess of what other providers bill for similar services

Other actions by HCFA include the following:[2]

- Home health agencies are being asked about related business interests before admission as a Medicare provider. This will help determine if there are any previous instances of fraud and abuse and will also serve to prevent unauthorized billings through nonexistent or nonapproved companies.
- Home health companies must have provided care to at least 10 patients before being allowed to provide care to Medicare beneficiaries. At least 7 of these patients must be receiving care at the time of survey for approval to receive a Medicare provider number.
- Claims review has increased to 25% of claims submitted. HCFA has set aside $10 million to perform audits. This is nearly double that of the past.
- Fiscal intermediaries have hired medical directors to advise claims processors and providers on medical necessity of care.

The Balanced Budget Act of 1997 also included proposals that attempt to reduce the cost for home health services. These proposals included the following:

- A prospective payment system (PPS) would be established. This would replace the cost reimbursement system. HCFA will determine what will be paid for a unit of service, how many visits will be included in the unit, and what mix of services will constitute the unit of service.
- Felons will be barred from participating in the Medicare program.
- Medicare Part A and Medicare Part B benefits for home health services will be established.
- Periodic interim payments will be eliminated.
- Billing will be by service location rather than by agency office locations. This is an attempt to prevent agency offices in a higher reimbursement urban setting from billing for services provided in a lower reimbursement rural setting.
- Guidelines for service unit frequency and duration will be established. Those service units in excess of the guidelines would not be reimbursed.
- There will be clarification of the terms *intermittent* and *part-time*.

MEASURING QUALITY IN HOME CARE SERVICES

The Clinton administration is aggressively pursuing initiatives to measure and improve the quality of home care services. Two proposed rulings announced in March 1997 would impact the home care industry. The first proposal would revise Medicare's Conditions of Participation. These revisions would include

- a requirement that HHAs be subject to criminal background checks
- the expansion of existing HHA qualifications to include HHAs who have completed nurse aide training or competency evaluations
- active involvement of patients in the planning and conduct of their care by discussing expected outcomes of care
- a requirement that home care agencies coordinate all the physician-ordered care for patients

The second proposed regulation requires that home health agencies use the Outcomes and Assessment Information Set (OASIS). This standardized system is designed to monitor patients' conditions and levels of satisfaction. This system would require that each new patient receive a standardized assessment within 48 hours of admission. This assessment is designed to determine the care and support needs of each patient. It would be updated continually to monitor and track changes in the patient's condition. This continuous assessment would end upon discharge of the patient from the home health agency. Home health agencies would be required to evaluate the OASIS assessments, track this information, and incorporate changes in their quality improvement programs. These data sets would also be used by inspectors and surveyors to standardize the agency surveys and to identify improvement opportunities related to patient care and satisfaction.

EXAMPLES OF ADVANCED CLINICAL PRACTICES IN HOME CARE

Best home care practices are not well documented, yet there are examples of wide variations and innovations. For instance, West Coast agencies have been successful in managing post-total hip replacement care in 6 to 8 visits with outcomes similar to those realized from 8 to 12 visits on the East Coast.

Recognizing the high incidence of psychosocially driven emergency department (ED) visits, a very large Southern home health agency has become creative in working with a number of hospitals to manage their Medicare risk ED visits. It has developed a triaging program that identifies patients before processing at the hospital and refers them to an adult day care program with after-hours homemaker care to effectively decrease ED visits and their related admissions by 25%.

Disease state case management companies have entered the market with a home care model that combines in-home environmental assessments and routine visits with up to daily telephonic contact to maximize treatment compliance in chronic diseases such as congestive heart failure. These companies have shown the ability to significantly reduce ED visits, admissions, and overall costs associated with the disease.

An example of a procedure-specific clinical process that has been developed by another Southern city for post-lumbar laminectomy using a combination of accelerated postoperative teaching and two home care follow-up visits reduced inpatient hospital stays from five to six days, to two days.

REFERENCES

1. Health Care Financing Administration, US Department of Health and Human Services, Bureau of Data Management and Strategy. *HCFA Statistics*. Publication no 03394. Washington, DC: Health Care Financing Administration; 1996.
2. Health Care Financing Administration. Press Release. January 13, 1998.
3. Schworm K, Gruenwedel E. The industry's facts and figures. *HomeCare*. July 1997:36.
4. Health Care Financing Administration—Medicare and Medicaid, US Department of Health and Human Services. *Medicare and Home Health Care*. Publication no 10969. Washington, DC: Health Care Financing Administration; 1996.

PEGGY H. RODEBUSH, RN, MSN, is a senior manager in Ernst & Young's health care business transformation service line. In this role, she works with leading health care and home health clients across the United States. She is a nationally recognized post–acute care and medical management expert and is a frequent speaker at national conventions.

KATHLEEN M. L. POPPER, PHD, is a health care strategy senior manager in Ernst & Young's Washington, DC, practice. She has spent over 20 years in health care operations and strategy, including 7 years in home care operations as CEO and COO for several subsidiaries of National Medical Enterprises and 3 years of managed care experience as director of strategic planning with Humana, Inc. Her experience crosses many aspects of health care delivery from critical to long-term care, neonates to the frail elderly, and from both the provider and payer perspectives. Dr. Popper received a PhD in marketing and international business from Michigan State University, an MS in administration from Pepperdine University, and a BSN from the University of the State of New York.

BARRY K. MORRISON is a senior consultant for Ernst & Young's health care business transformation line.

CHAPTER 23

Subacute Care

Kathleen M. Griffin

Chapter Outline

- Introduction
- Subacute Care Defined
- Subacute Care Categories
- Subacute Patients
- Subacute Providers
- Subacute Care Within a Continuum of Care
- Payment for Subacute Care
- Selecting a Quality Subacute Care Provider
- Conclusion

INTRODUCTION

Subacute care has emerged in response to pressures from third-party payers to provide a less costly alternative treatment setting to acute hospital care. Subacute care is provided both in specialty hospitals and in subacute skilled nursing facilities and units. In 1994 it was estimated that there were approximately 720 freestanding subacute providers with 27,050 beds. These providers reportedly admitted 270,000 patients in that year, accounting for 8.1 million patient days and $3.4 billion in revenues. Approximately 73% were Medicare beneficiaries. Most of the remainder were covered by managed care plans.[1] Although the national subacute market size has not been updated since 1994, it is certain that the number of providers with dedicated subacute units in hospitals and in freestanding nursing facilities has grown significantly since that year. In 1996, there were 2,084 hospital-based skilled nursing facilities, the vast majority of which were subacute providers.[2]

SUBACUTE CARE DEFINED

Definitions of subacute care have been prepared by a number of organizations. The definitions developed by two organizations, the National Subacute Care Association (NSCA) and the Joint Commission on Accreditation of Healthcare Organizations (Joint Commission), shown in Exhibit 23–1, appear to contain the key components reflected in most other definitions.

SUBACUTE CARE CATEGORIES

In spite of the promulgation of definitions of subacute care by NSCA and the Joint Commission, there remains a great deal of confusion about exactly what subacute care is. This confusion is due in part to the lack of a federal definition of subacute care, and in part to the fact that subacute care is commonly provided in three dif-

---

This chapter is adapted from KM Griffin, Subacute Care and Managed Care, in *The Managed Health Care Handbook*, 3rd ed, PR Kongstvedt, ed, pp 388–401, © 1996, Aspen Publishers, Inc.

Exhibit 23–1 National Subacute Care Association and Joint Commission on Accreditation of Healthcare Organizations Definitions of Subacute Care

The definition developed by NSCA is as follows:*

Subacute care is a comprehensive, cost-effective inpatient level of care for patients who

a) have had an acute event resulting from injury, illness, or exacerbation of a disease process
b) have a determined course of treatment, and
c) though stable, require diagnostics or invasive procedures but not intensive procedures requiring an acute level of care.

The severity of the patient's condition requires:

a) active physician direction with frequent on-site visits
b) professional nursing care
c) significant ancillary services
d) an outcomes-focused interdisciplinary approach utilizing a professional team, and
e) complex medical and/or rehabilitative care.

Typically short term, subacute care is designed to return patients to the community or transition them to a lower level of care.

The definition developed by the Joint Commission is as follows:**

Subacute care is comprehensive inpatient care designed for someone who has an acute illness, injury, or exacerbation of a disease process. It is goal-oriented treatment rendered immediately after, or instead of, acute hospitalization to treat one or more specific active complex medical conditions or to administer one or more technically complex treatments, in the context of a person's underlying long-term conditions and overall situation. Generally, the individual's condition is such that the care does not depend heavily on high-technology monitoring or complex diagnostic procedures. Subacute care requires the coordinated services of an interdisciplinary team including physicians, nurses, and other relevant professional disciplines, who are trained and knowledgeable in assessing and managing these specific conditions and in performing the necessary procedures. Subacute care is given as part of a specifically defined program, regardless of the site. Subacute care is generally more intensive than traditional nursing facility care and less intensive than acute care. It requires frequent (daily to weekly), recurrent patient assessment and review of the clinical course and treatment plan for a limited (several days to several months) time period, until the condition is stabilized or a predetermined treatment course is completed.

*Courtesy of National Subacute Care Association, Bethesda, Maryland.
**Source: © *CAMH*. Oakbrook Terrace, IL: Joint Commission on Accreditation of Healthcare Organizations, p 18. Reprinted with permission.

ferent settings: specialty hospitals, hospital-based skilled nursing facility units, and freestanding skilled nursing facilities. Each setting tends to focus on one or two of the four different categories of subacute care. These categories are

- transitional subacute care
- general subacute care
- chronic subacute care
- long-term transitional subacute care

Hospital-based subacute skilled nursing units typically focus on the first category, transitional subacute care. Nursing facility subacute units usually can be classified as general subacute or chronic subacute care. Specialty hospitals (most often, long-term care prospective payment–exempt hospitals) would focus on long-term transitional subacute care. Exhibit 23–2 depicts the categories of subacute care, explaining the key differences in service intensity and length of stay parameters.

SUBACUTE PATIENTS

Subacute patients vary in acuity levels and exhibit different problems. Subacute patients generally include the following:

Exhibit 23–2 Types of Subacute Care

Transitional Subacute Care

Transitional subacute care can be described as short-stay (under 20 days) hospital step-down care. Nursing staffing averages 5.0 to 6.5 hours of direct care per patient day. About 50% to 70% of the direct nursing care is provided by licensed nurses. Transitional subacute units are utilized for patients who require daily medical care and monitoring; highly skilled nursing care; an integrated program of therapies, both rehabilitative and respiratory; and frequent utilization of pharmaceutical and laboratory services. Days in this type of subacute care unit serve as replacement hospital days, to effect a reduction of acute hospital days. In other words, a transitional subacute unit actually serves as a substitute for continued hospital stays, not as an alternate hospital discharge placement. For example, stroke patients may be transferred to a transitional subacute unit on day 4 or 5 of hospitalization in the acute hospital, and coronary bypass patients who are not off the ventilator within 4 or 5 days may be transferred for a weaning program. Transitional subacute units typically have a variety of physician program directors or consultants, a dedicated staff of acute or critical care nurses, 24-hour respiratory therapy, and 7-day-per-week rehabilitation therapies.

General Subacute Care

General subacute units are most often utilized for patients who require medical care and monitoring at least weekly, short-term nursing care at a level of approximately 4.0 to 4.5 hours per patient day, and rehabilitative therapies that may extend from 1 to 3 hours per patient day. Short stay in nature (averaging 25–30 days), general subacute care units focus on patients who require rehabilitation, wound care, or intravenous therapies, often with other medical complications. Although there is some overlap in the clinical programs between the transitional subacute units and general subacute care facilities, the key difference is the acuity level of the patients. A sizable number of patients in the general subacute units are geriatric because younger patients at these acuity levels tend to be cared for by home health services. The goal of both transitional subacute units and general subacute units is to manage the patient's recovery or rehabilitation in a cost-effective manner and to discharge the patient home, or in some cases, to a less expensive level of care such as long-term care or an assisted living facility.

Chronic Subacute Care

Chronic subacute units manage patients with little hope of ultimate recovery and functional independence, such as ventilator-dependent patients, long-term comatose patients, and patients with progressive neurological disease. Typically, these patients require nursing staffing at the level less than the general subacute unit (3 to 5 hours per patient day), medical monitoring biweekly to monthly, and restorative therapies, usually provided by nursing staff with guidance from rehabilitation therapists. These patients either will eventually be stabilized so that they can be discharged home or be cared for in a long-term care facility, or they may expire. Their average length of stay is 60 to 90 days.

Long-Term Transitional Subacute Care

Long-term transitional subacute facilities most often are licensed as hospitals rather than as nursing facilities. They usually are exempt from the Medicare prospective payment system as long-term care hospitals and have average lengths of stay of at least 25 days. Overall average length of stay for long-term transitional subacute care is 28 to 42 days. Typically, these facilities provide care for acute ventilator-dependent or medically complex patients. Because these facilities are hospitals, attending physicians visit the patients daily. Nursing staff tend to be primarily registered nurses, and nursing hours per patient day may range between 6.5 and 9.0 depending on the types and acuity levels of patients.

Courtesy of Health Dimensions Consulting Group, Scottsdale, Arizona.

- medically complex patients who are chronically ill or have multiple medical problems or disorders; these patients need medical monitoring and specialized care but can be managed in a subacute setting
- respiratory care patients who require ventilator weaning or ventilator care programs as a result of a respiratory disease, injury, or impairment or who require medical and nursing care as well as therapies to recover from an acute respiratory episode
- recuperating surgery patients who need rehabilitative therapy but no longer need intensive care services
- patients who require rehabilitation for a variety of reasons, most frequently after orthopaedic surgery or a stroke
- patients with head injuries
- patients who have brain injuries as a result of ischemic or hemorrhagic stroke, blunt trauma, or penetrating trauma
- cardiovascular patients who require a cardiac recovery or rehabilitation program, often related to congestive heart failure or cardiovascular surgery
- patients with such medical conditions as septicemia or osteomyelitis who require short-term intravenous therapy
- oncology patients who require radiation oncology services, chemotherapy, pain management, and rehabilitation
- wound management patients with chronic wounds (eg, pressure ulcers, necrotic wounds, or peripheral vascular disease ulcerations) related to diseases that need management before the wounds will heal

Although patients of all ages may suffer one or more of these disorders, the vast majority of subacute patients are geriatric patients.

SUBACUTE PROVIDERS

Although managed care organizations are increasingly becoming payers for subacute care, especially with the growth of Medicare risk health maintenance organizations (HMOs), Medicare continues to be the major payer for subacute services. As a result, provider settings for subacute care, to a great extent, reflect the idiosyncrasies of the health care reimbursement system.[3] The three most common types of settings for subacute care are hospital-based skilled nursing facility subacute units, subacute units in freestanding skilled nursing facilities, and long-term care hospitals.

Hospital-Based Subacute Skilled Nursing Facility Units

Hospital-based subacute skilled nursing facility (SNF) units allow the hospital to create a continuum of care. Patients who no longer require the intensity of services typically found on the medical/surgical floor of an acute care hospital can be transferred to a subacute unit where the sophisticated diagnostic, monitoring, and emergency response capabilities are available, but the intensity of services is less. Moreover, the programs in the subacute unit are oriented toward a patient's optimal functional independence at the time of discharge.

In order to be eligible for favorable reimbursement by Medicare, the hospital-based subacute unit must be licensed as an SNF unit. The result is that the hospital's performance under the Medicare prospective payment system (PPS) is improved. Hospitals may reduce their inpatient lengths of stay for Medicare patients by utilizing the subacute SNF unit as a step-down or transitional facility for Medicare patients.

Under Medicare payment prior to PPS for SNFs, a hospital was able to reallocate certain Medicare expenses from the hospital to the subacute SNF unit as a new cost center. As a result, a portion of Medicare costs previously allocated to an inpatient area subject to Medicare's PPS could be distributed to a cost-based, extended care reimbursement area. However, the Balanced Budget Act of 1997 changed the Medicare reimbursement system for SNFs to a PPS. Beginning with the first cost reporting period after July 1, 1998, subacute and SNF providers will be subject to a case-mix, adjusted per diem, prospective payment for covered services. There will be no exemptions or exceptions from cost caps. The per diem PPS rates will be calculated utilizing the estimated costs of SNF services derived from fiscal year 1995 Medicare cost reporting periods, subject to certain adjustments. For SNFs that filed a 1995 Medicare cost report, there is a 4-year transition period that includes a blend of federal payment rates and facility-specific payment rates (Figure 23–1). For newer facilities, those that did not file a 1995 Medicare cost report, there will not be a phase-in period. The subacute per diem will be based entirely on the federal rate.

For managed care organizations, hospital-based subacute units provide a lower cost alternative setting for patients who are not medically stable enough to be transferred to a subacute unit in a freestanding nursing facility, or for patients who simply require a few additional days of inpatient care prior to being discharged home. The location of the subacute unit in the hospital facilitates patient–physician interaction and enhances the integration of services between the subacute unit and the hospital. For example, although the subacute unit's nursing staff usually will be different from the nurses who cared for the patient on the medical/surgical floor, rehabilitation and respiratory staff members who provided services to the patient while he or she was in a hospital bed may continue to provide services to the same patient in the hospital-based subacute unit. The subacute unit also can benefit from the hospital's quality improvement programs, infection control procedures, and management information system.

Although it is clear that there are many system and patient management benefits to hospital-based subacute units, the costs of patient care in these units typically are greater than the costs for care in subacute units in freestanding nursing facilities. In 1994, the average cost per day for Medicare patients in hospital-based skilled nursing facilities was $443; for Medicare patients in freestanding SNFs, it was $235.[2]

Subacute Units in Freestanding Skilled Nursing Facilities

The creation of a subacute unit in a freestanding SNF usually involves the establishment of a distinct area within the facility that is separated from the areas of the building dedicated to long-term care services. Subacute units in freestanding SNFs have separate nursing stations, patient rooms, and common areas, so that subacute patients and long-term care residents and their families do not mix.

Subacute units in freestanding SNFs typically are positioned as a low-cost alternative to the hospital setting. Although more recent data were not found, managed care reimbursement as of 1994 for patients in subacute units in freestanding SNFs ranged from $250 to $550 per day.[3] When Medicare PPS for SNFs is implemented, it is expected that managed care rates will be comparable to federal per diem rates, which will be case-mix based.

From the provider perspective, the greatest challenge to the freestanding SNF that has created a subacute unit is to ensure that there is a cultural paradigm shift from a long-term care, custodial focus to a short-term recovery and rehabilitation focus, wherein the patient will be discharged home or to a less costly level of care in 2 to 4 weeks. To achieve this conceptual shift, the most successful subacute units in freestand-

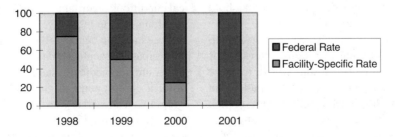

Figure 23–1 Phase-In of Prospective Payment for SNF (Subacute) Payment. Courtesy of Health Dimensions Consulting Group, Scottsdale, Arizona.

ing SNFs have a staff that is dedicated to the subacute unit, that is separate from the nursing, rehabilitative, and social services staff for the long-term care residents. In addition, the effective subacute unit in a freestanding nursing facility employs a medical director, who is different from the administrative medical director for the long-term care facility. Other components of successful subacute units are specific programs of care, outcome measures, subacute unit–specific admission and discharge criteria, and care protocols that help ensure that patients in the subacute unit receive the services they need in a cost-effective manner.

Long-Term Care Hospitals

Long-term care hospitals are one of five types of hospitals that may be excluded from the Medicare PPS reimbursement. Instead of being paid prospectively on the basis of diagnosis-related groups (DRGs), the PPS-exempt long-term care hospitals are paid a specific amount per Medicare discharge. The amount is established based on the individual hospital's costs during its initial year of PPS-exempt operations.

The Balanced Budget Act also affected Medicare payments to long-term care hospitals by placing a cap on the amount per Medicare discharge paid to the PPS-exempt long-term care hospital. For existing PPS-exempt long-term care hospitals, as of October 1, 1997, payments are capped at the 75th percentile of the per discharge payment amount for all long-term care hospitals. Those hospitals with per discharge payments that are at, or below, the 75th percentile threshold retain their old payment, while those that exceed the 75th percentile threshold are capped at that threshold amount.

Long-term care hospitals provide services to patients who continue to require intensive or other acute inpatient care and whose average length of stay is 25 days or more. The patients in long-term care hospitals usually have complex medical conditions and multisystem failures that require more intensive care, monitoring, and emergency back-up resources than are available in free-standing SNF subacute units. Patients may be admitted to long-term care hospitals directly from the intensive care unit of an acute care general hospital.

Subacute programs in long-term care hospitals provide more hours of nursing per patient day (6.5 to 9.0 hours) than typically are provided in subacute programs in hospital-based or freestanding SNFs, and average lengths of stay are longer than those in SNF subacute care units. In 1994, patients in subacute programs in long-term care hospitals had an average length of stay of 29 to 42 days, depending on whether the patient had a prior PPS hospital stay.

While the costs of subacute care and long-term care hospitals usually are higher than the costs for subacute care in SNF subacute units, costs of care in long-term care hospitals can be considerably less than the costs of care in an intensive care unit in an acute care general hospital. It is likely that managed care organizations will attempt to match the new Medicare payment limits when contracting with long-term care hospitals in the future.

Specialty Hospital-Based Subacute SNF Units

Both long-term care hospitals and PPS-exempt rehabilitation hospitals may create subacute SNF units within the hospital. The subacute unit within a long-term care hospital would focus on the medically complex patients who have met certain goals in the long-term care hospital and who no longer need the same intensity of services. However, such patients would require continued inpatient care for their medical conditions, in order to be discharged home or to a long-term care facility.

Freestanding acute rehabilitation hospitals may create subacute SNF units for patients who either are not medically stable enough to benefit from a comprehensive physical rehabilitation program or are unable to tolerate the comprehensive rehabilitation program (ie, 3 hours or more of rehabilitation daily) but can benefit from 1 to 2 hours of physical rehabilitation daily.

While the average length of stay for patients in the acute rehabilitation hospital may be 18 to 20 days, the average length of stay for patients in the slower paced, less intensive rehabilitation program in the subacute SNF unit within the rehabilitation hospital may be 20 to 30 days. Typically, the costs of care in the subacute SNF unit of the specialty hospital would be less than the costs for acute care in the specialty hospital.

SUBACUTE CARE WITHIN A CONTINUUM OF CARE

Subacute care cannot be viewed as independent from other levels of care within the care continuum. Appropriate subacute care utilization requires an effective case management system that ensures that the patient receives the right care, at the right time, in the right setting, and for the right cost. The case management system must focus on the patient's condition and medical needs, level of family and/or other social support systems available, services that are available within the continuum, location of those services, and health benefits available to the patients. Table 23–1 shows how transitional subacute care and general subacute care fit into a care continuum and contrasts the subacute care levels with other components of the care continuum such as intermediate/custodial care, skilled nursing care, acute rehabilitation, and acute care.

Table 23–1 Subacute Care Within the Care Continuum

	Lowest Acuity					Highest Acuity
	Nursing Facilities			Hospital		
	Intermediate Care	Skilled Nursing	General Subacute	Acute Rehabilitation	Transitional Subacute	Acute Care
Patients (residents)	Restorative care	Medically stable/ rehabilitation	Medically stable/ rehabilitation	Medically stable/ need acute rehabilitation	Medically sick/ complex care	Medically unstable/invasive procedures/most complex care
Physician visits	Monthly	Monthly	Weekly to biweekly	Daily	3 to 7 times/ week	Daily
Nursing (HPPD)	<2.5, LPN/CNA	2.5 to 3.5, 1 RN/LPN/CNA	4.0 to 4.5, RN/LPN/CNA	5.5 to 7, RNs and nursing assistants	5.0 to 6.0, RNs and CNAs	6.5 to 9, RNs
Respiratory therapy	No	Rarely/prn if any	Rarely/prn if any	On-site 24 hours	On-site 24 hours	On-site 24 hours
Rehabilitation	Rare	3 to 5 times per week	5 times per week	5 to 7 times per week, 3 hours/ day	Daily PT, OT, ST	Daily PT, OT, ST
Pharmacy, lab	Contract	Contract	Contract	Pharmacology: On-site 24 hours Laboratory: May be contract	On-site 24 hours	On-site 24 hours
Average length of stay	2 years+	34 days	25 days	17 to 19 days	17 days	
Discharge	Death	LTC or home	LTC, home, or acute rehabilitation	Home or general subacute care	Home (LTC rare)	Home or SNF

Note: CNA, certified nursing assistant; HPPD, hours per patient day; LPN, licensed practical nurse; LTC, long-term care; OT, occupational therapy; PT, physical therapy; RN, registered nurse; ST, speech therapy.

Courtesy of Health Dimensions Consulting Group, Scottsdale, Arizona.

As many health care providers in the United States convert from nonaffiliated, independent provider entities into integrated delivery systems, the four categories of subacute care are expected to be owned or related components of every system. However, during the current transition period from multiple independent providers to integrated provider networks, utilization of subacute care, like other post–acute health care levels, has tended to be stratified and fragmented. The regulatory requirements for subacute providers within SNFs, whether hospital-based or free-standing, have served as barriers to easy transition of patients between the acute and subacute settings. For example, in order to transfer a patient from an acute hospital bed to a subacute SNF bed in an adjacent unit within the hospital, the patient must be formally discharged from the hospital and then admitted to the subacute care unit. The admission procedures to the subacute care unit must comply with federal and state nursing facility regulations. Compliance with these regulations often means the completion of a substantial amount of paperwork related to the admission process.

Nevertheless, active case management, within the integrated delivery system wherein an individual patient's care is managed by the same case manager throughout the continuum, can help ensure that the transfer of a patient to the most appropriate level of care within the continuum occurs as seamlessly as possible.

PAYMENT FOR SUBACUTE CARE

Although the majority of subacute patients have Medicare as a primary payer, increasingly, managed care organizations are including subacute care in their hospital or health care system agreements.

Managed care organizations and subacute providers negotiate payment under a variety of arrangements:

- *Discounted fee for service*: The provider typically agrees to furnish subacute care services at a discount from its standard charges. The discount may be a percentage of the standard charge for all services, or the discount may be specific to the service or category of service.
- *Per diem*: The managed care organization pays the provider a fixed rate for each day that an enrollee is treated within the provider's subacute care facility or unit. The per diem rate may be specified in a contractual arrangement or may be negotiated for each patient admission.
- *Per case*: The managed care organization pays the provider a fixed rate for each case of inpatient treatment. The rate will vary depending on service category or patient category. This payment methodology would be similar to the hospital DRG payment under Medicare.
- *Capitation*: In this arrangement, the provider receives from the managed care organization a fixed payment per enrollee per month. For that monthly fee, the provider agrees to furnish specified subacute care to the payer's enrollees. The number of enrollees, as opposed to the utilization of services, controls the providers' revenues.

Today, the most common payment arrangement between managed care organizations and subacute providers is the per diem payment. In the contract between the subacute provider and the managed care organization, certain items and services typically will be included in the per diem rate, while items or services over which the provider has less control often will be excluded. Exhibit 23–3 lists usual inclusions and exclusions from a per diem rate negotiated between the managed care organization and the subacute care provider.

Per diem rates tend to vary based on patient acuity as well as resources required by the patient. Often, subacute care providers utilize a patient acuity measurement system to define subacute care levels, and each level has a different per diem payment amount. An example of subacute care per diem payment levels is shown in Exhibit 23–4.

Exhibit 23–3 Items and Services Usually Included in or Excluded from a per Diem Rate for Subacute Care

---

INCLUSIONS
- Room and board (semiprivate)
- Nursing and personal care
- Medical social services
- Recreation/activities program
- House toiletries
- Patient/family education
- Surgical dressings
- Dietary consultation
- Case management

EXCLUSIONS
- Special beds
- Ventilators
- Respiratory therapy
- Intravenous antibiotics
- Third-generation pharmaceuticals
- Traction equipment
- Prosthetic devices
- Laboratory tests
- Radiology services
- Parenteral formulas, suppliers, equipment

Courtesy of Health Dimensions Consulting Group, Scottsdale, Arizona.

Subacute care providers may include a stop-loss provision for patients whose acuity levels significantly increase during their inpatient stay in the subacute care unit or facility. Conversely, the managed care organization may include stipulations in the agreement that the patient will be reviewed weekly to determine whether a less expensive level of subacute care or discharge home or to a long-term care facility is appropriate.

SELECTING A QUALITY SUBACUTE CARE PROVIDER

In most areas of the United States, managed care organizations have an array of subacute providers from which to select. The indicators of quality discussed below may be used as benchmarks in the selection process.

Accreditation

The size of the subacute provider marketplace and the number of alternative settings for managed care organizations have spurred the need for an agreed-upon set of national standards against which to judge performance, monitor service delivery, and determine the outcomes of care. Although some states are exploring or have special licensing categories for subacute care, Medicare does not differentiate subacute care from the skilled nursing benefit for Medicare beneficiaries. During the past several years, however, two accrediting organizations have created standards for subacute providers: the Joint Commission and the Commission on Accreditation of Rehabilitation Facilities (CARF).

The Joint Commission has created a protocol for accrediting subacute programs.[4] The Joint Commission took existing standards for long-term care and tried to tailor those standards to the needs of subacute patients, particularly in areas related to time frames, staff qualifications, organizational structure, leadership and safety, and equipment management. In addition, standards for comprehensive rehabilitation, medical credentialing and privileging, and respiratory care have been added to form the Joint Commission's subacute accreditation protocol. Although the protocol uses the term "residents," the Joint Commission considers the term "patients" appropriate for recipients of subacute care.

The subacute protocol incorporates the following major sections:

- resident rights and organization ethics
- continuum of care
- assessment of residents
- care and treatment of residents
- education of residents
- improving organization performance
- leadership
- management of the environment of care
- management of human resources
- management of information
- surveillance, prevention, and control of infection

Exhibit 23–4 Subacute Care/per Diem Payment Levels

Subacute care: special	Special arrangements. Patients with specialized care needs. Averages 6.0+ nursing hours per patient day, and 0 to 2.0+ hours of therapies per patient day.
Subacute care: tier III	Patients requiring intense medical, nursing, and/or rehabilitative interventions and procedures.
	Definition of intense: 4.5 to 6.0 nursing hours per patient day (with up to 50% professional nursing time) and 0 to 2.0 hours of rehabilitation therapies per patient day.
Subacute care: tier II	Patients requiring moderate to minimal medical and nursing procedures and moderate rehabilitative interventions.
	Definition of moderate: 4 to 4.5 nursing hours per patient day (with up to 45% professional nursing time) and 0 to 1.5 hours of rehabilitation therapies per patient day.
Subacute care: tier I	Patients requiring minimal medical, nursing, and rehabilitative interventions.
	Definition of minimal: 3.5 to 4.0 nursing hours per patient day up to 1.0 hour rehabilitation therapies per patient day.
Skilled nursing care	Patients requiring skilled care with minimal medical and rehabilitation intervention. Averages 2.5 to 3.5 nursing hours per patient day, less than 30% licensed nursing professional time, 0 to 2.0+ rehabilitation therapies per patient day.

Courtesy of Health Dimensions Consulting Group, Scottsdale, Arizona.

CARF is the national accrediting agency that establishes standards for organizations serving persons with disabilities. Subacute providers may be accredited if they demonstrate compliance with the standards for one of the categories of comprehensive inpatient medical rehabilitation.[5] Comprehensive inpatient medical rehabilitation programs may seek accreditation in one or more of the three categories depending on the licenses they hold. Category 1 is reserved for acute rehabilitation programs within facilities licensed as hospitals. Categories 2 and 3 are reserved for subacute rehabilitation.

In selecting subacute providers, managed care organizations may wish to ascertain whether or not the provider is accredited according to the Joint Commission subacute protocol. If the subacute unit includes a rehabilitation program, it would be desirable to determine whether the unit has obtained CARF accreditation as a medical rehabilitation program.

Programs of Care

Subacute providers should have clearly defined protocols, care tracks, or programs for the key categories of patients whom they serve. Admission criteria, continuing stay criteria, and discharge criteria should be delineated for each program. Programs may include one or more of the following:

1. *Medically complex/postsurgical*: Patients in this program may require the following types of care:
   - active treatment of disease under direction of physician (administering intravenous medications, epidural medications, continuous infusion pumps, and hyperdermiclysis; monitoring/evaluating signs and symptoms of condition change; teaching care to patient and/or significant others; providing respiratory therapy and care; performing hemodialysis and peritoneal dialysis; evaluating

effective intervention through laboratory values, signs, and symptoms)
- postsurgical care (managing and evaluating drains and tubes; complex dressing changes; evaluating and assessing changes in wounds)
- pulmonary care (managing tracheotomized patients)
- nutrition management (enteral and parenteral feedings; monitoring the effect of intervention and therapeutic diets through weight, tissue turgor, wound healing, and laboratory values)

2. *Wound management*: Patients in this program may need complex treatment and dressing procedures; whirlpool treatment and debridement; electrical stimulation; specialty beds and pressure-reducing devices; frequent laboratory evaluation; teaching care to patient and/or significant others; ongoing assessment of the effective treatment by changes in wound status.

3. *Rehabilitation:* These patients typically have medical complications or frailties that preclude their ability to tolerate or benefit from acute rehabilitation services. Patients with orthopaedic conditions, strokes, degenerative neurological disorders, and other medical complexities may require the combination of subacute nursing care and a low-intensity rehabilitation program.

4. *Cardiopulmonary recovery/rehabilitation*: Patients in this program may have been hospitalized because of congestive heart failure or suspected myocardial infarction, or for cardiovascular surgical procedures. These patients typically are deconditioned as both cause and effect of acute treatment, possibly exacerbated by their stay in the intensive care unit or by their course of treatment resulting in malnourishment, weakness, frailty, and poor physical stamina. Patients also may have complicating comorbidities that require that the subacute services be provided in an environment that allows immediate access to the high-technology equipment and services of the acute hospital.

5. *Respiratory*: Patients for subacute care typically exhibit respiratory infections, pneumonias, or chronic obstructive pulmonary disorder (COPD) with medical complications. Some respiratory patients will be on ventilators and admitted to the subacute unit for weaning. These patients may receive intravenous antibiotics as well as rehabilitation in the subacute unit.

Clinical Staff

Clinical direction of a subacute program should be provided by a physician who is qualified by virtue of training and experience in the area(s) related to the program being offered. In addition to the medical program director, a medical staff of credentialed and privileged physicians should be created so that physicians may serve as either attending or consulting staff in the subacute unit or facility. A dedicated clinical staff for the subacute care unit or facility should report to a program director, who is responsible for the overall management of the subacute program. An interdisciplinary clinical team should include nursing, medical staff, social services, rehabilitation therapists, respiratory therapists, dietitians, pharmacists, and, as appropriate, psychologists and pastoral counselors.

Case Management

A case management system should involve appropriate coordination of care and allocation of resources, and an effective communication system with payers, families, physicians, and referral sources. The case management function usually is provided by a registered nurse. The objective of case management is to help the patient attain appropriate goals by the most cost-effective means. Case management is discussed further in Chapter 17.

Outcome Measurement System

An outcome measurement system should include an ongoing, organized, and systematic method of evaluating the results of interventions and services relative to patient and family goals and expectations. The outcomes to be achieved in a subacute program include the resolution of medical problems and functional improvement. A key outcome for subacute care is the reduction of rehospitalizations as well as reduced risk of utilization of health care services, following discharge from subacute care. (See Part XI for further discussion of outcomes measurement.)

Cost-Effective, Quality Care

The subacute program should incorporate admissions procedures that are as simple as possible, given the need to comply with regulatory requirements. Throughout the subacute care program, the focus should be on achieving optimal results in a reasonable time period so that the patient can be discharged home or to a less costly level of care. Operations should support patient and family dignity, realistic goal setting, and early preparation and planning for discharge.

CONCLUSION

The subacute industry has rapidly evolved into a recognized niche within health care. Its continued growth will be dependent on a clear demonstration of the cost-saving potential of moving patients out of higher-cost acute care hospitals and into lower-cost subacute care units and facilities, and of patient outcomes that confirm that subacute program treatment interventions have positive long-term effects. With the growth of managed care, cost-effective, high-quality subacute levels of care will continue to be important components in the continuum of health care.

REFERENCES

1. Ting HM. *Subacute Care: Analysis of the Market Opportunities and Competition.* Newport Beach, CA: Center for Consumer Healthcare Information; 1995.
2. Prospective Payment Assessment Commission. *Medicare and the American Healthcare System, Report to Congress.* Washington, DC: Prospective Payment Assessment Commission; 1997.
3. McDowell TN. An overview of provider reimbursement: Medicare, Medicaid, and managed care. In: Griffin KM, ed. *Handbook of Subacute Health Care.* Gaithersburg, MD: Aspen Publishers, Inc; 1995: 39–58.
4. Joint Commission on Accreditation of Healthcare Organizations. *1996 Accreditation Protocol for Subacute Programs.* Oakbrook Terrace, IL: Joint Commission on Accreditation of Healthcare Organizations; 1996.
5. Commission on Accreditation of Rehabilitation Facilities. *1997 Standards Manual and Interpretive Guidelines for Medical Rehabilitation.* Tucson, AZ: Commission on Accreditation of Rehabilitation Facilities; 1997.

KATHLEEN M. GRIFFIN, PHD, is national director of postacute and senior services, Health Dimensions Consulting Group, a member organization of the Benedictine Health System. Dr. Griffin is recognized as a pioneer in developing and operating successful subacute and rehabilitation facilities as components of integrated health systems. She is the editor of two textbooks on health care and aging, and is a nationally recognized author and lecturer on post–acute care and senior services. Dr. Griffin was founding chairman of the board of the National Subacute Care Association.

Chapter 24

Hospice Care in the United States: Issues and Emerging Trends

Anne C. Dye, Peggy H. Rodebush, and Geri Hempel

Chapter Outline

- Hospice Overview
- Financing and Reimbursement
- Size of the Hospice Industry in the United States
- Major Policy Issues
- Program Development
- Budget Development
- Future Integration and Affiliation Strategies

HOSPICE OVERVIEW

Hospice Philosophy

As defined by Flexner, hospice is a "medically directed, nurse coordinated program providing a continuum of home and inpatient care for the terminally ill patient and family. It employs an interdisciplinary team acting under the direction of an autonomous hospice administrator."[1] It is also a philosophy of care that accepts death as a natural part of life, seeking neither to hasten nor prolong the dying process, and existing solely to support the terminally ill person and family through the last stages of life. The primary objective of hospice is to provide supportive care and counseling to the dying patient and family. The clinical goals of hospice are palliative care oriented, with pain management and symptom control, not curative therapy, as the primary focus of treatment.

Senator James Randolph, in establishing National Hospice Week (SR 170, March 18, 1982), described hospice well. He stated, "Hospice is a place, people, and a philosophy. It is a system of care that seeks to restore dignity and a sense of personal fulfillment to the dying. The focus is on the patient and the family, rather than on the disease—and the aim is not to extend life, but to improve the quality of life that remains."

The first hospice in the United States opened its doors in 1974. It began as a grassroots reaction to the depersonalization of care and treatment for the dying patient. Early supporters of hospice recognized a need to isolate the terminally ill patient from the treatment-based philosophy of the acute care setting. Today hospice has developed into an integral component of the health care continuum.

The majority of hospices in the United States today are designed to provide care in patients' homes. Although services may be provided in a variety of settings and facilities, the home setting is a main component of the hospice philosophy. Providing care in this nontraditional setting also helps to contain the costs of care. Care for a terminally ill patient in the hospital setting is expensive, and hospice provides a cost-effective alternative to the high-technology, labor-intensive acute care setting.

Factors Influencing Growth of Hospice in the United States

During the last 50 years, modern medicine has made tremendous strides in the treatment of disease. As a result of this and other factors, the population in the United States has increased fairly rapidly. The number of older adults in particular has increased at a tremendous rate. In fact, the population aged 65 and over is expected to increase by 35% by the year 2015 (Figure 24–1). These demographic changes in the population, combined with a growing awareness of cancer and other terminal illnesses, issues surrounding cost containment in health care, an increasing need for individuals to take control over their own health care, and the changing views of death and euthanasia have influenced the hospice movement in the last 10 years.

Structure and Organization of Hospice

Hospices in the United States come in all shapes, sizes, and reimbursement models. Programs are located in office buildings, physician offices, and even churches. These programs may have contractual arrangements with other facilities to provide inpatient care. They may be freestanding with their own inpatient unit or may be affiliated with a hospital or an extended care facility. A program may be for profit or not-for-profit. Currently, in the United States, most hospices are not-for-profit. The staffing model may be all paid staff, a combination of paid staff and volunteers, or all volunteer. An all-volunteer model works cooperatively with agencies and other programs to provide the necessary services.

Regardless of the structure of the hospice, standards have been established by both regulatory agencies and the National Hospice Organization (NHO) that serve as the guiding principles for care of patients and families. These standards include requirements that care be available 7 days a week, 24 hours per day, with integrated inpatient and home care services available. Volunteers are used to assist with the patient and family during both the dying process and the bereavement process. An interdisciplinary team guided by a medical director plans and provides the care. The family members and

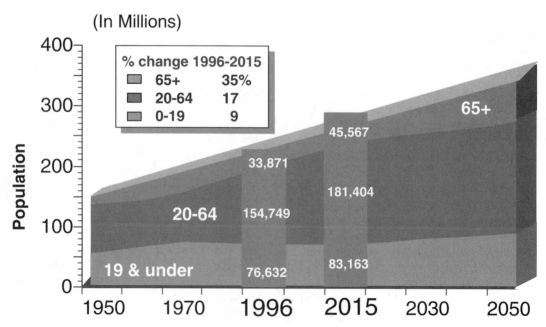

Figure 24–1 Elderly Population Is Growing Fastest. *Source:* Reprinted from U.S. Bureau of the Census, 1996.

anyone important to the patient participate in hospice care, working closely to support the patient during the final days.

FINANCING AND REIMBURSEMENT

Medical Coverage for Hospice Services

Hospice care is financed through several mechanisms: Medicare, Medicaid, private insurance, private pay, donations, and grants (Figure 24–2). While reimbursement for hospice services increased dramatically in recent years, Medicare remained the primary payer, representing 68% of hospice revenues, or $1.2 billion in 1994.[2] Medicaid hospice expenditures grew as well, totaling $197.6 million in fiscal year 1994, an increase of 53% over the $128.9 million spent in fiscal year 1993.[3]

The Medicare Benefit

The Medicare hospice benefit is available under Part A of Medicare. Medicare reimburses Medicare-certified hospices on a per diem basis by level of care, including routine home care, inpatient care for acute symptom management, continuous care, and respite services for durations of not longer than 5 days per episode. Persons electing hospice must have a terminal diagnosis with a life expectancy of 6 months or less, as certified by a physician. Care is provided in a variety of settings, including inpatient and at home.

Persons electing to use their hospice benefits under Medicare must select this benefit in lieu of traditional Medicare reimbursement for all treatments related to their terminal illness. Services provided include skilled nursing, physician services, home health aides, social workers, home medical equipment, palliative medications, laboratory testing, volunteer services, and bereavement counseling. These services are available 24 hours a day.

Managed Care

The key factors affecting hospice's success within a managed care environment include demonstration of quality, evidence of cost-effectiveness, and willingness to share financial risk.[4] Providers are developing strategies to address these factors, as increasing numbers of hospice programs have begun to compete for managed care contracts. For example, in Baltimore, Mary-

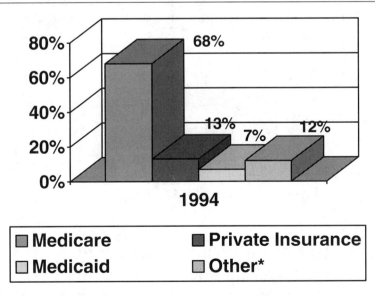

*Other denotes donations, grants, and private pay.

Figure 24–2 1994 Hospice Revenues by Payer. *Source:* Data from National Hospice Organization Fact Sheet, 1996.

land, hospice services for acquired immune deficiency syndrome (AIDS) patients covered by Medicaid are included in an AIDS care capitation program designed by Johns Hopkins AIDS Service, Johns Hopkins HealthCare LLC, the Maryland Department of Health and Mental Hygiene, and health maintenance organizations (HMOs) in Maryland.[5]

Eighty-two percent of managed care plans offered hospice services as part of their benefit package in 1993.[6] Managed care organizations (MCOs), such as Kaiser Permanente and Group Health Cooperative, continue to recognize the value of hospice and operate their own hospice programs that serve Medicare, Medicaid, and private clients. However, there is little information published on the managed care dollars spent providing hospice services. Additionally, hospice is still a carve-out for Medicare HMOs, and patients have to disenroll from Medicaid HMOs to receive Medicaid hospice benefits.

SIZE OF THE HOSPICE INDUSTRY IN THE UNITED STATES

Agency Characteristics

In 1995, the overall revenues for the hospice market were estimated at $2.8 billion, with Medicare revenues at about 68%, or $1.9 billion (unpublished data, AC Dye, Ernst & Young, 1997). According to the NHO, there were approximately 2,800 operational or planned hospice programs in all 50 states and Puerto Rico as of June 1996. HCFA reported that 1,857 Medicare-certified hospice programs provided hospice services to 309,336 Medicare patients in 1995.[7] The average length of stay for these patients was 59 days. Home health agency–based hospices made up 37% of the hospice market, while not-for-profit hospices represented 72% of the hospice industry (Figure 24–3).

Patient Information

In 1995, approximately one out of every seven individuals who died (14%) in the United States from all causes (not just terminal illness) received care from a hospice program.[2] HCFA statistics show that hospice patients are more likely to be older, married, and living with their spouse.[8] The most prevalent diagnoses at admission were related to cancer (71%), diseases of the heart and circulatory system (9%), and respiratory conditions (6%).[8] The number of hospice patients is expected to more than double between 1990 and 2000 (Figure 24–4).

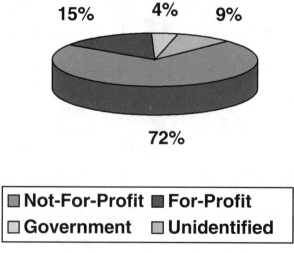

Figure 24–3 1995 Ownership Status of Hospice Programs. *Source:* Data from National Hospice Organization, 1996.

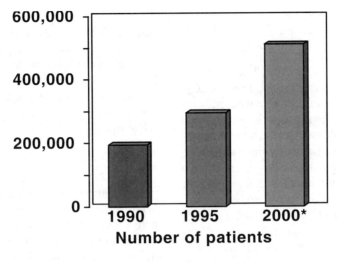

*Projections

Figure 24–4 Hospice Patient Growth: 1990–2000. Data from The Hospice Market, FIND/SVP, 1996.

Still, too few terminally ill persons receive care from hospice services. According to the Hospice Association of America, patients who received care other than hospice often died in the hospital instead of in the comfort of their own homes. Just 13% of hospice patients were admitted to the hospital in the second month prior to their death, compared to 41% admitted from other care providers during the same period of time.[9]

Growth Projections

The number of Medicare-certified hospices more than doubled between 1990 and 1995, largely as a result of the 1989 congressional mandate to increase reimbursement rates by 20% (Figure 24–5). The provider that emerged with clear market dominance was VITAS Healthcare Corporation. Fiscal year 1995 revenues for VITAS were $231 million, just over 8% of the US hospice market. It is expected that, with the aging of the "baby boomer" population and the increasing acceptance of hospice as a home- and community-based care treatment modality for the terminally ill, the number of hospice programs will increase rapidly. The House Ways and Means Committee projects an average annual growth rate for hospice at 25% through the year 2000.[10]

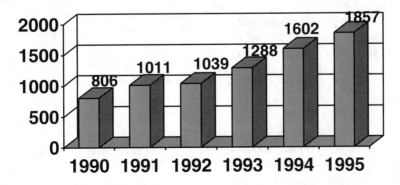

Figure 24–5 Medicare-Certified Hospice Growth by Year (1990–1995). *Source:* Reprinted from Bureau of Policy Development, Health Care Financing Administration, 1995.

MAJOR POLICY ISSUES

Ethics

Hospice began as a philosophy of care inspired by volunteer activity. As a philosophy, hospice is straightforward. It accepts death's inevitability and seeks to support the dying person and his or her family and friends through a coordinated effort of palliative symptom control, counseling, and support. Challenges arise when this philosophy is translated into a program of care that receives third-party reimbursement. The hospice must justify the terminal diagnosis of the population served, provide care and services at a lower cost than most programs oriented toward cure, and be responsible for providing many nontraditional services, such as bereavement counseling.

Any health care program that limits resources and aims to serve a select group of people must provide justification for the allocation of benefits. Traditionally, the allocation of benefits has been the responsibility of the government, third-party payers, or charities and not the responsibility of the provider. The Medicare regulations established for hospice have set criteria that the hospice must observe for patient selection and restriction of treatment modalities. However, it is the providers' responsibility to define which services a patient receives and which resources are used in caring for him or her.

By its very nature, hospice has the potential to be a target for ethical and moral dilemmas. The NHO has issued a code of ethics to guide the staff of hospice and palliative care programs through issues such as physician-assisted suicide, confidentiality, removal of artificial nutrition and hydration, and pain control.[11] In order to address these issues, hospices should support the development of internal ethics committees. Ethics committees are a key component in any health care organization and can assist in establishing baseline criteria regarding organizational policy for service provision, patient population, questions regarding suicide and assisted suicide, responsibility for resource conservation and allocation, and responsibility of care for those patients who do not qualify for services. As consumers of health care become more educated regarding the hospice philosophy and hospices develop a major role in the health care continuum, hospice ethics committees will play a vital role in how the medical community provides comfortable, compassionate, and palliative care to the terminally ill.

Legal Issues

In recent years, health care providers have been faced with a growing awareness and concern regarding the legal and regulatory issues surrounding the industry. Hospice providers may be at a particular disadvantage because of the type of care they provide. Legal issues may arise from a variety of areas, including, but not limited to, malpractice, wrongful death, negligence, and nontreatment. Believing that a hospice provides a valuable service does not necessarily protect it from potential legal issues. A successful hospice needs to understand the situations that could lead to litigation and have safeguards developed to minimize exposure to liability.

One of the most important safeguards a hospice can have to reduce its exposure to legal issues is a quality improvement program. Properly implemented, a quality improvement program will provide the hospice with tools for continuous improvement throughout the organization, thus reducing potential liability issues. Equally important is a risk management program. This program is a formal process designed to reduce liability exposure and foster an awareness within the organization regarding legal liabilities. While risk management programs must be tailored to individual organizations, several basic elements should be included:

- continuing review of insurance to determine adequacy of coverage
- ongoing review of the physical premises and equipment to discover and correct defects
- ongoing personnel performance appraisal review and revision of hospice policies so

that those policies reflect adequate quality of care measures
- maintenance of systems for investigating adverse incidents to prepare a defense and to develop procedures for avoiding future occurrences
- support of patient–family grievance procedures to handle complaints, solve problems, and prevent litigation[12]

Care Provision

The advent of Medicare certification in 1983 created extensive requirements to which hospice programs must comply to be eligible for federal reimbursement. Currently, Medicare requires hospice to be responsible for providing certain core services utilizing employees. These services include skilled nursing, social work, and counseling. Noncore services may be provided by contract employees and include physician services, home care aide/homemaker services, physical therapy, speech therapy, occupational therapy, volunteer services, and bereavement counseling. Additionally, the hospice is required to provide all medications, laboratory work, medical equipment, and supplies that relate to the terminal diagnosis.

While the Medicare program dictates the scope of services to be provided, the hospice defines how and to what extent services will be provided. Following an in-depth admission process, the hospice admits the patient into the program. Next, during an interdisciplinary team conference, a plan of care is established outlining the services the patient will receive. The care plan is then modified based on the patient's needs throughout the course of care. Services may be provided in the home or in an inpatient setting.

The hospice recognizes the special needs of the terminally ill patient, and all programs and services are developed to meet those needs. Although hospices may differ in how the services are provided, there are certain fundamental guidelines in developing the care delivery model. The following guidelines distinguish hospice from other programs. Hospice care is

- exclusively for the terminally ill
- focused on the patient and family
- provided to the family through the bereavement period
- provided by an interdisciplinary team
- medically directed
- available 24 hours a day, 7 days a week
- a service that uses volunteers as an integral part of the program

PROGRAM DEVELOPMENT

Service Models

Hospices may be licensed in several ways, depending on the affiliation of the provider. It is important to model potential cost report and other financial implications before choosing the licensure category for newly licensed programs. Additionally, there are criteria that must be satisfied for each licensure classification. The Government Accounting Office classifies hospice providers into the types discussed below.

Freestanding

The freestanding hospice is a separate, distinct facility providing both inpatient and home hospice services. Inpatient services may be provided by the hospice or contracted with a local hospital or nursing home. The start-up costs for a freestanding hospice and the continued operating expenses require aggressive financial planning.

Hospital Based

Hospital-based hospice programs are a distinct unit of a hospital that provides inpatient hospice services, also known as the palliative care unit. The program may provide home hospice services through its own hospital-based hospice or through a contracted arrangement with a freestanding program. The hospital unit generally requires remodeling of the physical plant to adapt to the hospice concept. A hospital-based program may have less autonomy than a freestanding program. However, it does have increased access to hospital resources and the medical community. The hospital-based hospice is guided by the governing board of the hospital, and the mission and philosophy of the hospice are generally those of the hospital.

Reimbursement is generally provided through the Medicare hospice benefit and other third-party payers. Due to the hospital affiliation, there may be an enhanced opportunity for inclusion of the hospice in managed care contracts.

Hospice Affiliated with an Extended Care or Skilled Nursing Facility

In this situation, the hospice program is a distinct part of a skilled nursing facility (SNF) or an extended care facility (ECF). Home hospice arrangements are generally provided through a community-based or a facility-based hospice. Many patients in a nursing home have a terminal illness, and the hospice provides the opportunity for the patient and family to take advantage of additional services. The hospice improves the continuity of care offered to the nursing home patient.

The mission and philosophy of the hospice complement that of the ECF or SNF. The hospice is governed by the facility board. Reimbursement is provided through the traditional Medicare hospice benefit and some limited third-party payers. A facility-based hospice may have some opportunities for recruitment of staff and volunteers depending on the community reputation of the facility.

Hospital-Based Hospice Home Care

This type of hospice is a hospital-based home health agency that provides hospice services. Inpatient services are provided either through the hospital's separate and distinct part or through a contracted arrangement with an ECF or SNF.

In this arrangement, the mission and philosophy of the hospice complement those of the home health agency and the hospital. The hospice may function as a semiautonomous program of the home health agency. If the inpatient unit is with the hospital, continuity of care is enhanced through the availability of the various programs. This arrangement provides patients with the opportunity to transfer among programs with little impact on patients. There is the potential, however, for home care and hospice programs to compete for referrals with common hospice diagnoses such as cancer, and to question when to refer patients from curative treatments in home care to more palliative hospice programs.

Reimbursement is provided through the Medicare hospice benefit and other third-party payers. The hospital-based hospice has an improved opportunity to obtain other third-party contracts due to the affiliation with the home health agency and the hospital.

Community-Based Home Health Agency Hospice

Part of a community-based home health agency, this type of hospice requires an agreement with a facility to provide inpatient services. The mission and philosophy of the hospice complement that of the home health agency, and the governing board of the agency provides the direction for the hospice. The hospice could function as a semiautonomous program that enhances the services offered through the home health agency. The home health–based hospice can provide services to a patient through a terminal care program of the home health agency prior to admitting the patient to the hospice. Reimbursement of the hospice is generally through the Medicare hospice benefit and other third-party payers.

Prior to determining the hospice licensure category suited for an organization, careful planning must occur. There are specific advantages and disadvantages to each model. The community or organization must address all planning issues prior to determining which hospice is best suited for them.

BUDGET DEVELOPMENT

The budget structure for hospice is unlike many other levels of care, primarily because reimbursement is both per diem and all inclusive of services provided for the terminal illness. There are similarities as well, such as the direct costs: employee salaries and fringe benefits, transportation, equipment, and supplies. Indirect costs include public relations, fundraising activities, volunteer recruitment and training, staff education, and space considerations. Key statistics to include when developing the budget for a hospice include the following:

- Average daily census: The number of patients that the hospice will care for on a daily basis.
- Average length of stay (ALOS): The average number of days a patient will stay on service. The most expensive time during the course of care for a hospice patient is during the admission process and when the patient is actively dying. If patients are admitted to service late in the course of illness, the costs to the hospice will be high. Also, if patients are admitted for a short period of time, the true value of the hospice for the patient and the family is not recognized.
- Payer mix: The Medicare hospice option pays a per diem rate. The average daily home rate is approximately $96. Many managed care companies may pay a per diem rate or break out the services.
- Staffing ratios: A critical component of determining the staffing ratio is the ALOS and the level of care needs of the patient. If a hospice's ALOS is less than 30 days, the level of care is greater and therefore the staffing needs will be higher than those for a hospice whose ALOS is greater than 60 days. Patients referred to the hospice who are close to death require more visits and services than patients who stay on the program longer. The NHO indicated that for programs with an ALOS of 60 days, approximately 34.5 visits are made. They were distributed as shown in Figure 24–6. The NHO recommends the staffing plan shown in Table 24–1.
- Expenses per patient per day for major costs: The hospice is required to provide all supplies, equipment, drugs, and treatments directly related to the terminal diagnosis. To accurately determine the cost of operating the hospice, the cost of medical supplies, equipment, drugs, and treatment must be monitored.
- Staffing productivity: The hospice is reimbursed at a per diem rate. However, it is still critical for the hospice to monitor the productivity of its field staff. Productivity standards are shown in Table 24–2.

Once the budget is developed, reimbursement can be projected. For most patients over 65, the Medicare hospice per diem rates by level of care can be utilized. The hospice should also evaluate various insurance and managed care contracts to determine the benefits provided.

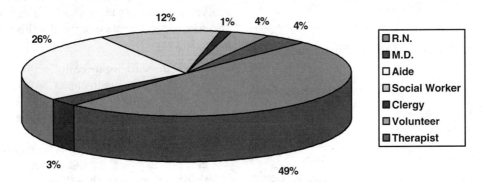

Figure 24–6 Distribution of Hospice Provider Visits. *Source:* Data from National Hospice Organization.

Table 24–1 Hospice Staffing Recommendations

Discipline	Daily Census	FTEs*
Registered nurse	8–12	1
Social worker	20–30	1
Chaplain	40–60	1
Home health aide	12–15	1
Volunteer coordinator	60–80	1

*FTE = Full-time equivalent

Source: Data from National Hospice Organization.

Specialty Programs

Hospice care continues to be a relatively new field of practice in our health care system. There are many innovative hospice programs that serve the terminally ill in unique and caring ways.

Zen Hospice Project Residence Program

This program operates a four-bed hospice residence. The primary goal of the project is to provide care and support to patients with terminal illnesses in a homelike setting. The residence is a restored Victorian home with high ceilings, fireplaces, and a patio/garden. Services are available to people with AIDS, cancer, and other life-threatening illnesses. Family and friends are encouraged to visit and actively participate in the patient's care. Medical services are provided 24 hours per day, 7 days per week, through a collaboration with Visiting Nurses and Hospice, a program of California Pacific Medical Center.

Table 24–2 Hospice Provider Productivity Standards

Discipline	Average Visits per Day
Registered nurse	3.7
Practical nurse	4.2
Social worker	2.5
Home health aide	4.5

Source: Data from National Association for Home Care, 1995.

Pediatric Hospice Programs

The death of a parent or a loved one is devastating. However, nothing is more traumatic for a family than the loss of a child. Pediatric hospices are being developed nationwide to provide support and services to this special population. The family of a pediatric patient may be more likely to use the services of a pediatric hospice during both the dying process and the bereavement process. These hospices are designed especially to provide the necessary support and services.

FUTURE INTEGRATION AND AFFILIATION STRATEGIES

The trend towards utilization of hospice care services has experienced tremendous growth over the last 10 years, primarily as a result of the implementation of the acute care prospective payment system in 1982 and the move to increase Medicare hospice reimbursement rates in 1989. Concern about escalating costs and overutilization of services has shaped current reimbursement trends, in both the governmental and private sectors. Accordingly, the market is beginning to change dramatically as network and provider consolidation continues, and strategic integration and affiliation trends accelerate. The next 5 years will see a dramatically changed business and health care environment within the post–acute care industry. The key challenge for hospice care providers will be to develop and implement effective strategies to address these changing factors in an environment increasingly dominated by managed care:

- Medicare shift from fee-for-service prospective pay reimbursement structures to Medicare HMO products
- selective managed care contracting strategies
- vertical integration strategies for post–acute care providers (eg, nursing homes, rehabilitation centers, home health, and hospice as integrated service lines)

- need for disease management product line development
- strong information technologies that bridge service lines

It is clear that hospice will continue to provide needed care to the terminally ill and that it will remain an important service to individuals and families, including those in managed care programs. It is equally clear that it will become more integrated with other modalities of care, and that the need for hospice will increase for the foreseeable future.

REFERENCES

1. Flexner JR. The hospice movement in North America—is it coming of age? *South Med J.* 1979;72:248–250.
2. National Hospice Organization. *Fact Sheet.* Arlington, VA: National Hospice Organization; 1996.
3. Hospice Association of America. *Hospice Facts and Statistics.* Washington, DC: Hospice Association of America; 1996.
4. Michal M. Managed care: the characteristics of a successful hospice. http://www.rbvdnr.com; accessed October 1997.
5. Kusinitz M. Johns Hopkins to announce AIDS capitated care program. http://hopkins.med.jhu.edu/newsmedia/press/1997/january/1997.htm; accessed January 1997.
6. Lewin-VHI, Inc. *Hospice Care: An Introduction and Review of the Evidence.* Arlington, VA: National Hospice Organization; 1994.
7. Beebe K. *Hospice State Summary.* Washington, DC: Health Care Financing Administration, Bureau of Data Management and Strategy, Office of Health Care Information Systems; 1996.
8. National Center for Health Statistics. *An Overview of Home Health and Hospice Care Patients: Preliminary Data from the 1993 National Home and Hospice Care Survey; Advance Data from the Vital and Health Statistics of the Centers for Disease Control and Prevention.* Publication No. 256. Washington, DC: National Center for Health Statistics; 1994.
9. Lemkin P. Hospice: can it work within managed care? *Caring.* August 1997:22–28.
10. House Ways and Means Committee. *1996 Green Book.* Washington, DC: House Ways and Means Committee; 1997.
11. American Health Consultants. Tips for deciding about a hospice ethics committee. *The 1996 Hospice Manager's Resource Bank.* New York: American Health Consultants; 1997.
12. Richards M. *Medical Risk Management: A Preventive Legal Strategy.* Rockville, MD: Aspen Systems; 1982.

ANNE C. DYE, MHSA, is a senior consultant in Ernst & Young's South/West Region Post Acute Health Care Consulting professional services practice. She holds a Master's degree in health services administration from George Washington University and has over 13 years of operational, marketing, and business development experience in health care, including ambulatory, home health, hospice, and long-term care. Ms. Dye has been director of business operations for the nation's largest hospice company with responsibility for strategic planning, nonclinical operations fiscal management, budget preparation and maintenance, service line development, and new site development.

PEGGY H. RODEBUSH, RN, MSN, is a senior manager in Ernst & Young's health care business transformation service line. In this role, she works with leading health care and home health clients across the United States. She is a nationally recognized post–acute care and medical management expert and is a frequent speaker at national conventions.

GERI HEMPEL is a manager for Ernst & Young in Tampa, Florida.

PART IX

Ancillary Services

Ancillary services include diagnostic and therapeutic services outside of the acute care setting delivered by nonphysicians on the orders of physicians. A special form of ancillary service is pharmacy. Traditional ancillary services are best managed in the traditional ways (traditional for managed care) that are discussed here, but pharmacy is unique. Drug benefits costs are significantly higher than other forms of ancillary services, and they are difficult to manage well. For this reason, as well as because of the connection between pharmaceutical services and other forms of care management, this topic must be discussed on its own.

Chapter 25

Ancillary Diagnostic and Therapeutic Services

Peter R. Kongstvedt

Chapter Outline

- Introduction
- Ancillary Services
- Physician-Owned Ancillary Services
- Data Capture
- Financial Incentives
- Feedback
- Control Points
- Contracting and Reimbursement for Ancillary Services
- Conclusion

INTRODUCTION

This chapter addresses those medical services that are generally considered ancillary services by most managed care plans. These services are provided as an adjunct to basic primary or specialty services and include most everything other than institutional services (although institutions can provide ancillary services).

Parts of this chapter are adapted from PR Kongstvedt, Managing Utilization of Ancillary and Emergency Services, in *The Managed Health Care Handbook*, 3rd ed, PR Kongstvedt, ed, pp 330–340, © 1996, Aspen Publishers, Inc.

ANCILLARY SERVICES

Ancillary services are divided into diagnostic and therapeutic services. Examples of ancillary diagnostic services include laboratory, radiology, nuclear testing, computed tomography (CT), magnetic resonance imaging (MRI), electroencephalograms (EEGs), electrocardiography, cardiac testing (including plain and nuclear stress testing, other cardiac nuclear imaging, invasive imaging, echocardiography, and Holter monitoring), and so forth. Examples of ancillary therapeutic services include cardiac rehabilitation, noncardiac rehabilitation, physical therapy (PT), occupational therapy (OT), speech therapy, and so forth.

Pharmacy services are a special form of ancillary services that account for a significant measure of cost and have been subject to tremendous inflation. This topic is discussed in detail in Chapter 26. Mental health and substance abuse services may also be considered ancillary from a health plan's standpoint, but they are really core services, albeit discretely defined. Those services are discussed in Chapter 32.

Ancillary services are unique in that they are rarely sought out by the patient without a referral by a physician. For example, it is certainly possible that an individual could self-refer to a rehabilitation center, but it is likely that the center would require a referral from a physician before accepting the individual into the program. Diagnostic studies almost universally require physician referral. One exception is the free-standing diagnostic center that has medical staff whose sole purpose is to guide a patient through the diagnostic work-up that the patient seeks (eg, a free-standing cardiac testing center whose advertisements appeal to people who want those tests done). Because those types of centers are out of a plan's control, as are freestanding urgent/convenience care centers, the only real way to control them is economic. If those centers do not have a contract with the plan, or if the plan requires authorization from a contracted physician to pay in full, then the plan does not have to pay such freestanding centers. In the case of a health maintenance organization (HMO), the plan does not have to pay at all. For a preferred provider organization (PPO), a point-of-service (POS) plan, or a managed indemnity plan, the plan may or may not have a partial payment liability, depending on the service agreement and schedule of benefits.

Because most ancillary services require an order from a physician, it is logical that control of such services is dependent on changing the utilization patterns of physicians. As discussed below, the other primary method of controlling costs of ancillary services is to contract for such services in such a way as to make costs predictable. Even with favorable contracts, however, controlling utilization of ancillary services by physicians remains an essential ingredient to long-term cost control.

PHYSICIAN-OWNED ANCILLARY SERVICES

There is compelling evidence that physician ownership of diagnostic or therapeutic equipment or services, whether owned individually or through joint ventures or partnerships, can lead to significant increases in utilization of those services. There are several studies that have documented this phenomenon in diagnostic imaging,[1] laboratory services,[2] and a remarkably wide range of other services.[3] Physician self-referral is now restricted by the Health Care Financing Administration (HCFA) for Medicare services,[4] and many private plans have followed suit, especially if they are enrolling public sector (ie, Medicare or Medicaid) members.

Actually tracing ownership or fiduciary relationships is not always easy to do. The ancillary services may have a completely separate provider name and tax identification number, may have a separate billing address (perhaps not even in the same geographic area), and may otherwise appear to be an independent vendor. Tracking unusually high rates of referral to a given provider of ancillary services (see Chapter 38) may be the only clue to such potential utilization abuse. Many plans are also clearly prohibiting physician self-referral in their provider contracts (unless expressly allowed by the plan) and are requiring the physicians to disclose any fiduciary relationship with such providers.

However, it is neither practical nor desirable to place too heavy a restriction on physicians' abilities to use appropriate services or equipment that they own in order to deliver routine care within their specialty. For example, orthopaedists cannot properly care for their patients if they cannot obtain radiographs. In some cases, a physician may be the only available provider of a given service (eg, in a rural area). In other cases, it may actually be more cost-effective to allow physicians to use their own facility. The point here is that physician-owned services must not be allowed to become a lucrative profit center, one that is subject to abuse.

Managed care plans deal with this issue in a number of ways. One method is to have an outright ban on self-referral other than for carefully designated services. For example, a cardiologist may be allowed to perform in-office exercise tolerance testing but be prohibited from referring to a freestanding cardiac diagnostic center in which he or she has a fiduciary relationship. Another method is to reimburse for such physician self-referred services at a low margin (not so low as to cause the physician to lose money but low enough to prevent any profit) or to include it in the capitation payment. The last common method is to contract for all ancillary services through a very limited network of providers and require the physicians and members to use only those contracted providers for ancillary services; this is discussed later in this chapter.

The advent of integrated delivery systems (IDSs) has complicated this issue somewhat. It is not always clear if the ancillary services are owned by the physician or the IDS, and, in any event, those services may be included in an all-encompassing global capitation rate. However, the regulatory environment is changing in this arena, which is particularly important for those MCOs that are contracting for public sector business (Medicare and Medicaid).

DATA CAPTURE

The ability to manage utilization of ancillary services will be directly related to an organization's ability to capture accurate and timely data (see Chapters 37 and 38). If you have a tight authorization system (see Chapter 20), you may get prospective data. If your claims management system is capable, you should be able to get retrospective data. If you have no way to capture data regarding ancillary services, you will have great difficulty controlling utilization. Lack of data will also make contracting problematic because no vendor will be willing to contract aggressively without having some idea of projected utilization (at least not on terms that will be beneficial to the plan or medical group responsible for the cost).

Data elements that you need to capture include who ordered the service (this is sometimes different than the physician of record; for example, a member may have signed up with a primary care physician [PCP] but a referral physician ordered the tests), what was ordered, what is being paid for (in other words, are you paying for more than was ordered?), and how much it is costing.

The ability to look at patterns of usage in ancillary services is quite valuable. For example, it would be useful to know that of 10 family practitioners there is 1 who routinely orders twice as many radiographs as are ordered by the other 9. There may be a perfectly good reason for this, but you will never know unless you can identify that pattern and look for the reasons.

FINANCIAL INCENTIVES

Ancillary services utilization is commonly incorporated into primary care reimbursement systems that are performance based (eg, capitation or performance-based fee for service). In one study, capitation with risk sharing, combined with education and feedback (see below) led to a clear reduction in the use of ambulatory testing, while having no adverse impact on outcomes.[5] (The topic of financial incentives is discussed in *The Managed Health Care Handbook*, 3rd Edition, and is beyond the scope of this text.)

FEEDBACK

The issue of monetary gain leading to excessive use of ancillary services has been discussed earlier in this chapter, but there are a number of nonmonetary causes of excessive testing: the quest for diagnostic certainty, peer pressure, convenience, patient demands, and fear of malpractice claims.[6]

There is evidence that physicians will modify their use of ancillary services when given feedback on their performance. Simple feedback regarding test ordering behavior has led to modest reductions in use.[7] This response has been confirmed for simple feedback, and somewhat greater decreases have been seen when feedback was combined with other written guidelines or peer review.[8,9]

Feedback to physicians regarding their use of ancillary services is therefore a worthwhile endeavor. Feedback should include comparisons to their peers and should be properly adjusted for factors that affect utilization (eg, age and sex of patients, specialty type, and the like). Feedback should also contain adequate data to allow a physician to know where performance may be improved. See Chapters 38 and 39 for further discussion about using reports and practice profiling.

CONTROL POINTS

Irrespective of physician self-regulation of the use of ancillary services, many plans apply additional controls over ancillary utilization. The most common of these are briefly discussed below.

Indications for Use

The first control point to discuss is indications for use of services. This is not an easy means of controlling ancillary services, but it has the potential of producing the best control and fostering high quality. In essence, this means using standards of care. Like protocols and clinical pathways (see Chapter 18 and Part X), standards of care outline the events and thought processes that should occur before physicians refer for ancillary or consultant services.

Standards of care are especially useful in certain types of services. Theoretically, one could develop standards of care for virtually any service, but because review of such standards is time consuming, it is not worthwhile in all cases. For example, unless a plan is experiencing a tremendous cost overrun connected with urinalyses, there will be no marginal benefits to developing a protocol for when a urinalysis is required and when a urine dip test will do.

Cardiac testing is another matter. Cardiac testing, particularly stress testing and imaging, is quite expensive and highly common. Indications for cardiac testing have been published in medical journals, and texts and algorithms are available, but the ordering of cardiac testing sometimes defies rationality. As mentioned earlier in this chapter, some physicians may use a scattershot approach, ordering tests simply to try to uncover some piece of information. Concentration on this service via chart reviews for appropriateness may yield interesting results and give an organization direction in developing standards for ordering.

There are now multiple sources for clinical protocols. In the example of cardiac testing, a reasonable approach is to enlist several highly respected cardiologists to use published protocols as a beginning, and then tailor the algorithms, protocols, or standards rather than simply impose the protocol without input from plan physicians. A well-reasoned, well-researched, and well-presented approach to cardiac disease will benefit the patient and result in lower costs.

The problem with using standards of care is that it exposes you to charges of practicing cookbook medicine. If you are imposing arbitrary requirements on physicians, that charge may be true. If, however, you are using the best and latest in medical intelligence as well as respected journals and experts to develop the standards, then you are simply expecting high-quality medical practice and thoughtful care of the patient. Some plans have found that adherence to good protocols has such a beneficial effect that those plans require specialists to agree to follow such protocols and guidelines as a condition of the specialists' participation in the health plan.[10]

Test of Reasonableness

If you do not have standards developed, or if you choose not to do so, there are still other approaches. The first is a continual test of reasonableness: Will the test or therapy help? In other words, will the test provide a piece of information that will have an effect on the care of the patient, or at least on the diagnosis or prognosis? In too many cases, tests are ordered only because they have always been ordered. A good example of that is the routine admission chest radiograph. Despite multiple articles in the medical literature,[11–13] admission chest radiographs get ordered for many people who do not need them. The same issue may apply to many other routine studies (eg, preoperative electrocardiograms[14] or laboratory screening[15] for otherwise healthy patients).

Another example is long-term PT for patients who no longer show improvement but who continually complain to their physician. For example, a patient may complain of lower back pain, and a diagnostic work-up has yielded a negative result. The patient may not be losing weight or exercising as instructed but is still demanding that something be done. The physician orders PT because it is easy to do and because the patient likes the attention. This is clearly not cost-effective, but it happens.

Limits on Authority To Authorize

Limiting the authority to authorize ancillary services will also help control their use. An HMO can limit the authority to authorize services to the PCP only. In that case, a consultant must discuss the case with the PCP, and the PCP must actually order the test or therapy. This is not always practical, and there are legitimate reasons in some plans to allow certain consultants to order ancillary services; for example, orthopaedists need to be able to order X-rays, cardiologists need to be able to order electrocardiograms, and so forth. Further discussion of this issue may be found in Chapter 20.

On the other hand, as discussed earlier in this chapter, you need to watch out for the physician who has purchased an expensive piece of equipment and is hoping to increase revenue from its use. In those cases, allowing the physician to bill the plan for tests or procedures done with that equipment may cause problems. Again, one must be reasonable in this. Certain specialists use certain pieces of equipment routinely (eg, gastroenterologists use colonoscopes), and you may not want to hamper that unduly. What you do want to avoid is paying for someone else's amortization needs.

Limits on Services Authorized

Another standard feature of managed care is limiting the number of visits for therapy without prior approval. This refers not only to having a limited number of visits that are covered in your schedule of benefits but to having a limitation on the number of visits that a member may receive without reauthorization.

For example, you may allow up to three or four visits to PT, but for any more the PCP must receive a case report or the therapist must discuss the case with the physician or the plan's case manager. At that point a treatment plan is developed and the correct number of visits is authorized.

There will be exceptions to this last technique. In cases where the absolute treatment need is known, proper authorizations for the entire course of treatment may be made. Examples include radiation therapy or home intravenous treatments. In such cases, the treatment plan is worked out in detail before therapy is initiated. The number of treatments required and their duration are known and may be authorized at the beginning.

Failure to control prospectively the use of ancillary therapy may result in the number of treatments or visits required in a particular type of therapy exactly equaling the level of benefits your plan offers. Much preferred is a rational approach to treatment with review of the case by the member's physician or the plan's case management function (as appropriate) and a definite treatment plan with periodic reassessments required.

CONTRACTING AND REIMBURSEMENT FOR ANCILLARY SERVICES

Contracting and network development are topics that are beyond the scope of this book. However, since in the case of ancillary services, contracting is often one of the first approaches a MCO takes to dealing with costs in this area, a few comments are in order. Many ancillary services are among the first to be "carved out" of the main medical delivery system, with the risk transferred to another organization that is able to achieve economies of scale and manage the overall cost and quality. Therefore, a brief discussion of contracting is warranted here.

Closed panel plans, large medical groups, and IDSs have the option of providing certain ancillary services in house. It is up to management to do the cost benefit analysis to determine whether that is the best course of action. One thing to keep in mind, though, is that controlling utilization is no less difficult when the service is in house; then, referral for that service is often seen as free and certainly as convenient.

For open panel plans or closed panels that do not have the services in house, the services must be contracted for. A plan usually has its choice of hospital-based (sometimes that is the only choice), freestanding or independent, or office-based service. The choice will be dependent upon a combination of factors: quality, cost, access, service (eg, turnaround time for testing), and convenience for members. Unlike physician services, ancillary services usually may be limited to a small subset of providers. This allows for greater leverage in negotiating as well as greater control of quality and service.

In HMOs or plans that have absolute limitations on benefits for ancillary services, ancillary services often lend themselves to capitation. When capitating for ancillary services, you need to calculate the expected frequency of need for the service and the expected or desired cost and then spread this over the membership base on a monthly basis. Plans that allow significant benefits for out-of-network use (eg, a POS plan) may still capitate, but only for the in-network portion; out-of-network costs will have to be paid through the regular fee allowances. If the capitated provider strictly limits access or cannot meet demand, the plan could end up paying twice—once through capitation and a second time through fee for service. It is possible though very uncommon for a POS plan to have no out-of-network benefits for some ancillary services, thus more easily allowing for capitation; this may be difficult from a regulatory standpoint if the ancillary services are clearly part of the basic medical benefit. Simple PPOs generally are unable to capitate and must therefore depend on fee allowances or other forms of episode-related reimbursement.

Capitating for ancillary services clearly makes the provider of the service a partner in controlling costs and helps organizations budget and forecast more accurately. The benefit to the service provider is a guaranteed source of referrals and a steady income. In diagnostic services, great economies of scale will often be present (this is especially true for diagnostic laboratory services). In those services where the provider delivering the service may be determining the need for continued services (eg, PT), capitation will remove the fee-for-service incentives that may lead to inappropriately increased utilization. As with all capitation contracts, organizations must take care that the service is not seen by the providers as free, which may lead to uncontrolled utilization. Again, as with all capitation arrangements, an organization must be sure that it can direct all (or at least a defined portion) of the care to the capitated provider and not allow referrals to noncontracted providers.

Certain types of ancillary services require greater skill in capitating than others. If an ancillary service is highly self-contained, then it is easier to capitate; for example, PT usually is limited to therapy given by the physical therapists and does not involve other types of ancillary providers. Home health, on the other hand, is often a combination of home health nurses and clinical aides, durable medical equipment (DME), home infusion and medication delivery (which includes the cost of the drug or intravenous substance as well as the cost to deliver it), home physical therapy, and so forth. A number of plans have successfully capitated for home health services, although those have tended to be larger plans with sufficient volume to be able to accurately predict costs in all of these different areas. Other plans have been able to capitate only parts of home health (eg, home respiratory therapy) but have had less success in other forms. In those cases, a combination of capitation and fixed case rates (eg, for a course of chemotherapy) may yield positive results.

A recent variant on capitation is similar to the single-specialty management organization or specialty network manager. In this case, a single entity accepts capitation from the plan for all of a particular ancillary service (eg, PT). That organization then serves as a network manager or even an independent practice association (IPA). The participating ancillary providers may be subcontractors to the network manager and be paid either through subcapitation or through a form of fee for service, but in all events, the network manager is at risk for the total costs of the capitated service (the participating ancillary providers are usually at risk as well through capitation, fee adjustments, withholds, and so forth).

Some plans that capitate for ancillary services are employing risk and reward systems to ensure high levels of quality and satisfaction. For example, a plan may withhold 10% of the capitation or set up an incentive pool to ensure compliance with service standards such as accessibility, member satisfaction, responsiveness to referring physicians, documentation, and so forth.

Plans that do not have the option of capitating may still achieve considerable savings from discounts. Because ancillary services are often high-margin businesses, it is usually not difficult to obtain reasonable discounts or to have a negotiated fee schedule accepted for ancillary services. Related to that for therapeutic ancillary providers are case rates or tiered case rates. In this form of reimbursement, the ancillary provider is paid a fixed case rate regardless of the number of visits or resources used in providing services. For home health that includes high-intensity services such as chemotherapy or other high-technology services, the plan may pay different levels of case rates depending on which category of complexity the case falls into. These types of reimbursement systems are appealing but are often quite hard to administer, requiring manual administration by both the plan and the provider.

The only situation in which it is harder to obtain substantial discounts and savings is when there are a limited number of providers offering the service. Outside of exotic testing and therapy, this is usually not the case unless the plan is located in a rural area. In general, very high savings can be achieved through good contracting.

CONCLUSION

The management of ancillary diagnostic and therapeutic services requires a multifaceted approach. The first issue is the behavior of the physicians ordering the ancillary services. Through the use of profiling and feedback, direct discussions between the medical director and the physician, and the use of capitation, reasonably effective results may be obtained. The second issue is the ability of management to contract for these services on a favorable basis. Lastly, integration of these services into the overall constellation of services offered by large, organized medical groups is highly effective, because the physicians in the group are best able to balance the issues involved.

REFERENCES

1. Hillman BJ, Joseph CA, Mabry MR, et al. Frequency and costs of diagnostic imaging in office practice—a comparison of self-referring and radiologist-referring physicians. *N Engl J Med.* 1990;323:1604–1608.
2. Office of the Inspector General. *Financial Arrangements Between Physicians and Health Care Businesses: Report to Congress.* Department of Health and Human Services Publication no OAI-12-88-01410. Washington, DC: Department of Health and Human Services; 1989.
3. State of Florida Health Care Cost Containment Board. *Joint Ventures among Health Care Providers in Florida.* Tallahassee, FL: State of Florida; 1991.
4. The Ethics in Patient Referrals Act—Omnibus Budget Reconciliation Act of 1989.
5. Murray JP, Greenfield S, Kaplan SH, Yano EM. Ambulatory testing for capitation and fee-for-service patients in the same practice setting: relationship to outcomes. *Med Care.* 1992;30(3):252–261.
6. Kassirer JP. Our stubborn quest for diagnostic certainty: a cause of excessive testing. *N Engl J Med.* 1989;320:1489–1491.
7. Berwick DM, Coltin KL. Feedback reduces test use in a health maintenance organization. *JAMA.* 1986;255:1450–1454.

8. Marton KI, Tul V, Sox HC. Modifying test-ordering behavior in the outpatient medical clinic. *Arch Intern Med.* 1985;145:816–821.
9. Martin AR, Wolf MA, Thibodeau LA, et al. A trial of two strategies to modify the test-ordering behavior of medical residents. *N Engl J Med.* 1980;303:1330–1336.
10. Atlantic Information Services, Inc. *Provider Contracting & Capitation.* Washington, DC: Atlantic Information Services, Inc; 1993.
11. Tape TG, Mushlin AI. The utility of routine chest radiographs. *Ann Intern Med.* 1986;104:663–670.
12. Hubble FA, Greenfield S, Tyler JL, et al. The impact of routine admission chest x-ray films on patient care. *N Engl J Med.* 1985;312:209.
13. Food and Drug Administration. *The Selection of Patients for X-Ray Examinations: Chest X-Ray Screening Examinations.* Department of Health and Human Services Publication no 83-8204. Rockville, MD: National Center for Devices and Radiological Health; 1983.
14. Gold BS, Young ML, Kinman JL, et al. The utility of preoperative electrocardiograms in the ambulatory surgical patient. *Arch Intern Med.* 1992;152:301–305.
15. Narr BJ, Hansen TR, Warner MA. Preoperative laboratory screening in healthy Mayo patients: cost-effective elimination of tests and unchanged outcomes. *Mayo Clin Proc.* 1991;66:155–159.

CHAPTER 26

Pharmaceutical Services in Managed Care

Henry F. Blissenbach and Peter Penna

Chapter Outline

- Cost of Drugs
- The Pharmacy Benefit
- The Providers
- Determining Pharmaceutical Benefit Costs
- Managing the Pharmacy Benefit
- Ingredient Cost
- Quantitative Drug Utilization Review
- Audits
- Management of Quality
- Qualitative Drug Utilization Review
- Measurement of Success
- Pharmacy Benefit Management: Next Phase
- Conclusion

Before 1973, pharmacy, as a covered benefit, was not a significant part of the benefit dollar. Often it was not even a standard component of health benefits. The trend toward inclusion of a prescription drug benefit as part of a managed care benefit package, however, has evolved. At present, prescription drug benefits are a standard component of health benefits.

This chapter is adapted from HF Blissenbach and P Penna, Pharmaceutical Services in Managed Care, in *The Managed Health Care Handbook*, 3rd ed, PR Kongstvedt, ed, pp 367–387, © 1996, Aspen Publishers, Inc.

In tandem with this desire to include drug coverage as a benefit has been the growing number and complexity of medications available to improve the quality and length of life. As with all components of health care, drug prices increase annually. Throughout the entire health care industry, prescription costs are placing a financial stress on payers and budget managers of health care plans. To the individual who has health care coverage and a prescription drug benefit as part of that coverage, medications are considered an entitlement. The economics of a prescription drug benefit, however, require continued assessment of the appropriateness and necessity of drug use and subsequent aggressive, and sometimes controversial, interventions to manage cost.

The challenge to an appropriate pharmaceutical management program is to control costs without adversely affecting the quality of care and, equally important, providers' and recipients' perceptions of the quality of care. Decreasing, cutting back on, not covering, or omitting something previously perceived as a benefit is not well accepted by plan members. Additionally, providers often perceive these same changes as a threat to their independence to practice medicine or pharmacy.

Managing a pharmaceutical benefit requires an understanding of the components of that benefit. Contracting with members of managed care organizations (MCOs) to provide a quality drug benefit means promising to allow physicians to prescribe medicines that will cure acute illness, increase the length of life, or improve the quality of life. Organizations must contain the cost of these medicines without depriving individuals of necessary medicines, while at the same time improving quality (or at least not degrading it).

Unlike most other topics in this book, the management of pharmacy costs is very dependent on benefit structure and delivery structure. Therefore, discussion of these topics is appropriate here.

COST OF DRUGS

The percentage of the total health care expenditure that pharmaceuticals represent is a highly scrutinized area of economic concern to the public, the payers, and the policy makers. The pharmaceutical industry as a whole, including the manufacturers, wholesalers, and dispensers of the product, has been widely criticized because drug products are perceived to be expensive without adequate evidence of cost-effectiveness. Yet, as P. Roy Vagelos, past chair and chief executive officer at Merck and Company, states, "even if each of the medicines that may eventually be found to prevent or treat diseases become tremendous commercial successes, patient cost for the medicines would be far less than the cost of the diseases."[1]

The consumer price index (CPI) measures the average change in retail prices paid by consumers for products. The CPI further differentiates drug products according to their product type. Prescription drugs are reflected in the CPI-Rx. Between 1981 and 1986, this component increased by almost 80.0%, with an average rate of 10.2% per year. The CPI-Rx average dropped during subsequent years. After a slight increase in 1989 to 9.5%, the CPI-Rx had maintained at about 9.0% for several more years until further erosion in 1994. However, as this book is being written, pharmacy benefits costs are once again rising in excess of any other segment of health care costs; we encourage readers to research this information on their own.

What does this mean in terms of overall cost to the MCO when providing a drug benefit program? As Table 26–1 shows, pharmacy benefits costs have generally remained in the region of 10% of operating costs (varying by type of MCO). MCOs, however, have often been reluctant to charge the premium payer an amount equivalent to the percentage of operating expense that the drug benefit consumes. Hence, for most MCOs offering a pharmacy benefit, the drug benefit program has frequently resulted in losses.

As we will see throughout this chapter, it is becoming more important to manage the cost of the pharmaceutical benefit than to save money. If MCOs choose to continue to operate at a loss for the drug benefit program, managing the amounts of these losses becomes paramount.

THE PHARMACY BENEFIT

Before discussing policies, procedures, and services necessary to ensure successful management of the pharmacy benefit, we need to review what a managed care pharmacy benefit includes. Typically, each member of an MCO that offers a prescription drug benefit can receive prescrip-

Table 26–1 Drug Expenditures as a Percentage of Operating Expenses

	Type of MCO				
Year	Total (%)	Staff (%)	Network (%)	IPA (%)	Group (%)
1988	10.0	5.0	12.0		11.0
1989	10.0	5.0	10.0		11.0
1990	9.0	6.0	10.0		9.0
1991	11.0	9.0	10.0		11.0
1992	9.0	8.0	10.0	10.0	8.0
1993	12.0	8.0	9.0	13.0	11.0
1994	10.0	8.0	9.0	11.0	12.0
1995	9.4	9.2	10.1	9.2	10.0
1996	10.4	9.1	10.8	10.7	9.9

Note: IPA = independent practice association

Courtesy of SMG Marketing Group, Inc, Chicago, Illinois.

tions as a covered benefit as long as the following criteria are met:

- The individual must be eligible for coverage by the MCO. An eligible member is the primary cardholder or dependent of the cardholder. The eligible member or employee usually must present identification designating that he or she is a member of that MCO.
- In some cases, the prescription must be written by a contracted prescriber (ie, an eligible prescriber on record with the MCO). When the MCO closes its physician prescriber list and accepts only prescriptions written by contracted physicians, the pharmacist must determine eligibility.
- Prescriptions for over-the-counter medications are ordinarily not covered; only prescriptions that are legend will be covered. (A legend drug is one labeled "Caution: Federal law prohibits dispensing without a prescription.") Even if the medication is a legend drug, however, that does not necessarily mean that it is covered.
- Most MCOs now have formularies. If a formulary is "open," it is merely a list of preferred drugs; drugs prescribed but not on the list will still be covered. If the formulary is "closed," then only drugs on the formulary will be covered.
- Many MCOs require that specific guidelines be met before certain drugs will be covered (a common example is growth hormone).
- Prescriptions must be filled at designated pharmacies—pharmacies that have a contractual agreement with the MCO. The covered member cannot take the prescription into any pharmacy to have it filled but must remain within the network.
- If the medication is available generically, it will be reimbursed at a generic rate and probably will be dispensed as a generic equivalent. Often, the member has the option of paying the difference between the generic and the branded products.
- For the member to receive the prescription, a deductible and/or copayment is usually required (eg, a $100 deductible must be met, after which coverage with copayments begins). Members are expected to pay a portion of the cost of their prescriptions.
- There is usually a different level of copay for generically available drugs and for brand name drugs (eg, $5 for generic and $10 for brand name).
- Recently, some plans have been responding to the marketplace's demands for broad access by having three levels of copayment:
  - low (eg, $5), for generic drugs
  - medium (eg, $10), for name brand drugs that are on the formulary
  - high (eg, $20), for name brand drugs that are not on the formulary and for which a formulary drug is available

Certificate of Coverage

The pharmacy benefit is typically defined in a document called the certificate of coverage or certificate of benefits that the MCO provides to members to describe their covered health care benefits. Before any cost management or cost containment procedures can be implemented, the benefit certificate must have language to allow these procedures. Once benefit language changes are in place, these need to be communicated and explained to members and to providers. This entire process often takes considerable time for approval and implementation. Many cost management efforts can be accomplished without changes being required in the certificate of coverage, however.

The certificate typically addresses the fact that medications are eligible for coverage if they meet certain criteria and are medically necessary and appropriate for treatment of the illness. Generally, the treatment must also be consistent with medical standards of the community and prevent the patient's condition from worsening. The fact that a provider recommends a certain medication or service does not necessarily mean that it is eligible for coverage under the contract.

Typically excluded from pharmacy benefit programs are services or prescription drugs that the MCO determines to be experimental or unproven, services or prescription drugs that are not generally accepted by the medical community as a standard of care, and others. Typical exclusions include anorexant drugs, cosmetic medications, and vitamins. All MCOs allow the member an appeal process should there be a disagreement with a coverage decision.

Do therapeutic qualifications alone automatically qualify a drug for coverage? Covered drug decisions can also be based on a determination that an individual's life will be longer or of higher quality. In other words, quality and outcome qualifications can be included when coverage of a medication is determined.

Managed Health Care and the Pharmacy Benefit

When one refers to a prescription drug benefit, ordinarily the implication is that someone other than the recipient is paying for the benefit. In other words, the receiver of the service does not pay for the prescription. Many individuals still pay for their prescriptions out of their own pocket, but the percentage of the population that has partial or total prescription drug coverage is increasing yearly. The largest group without a benefit is retirees.

How the Benefit Is Received

There are several ways that prescription services are obtained, and each of these has its own characteristic method of payment.

Recipient of Service Pays Entire Cost of Prescription

Until recently, this was the most common way that prescriptions were obtained. The recipient would call or visit the physician, the physician would write a prescription, and the recipient would take the prescription to a pharmacy, have it filled, and pay the cost of the product plus the service. Competition then entered the pharmacy marketplace, driving some of the product and service fees downward and somewhat decreasing prescription costs.

Partial Pay for Both Recipient and Third Party

Partial payment plans for drug benefit programs usually require an identification card designating eligibility. These programs are further classified as managed or unmanaged. The managed card program traditionally has been associated with MCOs. More recently, for quality and cost reasons, self-insured employers and even indemnity insurance plans with prescription drug riders are moving from unmanaged to managed card programs.

Prescription drug benefit programs with a partial payment requirement on the part of the recipient are increasing in popularity, and variations in the partial pay amount are significant factors in enabling the payer to manage the drug benefit cost. The common variations are discussed below.

Copayments. Typically, copayments are handled at the point of service. This mechanism requires a designated dollar amount in exchange for the product or service. In other words, a prescription is presented at the pharmacy, and upon delivery of the prescription to the recipient, the recipient furnishes a copayment amount. Sometimes the copayment is the same for a branded or generic, formulary or nonformulary prescription; other times there is a higher copayment for branded than for generic drugs. The copayment may vary from $3 to $20 per prescription, with lower copayments being more common. As noted earlier, there may be up to three tiers of copayments within the same benefits plan.

Deductibles. Deductibles are typically associated with indemnity insurance plans and sometimes with self-insured employer groups. They are gaining popularity in health maintenance organizations (HMOs) and preferred provider organizations (PPOs), particularly now that calculation and notification of up-to-date deductibles via on-line point-of-service claims processing systems are common. The prescription deductible, like any other medical service deductible, requires a designated out-of-pocket expenditure before the pharmacy benefit coverage comes into effect. Although the deductible should be approximately 25% to 35% of the annual drug cost, because these are prospectively determined amounts they most often are underestimated and rarely reach an appropriate percentage of partial payment. In the past, insurers and other payers have gambled that recipients would "shoe box" the receipt for services and would not file a claim for the eligible amount. With the increasing cost of prescription drugs, the decreasing comparative percentage of salary increases compared to prescription cost increases, and the ease of recordkeeping via on-line point-of-service claims processing systems, however, the shoe box effect is becoming less and less apparent.

Coinsurance. The coinsurance system is most common with indemnity insurance plans. Each time the benefit is used, a designated percentage is applied to the total cost of the prescription. In other words, a drug benefit plan with 20% coinsurance would require the recipient to pay 20% of the cost of the prescription each time it is obtained. Again, because they once relied on the shoe box effect, indemnity insurance plans are finding that unmanaged drug benefit riders with coinsurance applications are experiencing high costs.

Recipient Has No Partial Payment: Third Party Pays All

This method of payment typically is associated with state and federally financed programs. In these Medicaid-type programs, the recipient is not required to pay out of pocket any part of the drug benefit. There are a few exceptions to this. Some states have initiated minimal copayments ($0.25 to $1) for Medicaid recipients. Government-funded programs are typically managed by legislative regulations, and special interest groups have made managing a drug benefit system for state Medicaid programs difficult at best. Provider reimbursement fees are usually legislated, and discounts off the average wholesale price (AWP) of the product are determined by Congress. Because federal- and state-funded programs have been experiencing higher drug expenditures than the private sector, however, both levels of government are requiring more management applications for these programs.

Components of a Pharmacy Benefit

A prescription drug benefit has several components. These components depend on whether the benefit is unmanaged or managed. An unmanaged program is simple to facilitate and, with minor exceptions, allows the eligible recipient to have prescriptions filled, with the pharmacy collecting the designated copayment, deductible, or coinsurance.

A well-managed prescription drug benefit, on the other hand, can be complex and includes the following characteristics:

- appropriate benefit design
- point-of-service claims adjudication and processing
- a contracted and discounted pharmacy network
- an aggressive generic substitution program
- a cost-effective drug formulary program
- discounts from manufacturers via volume purchase or market share programs
- financial and utilization management reporting
- budgeting appropriateness based on accurate information

THE PROVIDERS

Staff Model or Closed Panel Managed Care Organizations

This type of MCO often employs its own pharmacists and owns its in-house pharmacies. The MCO assumes all the risk for the prescription drug service. This is the oldest form of prepaid pharmaceutical services in the country. The MCO-employed pharmacists dispense medications to plan members at MCO-owned pharmacies. The primary advantages of a staff model MCO prescription benefit are as follows:

- The MCO saves administration cost because there are no claims processed for reimbursement.
- Program changes (eg, drug formularies, copayment) are made easily because all affected providers are employed by the MCO.
- The MCO can take advantage of volume purchasing because of a large in-house prescription volume.
- Since physicians and pharmacists work for the same organization, it's easier to develop consensus on benefit management strategies.

There are also some disadvantages:

- This system requires a considerable capital investment by the MCO to provide pharmacy space, drug inventory, and staff.
- Lack of evening and after-hours emergency service and convenient accessibility often creates problems for plan subscribers.
- Difficulty in establishing pharmacist–patient relationships is sometimes experienced.

Some staff model MCOs also agree to cover over-the-counter (nonprescription) medications.

Independent Practice Association or Open Panel Managed Care Organizations

The base of pharmacy benefit programs in independent practice associations (IPAs) and open panel MCOs is contracted provider networks. Pharmacies are not owned, nor is the pharmacist's salary paid by the MCO. Instead, these are established, freestanding community pharmacies. Pharmacy participation in the limited pharmacy network is, for the most part, determined by the MCO.

Advantages include the following:

- Pharmacies are conveniently located for patient/member accessibility.
- The MCO can provide pharmaceutical benefits without a considerable investment in facility space, drug inventory, and pharmacy staff.
- The pharmacy network can expand easily as growth requirements emerge.
- The MCO can take advantage of competition in the marketplace to generate discounts.

There are also disadvantages:

- Administrative expenses increase as a result of claims processing and reimbursement.
- This decentralization of pharmaceutical services makes it more difficult to implement program, policy, and procedural changes.
- Criteria are necessary for selection of participating pharmacies to ensure nonviolation of existing laws.
- Managing the benefit is more difficult because physicians, pharmacists, and administrators have few common interests.
- Policies regarding reimbursement for pharmacy services must be determined and established.

Preferred Provider Organization

This benefit may look like a traditional MCO benefit with an IPA flair because there is a pharmacy network that is typically contracted and limited. A PPO benefit may also resemble an indemnity insurance benefit if it is not tightly managed, although loosely managed benefits are losing favor. Most PPOs have not been able to manage their pharmaceutical costs as well as MCOs, primarily because PPOs tend to be more provider sensitive and have been reluctant to implement aggressive cost management applications, as MCOs have.

Indemnity Insurance Plans

Typically unmanaged, the pharmacy benefit programs of indemnity insurance plans may utilize a prescription card program within a relatively large pharmacy network. Under this model, all pharmacies located in the geographic service area are generally afforded the opportunity to provide pharmacy services to the indemnity insurance subscriber. Ordinarily, these operate under a pay-and-submit approach with little or no benefit restrictions. Mail-order pharmacy services may be a component. Some indemnity plans function in a major medical approach, in which the subscribers pay out of pocket and then submit claims to the insurance plan for reimbursement (after deductible and coinsurance).

Advantages of this program include the following:

- Card programs deliver some level of control over ingredient cost and dispensing fee.
- Such programs maintain a strong freedom of choice concept, preserving long-standing pharmacist–patient relationships.
- Subscribers are not forced to drive considerable distances to have their pharmaceutical needs fulfilled.
- Mail-order programs achieve good control of ingredient cost and dispensing fee and are convenient for members on long-term medications.

The following are some disadvantages:

- As one might expect, the costs associated with operating an open pharmacy network are much greater than those of the other alternatives.
- Plans that use card programs must print and distribute administration manuals, participating pharmacy agreements, claims reimbursement forms, and the like, all of which contribute to total administrative cost.
- Such plans are unable to take advantage of competition in the marketplace to generate significantly discounted fees.
- Mail-order programs may result in waste when a prescription is changed in midcourse or when a member loses eligibility shortly after receiving a 90-day supply.

Self-Insured Benefits

The advantages and disadvantages are similar to those for indemnity insurance.

Government/Medicaid Programs

Traditional non–managed care public sector programs utilize contracted pharmacy networks and have the same advantages and disadvantages discussed above, depending on how the benefit is constituted. They are usually card and point-of-service programs and are often unmanaged. Many public sector programs, however, are moving to managed care and operate much the same way HMOs do.

DETERMINING PHARMACEUTICAL BENEFIT COSTS

How does one determine the true cost of a pharmaceutical benefit? How should that benefit be priced? What is its overall value? How does your cost compare to those of other MCOs and competitors? Trying to provide a pharmacy benefit program without knowing the answers to these questions puts managers at a distinct disadvantage.

Before management approaches can be initiated to control pharmaceutical expenditures, it is necessary to understand the cost of the program and the degree of responsibility that each of the components of that cost has to the bottom line.

The cost of pharmacy benefit can be determined by applying the following formula:

Total drug cost = (ingredient cost + dispensing fee − copay) × number of prescriptions

Total drug costs can be calculated either as per member per month (PMPM) or per member per year (PMPY) expenditures. The actual prescription cost is represented by the values in parentheses (ingredient cost + dispensing fee − copay). If they intend to decrease overall pharmacy benefit expenditures, organizations need to determine the percentages that each component represents. Although the prescription cost is often the cost

Exhibit 26–1 Illustration of PMPM Drug Cost

> Assume:
>   Ingredient cost = $21.00
>   Dispensing fee = $2.50
>   Copay = $7.00
>   Number of prescriptions = 0.6 PMPM
> Then:
>   PMPM drug cost =
>   ($21.00 + $2.50 − $7.00) × 0.6 = $9.90

indicator, PMPM costs are a more accurate indicator. A calculation example is provided in Exhibit 26–1.

The next step is to determine high or low status and to react accordingly. As evidenced by the above formula, there are several ways to reduce or control the PMPM cost:

- *Reduce ingredient cost:* This is accomplished by maximizing generic substitution, reimbursing for generics only according to a maximum allowable cost (MAC) list, implementing a drug formulary managing utilization, and using volume purchase (rebate) or discount contracting.
- *Decrease dispensing fees*: Take advantage of the competition in the marketplace to ensure the lowest acceptable dispensing fee.
- *Increase copays*: Increase the member's (or subscriber's) out-of-pocket responsibility for a portion of the drug benefit. This can act as a disincentive for utilizing the drug benefit; therefore, total costs could increase if members do not get the necessary prescriptions to manage their disease.
- *Decrease the number of prescriptions*: The number of prescriptions written by physicians affects the prescription cost. Once they are identified, physicians who write too many prescriptions can be evaluated for cost-effectiveness and notified (if appropriate) to try to bring them toward the norm.

MANAGING THE PHARMACY BENEFIT

Adequately and appropriately managing a pharmacy benefit consists of two integral components: management of the cost and management of the quality of that benefit. Successful pharmacy benefit management applications have proven that drug costs can be managed without adversely affecting quality of care.

Benefit Design

The pharmacy benefit design determines how the pharmacy benefit works. Simply stated, the benefit identifies for both members and providers the terms and extent of the coverage. All determinants of coverage hinge on the benefit design. The actual benefit design depends on several factors: competition, government regulations and requirements, union or employer specifications, dollars available, and the like. The real art of prescription benefit design is choosing where to save money and where compromises are possible. The benefit design should define prescription medications, describe refill restrictions (if any), list products or services excluded from the benefit, state payment responsibilities of the member, specify limits on the amount of medications allowed with each transaction, and identify approved prescribers and providers. Also, generic and formulary requirements as well as allowances for investigational or experimental medications should be listed.

Claims Adjudication

Once the benefit design has been finalized, a process must be implemented to reimburse for benefit coverage, unless of course the prescription is filled in a pharmacy owned by the managed care plan. Whether the pharmacist adjudicates the claim electronically or a claims processor at the plan performs this task, this procedure includes the following steps:

- verification of eligibility on the basis of enrollment information provided by the payer
- verification of coverage on the basis of the benefit design of the group
- verification of copay
- verification of reimbursement amount to the pharmacy in accordance with prearranged or contracted specifics

Enrollment Information/Eligibility Verification

Of utmost importance is the verification of eligibility before a claim is paid. Until recently, eligibility verification at the point of sale was not required or even possible. In fact, it was not unusual for many plans to pay pharmacy claims without having adequate eligibility or enrollment information to determine whether the submitted claim was eligible for reimbursement. Hand in hand with member eligibility goes prescriber (ie, physician) eligibility. Although still not the standard, a requirement to determine prescriber eligibility and to enter a prescriber identification number as part of claim processing are important parts of managing pharmaceutical costs.

Eligibility verification is accomplished simply: The member presents an eligibility card, and the provider verifies that the member is eligible. Although some plans still use printed eligibility lists, most pharmacies have moved to on-line point-of-service eligibility verification and claims processing.

Electronic Claims Adjudication

Not so long ago, all pharmacy claims were submitted on paper. The primary disadvantage was that, although the recipient of the prescription could present an identification card indicating eligibility for coverage, often eligibility had terminated without adequate notification to the provider, or the pharmacist would have a claim returned without payment because of a change in eligibility, or incorrect payment was received by the pharmacist, or the wrong amount of copayment was collected. All these increase the frustration level of the pharmacist and often put members at odds with the pharmacist.

Electronic claims processing reduces all these frustrations and allows for the point-of-service coordination of benefit services such as deductible, copayment, and coverage limits. When the pharmacist enters the prescription on line, that pharmacist receives up-to-date eligibility status and knows that acceptance by the on-line system ensures payment. Additionally, the delay in receiving payment for the prescription is decreased significantly, and rejected claims are eliminated.

Interestingly, the driving force behind point-of-service eligibility systems has not been the pharmacist but the payer. Cost containment pressures are forcing health care plans to take a hard look at the cost of paying for bad claims. Most payers have included a point-of-service requirement as part of pharmacy network contracting.

Pharmacy Provider Networks

Managed care plans often limit the number of pharmacies that provide services for enrolled members. Like hospital and physician networks, limited pharmacist networks allow managed care plans to ensure high volumes of business to pharmacies in exchange for lower prices. Limiting the pharmacy network allows the MCO to accomplish two objectives: to lower dispensing fees and to improve compliance with policies and procedures. In most large cities, the available pharmacy network is generally larger than necessary to fill the prescriptions of the plan's membership. MCOs will take advantage of that competitive marketplace to obtain discounts. Reimbursement is a function of supply and demand.

For a contractual arrangement to be successful, the payer must be willing to restrict covered members' access to pharmacies. When this happens, there may be an initial negative reaction. If the plan is large enough, one can also expect the local pharmacist associations to organize against the plan's decision. When a plan is deciding to decrease the pharmacy network, the negative reaction should be weighed carefully against the benefit. The standard within the managed care industry, however, is to provide the pharmacy benefit through a restricted pharmacy network.

Mail-order pharmacy is increasing in popularity nationally, such that 55% of managed care plans offer a mail-order component.[2] Employers offering a self-insured pharmacy benefit have offered mail order usually as an option. This has also been an especially popular method for retirees to receive prescriptions at a discounted rate. Those MCOs offering mail order as a component of the pharmacy benefit should require the mail-order dispenser to follow the same policies and procedures as the rest of the pharmacy provider network. Formularies, MAC reimbursement, eligibility verification, copay collections, and all other procedures must be followed. Usually, the mail-order companies are willing to compete even more aggressively than the members of the pharmacy network. Mail-order pharmacies may be especially good at ensuring generic and therapeutic substitution.

The final type of prescription vendor is the physician dispenser. Several companies offer repackaging services to physician offices as part of a system to dispense prescriptions. Some MCOs allow physician dispensers as part of the pharmacy benefit system, but the physician must accept the same discounted reimbursement as the rest of the pharmacy network. This includes a percentage discount from the AWP of the product and the discounted dispensing fee. Physician dispensers primarily dispense short-term medications and usually have little or no refill capabilities. The popularity of this system in MCOs is low, and usually there is little interest on the part of the physician to fill prescriptions for third-party payers; however, as pressure increases on physicians to accept lower capitation and fee rates, some may look for ways to provide more services, and hence, get more reimbursement.

INGREDIENT COST

There are several approaches to managing this significant cost portion of the equation. There are multiple approaches to managing ingredient cost; each method is dependent on the design of the drug benefit.

Generic Drug Policy

When the patent expires on a previously brand-only medication, usually other manufacturers competitively distribute the same drug. (The quality indicators of a generic program are covered later in this chapter.) Generic brands are significantly less costly than brand name medication. The average generic cost is anywhere from 40% to 70% less than the equivalent branded product cost. Almost 90% of MCOs require use of generics,[2] and approximately 40% of MCO prescriptions are filled with generic drugs.

The components of an aggressive generic program include generic reimbursement according to a MAC reimbursement rate. Because there are multiple manufacturers of generic medications, each pricing at different AWPs, and because most pharmacies participate in some form of purchasing group arrangement, the difficulty in identifying the true average price of a generic medication has created the MAC reimbursement process. This process allows the payer to set a price for a specific generic medication and indicates to the pharmacist the maximum amount that will be reimbursed as the ingredient cost. The determination of the MAC is highly technical and labor intensive.

Remember that generic utilization numbers can be misleading. An MCO could have an extremely high generic utilization rate and yet not maximize generic cost savings. This is exactly what happens when a MAC list is not part of the reimbursement policy.

If exceptions are included in the benefit design that allow the pharmacist to be reimbursed for prescriptions at other than the MAC, benefit costs will increase. These exceptions are a benefit design allowing the physician and/or member to request the branded product at the expense of the plan. Commonly called a dispense-as-written (DAW) policy, this request may be generated by the physician by writing "dispense as written" on the prescription. It may also be generated by a verbal request on the part of the member to receive the branded product rather than the generic. This will decrease the number of prescriptions dispensed generically and will cause a significant increase in the average ingredient cost. A well-managed pharmacy benefit program allows for member payment of the difference between the generic and the branded product should either the physician or the member request this option. Anything short of this will unnecessarily cost the plan money.

Average Wholesale Price Discounts

The AWP of a medication should be the purchase price of the medication or ingredient from a drug wholesaler. Little is more confusing or more difficult to determine than the purchase price of a medication. Hence the claims processor or the third-party payer utilizes an independent source, or pricing vendor, to determine the AWP of the medication. This AWP reference has become the standard of payment for the ingredient, and this reference source is usually part of the pharmacy contract.

To complicate the issue further, there are usually discrepancies between the purchase price of the ingredient by the pharmacy and the designated AWP per the pricing source. Like sticker prices on automobiles, the reference source purchase price and the actual purchase price are typically different. Hence a negotiated discount off the referenced AWP is a standard part of the pharmacy contract. This discount is often more important to the pharmacist than the dispensing fee because the AWP of the ingredient will continue to inflate over time whereas the dispensing fee is generally the same over time. The current marketplace allows the AWP discount for branded products to be in the 10% to 18% range. The differential factor is the competition within the marketplace. The AWP discount for generic drugs is significantly higher (estimated to be in the 40% to 60% range). Managers should not concentrate on AWP discounts for generics but rather should utilize a MAC rate.

Flat Rate

Recently a few plans have adopted a system of flat payments that do not vary by prescription. This type of system is only feasible when volume is high. This system makes budgeting easier and enlists the help of pharmacies.

Drug Formularies

The decision to require a drug formulary in a managed care environment is one that mandates careful planning. More and more MCOs are realizing the value of the drug formulary in managing costs and are moving toward aggressive formulary management. Most MCOs (96%) are using formularies, and almost 50% of plans have closed formularies.[2]

A drug formulary is best defined as a dynamic, comprehensive list of drugs designed to direct physicians to prescribe the most cost-effective medications. The list is organized by therapeutic class; the selection criteria for the drugs on the formulary are, first, patient care (therapeutics), and second, cost.

A drug formulary must meet three criteria to be successful:

1. It must reflect the practice of medicine in the community. Restricting physicians from using medications that have become a standard of practice in the community will be a difficult endeavor indeed.
2. It must be responsive to the therapeutic needs of the physicians. If physicians are not able to find medications that are necessary to treat patients and are continually requesting exceptions to the formulary, the effort to enforce a formulary will serve neither the physicians nor patients. In other words, it must be therapeutically appropriate.
3. It must be representative of cost-effective therapy. This is where most formularies that are nothing more than drug lists fall short. The true differentiating criterion among formularies is the ability to meet community standards and therapeutic necessities in a cost-effective manner.

When a drug formulary is used in an appropriate manner, quality of care is improved. Furthermore, by moving toward a closed or mandatory status and maximizing volume purchase contracts, a drug formulary can save 10% or more on the pharmaceutical benefit cost.

The formulary development process is extremely important to the success of a formulary system. Educating physicians that the drug formulary is coming ensures implementation without undue delay. A simple statement in the physician newsletter that the MCO has decided, via its medical staff advisory committee, to implement the drug formulary is useful.

A formulary committee or pharmacy and therapeutics committee comprising physicians, clinical pharmacists, and sometimes health plan administrators is necessary to give adequate input to the drug formulary process. Certain physician specialties are a must for this committee, including family practice, internal medicine, pediatrics, and gynecology. These physicians prescribe the most medications for health plan members and thus deserve the largest representation on the committee. Often, for various reasons, other specialty areas are represented (eg, psychiatry, dermatology, and surgery). Usually the internal medicine representatives on the committee can also provide input on their subspecialty areas. When no committee member represents an area of expertise (eg, infectious disease, rheumatology, cardiology, and so forth), the committee members can ask representatives of that area to attend on an ad hoc basis. Maximum success can be ensured if the formulary is developed at the local level, but with oversight, coordination, and some direction from the "central office." Creating a written protocol addressing the process to be used for adding to the drug formulary is beneficial.

After the formulary document has been approved, it is ready to be sent to the providers and promoted as the cost-effective, high-quality document that it is. Directions explaining how to use the document need to be included. The document should be formatted to be as simple and easy to follow as possible. There needs to be an index to which providers can turn to find immediate formulary information and a therapeutic categorization that facilitates identification of drugs available for certain disease entities. Currently, some electronic formularies are being developed for physicians' personal computers.

The promotion of the formulary also needs to include information about what happens if providers do not follow the formulary. This can be part of the endorsement on the front end, simply stating that there will be a monitoring process in place that will identify physicians who are continually not complying with the drug formulary, that these physicians will be contacted if they do not follow the formulary, and that consistent outliers (without justification) will be dealt with.

Drug formularies in staff model MCOs are generally followed without question. In the IPA model MCO, however, providers are typically private practice physicians and pharmacists who see the formulary as a hindrance or constraint on their ability to practice their profession. Furthermore, the providers may participate with multiple plans, each with a slightly different formulary. Therefore, the plan should expect provider pharmacies to call physicians about nonformulary medications, and the physicians should follow the advice of the pharmacist when they are called to change to a formulary drug.

Last comes the question of assessing the success of the formulary. This is easier if you determine the percentage of prescriptions that are written in compliance with the formulary than if you apply financial information to that formulary retrospectively. If cost-effective guidelines were followed in developing the drug formulary, however, then the logical assumption is that the higher the formulary compliance, the more cost-effective the drug formulary.

In those environments where there is a voluntary formulary, a compliance rate of greater than 95% should be expected. In an open formulary environment, however, a high compliance rate does not necessarily mean cost-effectiveness. Obviously, the easiest way to obtain 100% compliance is to put all medications on the formulary. A mandatory closed formulary with high compliance will achieve the greatest savings.

The institution of a drug formulary system also requires notification of the members of the plan that their medications will now be required to be prescribed per a drug formulary. Often, if this is a new policy, a period of grandfathering can be put in place so that individuals who are stabilized on a medication that is not part of the drug formulary can continue to use that medication. It is important to understand that the intent of the drug formulary is not to restrict medications from individuals who need them but rather to change physician prescribing behavior to the most cost-effective therapeutics.

Volume Purchasing and Rebates

The fourth mechanism in managing ingredient cost is volume purchase contracting, commonly called rebates. This is the mechanism by which the pharmaceutical manufacturer agrees to a volume-driven discount contract in exchange for formulary considerations. Most pharmaceutical companies have formed a managed care department to understand and interface with MCOs. Many companies have contractual relations with MCOs already and share utilization of their products. Although a couple of the manufacturers have fought the MCOs' attempts to manage cost, this tendency to gamble that their freedom of product choice philosophy will outlast cost containment is not prevalent. The need for MCOs and the pharmaceutical industry to work as allies is becoming more obvious. Both industries have the pharmaceutical product as their focal point, and both have much to gain by cooperative efforts in proving the value of their product.

Why should pharmaceutical companies agree to contract with MCOs? Why should they discount their products? There are a number of important reasons.

- It often is the only way the MCO will accept the company's product on the drug formulary. Most medications newly marketed today are therapeutically equivalent to an existing product that is probably already on the formulary.
- The MCO, in essence, becomes an extension of the pharmaceutical company's sales force. The product's formulary status serves as an endorsement for the product.
- Once a relationship exists, the MCO will preferentially review the pharmaceutical company's newly marketed products in a way that ensures the partner company the greatest opportunity for inclusion on the formulary.
- Most closed panel plans will cooperate with the partner pharmaceutical company to facilitate local representatives' accessibility to providers, at least for those products that are already on the formulary. The ability to see physicians and pharmacists is essential for pharmaceutical sales representatives.
- Formulary decisions provide a spillover effect; that is, physicians will tend to prescribe formulary products for all their patients, not just patients belonging to the MCO.

QUANTITATIVE DRUG UTILIZATION REVIEW

An integral part of managing pharmaceutical costs is the development of drug utilization review (DUR) programs. DUR and drug utilization evaluation programs offer the prospect of saving money both by restraining the use of unnecessary or inappropriate drugs and by preventing the adverse effects of misused medications.[3] DUR programs assess the appropriateness, safety, and efficacy of drug use. In utilization review efforts, cost and quality considerations in managing pharmacy benefits have been blended together. Realistically, the emphasis has been on the cost side; there are various reasons for this, including convenient access to cost data and the completeness of those data. Because plans are effectively managing the financial aspects of cost utilization, the demand for proof that the therapeutics/quality of care considerations are not being affected by these cost considerations continues to arise. Hence it is best to separate the DUR process into quantitative and qualitative elements. (Quality is discussed later in this chapter.) Realistically, quantitative DUR answers the questions, How costly? How often? For whom? By whom? The properties of quantitative DUR are as follows:

- It describes patterns of drug utilization and cost.
- It quantitates drug utilization and cost.
- It identifies areas and categories to be used for qualitative DUR.
- It identifies areas for education.
- It is not based on any predetermined criteria for standards.
- It can be used to describe the quality of drug use.

In essence, quantitative DUR selects the therapies to be reviewed. Data are collected, and those data are analyzed and reported. Based on findings, certain management and educational applications are then put into effect. To determine the significance of the quantitative information, a comparative analysis can be used. In other words, for each of the therapeutic categories indicated, an organization can compare its data with local or national utilization data in that therapeutic category to determine whether that organization's data falls within acceptable limits.

Success with any program of DUR demands a management information system capable of providing thorough and accurate information. The ability to tie in all components of the information, not just information from the pharmacy, to analyze the entire picture will ensure therapeutically and financially beneficial decisions. Differences in therapeutic utilization are driven by various factors; it should not be inferred that inappropriate utilization is always the cause. Both local and national dynamics, and patient demographics need to be considered before assumptions are made and action taken.

AUDITS

Often receiving less attention than more common cost management methods, the auditing process is extremely important to the managed care pharmacy benefit. The auditing function is performed essentially for fraud and abuse detection. Fraud can be perpetrated by members as well as providers. Reports focusing on the following should ensure that reasonable attempts to identify fraud are in place:

- generic utilization by pharmacy
- number of prescriptions dispensed costing more than $100 per prescription
- number of prescriptions dispensed indicating DAW

Although abuse generally is unintentional, sometimes it is not. From a quality of care standpoint, and certainly from a cost management perspective, providers and members abusing the system need to be identified and dealt with. Thanks to today's on-line electronic claims processing systems, abuse is becoming increasingly difficult to commit. Most MCOs are requiring pharmacies to have the on-line capability of checking for duplicate prescriptions, prescriptions filled too soon, and multiple providers.

Organizations should also conduct audits to ensure the integrity of the volume purchase or rebate contracting program. The pharmaceutical industry is aware of the possibility of fraud on the part of the provider and the potential for paying rebates for medications that are not dispensed. A successful total audit program should include detection of fraud or abuse by providers and members and protection when pharmaceutical industry rebate contracts exist.

MANAGEMENT OF QUALITY

Quantitative DUR deals with generics, formularies, dispensing fees, and other efforts to ensure cost-effective prescription drug benefits. One necessity is the ability to reduce pharmacy costs without compromising quality. Accomplishing this requires an efficient and reliable data system, quality assurance and utilization review processes, and assessment according to standards.

Defining quality has always been difficult. Most often it is a subjective rather than an objective measure. MCOs must ensure the provision of safe and effective drug therapy to health plan members. A structured program with continuous collection and analysis of information, in conjunction with authority to compare this information against a previously established standard, ensures the quality of the pharmaceutical benefit program. While many of today's MCOs seem to focus only on cost, the most successful MCOs manage cost by focusing on the quality of care as well.

Therapeutics

Drug Formulary

A well-managed drug formulary process can ensure the quality of the drug formulary document and is a critical component of the overall quality process. Drug formulary decisions should compare the therapeutic advantages of products before considering their relative costs. This review process includes the following:

- *Product therapeutic review*: The comparative review of the therapeutic advantages of one product over another (ie, the indications, the uniqueness, and the value of this product compared to the therapeutic alternatives available to physicians). Those drugs offering little or no therapeutic advantage may be rejected unless there is a significant cost advantage.
- *Pharmaceutics*: The characteristics of the drug in terms of its absorption and metabolism. The therapeutic advantage of a long-acting versus a short-acting drug preparation needs to be determined. The therapeutic evaluation should consider dosing frequencies; once-a-day therapy is typically more expensive than multiple daily dosing. If, in fact, dosing several times throughout the day will not affect the quality of the care, this determination can then be part of the cost containment strategy.
- *Side effects/adverse effects*: The likelihood of adverse effects for each product should be compared. Patient tolerance or intolerance to the medication means that compliance will be questionable. The drug formulary should assure the prescriber that the adverse effect profile of this medication has been considered and that a determination of appropriateness for drug formulary status has been attained. These types of formulary assessments are relatively easy to make, and the literature comparing products is readily available.
- *Effectiveness*: For some products in new therapeutic categories, there are serious concerns about overall effectiveness. Typically, these are biotechnology products, or those for previously untreatable conditions. Many of these are released with poor or limited documentation of efficacy (and sometimes safety), because of public pressure to make available something that "might help." Formulary committees have significant challenges in dealing with these products. They need to balance patient and provider demand with the possibility that for some patients, these drugs may do more harm than good.

Step Therapy

Step therapy is a mechanism often employed successfully within staff model MCOs but more difficult to institute in IPA models. Step therapy refers to the steps that a physician is encouraged to follow when prescribing medications to treat a specific illness: for example, unless the treatment modality is part of step 1, it should not be instituted without justification. Step 1 for hypertension could be salt restriction, weight reduction, and exercise. If this fails to lower blood pressure, step 2 could be choosing any medication within the therapeutic categories of thiazide diuretics, or beta blockers. Step 3 might include angiotensin-converting enzyme inhibitors or calcium channel blockers. If these fail, step 4 would be the addition of another drug from the step 2 category, and step 5 could be the introduction of medication choices from other therapeutic categories.

Step therapy typically is designed according to nationally or community-accepted criteria, often developed by the National Standards Committee on Therapeutic Modalities. These step therapies can also be adapted institutionally and often become a standard of practice for the community. The difficult political aspect of step therapies is that physicians often interpret them as dictatorial, imposing on their freedom to practice medicine. Claiming that individualization of patient care often runs counter to step therapy, some physicians will refuse to follow or even acknowledge step therapy but rather will insist on practicing medicine according to the standards and guidelines with which they are more familiar. Step therapy is being incorporated into prescribing according to outcome criteria.

The concept of disease management (see Part X) is related to step therapy in that experts determine the best approach to a disease, outlining successive strategies that can be used to control increasingly resistant candidates. Members of the pharmaceutical industry are intensely interested in disease management because they hope that it can be their entry point into more sophisticated relationships with managed care systems. To date, results of pharmaceutical companies' efforts to enter the disease management business have been mixed, primarily because of mistrust on the part of some MCOs.

Community Standards

Like step therapies, community standards imply an identifiable standard by which physicians are to prescribe. Unlike step therapy, however, community standards are often more subjective than objective. It is difficult to determine how one establishes a community standard. These standards may be determined according to accumulated data, which essentially means that community standards are similar to the community norm, or they could be determined by a representative group of specialists in a particular area who blatantly state that treating a medical problem in a manner different from their recommended way does not meet an acceptable standard of care.

Ensuring the quality of a managed pharmacy benefit program requires attention to community standards. Possibly more from a feasibility and dependability perspective, utilizing expertise in the community to determine standards allows the MCO to defend its decisions. Many physicians and attorneys discourage the use of prescribing according to community standards. They point out the lack of organization in determining these standards and the potential inappropriateness of this method. Nonetheless, the practice of medicine according to community standards utilizes patterns that the community has deemed credible.

Outcomes Management

Outcomes management measures and compares the effect of ordinary medical care on a patient's quality of life. Undoubtedly, outcome information will be part of both cost management and quality of care programs within MCOs. Decisions will be easier, and much more defensible, with enhanced credibility if they are based on outcomes. The public will be better assured that the pharmacy benefit not only is safe and effective but will result in a more positive outcome. To date, little is known about how expenditures for pharmaceutical therapeutic agents can positively affect health care outcomes compared to other treatments. As the information accumulates, the data are analyzed and the results disseminated, but progress has been disappointing.

It is anticipated that the results will show the pharmaceutical logic of interventions that improve both cost and the outcomes of health care. As new medications emerge, the value of the outcome will be weighed against the cost of the therapy. Reimbursement for new and expensive agents may be denied unless the quality of therapeutics based on outcome has been demonstrated. Justification for coverage of high-cost drugs will be an increasingly difficult and data-intensive task but will ensure quality of care. Outcomes are discussed in detail in Part XI.

Patient/Member Expectations of the Pharmacy Provider

The primary expectation of an MCO's members is that, when they present a prescription to the pharmacist, the prescription will be filled accurately and is indicated as a treatment modality for the problem with which they presented to their physician. Although members are not directly involved with the quality assurance process that ensures that these expectations are met, they believe there is a process in place to protect the quality of that service. Physician credentials dictate whether they are eligible to participate in health plans, but health plans check the credentials of pharmacies, not pharmacists. The regulatory agencies appointed by the state ensure the competency of the practitioner pharmacist.

Similarly, the assurance of the quality of the pharmacy is also often overseen by a state regulatory agency. Within the pharmacy practice acts of each state, specific qualifications are described for a pharmacy to meet the licensing requirements. Some plans have elected to go beyond this, requiring certain quality of care enhancements such as 24-hour service, and on-line utilization review programs. Each of these enhancements forces the plan to walk a tighter line between deeply discounting a pharmacy network and increasing the services required of the pharmacist and at the pharmacy. The best indicators of lack of quality in pharmacy services are obtained by audits, as addressed earlier in this chapter, and by encouraging member feedback concerning service at the participating pharmacy.

Managed Care Organization Expectations of the Pharmacy Provider

Like the member, the plan expects the pharmacist to dispense the prescription accurately and in a cost-effective manner. Additionally, the plan requires the pharmacist to follow all aspects of the contract between the plan and the pharmacy. In other words, all policies and procedures addressed in the pharmacy contract must be adhered to.

The plan also often expects the pharmacy to participate in a utilization review program, audit processes, and other services of value to the plan. If this is the case, the plan will have expectations of the pharmacy beyond the normal dispensing of prescriptions in a quality manner in exchange for an agreed-upon reimbursement rate.

Point-of-Service Review

The increasing popularity of point-of-service claims adjudication has made it more likely that utilization review will soon go on line. One does not have to think too far ahead to imagine a situation where a prescription will be entered into an on-line claims adjudication system, the reason for the medical intervention will be checked via compatible information systems, and the appropriateness of the medication prescribed for that medical intervention will be analyzed. Currently, on-line point-of-service systems at least check for drug–drug interactions; age, sex, and pregnancy interactions; therapeutic duplication; and allergies.

QUALITATIVE DRUG UTILIZATION REVIEW

Earlier in this chapter we addressed the quantitative aspects of DUR, which focus on cost containment. The other aspect is qualitative DUR. The properties of qualitative DUR are the following:

- criteria- or standard-based processing
- determination of the appropriateness of drug therapy prescribing and dispensing
- direct relationship between information generated and the quality of patient care

In starting the process of qualitative DUR, objectives need to be identified and stated. Criteria for drug use need to be created that define quality and standards for measurement. Data are then collected and analyzed. When there is failure to meet criteria, causes are identified. Subsequently, an intervention takes place, and there should be a reassessment of the results of that intervention. If necessary, the original objectives are modified. There is then documentation and dissemination of the DUR process and results.

As an example, consider a drug interaction. The objective is to perform concurrent DUR of a drug interaction and to inform pharmacies and prescribers of the presence of this interaction. By using criteria defining quality standards, an organization collects the information to identify patients who are receiving the drugs in combination and then notifies physicians who have prescribed this drug, informing them of the problem. Lastly, the organization monitors the results and then documents and disseminates this information.

Qualitative DUR can be directed at the member, physician, or pharmacy—and performed prospectively, concurrently, or retrospectively. Today, the approach is usually retrospective, primarily because of the lack of sophistication of on-line electronic point-of-service systems in providing the necessary information to do concurrent utilization and because the majority of the data currently are in a retrospective format. The exceptions would be for drug interactions, allergies, and duplicate therapy.

The following are the elements necessary to provide a qualitative DUR program:

- electronic point-of-sale review of drug therapy to alert the dispensing pharmacists of a potential problem
- retrospective data analysis (patient, prescriber, or pharmacy specific) to identify and evaluate concerns
- clinically based screening criteria that use decision-tree analysis
- evaluation of drug therapy for specific targeted populations
- definition of mechanisms for intervention and follow-up to identify problems
- definition of mechanisms to assess the impact of intervention
- integration of DUR with other databases providing medical diagnosis and financial cost

There are definitely some challenges to conducting a quality-driven DUR program. To utilize successfully the combination of quantitative and qualitative review to provide a safe and cost-effective pharmacy benefit program to members, the following must be addressed:

- Technology needs to be available to a plan-performed qualitative DUR, both concurrently and prospectively.
- There must be a shift from case review analysis to drug therapy process intervention.
- Too much time is spent analyzing cases; action must be taken more quickly.
- Currently, the patient and pharmacist are at the center of concurrent DUR intervention and managed care environments. The prescriber must be brought into the loop.
- We need to develop patient outcome–driven DURs. Outcome is the next logical step after quality assurance. Realistically, it is difficult to make cost-effective determinations without knowing outcomes.

MEASUREMENT OF SUCCESS

The success of a pharmacy benefit program's managers can be judged on two criteria: the overall ability to manage the cost of that program, and the consistency of the quality.

Pharmacy benefit program managers must manage costs based on their ability to maintain pharmaceutical expenditures within a predetermined budget. Without a doubt, their emphasis should be not only on managing costs but on reducing costs. Cost containment programs drive the budget each year. A portion of the pharmaceutical expenditure, the manufacturer's cost, is becoming more predictable. The utilization factor, that is, the shifting in utilization trends from less expensive to more expensive therapeutics to treat the same illnesses, is becoming more difficult to predict and typically has a bigger impact. You can consider that you are practicing successful cost management, or cost containment, if in fact you continue under budget in a pharmacy benefit as well as maintain pharmaceutical indicator costs (PMPM, ingredient costs, and prescription costs) at or under the national average for an MCO like yours. Anything less than this should be considered an inability to manage appropriately and should give the plan manager an incentive to find new management support for the pharmacy benefit program.

Some leading-edge plans now look at pharmacy expenses in light of total health care expenses. The emphasis is not on reducing each line item cost (eg, drugs, laboratory, radiology, emergency visits, etc), but on the bottom line. They have recognized that the goal should be to maximize the return on investment made in each cost center. As such, drug costs may go up, but if managed appropriately, total costs will go down because effective drug use will decrease hospital stays, emergency visits, and so on.

Quality is a much more difficult parameter by which to measure success. Certainly, the DUR programs addressed earlier in this chapter will help and, if followed, will provide the documentation for any internal or external agency requiring it. Because quality is often such a subjective entity, however, the development of subjective criteria to determine quality is helpful. A program's success can be determined in part by these subjective criteria. Again, utilizing the averages or norms found in similar plans for member utilization, beyond the cost of the service, will help ensure and document a successful, quality of care–driven pharmacy benefit program. Simply taking the information available, via a retrospective information system, comparing it with similar information from other plans, and then documenting action taken to investigate, and change if necessary, inappropriateness in the pharmacy benefit will ensure that high quality.

PHARMACY BENEFIT MANAGEMENT: NEXT PHASE

This chapter has attempted to point out the future of pharmacy benefit programs. There will be three core trends, each of which will significantly affect the success and even the continuance of coverage of prescription drugs in the future.

We Will Be Paying More Attention to Truly Managing Costs, Not Cost Shifting

In the past few years, we have implemented many successful methods for managing the pharmacy benefit cost profile. We have moved to an on-line claims and adjudication system, we have increased significantly the utilization of generics, we pay pharmacists according to a MAC schedule for generic medication, we have instituted drug formularies, we have successfully negotiated discounts from the pharmaceutical manufacturers, and we have discounted our pharmacy networks. Even so, drug costs continue to increase at percentages that are considered inappropriate. The reason is, quite simply, cost shifting. For example, the increase in the numbers of drugs within each therapeutic category is staggering. One only needs to look at the angiotensin-converting enzyme inhibitor category, the calcium channel blocker drugs, or the cephalosporin category to realize that the list of medications available to treat the same medical problems can sometimes read like a menu in a restaurant.

Statistics indicate that with each new therapeutic entity within a category, the utilization does not just divide among the group but actually increases overall. In other words, with each new drug that is marketed within a therapeutic category, utilization of medications within that therapeutic category increases manyfold. We can no longer continue to add therapeutic entities of all kinds to our drug formularies. Medications that offer no therapeutic benefit will not be allowed formulary status, and as the utilization begins to increase, criteria will be developed by which the offending medication will be eliminated.

Prior Authorization Will Increase, and Usual and Customary Prescribing Will Fade Away

As medication types, medication capabilities, and medication expenses all increase, the only way to manage the utilization of the most expensive medications is by the prior authorization process. Many drugs today, all of which are presumably better than previously available medications to treat similar medical problems, do not need the formulary or nonformulary status. Many medications are valuable for a certain population, and our current system of a product being either covered or not covered is becoming inappropriate. Hence, there is a need for a prior authorization process for many of these medications.

To make the prior authorization process feasible, from both an administrative and a compliance standpoint, we must be able to develop an acceptable and easy system. On a local level, this means accessibility to MCO case managers to ensure the appropriate application of the prior authorization process. On a national scope, this means telephone access by toll-free numbers to centrally located case managers. In both cases, the cooperation of the provider, including the pharmacist and the physician, is a must. We will not be able to continue using our current approach.

Outcomes Information Will Be Used To Make Decisions

Adequate resources will be available to develop sound outcome methodologies. Large-scale measurement of health outcomes, with feedback to all decision makers, will help ensure that quality is maintained and costs are managed. Drug costs are increasing at a faster rate than other health care costs, and these inflationary trends are not compatible with the continuance of coverage for a pharmacy benefit service. Therapeutic decisions in our managed care environment will be based on results as identified in outcomes.

CONCLUSION

The purchasers of the managed care benefit seek both quality and price. Expectations run high, and pressure is tremendous to keep the costs at a minimum while meeting these high expectations. Reimbursement for services continues to be a focal point of disagreement between the MCO and the provider. The pharmaceutical industry has recently experienced for the first time hands-on intervention by the federal government into its pricing policies. The past years have noted significant efforts to manage the costs of the pharmacy benefit. DUR, subsequent outcome results, action plans, and implementation of these action plans will dictate the future.

REFERENCES

1. Vagelos PR. Are prescription drug prices high? *Science.* 1991;252(5010):1080–1084.
2. Ciba-Geneva. *Pharmacy Benefit Report, 1995, Facts and Figures.* Geneva, Switzerland: Ciba-Geneva; 1995.
3. Atlas R. Editorial. *Drug Benefit Trends.* 1992;4:3.

HENRY F. BLISSENBACH, PHARMD, was president of Diversified Pharmaceutical Services, a subsidiary company of SmithKline Beecham Corporation in Minneapolis, Minnesota. He also holds an academic appointment in the College of Pharmacy at the University of Minnesota. Dr. Blissenbach is a member of the American Society of Hospital Pharmacists, the American Pharmacy Association, and the American College of Clinical Pharmacy, and has been actively involved in an advisory capacity with many pharmaceutical manufacturers and managed care entities. He has published numerous articles on the cost containment of pharmaceuticals and disease management with therapeutics.

PETER PENNA, PHARMD, is vice president of managed pharmacy for CIGNA HealthCare, based in Hartford, Connecticut. His area of expertise is pharmacy benefit design and management as part of comprehensive health care systems in staff, IPA, and PPO models.

Part X

Disease Management and Selected Clinical Conditions in Disease Management

The chapters presented in Part X fall into three basic categories. First is an overview of disease management. Many activities claim the title, but there is a constellation of coordinated care management that truly defines disease management. The second broad category of chapters is a discussion of selected diseases or clinical conditions that are effectively managed through disease management. There are clearly many more conditions than are discussed here, but for space reasons we have limited our discussion to three. Lastly, there is a chapter devoted to the issue of how the effectiveness of disease management is actually measured. Much of disease management has taken place with the belief that the benefits are self-evident, and this may not always be the case.

Part X also contains a discussion of the management of behavioral health and chemical dependency services. In general, these areas are amenable to disease management, though by no means are they clearly delineated. Therefore, attributes of both disease management and more traditional approaches to medical management are represented here.

Chapter 27

Fundamentals and Core Competencies of Disease Management

David W. Plocher

Chapter Outline

- Definition
- Definition Clarification
- Barriers and Drivers for Disease Management
- Business Plan
- Survey of Disease Management Programs
- Important Linkages
- Case Study
- Conclusion

DEFINITION

Disease management is a prospective, disease-specific approach to delivering health care that spans all encounter sites and augments the physician's visits with interim management through nonphysician practitioners, emphasizing education of members (through self-care) and physicians (through guidelines) and applied to chronic illnesses managed medically.

I thank several colleagues for their role in the survey used to create Figure 27–5: Linda Davis, Walter Elias, Nancy Spangler, and Mary Ann Huseth.

This chapter is adapted from DW Plocher, Disease Management, in *The Managed Health Care Handbook*, 3rd ed, PR Kongstvedt, ed, pp 318–329, © 1996, Aspen Publishers, Inc.

DEFINITION CLARIFICATION

Disease management has been the subject of hundreds of publications and conferences since the publication of a chapter on this topic in *The Managed Health Care Handbook,* 3rd Edition. This chapter will not attempt to review or summarize that information. Instead, I will refer readers to two excellent metaanalyses: a recent text on disease management, edited by Todd and Nash,[1] and a peer-reviewed document on chronic illness management by Von Korff et al.[2]

Disease management differs from conventional medical management and conventional hospital-based case management. Characteristics specific to disease management include the following:

- Physicians are no longer the center of caregiving. Instead, they are members of a caregiving team.
- Nonphysician practitioners deliver most of the care.
- Nearly all care is delivered in the ambulatory care setting.
- Guidelines and outcome measures are more condition specific than body system specific.
- Care is delivered more often over the telephone (including interactive voice response) and the Internet and less often in home and office visits. Medicaid subscribers may be

an exception to this type of care if they have limited access to telephones.
- To produce positive changes in members' health status, organizations focus more on education—member and physician behavior change—and less on highly advanced, highly technical, invasive medical procedures.
- Conditions that show modifiable variability in resource use (eg, prescription drug nonadherence) or morbidity (eg, emergency department visits for asthmatics) are preferred for disease management.
- Data must be collected from all sites of care annually (certain conditions may have shorter episode definitions).
- Fee-for-service physicians and hospitals are not financially rewarded for good disease management in most environments, though satisfied patients are less likely to switch physicians, and the contracting arms of purchasers and payers view these lower-cost providers as a better buy.

This list does not mention all components of disease management, such as the fundamentals of guidelines and outcomes. These components, reviewed in the above references, existed long before the term *disease management* was coined. As this list may suggest, renal dialysis centers and certain managed behavioral health services have displayed most of the features of disease management long before the term was conceived.

Disease management is not primary prevention, population health, or community health. The goal of disease management is more modest: to reduce frequency and severity of exacerbations of a chronic illness so that readmission costs are reduced.

Two historic phenomena may clarify the origin of some of disease management's distinguishing features. First, managed care organizations have struggled to improve their medical loss ratios. Our half-century-old group and staff models believed in the virtue of primary prevention, but added major emphasis on secondary and tertiary prevention over the past 10 years, for economic reasons (Figure 27–1). Secondary and tertiary prevention efforts can yield greater savings than primary prevention efforts.

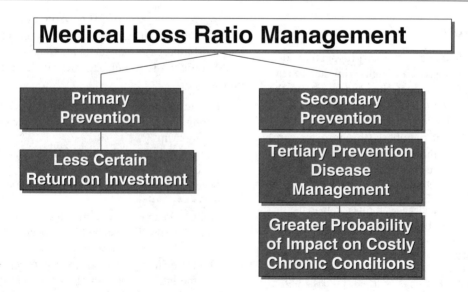

Figure 27–1 The Origins of Disease Management Medical Loss Ratio Management

Second, there has been a long-standing tendency to focus medical management on the acute inpatient stay, leaving ambulatory utilization costs unchecked. Figures 27–2, 27–3, and 27–4 offer three separate perspectives supporting this contention. Costs of noncatastrophic recurring care, diagnostic X-ray charges, laboratory charges, and other costs outside the acute inpatient stay have risen significantly over the past few decades.

In fact, ambulatory visits result in many more physician–member encounters than inpatient hospitalizations do. The probability of interacting with a member is shown by a mathematic ratio of encounter sites. The average annual interaction with providers is:

- for hospitalization: 70 admissions/1,000 members/year
- for ambulatory MD office visits: 4,000 encounters/1,000 members/year

In addition to learning to focus on ambulatory as well as inpatient care costs, disease management experts are finally learning from models in general industry that describe supply chain management with concentration more on annual cost than on unit cost. For example, a heart failure program's prescription drug costs may rise slightly but be more than offset by the larger decrease in total care costs.

BARRIERS AND DRIVERS FOR DISEASE MANAGEMENT

Todd and Nash[1] and Von Korff et al[2] offer thorough discussions of the barriers to and drivers of disease management programs. Some of the most important drivers include

- fragmented delivery system
- reimbursement favoring component care delivery
- information system incompatibility

There are many important drivers for disease management programs as well.

- a rise in risk sharing contracting
- information systems that are beginning to collect data across all settings
- a desire for more useful guidelines
- a desire to improve continuous quality improvement techniques
- purchaser and payer interest in and requirements for proof of value

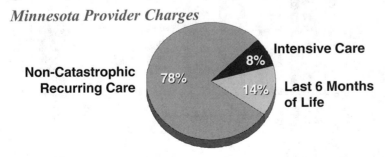

"Rising health care costs may stem more from the proliferation of laboratory tests than from the often-cited budgetary burdens of technological advances or treatment of the gravely ill."

Minnesota Provider Charges

Figure 27–2 The Origins of Disease Management (Analysis in 1983 by Minnesota Medical Association)

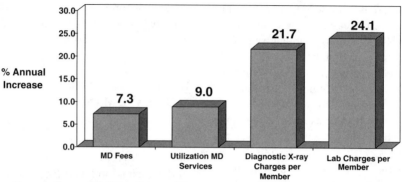

Figure 27–3 Physician Spending, Private Health Insurance. *Source:* Reprinted from Z Dyckman, Physician Cost Experience under Private Health Insurance Programs, *Health Care Financing Review*, Vol 13, No 3, pp 85–96, 1992, Health Care Financing Administration.

BUSINESS PLAN

A list of key program elements to remember while composing the business plan for the disease management initiative is shown in Exhibit 27–1. From strategic plan/governance to benefit design, marketing and sales issues to education, there is much to consider.

SURVEY OF DISEASE MANAGEMENT PROGRAMS

A group of researchers and I recently interviewed the operators of 24 disease management programs. Our questions searched for the characteristics of each site that contributed to its success. Here is a summary of the composite of proficien-

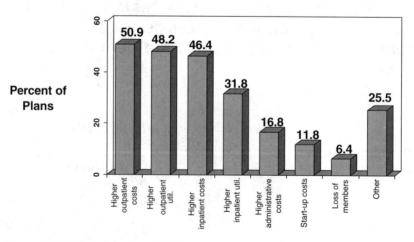

Figure 27–4 Reasons for 1988 Net Loss from Health Maintenance Organization Operations. Courtesy of Interstudy.

Exhibit 27-1 Program Elements for Disease Management Business Plan

- Strategic plan/governance
- Provider network development
- Capitalization/ownership
- Benefit design
- Structure/model
    - Emergency department/management observation rooms
    - Inpatient (hospital) management
    - Ambulatory clinic management
    - Pharmacy management
- Marketing and sales
    - Employer groups
    - Local health plans
        1. Fee for service
        2. Capitation
    - Medicaid/Medicare
    - Individuals
- Enrollment, billing, and collection
    - Member verification
    - Claims submission and collection
- Patient access to services
    - 24-hour nurseline
- Education
    - Telephone-based and mailed information
    - On-site intervention
- Community intervention
    - Community programs
    - Worksite programs
    - School programs
- Case management and clinical guidelines
    - Inpatient
    - Ambulatory
- Entry/discharge from program
    - Identification/patient profile
    - Education
    - Follow-up
    - Outcome definition
- Information management
    - Ability to identify targeted members through claims, pharmacy data, and risk surveys
    - Disease-specific provider databases
    - Ability to automate reminders
    - Automated tracking of members
- Data collection and outcome evaluation
    - Emergency department visits and hospital days/1,000 members
    - Patient clinical status indicators
    - Patient functional status indicators
    - Patient knowledge and self-management skills
    - Physician/patient compliance with treatment guidelines
    - Patient's perceived value of mailed materials
    - Patient satisfaction
- Reporting
    - Clinical outcomes—ability to generate provider reports
    - Financial outcomes

Courtesy of Ernst & Young LLP.

cies. (Within each proficiency, we have developed detailed scoring criteria with numeric thresholds, but these details are not presented here.)

- implementation: speed to market, successful implementation
- management tools: automated tracking, ticklers, guidelines, surveillance for outcomes, provider profiles
- staff: adequate staffing ratios for nonphysician practitioners managing a given cohort of patients
- organizational integration: roles and processes defined, no duplication of effort, few handoffs, no silos (eg, case managers, utilization managers, disease managers, and demand managers work together and have systems and tools that connect to each other's activities)
- marketing and sales: successfully sold to multiple groups, regionally or nationally
- targeting tools: accuracy, predictive validity independently established, automated; optimal use of surveys and pharmacy and claims data
- stratification tools: accuracy, predictive validity independently established, designed to prompt interventions for optimal outcomes
- guideline validity: high quality of evidence

- member behavior change: method based on behavior change models including learning style, readiness to change, and efficacy; interventions targeted and customized; maintenance strategy
- physician behavior change: behavior change based on research including aligned incentives, academic detailing, feedback
- outcomes collected: automated collection, both process and endpoints, including utilization, satisfaction, functional status, and clinical indicators
- reported outcomes: results frequently reported, sustained or improved outcomes
- return on investment (ROI): costs and benefits measured, positive return within fewer than 3 years

When studying a new program, a snapshot of strengths and weaknesses can be assembled in the form of a spider diagram, as in Figure 27–5. The spider diagram is an easy and clear way to compare health care providers against "best of breed" performance.

We see the next generation of disease management programs evolving with two added characteristics:

1. Care managers will improve coordination of services for a patient with *multiple* chronic diseases.
2. Care managers will become more reluctant to carve out services to a separate, outsourced vendor, believing that the continuity of care for these complex patients is better served with a carved-in model.

IMPORTANT LINKAGES

In Figure 27–6, the fit for disease management within the spectrum of services following member enrollment is summarized.

The operational detail inside the disease discovery and follow-up processes is exemplified as follows. After the disease is discovered, it should be classified by risk level (mild, moderate, or severe), and appropriate intervention should follow. Risk level is determined by

- how well the patient understands the disease
- how well the patient learns
- how well the patient cooperates with the provider
- severity of illness measures (International Classification of Diseases, Ninth Edition, Clinical Modification [ICD-9-CM] codes)

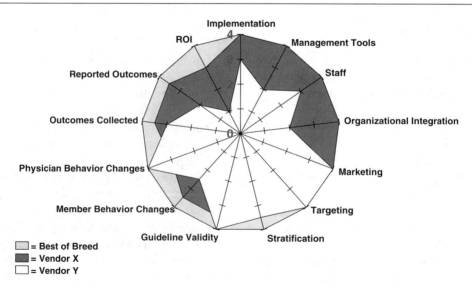

Figure 27–5 Disease Management Capabilities. Courtesy of Ernst & Young LLP.

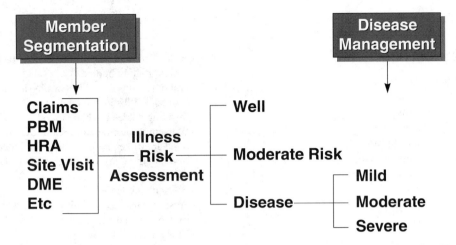

Figure 27–6 Important Linkages. *Note:* DME, durable medical equipment; HRA, health risk appraisal; PBM, pharmacy benefits management. Courtesy of Ernst & Young LLP.

- the patient's resource use patterns (incorrect administration of medications, excess emergency department use)
- modifiability of course of disease

Next, in an outbound phone call to the patient, the caller should interview the patient. The number of questions can vary greatly; up to 180 questions (45-minute duration) can occur. The caller should try to determine the patient's level of knowledge and then educate the patient about self-care techniques, symptoms and signs to watch for at home, and who to call or where to go for help as certain changes occur.

Several types of intervention are possible:

- mild risk—mail education materials
- moderate risk—phone and mail communication to provider
- severe risk—dedicate home care team specializing in the disease

CASE STUDY

A congestive heart failure (CHF) program that I recently designed with other professionals is summarized in Exhibit 27–2. See Chapter 28 for additional perspectives on disease management of CHF.

In this case, we were asked by a private, 420-bed hospital in the northeastern United States to assist in formulating its response to new market pressures. The payers were no longer as concerned about length of hospital stay for CHF as they were about annual care costs. The chief executive officer met with us and agreed to fund the start-up of an expanded case management program with a home care emphasis for CHF.

We conducted multiple site visits for discussions with physicians, nurses, and ancillary care services, including training on disease management fundamentals. We then moved from these fundamentals into specifications that were unique for CHF and agreed on the following program elements (a partial list):

- structure
- practice guidelines
- data elements
- functional status scale
- behavior change techniques

Initially, the referring physicians were not supportive. The fee-for-service environment would result in loss of revenue to them whenever they referred a patient. However, after further educational sessions, some movement began to occur in their attitudes.

Exhibit 27–2 Design of a CHF Program

THE BEGINNING

- Began in August 1996
- Referral sources:
  - Physicians
  - Discharge planners
  - Home health care
- Multidisciplinary team
  - Pharmacist
  - Dietitian
  - Social worker
  - Chaplain

THE PROCESS

- Initial assessment
  - Registered nurse (RN) collects recent data on patient's use of hospital, emergency department, physician office
  - RN administers the Minnesota *Living with Heart Failure* questionnaire
- Concurrent care
  - RN on call 7 days/week, 12 hours/day
  - Patient calls RN directly
  - RN can do in home
    1. Pulse oximetry
    2. Blood draws
    3. ECG
    4. IV Lasix or Bumex
  - The CHF hotline
  - CHF support group

HOTLINE TIPS FOR URGENT CARE

(*not* a substitute for 911 for extreme, catastrophic emergencies)

- Given detailed home diary for events to track and triggers for dialing hotline
- Excerpt of reasons to call RN or physician
  - Gained 2–5 lbs in 2–4 days
  - Swelling ankles or abdomen
  - Worsening shortness of breath (SOB)
  - Sudden awakening from sleep with SOB
  - Needing more pillows to raise head when trying to sleep
  - Worsening cough
  - Persistent nausea, vomiting, diarrhea
  - New or worsening dizziness
  - New fatigue with exertion
  - Loss of appetite

CASE STUDY

- 86-year-old female with CHF
- Prior to CHF program (6 ER visits in 6 months)
- Following entry into CHF program (no ER visits in 3 months)
- Typical intervention
  - Case manager found 4-lb gain and worsening SOB
  - Home visit did ECG, blood work, oximetry, and IV Lasix

RESULTS

- Patients like it (more comfortable calling in a question to the RN than their physician)
- Physicians liked it—eventually
  - Now referring "difficult" patients
  - Phone call volume to physician reduced
  - Perceived as an extension of physician office rather than a separate home health care or hospital program

---

The results are encouraging. Over 75 patients have been through the program. Preliminary analysis shows that there is value in directing staff and resources toward the more severely ill CHF patients. Using the New York Heart Association classification, we found that the 25 Class III patients showed the largest improvement, reducing by over 50% their hospital admits and total hospital days. Interestingly, the 25 Class IV patients did not reduce resource use, perhaps confirming one of the requirements for disease management offered earlier in the chapter: the circumstances of the patient must be *modifiable*. Similarly, Class I and II patients (the remaining 25) did not change hospital use, as mildly ill patients are usually managed in the ambulatory setting.

CONCLUSION

A final caution for the attendee of the next disease management conference. Beware the vendor that dusts off its guidelines or outcome database and repackages it in a presentation titled "disease management." Practice guidelines and outcome measurement have been around for decades. Beware the promotion of a single pharmaceutical agent as the only indicated treatment for the condition. Disease managers will allow for continuous innovation, prompt adoption of blockbuster drugs, and continuous reassessment using pharmacoeconomic analyses. Please skip the lecture on the pathophysiology of the disease for training physicians to manage the patient in the acute hospital setting. Disease management does not occur in the acute inpatient setting; patients are not available for teachable moments while they are intubated. Disease management also does not occur during the 8-minute physician office visit, crammed with the technology of laboratory work, imaging, and so on.

Disease management can occur just about everywhere else. Communication technology is the most important kind of technology; multiple media are available for information transfer 24 hours a day, 365 days a year. The most successful caregivers (many of them nonphysicians) are making a difference through their skill in member assessment and member behavior change techniques.

REFERENCES

1. Todd W, Nash D, eds. *Disease Management: A Systems Approach to Improving Patient Outcomes*. Chicago: American Hospital Publishing, Inc; 1996.

2. Von Korff M, Gruman J, Schaefer J, Curry SJ, Wagner EH. Collaborative management of chronic illness. *Ann Int Med*. 1997;127(12):1097–1102.

Chapter 28

Disease Management of Congestive Heart Failure

George Mayzell

Chapter Outline

- Background
- Disease Management Programs
- Disease Care Continuum
- Population-Based Identification and Confirmation
- Validation and Confirmation
- Stratification and Prioritization
- Interventions
- Cardiac Nurses/Case Management
- ACE Inhibitors
- The Role of the Cardiologists
- Education
- Telemonitoring
- Home Visits
- Outpatient CHF Clinics
- Cardiac Rehabilitation
- Acute Care
- Incentives
- Measurement and Evaluation
- Cost Benefit Analysis
- Conclusion

BACKGROUND

Congestive heart failure (CHF) is one of the most important health problems in terms of morbidity, mortality, and cost.[1-3] Following are some statistics about CHF:

- It affects an estimated 4.8 million Americans and accounts for approximately 400,000 deaths each year.[1]
- It results in nearly 6 million inpatient hospital days each year.[4]
- It produced $17.8 billion in health care costs in 1993.[1]
- CHF is the most expensive medical disorder in the United States.[3]
- In one study, over 47% of CHF patients are readmitted within 90 days of discharge.[3]
- One in 10 people 70 years and older is affected with CHF.[1]

CHF is a condition in which the heart fails to maintain adequate cardiac output. It is usually caused by either a heart attack(s) or long-standing hypertension.[4] CHF usually affects older individuals and has approximately a 10% mortality at the end of 1 year.[1] Fifty percent of all people with CHF will die within 5 years.[1] The typical CHF patient has two to three comorbid conditions, and most are on more than six medications.[3] Of the percentage of CHF patients that visit the emergency department, approximately 90% will be admitted to the hospital.[4] As the US population ages, due to the "graying" of the baby boomer generation, the number of CHF cases is expected to increase to well over 5 million by the year 2030.[1-4]

CHF patients are high cost because of their multiple yearly admissions (usually about 1.5 admissions a year) and their high readmission rate (20% to 47% are readmitted within 90 days).[3] Approximately 35% of all patients with CHF are admitted annually[5] with an average cost of each admission of $6,000.[6] The average length of stay is 7.7 days, including 3 days in the intensive care unit (ICU).[7] There is a large potential for improving care of these individuals, while at the same time saving health care resources (Figure 28–1).[3,8-17]

DISEASE MANAGEMENT PROGRAMS

CHF disease management programs can conclusively provide a positive return on investment. Their success is measured by decreasing admission rates, readmission rates, length of stay, and cost, as well as improving quality of life. These programs seem to work best when they focus on avoiding hospital admissions (and readmissions) even if they increase outpatient care. For example, an Independence Blue Cross plan reduced hospital admission and emergency department (ED) visits by 50% and improved quality of life. This Blue Cross plan estimates it has saved over $1 million in hospital bills for the 250 patients enrolled.[8]

DISEASE CARE CONTINUUM

The CHF disease care continuum is illustrated in Figure 28–2. Disease management programs can start at any point in the continuum and be effective. However, the earlier in the disease process a program starts, the longer the time frame to see a return on investment. But most CHF disease management programs focus on the sickest patients, because in today's managed care environment, it is difficult to start a program early in the continuum. A positive cost benefit analysis or return on investment analysis needs to be seen quickly in this "early era" of disease management, even though focusing on the risk factors of CHF could save more money in the long run, in that fewer patients would develop CHF. Because most programs start with patients well into the disease process, the programs focus on compliance and complication management. As the National Committee for Quality Assurance (NCQA) and other accrediting bodies continue

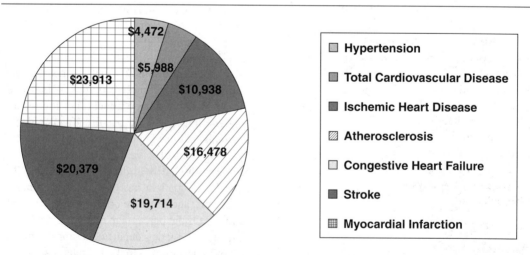

Note: Reported from claims data of $443 million from 1/93 to 12/93 of privately insured individuals. Totals represent hospital and ambulatory care costs combined and averaged among all patients (inpatient, outpatient, or both) with a diagnosis.

Figure 28–1 Average Heart-Related Health Care Claims per CHF Patient. *Source:* MarketScan Database, the MEDSTAT Group, Inc, Ann Arbor, Michigan.

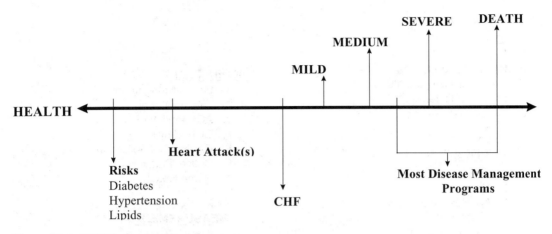

Figure 28–2 CHF Disease Continuum

to make accreditation more demanding, health plans will be compelled to expand these programs to focus on the entire CHF population and the disease-specific prevention arena.

As Figure 28–2 illustrates, starting with risk factor modification would appear to offer advantages. However, it would take several years to see results. Starting farther to the right in the diagram means a shorter time frame and more easily measurable short-term results. With resource limits as they are, most programs place their emphasis to the far right side of the diagram with the sickest of the CHF patients. These are the patients with multiple admissions, low quality of life, and high levels of morbidity and mortality. Currently, patients with mild and easily controllable CHF are often not part of disease management programs. This is changing as proof of program effectiveness is documented.

POPULATION-BASED IDENTIFICATION AND CONFIRMATION

The first step in any CHF disease management program is to identify patients with the disease (Figure 28–3). Using a population-based approach, this identification process is much more difficult than it sounds. Administrative data (ie, claims data) are most often used to make an initial determination.

Administrative data include all of the physician office encounter forms (usually HFCA 1500s with International Classification of Diseases, Ninth Edition [ICD-9] codes and CPT codes) and hospital Uniform Billing forms, which include diagnosis-related groups (DRGs). These forms are fraught with inaccuracy, partially because of the informality with which coding is usually done, particularly in physician offices. For example, a patient who comes in with symptoms suggestive of heart failure might get the diagnosis of "rule out CHF." When this diagnosis goes through coding, it might then be coded as CHF. It will be picked up in the identification process, even if it turned out the patient had some form of pulmonary disease. Also, the hospital DRG 127 may include some "shock" diagnoses that are not related to CHF. Coding on electrocardiograms and other cardiac tests such as echocardiograms, cardiac catheterizations, and stress tests tends to be presumptive and therefore is best not used.

Additionally, claims data are often not timely. It can easily take approximately 90 days to get claims reports out of the system (partly because claims do not usually come in to the health plan that quickly). Therefore, there is a significant time lag when trying to identify patients quickly and early in their disease course. And when new patients enter the plan with a significant history of CHF, there can also be a delay in available

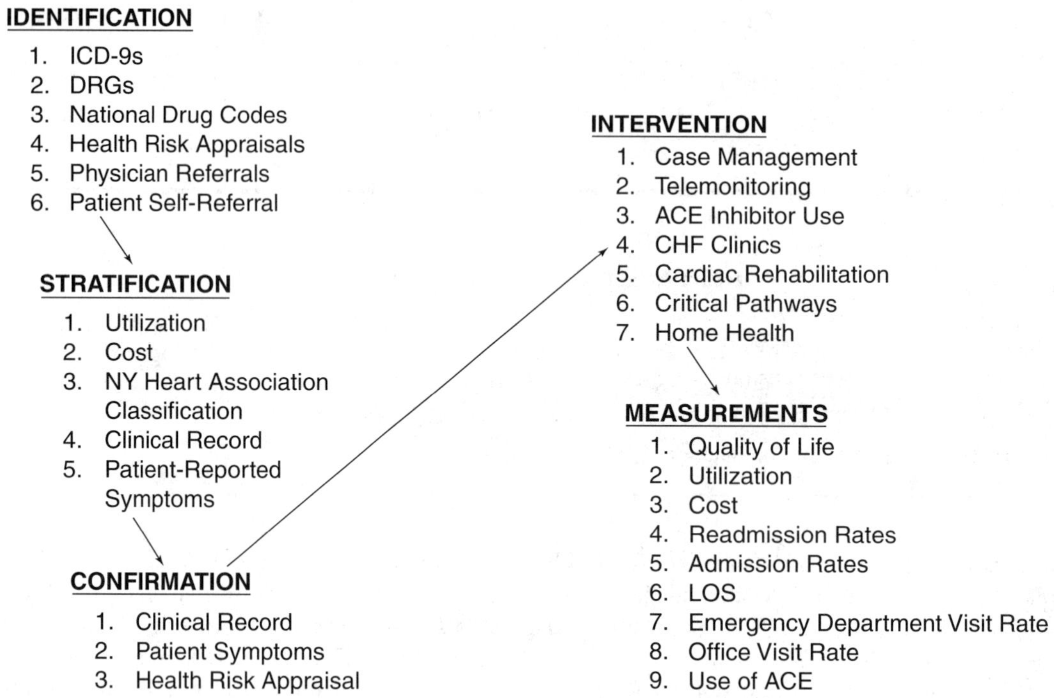

IDENTIFICATION
1. ICD-9s
2. DRGs
3. National Drug Codes
4. Health Risk Appraisals
5. Physician Referrals
6. Patient Self-Referral

STRATIFICATION
1. Utilization
2. Cost
3. NY Heart Association Classification
4. Clinical Record
5. Patient-Reported Symptoms

CONFIRMATION
1. Clinical Record
2. Patient Symptoms
3. Health Risk Appraisal

INTERVENTION
1. Case Management
2. Telemonitoring
3. ACE Inhibitor Use
4. CHF Clinics
5. Cardiac Rehabilitation
6. Critical Pathways
7. Home Health

MEASUREMENTS
1. Quality of Life
2. Utilization
3. Cost
4. Readmission Rates
5. Admission Rates
6. LOS
7. Emergency Department Visit Rate
8. Office Visit Rate
9. Use of ACE

Figure 28–3 Identification and Intervention of CHF Patients

and accurate claims data. Because they are new members, these individuals have no claims history in the system; the history lies in the previous plan's database.

Lastly, it is sometimes difficult to decide which ICD-9 codes to use. Many are straightforward, but it is unclear, for instance, whether one should use right-sided CHF or diastolic dysfunction as identifiers. Most providers have chosen not to use these codes because the treatment is markedly different.[18] Additionally, there is controversy about the diagnosis "cardiomyopathy." Some health plans have found that family practice physicians typically do not consider cardiomyopathy part of the CHF continuum, even though most cardiologists do.

Adding pharmacy data or national drug codes (NDCs) may not help in identification, because diuretics, angiotensin converting enzyme (ACE) inhibitors, and digoxin are used for many other conditions. Some health plans have looked at data with and without mention of each of these drugs (individually or in pairs) and did not find a significant increase in the sensitivity of CHF patient identification. Thus, pharmacy data may not be a strong identifier for CHF patients.

There are two additional ways to help identify patients that can be used in conjunction with, or in lieu of, the above-mentioned methods. The first is using direct patient referrals through health risk appraisals (see Part I). Surveys can be mailed to the entire population or selected population groups and patients self-report if they have CHF and are interested in the program. Surveying can be done in conjunction with other health risk appraisals that may help select patients for other disease management programs or case management. This method is often used in the geriatric population. Another way of identifying these patients is to get physician support and physician referrals. This works best in a tightly affiliated system where incentives encourage physicians to be directly involved in the program. Some programs have found that nurses and hospital financial officers are major referral sources as well.

VALIDATION AND CONFIRMATION

Once the CHF patients are identified, some form of confirmation will need to be done (particularly if administrative data were used to identify the population). The patient diagnosis is confirmed by checking with the physician or patient or looking at a chart review, echocardiogram, muga scan, or cardiac catheterization results. This confirmation is often done at the same time as the stratification and prioritization (Figure 28–4). This is a good time to obtain patient permission to participate in the program. In primary care physician–based managed care plans, permission of the primary care physician is also advisable; in some plans, the CHF patient may even be removed from a primary care physician's panel so that a cardiologist may serve as the patient's primary physician.

STRATIFICATION AND PRIORITIZATION

Typically, resources are the greatest limitation on the types of disease management programs implemented. At this writing, it is an unfortunate fact that more resources cannot be dedicated to these programs. Because of these limitations, most of the time and effort is spent on the sickest patients, since they have the highest and most measurable medical costs. Stratification is a critical part of a disease management program; it ensures that the maximum resources can be dedicated to the sickest patients who will need specialized attention with education, home visits, and case management.

There are several ways to select the "sickest of the sick." The first is to once again use administrative data. Often, the first stratification of the data will be in the form of utilization statistics and financial statistics. A ranking system is created using metrics such as admissions, ED visits, length of stay, cost per stay, outpatient visits, total cost of care, admissions

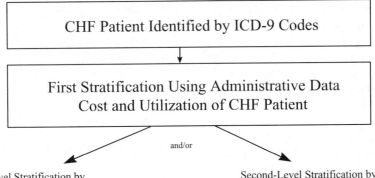

Figure 28–4 Stratification Methods

per year, and number of readmissions in 60 days.

For example, an admission with a diagnosis of CHF is one of the more significant stratification drivers, while a low total cost per patient per year and no admissions would be suggestive of a low-risk patient. Even using these parameters, there is much "noise" in administrative data, including non-CHF high-dollar diagnoses, faulty coding, patients who have died or disenrolled, and the issues of stratifying new patients who are admitted with their first episode of CHF.

This administrative evaluation can tentatively rank patients into low-, medium-, and high-risk categories, after which a telephone call to the patient or physician can confirm the actual clinical or functional status. One of the problems with using administrative data is that past high individual cost or utilization is not always predictive of future utilization or costs. This is a significant limitation in using claims data to stratify patients.

To stratify patients with or without using administrative data initially it is also possible to use clinical parameters. This step employs clinical data to validate that these patients have heart failure and to put them into a clinical or functional stratification. In some staff model health maintenance organizations (HMOs) or programs with close physician alignment, the physician and/or physician's records can give this information.

First of all, one must make sure that the diagnosis of CHF is accurate and that the patient has *systolic* dysfunction. This is difficult, since the symptoms of other diseases may be similar. Administrative data often will not make this differentiation. Chart review or physician input will be necessary for this identification and confirmation. The ejection fraction will be normal in diastolic dysfunction (or higher than symptoms would suggest), and a beta blocker or calcium channel blocker may be used.[18]

The next step is to quantify the clinical severity. One of the most commonly used methods to quantify patient function is to use the New York Heart Classification. This information could be obtained from the medical record, patient interview, or a health risk appraisal (written survey). The classification is as follows[19]:

- *Class I:* Includes patients with cardiac disease but without resulting limitations on physical activity. Ordinary physical activity does not cause undue fatigue, palpitations, dyspnea, or anginal pain.
- *Class II:* Includes patients with cardiac disease resulting in slight limitation of physical activity. The patients are comfortable at rest. Ordinary physical activity results in fatigue, palpitation, dyspnea, or anginal pain.
- *Class III:* Includes patients with cardiac disease resulting in marked limitation of physical activity. The patients are comfortable at rest. Ordinary activity causes fatigue, palpitations, dyspnea, or anginal pain.
- *Class IV:* Includes patients with cardiac disease resulting in inability to carry on any physical activity without discomfort. Symptoms of cardiac insufficiency or of the anginal syndrome may be present even at rest. If any physical activity is undertaken, discomfort is increased.

Another, more accurate way of quantifying the severity of CHF is by use of the cardiac ejection fraction. This is an accurate method clinically, but it is often very difficult to obtain this information. It can be in the cardiologist's chart, the primary care chart, or the hospital records. Furthermore, there may be no recent evaluations of cardiac function.

INTERVENTIONS

There are three broad areas in which an intervention can take place.

1. outpatient, which might include home care, physician education, outpatient CHF clinics, cardiac rehabilitation, telemonitoring, and cardiac case management
2. acute noninpatient cardiac care, which might include acute care in the home setting (see Chapter 22), subacute units that

are set up for acute cardiac care (see Chapter 23), and specialized ED observation units (see Chapter 14)
3. inpatient clinical pathways, with intensive coordination with outpatient care

In comprehensive disease management, several of these programs are often initiated at the same time. There has been little evidence to suggest which interventions work better than others, work best in combination, or are synergistic. A listing of reasons for readmission of patients with CHF is shown below.[20] Attention to these factors is required in the disease management program.*

- lack of compliance with overall treatment plan—64%
- lack of compliance with diet—22%
- lack of compliance with medications—6%
- lack of compliance with diet and medication—37%
- uncontrolled hypertension—44%
- cardiac arrhythmias—29%
- environmental factors—19%
- inadequate therapy—17%
- pulmonary infection—12%
- emotional stress—7%

The type of intervention that is selected often depends on who is setting up the program. In an independent practice association (IPA) model HMO, most programs are centered on case management, telemonitoring, clinical guidelines, and education. Staff model HMOs might be more centered on clinical pathways, CHF clinics, and inpatient care. Pharmacy benefit companies often focus on appropriate drug use and physician and/or patient educational programs (see Chapter 26). Physician incentives are important drivers in any program and will be briefly mentioned below but are beyond the scope of this book.

CARDIAC NURSES/CASE MANAGEMENT

Many programs center around coordinating care through specialized nurses trained in cardiac care. This is often done through case management programs. It can take several months to train a nurse to be an expert in cardiac care. These nurses are the initial intake point for the patient into the disease management program. They take a detailed cardiac history, coordinate with the primary care physician and/or cardiologist, assess the social needs of the patient, and coordinate cardiac education. The nurses often go out and visit the patient and provide hands-on care and physical evaluation. In an IPA model managed care environment, care must be coordinated with home health care nurses. Monitoring daily weight and compliance with diet and medications has been valuable in preventing admissions and readmissions.[21-24]

These specialized cardiac nurses must have a number of resources at their fingertips: access to social services, specialized drug programs, support groups, and other services to help these patients, who are often older and whose social needs heavily influence their medical needs. Many patients run out of medications because of financial limitations or lack of understanding of the medications' importance. Nurses and case managers must have the authority to waive copayments and pharmacy deductibles when appropriate. Transportation problems and loneliness can also contribute to hospitalization risk.

One unique program has mentally competent nursing home residents call CHF patients several times a week. They are trained to ask only two questions. One is about all weights since the last call, and the other is about medication compliance. They are given parameters for which they need to report through a dedicated nurse/case manager should there be medication problems or weights beyond parameters. The average phone call lasted over 20 minutes, suggesting

---

*This list is adapted with permission from J Gahli, Precipitating Factors Leading to Decompensation of Heart Failure Traits among Urban Blacks, *Archives of Internal Medicine*, Vol 148, No 9, pp 2013–2016, © 1988, J Gahli.

that these CHF patients have a significant social need. These patients' admission rates dropped significantly as a result of this simple intervention, which clearly gave residents at the nursing home an important purpose, as well as helping the patients with CHF.[25]

ACE INHIBITORS

Tracking compliance of ACE inhibitor use is critical to any heart failure program. These medications have been proven to improve morbidity and mortality in the CHF patient.[26] The medications save 50 lives and prevent 200 hospital admissions per 1,000 patients treated, and cost only $15,000 a year per life saved according to Dr Marc Thames from the University of Cleveland.[6] In evaluating the use of these drugs, it has been observed that only 30% to 45% of patients with heart failure are actually on these medications.[6] While some of these patients have contraindications (eg, hypotension or allergic reactions), one would still expect the percentage of patients on this medication to be higher. In addition, it is important to educate both the physician and patient on the proper use of these medications in order to increase compliance.

Use of ACE inhibitors is one of the common metrics in a CHF program. It clearly measures a process of care (see Chapter 33), which has been linked to improved outcomes in many studies.[26] Since use of ACE inhibitors can often be captured in the pharmacy claims system, it is an ideal metric that can be measured on the entire CHF population. This process will give you a true population-based improvement initiative. ACE inhibitors are also often prescribed at less than the maximal beneficial dose,[21] and it is felt by most that these medications differ little in terms of their efficacy. The dosing interval may also play a role in patient compliance. Formulary decisions must therefore be made carefully and with coordination of any disease management initiatives.

Other cardiac medication compliance is also important in managing these patients. It is estimated that more than $100 million could be saved annually if cardiac medications were used properly.[6]

THE ROLE OF THE CARDIOLOGISTS

One controversial area of CHF disease management is whether to focus management on the primary care physician or the cardiologist. One of the prime tenets of managed care is that coordination of care should be done through the primary care physician. This model of delivery is thought to lower costs and improve coordination of care.

In advanced CHF, this principle is not so clear cut. In one study, patients receiving care from cardiologists were more likely to have a baseline determination of left ventricular function (61% versus 44%), receive higher does of ACE inhibitors, and have a shorter hospital length of stay (4.4 days versus 5.6 days) than patients seen by primary care physicians. While this difference did not reach statistical significance, it did suggest the importance of integrating cardiologists into any program.[27]

In reviewing charts of CHF patients, it is often difficult to tell who is acting as the primary treating physician. Many of these patients jump back and forth from the cardiologist to the primary care physician. Because of this, some health plans reassign the role of primary care physician to the attending cardiologist for advanced CHF patients. At the very least, it is critical that any CHF disease management program assist in the coordination of care between primary care physician and cardiologist.

EDUCATION

Patient and physician education is a cornerstone of most CHF programs. Most studies have found that patients are poorly educated on their own disease process, including the importance of medication compliance and the symptoms of increasing CHF. Most programs center on some form of literature distribution, as well as physician education.

Specialized nurses are trained to educate patients on a one-on-one basis. This can be done through the physician's office or through a home health provider. Programs emphasize the importance of daily weights, acute symptomatology management, medication compliance, ACE inhibitor use, and, most important, whom to call and when to call when symptoms occur. In addition to learning about how better to detect changing symptoms, patients must be given an easy and comfortable route to report symptom changes. This can be done by the patient calling directly but is often a part of a telemonitoring program in which the patient is called regularly to give their weights and symptoms; telemonitoring is discussed below.

Physician education is more difficult, since physicians tend to be less accessible. It can be done by letter, lecture, or face to face through pharmacy detailers or medical directors. Rates of hospitalization, quality of life, and ACE inhibitor use can be reported back to the individual physician to provide feedback and improve adherence. These "report cards" can help inform physicians and assist in changing behavior.

TELEMONITORING

Telemonitoring is part of most CHF programs and can either be done internally through case managers and clinic nurses or externally through a dedicated telemonitoring service. These programs are used to collect follow-up data, including adherence with daily weights, diet, and medications, as well as quality of life assessments. The programs may provide scales so the patients can weigh themselves. There is even a specialized program in which patients punch in the digits of their weight on a touch-tone phone using a computerized answering and tracking system.[28]

Ongoing social interactions with the patient appear to be critical to a program's success. As noted earlier, social problems can severely influence medical problems, particularly in the geriatric population. Patients may have no social support at home or transportation to get to the store to pick up medications. They may run out of money before the month is out and be forced to choose between medications and food. It is more cost-effective for the managed care organization to pay for the digoxin and Lasix for a few months than to pay for an avoidable admission. Transportation can also be a problem. The nurse and/or case manager must have the authority to make decisions that allow flexing of benefits to provide specialized services such as transportation.

A program by Dr. Avitall with Advanced Medical Devices uses a home health monitor that transmits to a monitored station measurements of weight, blood pressure, pulse, and oximeter readings. This system alone, with a weekly nursing call, decreased readmission rate to 14% in a small study, compared with a national average of 42%.[28]

Monitoring is often done at various intervals, depending on the needs of the patient. Usually, a schedule is set up based on the original stratification discussed earlier and is modified to suit the individual patient's needs. Patients who are recently discharged from the hospital are called daily for a brief period, then placed into one of the other stratification groups. Because of the high readmission rates, it is critical to give this recent discharge group special attention.

HOME VISITS

It is useful to combine telemonitoring with a home visit. This allows the cardiac specialist to inspect the home environment and evaluate the family support. It allows the patient to put a face to a seemingly impersonal program. During a home visit, it is useful to inspect the medicine cabinet as well as the refrigerator. Medication noncompliance and polypharmacy are common. The patient may also be taking medications that are over the counter or were prescribed in the distant past. Many of these medications, such as nonsteroidal anti-inflammatory agents, can interfere with cardiac medications. Pickles, ham, and tomato juice in the refrigerator (signs of high salt intake) may also give a clue to poor dietary habits. While in the home, other aspects of preventive health can be evaluated, such as social support systems and fall prevention.

OUTPATIENT CHF CLINICS

Many large groups and integrated delivery systems are setting up their own outpatient CHF clinics. When patients are seen regularly, symptoms can be controlled and admissions averted. Many of these clinics are staffed by nurse practitioners or geriatric nurse practitioners. They can serve patient educational goals as well as social needs. Some physicians even see these patients in a group setting. These programs can be designed in concert with other geriatric initiatives.

Some CHF patients in these programs may have been poorly served by primary care physicians and they now have expert cardiac care, regular follow-up, and immediate access to medical interventions when symptoms exacerbate. Results can be excellent. Cass Hospital Clinic, for instance, had a 72% drop in admissions per patient per year and a 46% improvement in New York Heart Association functional status.[4]

CARDIAC REHABILITATION

Cardiac rehabilitation is part of many programs, particularly those that have an inpatient component or are hospital sponsored. These rehabilitation programs are used to set up an exercise and education program in a monitored, safe environment. Patients often enter them after hospital discharge from an acute event, but they can also be used in conjunction with outpatient programs. In a patient with significant ischemic disease, cardiac rehabilitation may be the only safe environment to increase the patient's functional endurance.[29] Usually these programs last from 6 to 12 weeks and can have an ongoing follow-up component. These programs allow patients to be discharged sooner and have the educational component as an outpatient. They help to prevent the rapid readmissions that are so common in CHF patients. Recent literature notes exercise to be beneficial in CHF patients.[24]

ACUTE CARE

Hospitals, staff model HMOs, and integrated systems frequently have an acute care component to their disease management programs. This might include an ED observation unit to manage CHF on an outpatient basis, specialized skilled nursing facilities (or subacute) units to treat heart failure, or a specially trained home health team to handle heart failure at home. Many of these programs feature intravenous infusions of inotropic agents, which have proven effective in decreasing admission rates.[3,30] Most symptomatic CHF patients who show up in the ED are admitted; therefore, easy-to-use access to an alternative may avert some of these admissions. Subacute units can be used to directly admit CHF patients from home or from the ED, or to transfer patients out of the hospital as soon as they are hemodynamically stable. Specialized training, staffing, and equipment are needed.

INCENTIVES

Incentives are important in any physician-driven program. These are difficult to align in many health systems and can be best accomplished by different mechanisms. While incentives are generally beyond the scope of this book, a brief mention of three examples is warranted here.

1. In global capitation incentives, physicians are at risk for the entire health care dollar and therefore have incentives to keep the patient out of the hospital and improve the long-range health and well-being of the patient.
2. In outcome-based incentives, physician bonuses are based on the outcomes of patient care. Decisions can be based on hospitalization rates, ACE inhibitor use, or quality of life and other scores.
3. In another type of incentive, the program adds value to the physician's work by providing care to the patient that would normally be provided by the physician or not at all. This enables the physician's practice to be more efficient in the care of these patients and to have more satisfied and compliant patients.

This last method is difficult since it relies on a certain level of trust. Physicians must believe that the program will result in time savings and better care. Since physicians' experience with most health plans may have been unfavorable, this trust building will be an uphill battle. In addition, these programs often take a significant amount of physician time in working with the nurses to coordinate care. The need for this time must be recognized, and the time must be optimized to the patients' benefit.

MEASUREMENT AND EVALUATION

In any disease management initiative, one must measure a number of parameters to show that the project is successful. This sounds fairly simple, but the data may be difficult to obtain. These measurements fall into two groups. First there is the external group, where measurements are used to showcase one's initiatives to external entities such as NCQA, large employers, and so on. External measurements focus on three areas: (1) quality of life, (2) process/outcome of care, and (3) satisfaction. (Quality of life and process/outcome of care are discussed in detail below.) Second, there is the internal group, where measurements are used to validate the financial success and cost benefit analysis of a project. Obviously, there is crossover in these measurements.

It is tempting to explore multiple metrics to evaluate and validate a CHF disease management program; however, it is preferable to pick a few key indicators and focus measurements on these items. It is useful to measure baseline information at the start of the program, rather than having to go back and re-create the baseline measurement on an unexpected variable. Some examples of useful items to measure include admits per year,[3,9,14,30-32] average length of stay,[3,9,30] quality of life scores,[3,8,14] annual savings,[3,14,30] global ejection fraction,[3] ACE use,[6,21] and readmission rates.[6,31,32] Compliance rates and functional status are also good measures. All of these metrics are compared to the baseline CHF population the year prior to the intervention or at the start of the program. Claims data and pharmacy data are relatively easy to obtain, while clinical data such as ejection fraction, quality of life, or functional status must be obtained from the physician, patient, or clinical record.

Quality of Life

Quality of life is difficult to quantify in a chronic disease state, in that the natural course of these disease processes results in a decreasing quality of life. Programs may or may not improve the quality of life, but hopefully they should slow its decline.[8] Since most disease management programs do not have the luxury of a control group, it is very difficult to prove that a decline in quality of life is less dramatic in the study group. Nevertheless, it is useful to measure quality of life; one validated instrument is the Minnesota Living with Heart Failure questionnaire.[32] Other quality of life tools that have been used include the Chronic Heart Failure questionnaire, SF-36 or SF-12, and various proprietary questionnaires. The SF-36 or SF-12 are more general in nature but have the advantage of being applicable to multiple disease processes. It is also important to track the patient's functional status with tools such as the New York Heart Classification.[19] Other more general quality of life tools include Sickness Impact Profile, Psychological Adjustment to Illness Scale, and Nottingham Health Profile.[33]

Process/Outcome of Care

Process of care and/or clinical outcomes are essential study metrics. As mentioned above, one of the most utilized indicators for CHF is the use of ACE inhibitors. According to medical literature, improving certain process of care, such as ACE inhibitor usage, results in improved outcomes. Other process measures include the decrease in use of certain calcium channel blockers (which may impair inotropic heart function), decrease in use of nonsteroidal anti-inflammatory agents (which may decrease the efficiency of diuretics), and increase in compliance with medications, daily weights, and exercise. Measuring decreasing admission and days in the hospital may also be interpreted as improved morbidity. The ultimate goal is to improve morbidity, mortality, and quality of life.

Satisfaction

Satisfaction should be measured from both the provider and the patient viewpoint. Satisfaction with disease management on the patient side typically has been quite high. It is difficult to know if this satisfaction is a result of the program or because of the personal contact and social interaction with medical staff. Generally, providers have been pleased with disease management programs if they have had participation in the development of the program. If physicians recognize the value to their patients, they will be strong advocates of a program. Physicians are likely to be the best referral source for new patients if the physicians have been involved in a program.

Internal Measurement

Internal measurements are easier and more straightforward. These includes total cost for each CHF patient per month, number of admissions per year, number of ED visits per year, average length of stay per admission, and readmission rates. Most CHF programs have shown an improvement in all of these measures.[3,8,9,14,30-32]

COST BENEFIT ANALYSIS

A cost benefit analysis should be done before, during, and after initiating any study. This topic is discussed in detail in Chapter 31 but will briefly be mentioned here as well. The cost of program implementation must be quantified and will be different for each program, depending on the delivery system structure and the programs implemented. The financial benefits are more difficult to evaluate; there are few benchmarks available. However, there are study data rapidly becoming available that will assist in estimating the savings of individual programs.[3,8,14,30] Some studies, particularly case management programs, have started by measuring the number of averted admissions, the average cost of those admissions, and the resulting savings. This may be effective in the short term.

As the program gathers momentum, it should prevent these patients from progressing to the acute admission stage. They stabilize (hopefully), and therefore it is difficult to track averted admissions over the long run. However, average admissions per patient per year should decrease. It is also helpful to look at the cost of an admission (not for the average heart failure patient but for the patient group the program is focusing on). In other words, patients with class IV CHF and an ejection fraction of 25% generally have more costly admissions than those who have mild CHF. Comorbidities also play a significant role, in that patients with comorbidities have higher utilization and medical costs.

The most common way to evaluate benefits is to look historically at admission and readmission rates for the population of heart failure patients. These rates can then be compared with rates during the postintervention period. They can be converted to cost data using local costs or national benchmarks (approximately $6,000 per admission). This will provide an estimate of potential savings.

Another value that might be calculated is the decreased morbidity that comes with increased use of ACE inhibitors. The improved quality of life and mortality are difficult to quantify financially but are an important footnote in any cost benefit analysis.

CONCLUSION

CHF disease management programs are becoming a standard for health plans and integrated medical groups. These programs have shown improvements in morbidity, mortality, and quality of life. Most programs up to this point have focused on the "sickest of the sick" in CHF. However, the trend is to begin the programs earlier in the disease process, so that they focus on risk factor modification and prevention. This type of population-based approach has the potential to improve care for a large group of individuals and begins to tap into the real potential of managed care.

REFERENCES

1. National Heart, Lung and Blood Institute. *National Heart, Lung and Blood Institute Data Fact Sheet.* Bethesda, MD: US Department of Health and Human Services; September 1996.
2. *Heart and Stroke Facts: 1995 Statistical Supplement.* Dallas, TX: American Heart Association, AHA National Center; 1994.
3. Ryan CC. Homecare therapy: a cost-effective alternative approach to the management of advanced heart failure. *Am J Managed Care.* 1996;2(10):1351–1355.
4. Cardiology Preeminence Roundtable. *Beyond Four Walls.* Washington, DC: The Advisory Board Company; 1994.
5. Young JB. Contemporary management of patients with heart failure. *Med Clin North Am.* 1995;79:1171–1190.
6. Weaver J. Managing congestive heart failure. *Pharmacoeconomics.* February 1997;16–21.
7. O'Connell JB. Economic impact of heart failure. *J Heart Lung Transplant.* 1994;13:s107–s112.
8. Independence Blues plan to expand CHF management. *Dis Manage News.* 1996;1(7):3–4.
9. Kornowski R, Zeeli D, Averbuch M, et al. Intensive home care surveillance prevents hospitalization and improves morbidity rates among elderly patients with severe congestive heart failure. *Am Heart J.* 1995; 129(4):762–766.
10. Debusk R. Kaiser said to be planning use of multifit CHF plan. *Dis Manage News.* 1996;1(18):6–7.
11. Guyatt G. Measurement of health-related quality of life in heart failure. *J Am Coll Cardiol.* 1993;22: 185A–191A.
12. NYL care SDMS CHF management program posts big initial gains. *Dis Manage News.* 1996;1(17):2–3.
13. Rich MW, Beckham V, Wittenberg C, et al. A multidisciplinary intervention to prevent the readmission of elderly patients with congestive heart failure. *N Engl J Med.* 1995;333(18):1190–1195.
14. Rich MW. Prevention of readmission in elderly patients with CHF. *J Gen Intern Med.* 1993;8:585–590.
15. Lewis B. Ralin Medical Inc report dramatic results in care of congestive heart failure patients. Presented at Managed Care Congress; January 22, 1997; San Francisco.
16. Hospital's education-centered CHF effort succeeds. *Dis Manage News.* 1996;1(23):2–3.
17. Strong CHF program results help propel new Humana DM efforts. *Dis Manage News.* 1996;2(2):1–6.
18. Bonow RO, Udelson JE. Left ventricular diastolic dysfunction as a cause of congestive heart failure. *Ann Intern Med.* 1992;117:502–510.
19. Criteria Committee of the New York Heart Association. *Diseases of Heart and Blood Vessels: Nomenclature and Criteria for Diagnosis,* 6th ed. Boston: Little, Brown & Co; 1964.
20. Gahli JK, Kadakia S, Cooper R, Ferlinz J. Precipitating factors leading to decompensation of heart failure traits among urban blacks. *Arch Intern Med.* 1988;148(9): 2013–2016.
21. Bilodeau A. Getting ACE inhibitors into the right hands. *Managed Care.* January 1997;31–32.
22. Brass-Mynderse NT. Disease management of congestive heart failure. *J Cardiovasc Nurs.* 1996;11(1):54–62.
23. Drugs for chronic heart failure. *Med Lett.* 1998;38(985): 92–94.
24. Dracup K, Baker D, Bunbar S, et al. Management of HF: counseling, education, and lifestyle modifications. *JAMA.* 1994;272(18):1442–1445.
25. US Department of Health and Human Services (DHHS). *Health United States 1994.* DHHS Publication no (PHS)95-1232. Hyattsville, MD: DHHS; 1995.
26. Consensus Trial Study Group. Effects of enalapril on mortality in severe congestive heart failure: results of the Cooperative North Scandinavian Enalapril Survival Study. *N Engl J Med.* 1987;1429–1435.
27. Haoranek E, Graham G, Pan Z, et al. Process of outpatient management of heart failure: a comparison of cardiologist and PCP. *Am J Managed Care.* 1996;2(7): 783–789.
28. Schieszer J. CHF: computerized home monitoring. *Intern Med World Rep.* 1996;11(21):9–10.
29. Wenger NK, Froelicher ES, Smith LK, et al. *AHCPR Guidelines for Cardiac Rehabilitation.* Clinical Practice Guideline no 17. AHCPR Publication no 96-0672. Rockville, MD: US Department of Health and Human Services, Public Health Service, Agency for Health Care Policy and Research and the National Heart, Lung and Blood Institute; 1995.
30. Chapman D. Development of HF center: a medical center and cardiology practice join forces to improve care and reduce cost. *Am J Managed Care.* 1997;3(3): 431–437.
31. Naylor M, Brooten D, Jones R, Lavisso-Mourey R, Mezey M, Pauly M. Comprehensive discharge planning for the hospitalized elderly. *Am Coll Physicians.* 1994;120(12):999–1006.
32. *Minnesota Living with Heart Failure Questionnaire.* Minneapolis, MN: University of Minnesota; 1994.
33. Grady K. Quality of life in patients with chronic heart failure. *Crit Care Nurs Clin North Am.* 1993;5(4): 661–670.

GEORGE MAYZELL, MD, MBA, is medical director for the Northern Geographic Business Unit of Blue Cross and Blue Shield of Florida. His responsibilities include care and quality management in the 18 counties surrounding the Jacksonville market. Prior to joining Blue Cross and Blue Shield of Florida in 1996, Dr. Mayzell performed consulting work as the associate director of PruCare. He also completed 10 years of private practice in the Jacksonville area. He received his MD from the University of Medicines in New Jersey and is board certified in both internal medicine and geriatrics. He received his MBA from Jacksonville University in 1993.

CHAPTER 29

Diabetes Disease Management

David K. McCulloch

Chapter Outline

- Introduction
- A Population-Based Approach to Diabetes Care
- Practical Changes Necessary To Have More Effective Diabetes Care
- Future Directions

INTRODUCTION

From the perspective of the whole health care organization, the primary care team, and the patient, diabetes is "bad news." From the point of view of the health care organization, diabetes is staggeringly expensive. About 4% of the population is known to have diabetes (with perhaps another 4% being undiagnosed), and yet they account for almost 15% of all health care dollars (Figure 29–1). An average person with diabetes enrolled in a managed care organization will cost four times as much as an age- and gender-matched enrollee without diabetes.

From the point of view of the primary care team, while patients with diabetes may present with many non-diabetes related problems, these patients also require the team to remember legions of routine diabetes-related tests and procedures that need to be incorporated into daily care. For patients, diabetes can be an ever-present burden requiring continual attention. Over a few years, patients are likely to have had dozens of visits to many different health care professionals. Patients may have been given conflicting pieces of information and advice, leaving them with the impression that there is no overall plan for care, that most of the problems are their fault, and that they ought to "try harder."

Traditional approaches to medical practice do not meet everyone's needs. Outpatient clinics are usually ruled by the "tyranny of the urgent" and are organized to respond quickly to acute patient problems but do not adequately serve the needs of those with chronic illness like diabetes.[1] Most patients with diabetes (>90%) receive their care from primary care providers who may not have a special interest in or up-to-date

---

The author especially thanks Ed Wagner, whose stimulating vision and energetic leadership have driven most of the diabetes improvement efforts at Group Health Cooperative of Puget Sound. In addition, I am surrounded by a team of dedicated and enthusiastic colleagues who constantly battle to sweep aside day-to-day problems to find ways to innovate and improve. These include Martha Price, Mike Hindmarsh, Brian Austin, Kristine Odle, Karen Artz, Melissa Parkerton, John Brebner, Matt Handley, Mike Stuart, Mick Braddick, members of the Diabetes Steering Committee, and the Clinical Planning and Improvement Division. Lastly, I thank the patients, who not only provide us with our purpose but are a great source of inspiration.

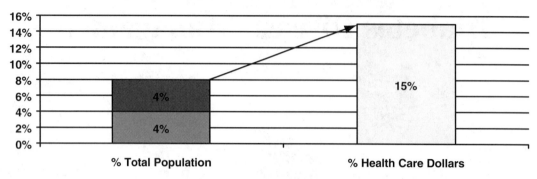

Figure 29–1 Incidence and Cost of Diabetes

information about diabetes, and who see their patients with diabetes during busy days filled with patient-generated visits for specific complaints, most of which are not diabetes related. If the last 15 patients a provider saw in a day did not have diabetes, and that provider was suddenly faced with a patient with diabetes who has a sore knee, it is asking a lot to expect the provider to remember that it has been over a year since this patient's last dilated retinal eye examination and 18 months since the last hemoglobin A1c test, and that doing a foot examination or checking for microalbuminuria might be a good idea, since this patient is not likely to show up again until the patient's next sports-related injury. There has been heated debate about whether the care for patients with diabetes would be better if done by individuals or teams with more expertise in diabetes management. Specialist physicians have been shown to be more knowledgeable about efficacious interventions for major chronic illnesses, tend to adopt new approaches more quickly,[2,3] and produce better outcomes in hospitalized settings.[4,5] When patients with diabetes see specialists in the context of organized programs like hospital-based clinics, outcomes are improved,[6,7] although it is difficult to disentangle how much of the improvement is due to the expert knowledge and how much to the systematic and organized approach.

Although hardly any health care plan is doing a great job with diabetes care, there is a huge potential for simultaneously improving outcomes for patients and reducing overall health care costs. In response to this situation, there has been a proliferation of commercial companies offering prepackaged solutions: guidelines, tracking software, or other types of support for disease management. It is unlikely that there is a single approach that will work in all situations. There are general principles and suggestions for approaches that will make diabetes care more efficient, better organized to meet everyone's needs, and more satisfactory for all concerned.

A POPULATION-BASED APPROACH TO DIABETES CARE

Population-based diabetes care is more than a fad that is suitable only for large organizations with dedicated computer networks and infrastructure. Its principles are straightforward and can be applied to various clinical practice settings (from small group practices that may have managed care contracts with several different companies, plus additional fee-for-service patients, all the way to large staff model health maintenance organizations [HMOs]). The following self-test should be applied by the practitioner: Can I identify all the patients with diabetes who are under my care? Do I know what services all those patients should be offered in any given year? Can I organize my care so that the right services are offered to the right patients? Do I have a system for tracking how I'm doing? While the principles are the same in all clinical settings, the practical details of how to use this approach will vary widely.

Identifying Those Who Have Diabetes

There are many ways to identify patients with diabetes. Each of these methods has advantages and disadvantages. Pharmacy data allow identification of those patients picking up prescriptions for diabetes-specific medications (for example, insulin, sulfonylureas, metformin, acarbose, or troglitazone). This will not identify the 20% or more patients with diabetes who are treated with lifestyle modification (diet and exercise) only and may occasionally identify people who do not have diabetes but are picking up the prescription for a friend, relative, or pet. (When we fixed the problem in our health plan tracking capability, an audit of our diabetes registry identified two diabetic cats!)

Laboratory data can identify those patients with high blood glucose or hemoglobin A1c levels. There are problems here, too. The international diabetes community has recently decided to change the criteria for defining diabetes.[8] It has been suggested that a diagnosis of diabetes requires two fasting blood glucose values of 126 mg/dl or two random blood glucose values of 200 mg/dl, without reliance on the level of HbA1c for diagnostic purposes.[3] This is not helpful for a patient who was brought into an emergency department unconscious, was given an empirical intravenous infusion of glucose, but then had a blood glucose level taken that is reported at 450 mg/dl. It is also not helpful to classify a patient who had a random blood glucose of 204 mg/dl and an HbA1c on the same day of 7.4% (with the normal range for the lab being between 3.8% and 6.1%). There must be a practical compromise that will identify most diabetic patients efficiently. For example, a plan may require two abnormal values during a 12-month period and insist that they be fasting or random blood glucose levels only (not HbA1c).

Practitioners should also access claims data, which use hospital discharge codes; outpatient treatment record forms (TRFs); or International Classification of Diseases, Ninth Edition, Clinical Modification (ICD-9-CM) codes. Practitioners can also use a manual list or card file of the patients, noting those with diabetes. The problems with any of these systems is that they fail to identify the 20% or more patients with diabetes who tend to avoid contact with the health care system. It is important to try to reach out to these patients and encourage their participation in programs of routine care (outlined below), or they will inevitably show up at a future date with much more advanced, less treatable, and more expensive consequences of their diabetes.

Subsequent to identification of the diabetic population (often from several of these sources), tracking must be done. This tracking can be done in a card file, but using a computerized spreadsheet or database is better. Although the ideal is to have a network of computers with interconnected and dynamic databases, where information can be continually updated, it is possible to make use of some simple freestanding desktop or laptop computers, with off-the-shelf software to help manage this population. The identification criteria used at Group Health Cooperative of Puget Sound is shown in Exhibit 29–1. Details of what information to keep and track for each patient will be discussed below.

Knowing What To Do for Your Diabetic Population

Although most health care professionals have been well taught about appropriate care for diabetic patients at some time during their training, there are two main problems of applying this in daily practice. First, it is hard to remember how to prioritize the various aspects of care, and second, it is difficult to stay abreast of important new developments (the value of microalbumin-

Exhibit 29–1 Criteria Used To Identify Diabetic Patients at Group Health Cooperative of Puget Sound

> A patient is identified as diabetic if *any* of the following conditions have been met:
> - A prescription for any diabetes-specific medication (insulin, sulfonylurea, metformin, acarbose, troglitazone, etc)
> - Two fasting blood glucose values of 126 mg/dl or two random blood glucose values of 200 mg/dl (or one of each) during the previous 12 months[3]
> - Any hospital discharge diagnosis of diabetes
> - Two outpatient codes for diabetes
>
> Courtesy of Group Health Cooperative of Puget Sound, Seattle, Washington.

uria screening and early treatment with angiotensin converting enzyme inhibitors for certain patients is a recent example of this). The biggest and most common mistake when observing primary care providers interacting with patients with diabetes is that there is too much time spent on a futile review of blood glucose levels in patients who are stuck at a certain HbA1c and not enough time spent on other aspects of care that would be of more benefit to the patient (such as cardiac risk reduction and screening and management of eyes, kidneys, and feet).

There are many ways to be reminded of the appropriate priorities and to keep up-to-date with changes in thinking. The American Diabetes Association (ADA) publishes an annual report on appropriate standards of care.[9] However, simply publishing recommendations is no guarantee that they will be followed. When 1,434 physicians in the United States were surveyed about how closely they were adhering to the nationally promoted, ADA-endorsed recommendations for routine care, only 50% reported performing semiannual neurologic and foot examination, and even fewer were performing routine eye examinations or urinary protein measurements.[10] Even when practice patterns in several academic medical training centers were evaluated 3 years before, the year of, and 3 years after the publication of the ADA's standards of care in 1989, there were no real signs of improvement, and most measures fell far short of the recommended care delivery (Figure 29–2).[11]

In an attempt to improve this situation, there has been a proliferation of published clinical guidelines in the past few years. The best of these are explicit evidence-based guidelines,[12] and many are available in large glossy notebook formats, or as interactive software. But even good guidelines will not result in improved care if they are purchased, then placed on an office shelf to gather dust (or behind a computer screen icon that is never clicked on). To be effective, the team that is expected to use these guidelines needs to believe in them. The team also needs to customize the guidelines to the individual practice setting, deciding which team members will be responsible for particular aspects of the process.[13,14]

Another approach to try to encourage more organized and appropriate diabetes care is to audit clinical practices for their adherence to published standards of care. The Health Employer Data and Information Set (HEDIS) from the National Committee on Quality Assurance (NCQA) is one attempt at this, but it includes only a few measures related to good diabetes care. The Health Care Financing Administration (HCFA) has also employed "watchdog" techniques with peer review organizations (PROs) helping to audit care. The Foundation for Accountability (FAccT) has a more extensive set of measures for diabetes care. The most comprehensive approach, launched jointly by the ADA and NCQA in the spring of 1997, is the Provider Recognition Program, which encourages individual health care providers, or larger groups of providers, to submit data on a random sample of their patients with diabetes, and which includes a wide range of measures of care. While even this effort has been criticized by some for not being rigorous enough, it represents an excellent starting point to allow a self-audit of diabetes care. A summary of the measures used is shown in Table 29–1.

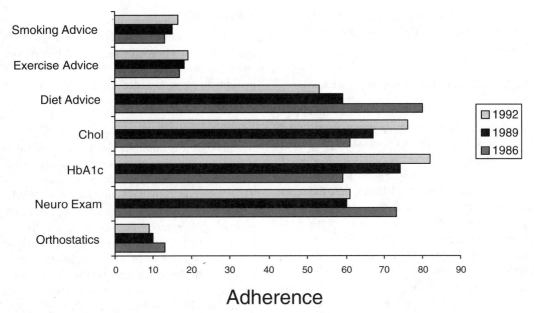

Figure 29–2 Effect of Publishing ADA's Standards of Care (in 1989) on Practice Patterns in Academic Settings. *Source:* Reprinted with permission from NW Stolar, *Diabetes Care,* Vol 18, pp 701–707, © 1995.

A pilot study involving over 20 clinical sites and about 2,000 patients was done to decide how many patients with diabetes would need to achieve the measures in order for the provider (or group) to obtain recognition for the quality of its diabetes care. These qualifying criteria are likely to change in the future, to encourage steady improvement in overall standards of care.

Table 29–1 Measures of Care Used for Adult Diabetic Patients in the ADA/NCQA's Provider Recognition Program

Test	Routine Screening Frequency	Notes
Smoking cessation counseling	Every visit	For smokers only
Blood pressure with diastolic below 90 mm Hg	Every visit	
Lipids	Annually	
Dilated eye exam	Annually	More often if significant diabetic retinopathy develops
Foot exam	Annually	Every visit, if peripheral vascular disease or neuropathy present
Microalbuminuria	Annually	
HbA1c % below 10% below 8%	Twice a year	Every 3 months until goal is reached
Education/self-management review	Annually	
Patient satisfaction	Annually	From patient survey

Source: Data from National Committee for Quality Assurance and American Diabetes Association.

(More details about this program may be obtained by calling the ADA at 703-549-1500, extension 2202.)

Having a System for Matching A with B

If an organization has identified its members with diabetes and has agreed upon a prioritized list of the services that this population needs, the organization must have an easy way to review these data to match people with services. The simplest display is a spreadsheet where the rows are individual patients and the columns are the data elements that you want to keep track of (such as the date of the last foot examination, HbA1c test, microalbuminuria result, etc). This can be kept as a hard-copy chart on which someone fills in the dates and results of tests as patients get them, so that blank spaces make it obvious which patients are overdue for particular tests.

Having this information on a spreadsheet or database program on a computer has several advantages. The lists can be sorted so that the practitioner might print specific subsets needing more attention. For example, it may be important to identify patients under 70 years of age who are not on an angiotensin converting enzyme inhibitor, but have not had a microalbuminuria screening test done, or to identify all those who are overdue for a foot examination, or all those who are on maximum doses of oral hypoglycemics but have HbA1c's over 9.0%. There are various ways to use this information, involving redefinition of team roles (discussed below). The most sophisticated system would have a dynamic and continuously updated registry of diabetic patients, which pulls in data from other databases and also allows data entry for information that can't be pulled in automatically. In the Group Health diabetes registry, we have information pulled in from the administrative, pharmacy, and laboratory databases and have created four additional data entry screens to capture important information that can't be routinely captured without chart review (Table 29–2).

Vital Statistics

This data entry screen allows capture of smoking status, height, weight, and blood pressure. This allows particular high-risk subsets of patients to be easily identified, so that they can be offered additional help.

Retinal Screening

Although it is possible to capture some information about which patients have had eye examinations, laser therapy, or vitrectomy from TRF/claims data, chart documentation is often indecipherable. We have therefore asked our ophthalmology/optometry teams to do direct data entry of important information that would be helpful to the primary care team. This includes the date of examination, the visual acuity in each eye, and the retinopathy status (none, background, macular edema, proliferative retinopathy, etc).

Foot Care

Group Health has introduced an explicit, evidence-based foot care guideline that gives a quick, easy, and standardized way to identify patients whose feet are at high risk for future foot ulcer or amputation (based on the presence of neuropathy and/or peripheral vascular disease). We have a simple data entry screen that captures the date and result of this examination, so it quickly allows the primary care team to identify how many of the patients with diabetes have had the annual foot screening and how many have "high-risk" feet (and therefore need additional teaching and attention).

Patient Education

Although most authorities acknowledge that patient education, behavior change, and self-management support are the cornerstone of diabetic management, traditional chart systems often fail to identify which patients have been taught what, when, and how far the patient has been able to move toward improved behavior in particular areas (exercise, diet, or blood glucose monitoring). We have therefore developed a data entry screen that allows someone to enter and track this information.

Table 29–2 Data Elements Captured on the Diabetes Registry at Group Health Cooperative of Puget Sound

Category	Data Elements	Source
Demographics	Name, gender, address, phone number, ID, date,* ID source,* consumer number	Administrative database
Vital signs	Smoking status, height, weight, blood pressure	Vital statistics data entry screen
Cardiac	Aspirin use, cholesterol, low-density lipoprotein, high-density lipoprotein, triglycerides	Pharmacy and laboratory databases
Renal	Angiotensin-converting enzyme inhibitor use, serum creatinine, urine alb:creat	Pharmacy and laboratory databases
Eye	Date and results of most recent dilated eye exam	Administrative database and eye data entry screen
Foot care	Date and results of most recent foot exam	Foot care data entry
Glycemic control	HbA1c, oral hypoglycemics, and/or insulin regimen	Pharmacy and laboratory
Patient education	Date of initiation of each element of self-management/behavior change	Patient education data entry screen
Service utilization	Outpatient visits, hospitalizations, phone, contacts	Administrative database

*The date on which the person was identified as having diabetes, and the source of that identification (laboratory database, pharmacy database, etc).

Courtesy of Group Health Cooperative of Puget Sound, Seattle, Washington.

Tracking Progress and Making Appropriate Changes

It is important to avoid feeling overwhelmed by trying to fix every aspect of diabetes care simultaneously. It is also important not to wait until there is a fully automated computer system to facilitate the work. For any health care organization embarking on quality improvement efforts (see Chapter 33), there are several practical decisions to be made. Having identified all the areas to improve diabetes care, organizations must then decide which areas are most important. Here, all sorts of practical and political issues arise. Should the focus be retinal eye screening rates because this is the main HEDIS measure and therefore one with which the organization may be compared to other competitors? Should the focus be on improvements that are most likely to result in reduced costs, such as identification of patients who are at high risk of developing foot ulcers in the near future, and on instituting programs to teach those patients protective foot care techniques? Or should the system choose areas likely to have the biggest impact on the future health of patients with diabetes, such as smoking cessation?

These choices may be influenced by the ease of collecting the relevant data for each area of diabetes care (discussed in more detail below). Having decided on the most appropriate area to target, practitioners should then develop and implement an evidence-based improvement strategy that is tailored to the strengths of the particular organization. Finally, the impact of the improvement effort should be continually evaluated. Although this may seem obvious, the ability to modify any improvement effort is dependent on collecting meaningful data that encompass the continuum of care.

In order to improve one aspect of care, it is necessary to positively influence several interconnected areas. It may be necessary to analyze different measurements to understand why an improvement is, or is not, being seen. These areas include patient and provider knowledge and behaviors, process measures, pathophysiologic measures, and measures of patient function and quality of life. For example, an organization may decide to reduce the morbidity and costs associated with diabetic foot ulcers and amputations. One of the easiest things to measure may be the amputation rate. However, since this is an insensitive measurement of the final stages of the pathophysiologic process, it may not help evaluate the improvement effort. If an organization measures only amputation rate, and if a new program is implemented to try to improve foot care, it is possible that when amputation rate is measured again a few years later, it will not have changed. The organization would not know why the improvement effort has apparently failed. A better approach would be to track some measurements in each of several interrelated areas (Exhibit 29–2).

1. *Patient and/or provider behaviors.* It would be instructive to take a random sample of providers and find out what they currently believe, and do, with regard to foot care. When we did this with a random sample of 40 primary care providers, the results were very instructive. Fewer than 50% of providers were confident about when to refer to podiatry or about their current diabetic foot ulcer management. Specifically, they were not confident about debridement techniques; two thirds were confident about when to use antibiotics in patients with diabetic foot ulcers, but almost 50% were not confident about which antibiotics to use. At least a third were not confident about how to diagnose osteomyelitis or when to refer to vascular or orthopaedic surgery. A similar survey should be done for patients to evaluate what they are currently doing for their feet. When we did a telephone survey of almost 400 diabetic patients, we found that, although the majority of them realized that foot care is an important part of diabetes self-management, many of them were doing inappropriate behaviors, or were incapable of doing effective self-evaluation. Specifically, over 50% walked around barefoot for more than 5 minutes, on a daily basis, and half of them cut their toenails straight across and did not file their nails afterward (thereby increasing their risk of developing injuries and ulcers on the adjacent toes). A third of patients were

Exhibit 29–2 Different Types of Measurements

Patient and/or Provider Behaviors	Process Measures	Pathophysiological Outcomes		Patient Function
		Early	Late	
What do patients do for their feet?	Number and quality of foot exams	Number of "high-risk" feet identified	Amputation rate	Physical function
What do providers think about preventive care?	Foot care education	Number of foot ulcers, etc		Days off work, etc
	Hospitalization			

unable to reach their feet easily, and almost half could not see the bottom of their feet easily.
2. *Process measures.* Many organizations do not have a standard way of performing or documenting diabetic foot examinations, but some attempt should be made (usually by chart review) to document how often foot examinations are being done and how many patients are being given foot care education.
3. *Pathophysiological outcomes.* It is important to document how many patients have been identified as having "high-risk" feet (due to neuropathy and vascular disease, etc), how many have previous or current foot ulcers present, and how many admissions there are for foot infections, reconstructive vascular surgery, amputations, and so on.
4. *Patient function.* Overall patient function and quality of life can be assessed using tools such as the SF-36. By taking this approach, it should be possible to identify why an improvement effort has been successful, and how to improve it. For example, it is possible that neither patients nor providers think that regular screening and prophylactic foot care are important; or that patients have incorrect notions about proper foot care. Or it may be that even though everyone believes foot examinations to be important, very few examinations are occurring. Or perhaps the program has improved the number of foot examinations that are occurring and the number of high-risk feet being identified, but the appropriate education is not being done, so the number of admissions and foot ulcers is not going down. In order to improve the most important outcomes (fewer ulcers and amputations, and healthier, more functional patients), it is important to understand which of the interrelated areas needs most attention.

A similar set of interrelated behaviors, attitudes, process measures, and pathophysiologic and functional outcomes can be developed for all of the important areas of diabetes care improvement.

PRACTICAL CHANGES NECESSARY TO HAVE MORE EFFECTIVE DIABETES CARE

Within the Health Care System

Traditional administrative structure, focused on relatively short-term goals (particularly in the current era of hard economic competition), does not make population-based care easy. Senior administrators must support a planned and proactive approach to care. This shouldn't be difficult, since it is well known that over 50% of the cost of diabetes care is for the inpatient management of potentially preventable end-stage complications (such as intravenous antibiotics, total contact casts and amputations for foot ulcers, or dialysis or transplants for end-stage renal disease). There is a growing body of data on the potential cost savings of employing microalbuminuria screening,[15] retinal eye screening,[16] and foot care education programs,[17] and of improving glycemic control.[18]

Administrative support at the clinic/practice team level needs to be translated into tangible changes in how teams are structured, scheduling is done, and various activities are valued and rewarded. For example, primary care teams need to be given regular, specified periods when they can meet as a team, review their diabetic registry, identify subsets of patients needing particular help, and then assign specific tasks and roles to team members.[14] For groups of providers working together managing diabetes, it should be possible for every provider to be freed up for at least half a day a week. During those times, other team members could cover the acute needs of that provider's patients while the provider could do other tasks, such as running group visits for patients with diabetes who have similar needs, or scheduling planned diabetes review visits for patients who have been called and invited to come in, not because they had a specific problem, but because they were overdue for routine diabetes health maintenance.

The organization should make sure that rewards and recognition are in line with appropriate goals. It is pointless to offer incentives to providers based solely on the volume of acute visits he or she can perform in a day, if, at the end of the year, most of their patients with diabetes are languishing in neglect, quietly developing foot ulcers, hypertension, and rising creatinines, which are destined to result in poorer health outcomes and higher costs in the near future. The organization should provide feedback to teams and reward those managing their diabetic (and other high-risk) populations well. Other systematic improvements might include helping develop better patient education and self-management support material (discussed in more detail below) or considering centralized consulting nurse phone service, to free up other team nurses to do planned diabetes phone calls, diabetes registry data entry, and registry review. Before adopting the latest slick software package, it is crucial to involve the end users in development, to ensure that what is chosen is really useful software that will facilitate planned care administration.

Within the Health Care Team

As mentioned above, redefining (or clarifying) the roles of physicians (MDs), registered nurses (RNs), physician assistants (PAs), licensed practical nurses (LPNs), and other team members can make regular diabetes care feasible. After deciding which area of diabetes work to focus on, the team members should break down their efforts into specific tasks and assign those tasks to different people. For example, who will review the registry to identify the patients who need a foot examination? Who will call these patients and invite them to come in? It may be worth trying to bring 8 to 12 patients (who all need foot examinations) in on the same morning. Perhaps an RN, LPN, or PA could see each of them briefly to identify which of them have high-risk feet. Those with low-risk feet could leave, but those identified as being at high risk could participate in some group education later in the morning. The team should then decide who should record the foot examinations, or enter the information on the diabetes registry.

Other studies have shown that the use of nurses to manage caseloads of diabetic patients under the supervision of diabetologists results in improved outcomes.[19,20] In one study, each nurse was the case manager for about 250 diabetic patients, with a diabetologist overseeing the care of 4 nurses.[19] With almost 15,000 diabetic patients in Group Health, this approach would require a substantial increase in both nursing and diabetologist staffing. Other organizations would face the same staffing problem. While we would not suggest that all diabetic patients can be managed in a primary care setting, we believe that substantial improvements in routine care can be achieved by the primary care teams. In many health care organizations, the criteria used to determine which diabetic patients are seen in a primary care setting, and which ones are referred to be seen by a diabetes nurse, or by an endocrinologist/diabetologist, are arbitrary, based more on patient preference than on objective evidence of the complexity of the patient's illness. By improving the routine aspects of diabetes care using the approaches outlined here, organizations should be able to identify subsets of diabetic patients, using objective criteria, who should be seen by nurse managers, or specialty teams.

For the Patient

There are few diseases that demand as much from patients as diabetes does; by what they do in their day-to-day lives, patients with diabetes strongly influence their destiny. Patients need to become the central person in the health care team. Coaching and educating patients—empowering them to be better able to make informed decisions about care along with the health care team—will pay big dividends.[21] The patient should have a clear idea about long-term goals as well as what to expect at every visit and should be encouraged to actively seek out the appropriate services, at the appropriate time intervals, throughout the year. It is difficult to get the balance right—patients should not feel that everything is their responsibility, and that if they don't get an eye exam on time, it is entirely their fault. However, if they truly understand the long-term goals, they can be immensely helpful in their care.

Engaging patients to become active partners in their health care can be challenging. In this era of information overload, several different approaches may be necessary. Letters informing patients of what services are available and which they should seek out may be effective for some patients. The ADA, as well as some commercial companies, have produced credit card-size summaries of essential information. These can be mailed to patients, can be available at the reception desk at the clinic, or can be available at the pharmacy, when patients pick up any diabetes-related drugs or equipment. Telephone information lines, patient newsletters or magazines, posters in the waiting areas, and the demeanor of clinic staff should all convey the same message to patients: patients' input and insights, desire and requests, are welcomed and will be an integral part of the health care plan that will be developed. A novel and effective technique is to encourage patients in the waiting room to use interactive media to identify particular areas of interest or concern. By the time patients get to see the health care team member, they have an individualized summary and assessment of their concerns (RW Glasgow, personal communication).

The traditional approach to education of patients with diabetes has been to offer them classes. While this approach may work for some people, there are several problems. Classes may be expensive (either directly, or because of lost wages while attending). It is often difficult to address the needs of a diverse group of people with different ages, social and educational backgrounds, and types of diabetes. Most adults do not learn well by being immersed in facts over a short period of time, with little or no follow-up. For group classes to be most successful, they should involve patients who are broadly similar (perhaps all on maximum doses of oral agents and anxious about starting insulin therapy, or all on insulin therapy but with HbA1c's over 8% and considering a more intensive insulin regimen). In addition, the classes should be practical and focused on behavior changes, and they should involve worksheets and homework assignments. In addition to classes, regular ongoing follow-up should be incorporated into routine clinic visits, where individualized feedback and support can be given to reinforce appropriate changes in self-management behavior. The goal of all patient-centered strategies should be to promote truly collaborative care management, which involves the four main stages described in Exhibit 29–3.

A large deficiency in the traditional approach to management of chronic diseases such as diabetes is the lack of an effective way to document and track the education/self-management support plan for a patient. Typically, if busy providers see patients, there is no way to know what the patients know, what they want to work on, how ready they are to make changes in particular areas, or what their goals and targets are in those areas. Having such a summary, whether

Exhibit 29–3 Four Stages to Collaborative Care Management

Stage 1:	Both the patient and the health care team define what they perceive the problems to be and focus on areas that both provider and patient consider important.
Stage 2:	Through shared decision making, the patient and provider agree on targets and goals of diabetes management, and on plans for achieving these goals, based partly on patient preferences and readiness.
Stage 3:	The patient chooses self-management training and support services that are most suitable for his or her ability and learning style.
Stage 4:	The patient should have a clear idea of the plan for further follow-up and support.

Courtesy of Group Health Cooperative of Puget Sound, Seattle, Washington.

in the form of a flow sheet, or printed from a computerized database, not only makes patients feel that their input is important but ensures that patients and providers could quickly remind themselves of where things were left at the last visit so that efficient use could be made of the time at hand. Group Health's diabetic patient education/self-management summary is shown in Figure 29–3.

FUTURE DIRECTIONS

I hope these remarks will stimulate innovative thinking about incorporating some of these approaches in day-to-day work with patients with diabetes. Some may criticize the concept of disease state management as being cookbook medicine that detracts from the individuality of the doctor-patient relationship. Certainly, when Group Health began trying to implement a whole set of supports for primary care providers (clinical guidelines, diabetes registries, patient education materials, feedback through report cards profiling process measures and patient outcomes, etc) there was concern that the primary care teams would find the support intrusive and time consuming.

Our experience has been just the opposite. Primary care teams have expressed increased interest and confidence in dealing with diabetes. Having gained easy tools to remind them of the appropriate priorities and needs for individual patients with diabetes, primary care teams report that they have more time to do what they are particularly good at, which is interacting with patients and helping them to live with diabetes.

Organizations need to continue moving, using existing and future technology to make it easier to do routine care well. Rather than relying on busy individuals to try to remember everything, organizations should make it easier to do the right thing than not to do it. For example, when a

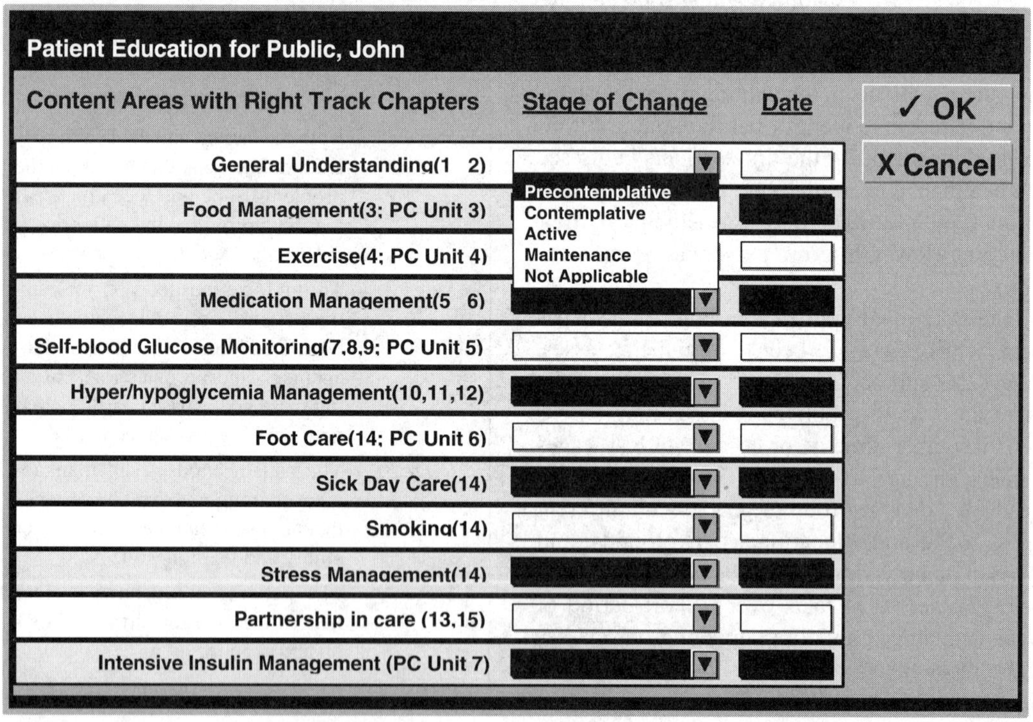

Figure 29–3 Sample Diabetic Patient Education/Self-Management Summary. Courtesy of Group Health Cooperative of Puget Sound, Seattle, Washington.

patient shows up for the first time in 9 months for an acute visit (eg, for a sprained ankle), as soon as the patient's health card (or registration number) is entered by the receptionist, this should identify that the patient has diabetes. If databases are truly interactive, then the health care system should know that the patient is perhaps overdue for microalbuminuria screening, HbA1c testing, and a foot exam, and was still a smoker at the last visit. In addition to a TRF form and some labels, a printout should be generated reminding the primary care team members that in addition to dealing with the sprained ankle, they might consider following up with the items that are overdue. It should even be possible for the relevant lab slips to be filled out, in anticipation that the primary care provider will want to approve them, sign them, and send them off.

Other innovative approaches to patient education should also be explored. With everyone feeling increasingly busy and stressed, organizations need to try to find teachable moments and situations wherever possible. Interactive computer programs (with touch-screen technology) can be effective, even for older patients who are less familiar with this medium. The Internet provides huge possibilities for connecting patients with relevant information and other people with similar needs, problems, and goals. This is an arena in which the continual advances in clinical care will be better served if matched with continual advances in the overall organizational approach.

REFERENCES

1. Wagner EH, Austin BT, Von Korff M. Organizing care for patients with chronic illness. *Milbank Q.* 1996; 74:511–544.
2. Ayanian JZ, Hauptman PJ, Guadagnoli E, et al. Knowledge and practices of generalist and specialist physicians regarding drug therapy for acute myocardial infarction. *N Engl J Med.* 1994;331:1136–1142.
3. Markson LE, Cosler M, Turner BJ. Implications of generalists' slow adoption of zidovudine in clinical practice. *Arch Intern Med.* 1994;154:1497–1504.
4. Horner RD, Matchar DB, Divine GW, Feussner JR. Relationship between physician specialty and the selection and outcome of ischemic stroke patients. *Health Serv Res.* 1995;30:275–287.
5. Brown JJ, Sullivan G. Effect on ICU mortality of a full-time critical care specialist. *Chest.* 1989;96(1):127–129.
6. Hayes TM, Harries J. Randomized controlled trial of routine hospital care versus routine general practice care for type II diabetics. *Br Med J.* 1984;289:728–730.
7. Verlato G, Muggeo M, Bonora E, Corbellini M, Bressan F, de Marco R. Attending the diabetes center is associated with increased 5-year survival probability of diabetic patients. *Diabetes Care.* 1996;19:211–213.
8. The Expert Committee on the Diagnosis and Classification of Diabetes Mellitus. 1997 report of the Expert Committee on the Diagnosis and Classification of Diabetes Mellitus. *Diabetes Care.* 1997;20:1183–1197.
9. The American Diabetes Association. Clinical practice recommendations–1997. *Diabetes Care.* 1997;20(suppl 1):S1–S70.
10. Kenny SJ, Smith PL, Goldscmid MG, Newman JM, Herman WH. Survey of physician practice behaviors related to diabetes mellitus in the U.S. *Diabetes Care.* 1993;16:1507–1510.
11. Stolar M. Clinical management of the NIDDM patient: impact of the American Diabetes Association guidelines, 1985–1993. *Diabetes Care.* 1995;18:701–707.
12. Handley MR, Stuart ME. An evidence-based approach to evaluating and improving clinical practice: guideline development. *HMO Practice.* 1994;8:10–19.
13. Handley MR, Stuart ME, Kirz HL. An evidence-based approach to evaluating and improving clinical practice: implementing practice guidelines. *HMO Practice.* 1994;8:75–83.
14. Payne TH, Galvin M, Taplin SH, Austin BT, Savarino J, Wagner EH. Practicing population-based care in an HMO: evaluation after 18 months. *HMO Practice.* 1995;9:101–106.
15. Borch-Johnsen K, Wenzel H, Viberti GC, Mogensen CE. Is screening and intervention for microalbuminuria worthwhile in patients with insulin-dependent diabetes? *Br Med J.* 1993;306:1722–1725.
16. Javitt JC, Aiello LP, Chiang Y, Ferris FL, Greenfield S. Preventive eye care in people with diabetes is cost saving to the federal government. *Diabetes Care.* 1994; 17:909–917.
17. Sinnock P. Reduced hospital utilization and cost savings associated with diabetes patient education. *J Insurance Med.* 1986;18:24–30.
18. Eastman RC, Javitt JC, Herman WH, et al. Model of complications of NIDDM, II: analysis of the health benefits and cost-effectiveness of treating NIDDM with the goal of normoglycemia. *Diabetes Care.* 1997;20: 735–744.

19. Peters AL, Legorreta AP, Ossorio RC, Davidson MB. Quality of outpatient care provided to diabetic patients: a health maintenance organization experience. *Diabetes Care*. 1996;19:601–606.
20. Legorreta AP, Peters AL, Ossorio RC, Lopez RJ, Jatulis D, Davidson MB. Effect of a comprehensive nurse-managed diabetes program: an HMO prospective study. *Am J Managed Care*. 1996;2:1024–1030.
21. Anderson RM, Funnell MM, Butler PM, Arnold MS, Fitzgerald JT, Feste CC. Patient empowerment: results of a randomized controlled trial. *Diabetes Care*. 1995;18:943–949.

DAVID K. MCCULLOCH, MD, FRCP, is currently a diabetologist with the Group Health Cooperative of Puget Sound and a clinical associate professor of medicine at the University of Washington. He has had a key role in diabetes improvement efforts at Group Health Cooperative of Puget Sound since 1994. Previously, Dr. McCulloch was a co-investigator in the Diabetes Control and Complications Trial. He has published over 100 articles and abstracts of original clinical research in the field of diabetes.

CHAPTER 30

Asthma Disease Management

Benjamin Safirstein, Joan Kennedy, and Barbara Barton

Chapter Outline

- Disease Management: An Innovative Concept
- The Suitability of Asthma for Programmatic Disease Management
- A Framework for Setting Program Objectives
- Nine Critical Components in the Oxford Health Plan
- The Four Most Critical Steps
- Industry Alternatives to a Comprehensive Disease Management Program
- Barriers to Program Implementation
- Conclusion

DISEASE MANAGEMENT: AN INNOVATIVE CONCEPT

Traditionally, health care delivery models have focused on the treatment of acute or infectious disease states. In this model, termed the *experience-based* or *episodic* model, it is the expectation of patient and provider alike that treatment will be followed by recovery. Patients present with symptoms. They are treated and recover. While this delivery model remains viable and appropriate for many situations, such as a case of chicken pox or a broken leg, it misses the mark when treatment must be provided to patients who never fully recover, patients who are chronically ill. For patients with chronic disease, the episodic model is inadequate because, even when symptoms are relieved, treatment does not lead to recovery. Patient satisfaction may decrease, and the cost of care may increase needlessly.

More recently, health care professionals have begun to recognize that episodic treatment models do not meet the needs of chronically ill patients. As a result of experimentation, evaluation, and innovation at some advanced managed care organizations (MCOs) and integrated delivery systems (IDSs), a new treatment paradigm for chronic disease has begun to emerge. (For a discussion of different types of MCOs and integrated provider systems, please refer to *The Managed Health Care Handbook*, 3rd Edition.) As discussed in Chapter 27, *disease management* is the term used to describe the new paradigm. Disease management is an integrated and comprehensive *system* for managing patients with chronic conditions through a coordinated approach to care. It is based on principles taken from both public health and business. Disease management is characterized as *integrated* because it brings together such diverse health care concepts as practice guidelines, provider networks, case management, patient and physician education, patient stratification, data systems, and other electronic technology. It is characterized as *comprehen-*

sive because through the act of coordinating these diverse concepts, disease management is able to produce positive clinical, financial, satisfaction, and quality of life outcomes.

Disease management integrates many operational and managerial concepts that were formerly considered distinct. And unlike episodic treatment, disease management focuses on a *population-based* model of health care delivery. In the population-based model, a concerted effort is made to link the various stages of a chronic disease with the levels of disease severity experienced in the patient population. The linking makes it possible to provide patients with appropriate strategies for controlling disease that lead to both improved patient outcomes and reduced costs. Thus, by a careful analysis of the patient population, which we term *patient stratification and classification,* disease management can be designed to intervene and prevent the advance of the disease to its next, more severe and costly stage.

THE SUITABILITY OF ASTHMA FOR PROGRAMMATIC DISEASE MANAGEMENT

The population-based approach of disease management programs begins with a complete understanding of the chronic disease to be managed—in this case, asthma. This section provides a brief overview of asthma, including its epidemiology and risk factors. (Space limitations prevent us from presenting a description of asthma and its treatment that is sufficiently comprehensive for the design of a disease management program. We advise readers to seek out longer and more in-depth descriptions before putting their own programs in place.)

Epidemiology

Asthma affects over 11 million Americans annually, creating $2.4 billion in direct health care costs.[1] From 1980 to 1987, the prevalence rate of asthma increased 29%, and death rates for asthma as the first-listed diagnosis increased 31%.[2] Asthma is also the most common chronic disease affecting children. Nationally, two thirds of asthma care dollars spent for children younger than 18 years old are for inpatient admissions and emergency department care.[1] In 1992, asthma was one of the 10 most frequently billed diagnoses at Oxford Health Plan (OxHP), affecting 5% of its members. Increases in asthma-related morbidity, mortality, and care costs are occurring despite recent scientific advances in knowledge about the disease and its therapies and the widespread use of practice guidelines. Experts suggest that the major factors contributing to these increases are under-diagnosis and inappropriate treatment.[3]

Definition, Complications, and Special Considerations

Asthma is a chronic inflammatory disease of the airways. In the Expert Panel Report II from the National Asthma Education and Prevention Program of the National Institutes of Health (NIH), asthma is defined as

> a chronic inflammatory disorder of the airways in which many cells and cellular elements play a role, in particular, mast cells, eosinophils, T lymphocytes, neutrophils, and epithelial cells. In susceptible individuals, this inflammation causes recurrent episodes of wheezing, breathlessness, chest tightness, and cough, particularly at night and in the early morning. These episodes are usually associated with widespread but variable airflow obstruction that is often reversible, either spontaneously or with treatment. The inflammation also causes an associated increase in the existing bronchial hyper-responsiveness to a variety of stimuli.[2]

A comprehensive review of complications and special considerations related to asthma is found in the NIH *Guidelines for the Diagnosis and Management of Asthma.*[2] This discussion is limited to the most frequently encountered asthma complications, which are emphasized in OxHP's Better Breathing program. Elements of that program are used for illustrative purposes throughout the remainder of this chapter.

With the increasing asthma mortality rate observed over the past decade, the risk of death from asthma exists for all asthmatics, regardless of severity level. Recent studies[2] revealed that the following factors are associated with an increased risk of asthma-related death:

- previous life-threatening exacerbations of asthma or recent hospitalization or emergency department visits for asthma
- ethnicity (The NIH[2] reports that the asthma death rate among African Americans of all ages is almost 3 times higher than the rate observed among Caucasians. In the 15-44 age group, the death rate for African Americans is about 5 times higher, especially in urban areas.)
- lack of adequate and ongoing medical care that provides appropriate follow-up and preventive therapy
- significant depression and/or psychosocial behavioral problems
- complacency or underestimation of the severity of the disease by the patient, patient's family, or health care providers

Asthma during pregnancy deserves special consideration. The most important goal for managing asthma during pregnancy is to maintain sufficient lung function and blood oxygenation to ensure that the fetus receives an adequate oxygen supply, while avoiding, as much as possible, drugs that pose a threat to the fetus. Poorly managed asthma during pregnancy can result in poor fetal outcomes, including low birthweight, increased perinatal mortality, and increased prematurity.

Treatment and Therapy

The treatment of asthma requires continuous care. In essence, its therapy has four goals.

1. Maintain normal activity.
2. Maintain near-normal pulmonary function.
3. Prevent chronic and troublesome symptoms.
4. Avoid adverse effects from medications.

Its therapy also has four components.

1. patient education
2. environmental control
3. comprehensive pharmacological therapy
4. objective measurement

Manageability

Asthma is a chronic disease that is well suited to disease management. By reducing the number of acute episodes or exacerbations provoked by the chronic condition, clinical outcome, patient satisfaction, and utilization measures are improved. The ability to investigate and, more precisely, to subdivide or *stratify* the treatment population by disease severity is at the heart of the population-based treatment method and makes the selection of appropriate therapies more feasible. Asthma patients can successfully be classified by the severity of their disease, educated to understand all stages in the continuum of asthma, and taught to recognize symptoms earlier. Early recognition can reduce the severity of the bronchospasm as well as the level of intervention required. Providers can be educated to recognize and apply all available resources, providing a broader range of care to the patient. Through the integration of care—the coordination of patients, providers, and resources into a single, coherent system—intervention can take place in time to prevent emergency department care or hospitalization. The discussion will now turn to the basic steps required to design and implement a disease management program for asthma.

A FRAMEWORK FOR SETTING PROGRAM OBJECTIVES

The advantage of an innovation such as disease management should now be clear. It leads to a win-win situation: Patient outcomes improve, and the costs of care are reduced. But if the disease management program is to succeed, the first step for management will be to provide the implementation team members with a set of objectives against which they can evaluate their progress. To illustrate this, at OxHP, each disease management program has four categories of objectives that are monitored. Improving in any of these areas without losing ground in the others confirms that OxHP has developed a value-added product line. Although specific measures may vary depending on the disease, the four categories remain the same for each program.

1. *Improvement in Clinical Parameters.* Improvement across clinical parameters could include increased member/physician compliance with treatment guidelines, enhancement of self-management strategies that teach patients better self-monitoring, reduction in the number of readmits and illness exacerbations, and minimization of complications.
2. *Improvement in Costs.* Depending upon the applicable MCO's or IDS's initiatives or philosophy, the financial goals will differ. Overall, the financial goals should be a direct result of the improved quality of care and patient empowerment strategies (see discussion below) central to every disease management program. For instance, cost savings could occur through decreases in inpatient admissions, lengths of stay, and emergency department visits, reflected in per member per month cost reduction.
3. *Improvement in Member/Physician Satisfaction.* Data derived from common sources, such as claims and lab tests, may be useful only for capturing financial outcomes. Gathering satisfaction information is necessary for evaluating the program and requires using more direct, self-reported data. Satisfaction indicators evaluate how members and physicians perceive the effectiveness of the disease management program. Satisfaction surveys should ask the following questions: Did the program meet both member and physician needs? Did members and physicians find educational materials effective? Was there an opportunity to receive continuous feedback?
4. *Improvement in Quality of Life and Functional Status.* The patient's perception of quality of life has been shown to be an important indicator of overall health status.[4] Including improved quality of life as an objective in a disease management program acknowledges that patients' psychosocial needs can be just as important as their clinical needs. Quality pertains not only to the skill with which care is delivered but to the appropriateness and consistency of the care. These indicators depict patient understanding and implementation of self-management strategies that result in the ability of patients to take better control of their lives and function better on a daily basis. Improvements in this area may include increased understanding of the illness (which in turn leads to better self-management), increased feelings of control over the illness, and improved daily living function brought about by increased education and self-monitoring.

NINE CRITICAL COMPONENTS IN THE OXFORD HEALTH PLAN

In the introduction, we alluded to the fact that a distinguishing feature of the disease management concept is the *integration* of diverse health care concepts and procedures. In this section, we provide more detail about what integration entails by describing the nine critical components in the OxHP disease management program for asthma, the Better Breathing program.

1. patient empowerment
2. member education
3. provider education
4. treatment guidelines
5. network development
6. case management
7. technological support

8. evaluation of outcome measures
9. continuous quality improvement

In the discussion that follows, we will describe each component along with its implications for asthma management.

Patient Empowerment

More than a specific set of procedures that belongs to asthma alone, patient empowerment is a policy and a way of doing business with patients. First, the concept of patient empowerment strives to change the patient's outlook from that of passive recipient of care to one of proactive participant. It relies upon the policy that health care delivery can be much more effective if patients become respected participants in the design of their own treatment plans, and that patient observations and opinions will be heard. Therefore, a sound disease management program attempts to restructure the health care delivery system by emphasizing the patient's role, especially when the objective is behavior change. Wherever possible, patients are educated and encouraged to self-manage their illness. The goal is to empower patients and family caregivers so that they play a large part in determining outcomes.

Member Education

In order for patient empowerment to occur, members must first be educated. Patients often do not have all the information needed to manage their condition. Providing them with continuous education throughout the course of treatment is a necessary component of every disease management program. Education provides patients with the opportunity to become active members of their treatment team; it enables them to make knowledgeable decisions regarding how they want their treatment to occur. Education also fosters behavior change that can be translated into improved health and reduced cost. Education can take place in the form of written materials, face-to-face or telephone-based case management, and active learning (eg, sending a visiting nurse to a member's home to teach the member how to use the peak flow meter).

When educating patients, it is important to keep in mind that just because patients have the same illness does not mean they will respond the same way to an education technique. Education must be individualized. Teaching strategies must vary with the individual patient's personality, age, capability, functional status, and capacity to cope with the stress resulting from the disease. Being sensitive to how an individual experiences the disease will make it more likely that the patient will become engaged in the care process.[5]

In OxHP's Better Breathing program, members are educated about their disease and its management and are provided with and taught how to use monitoring equipment, such as peak flow meters. OxHP employs targeted intervention. That is, the level and type of education is determined by the patient's disease severity and coverage type (ie, commercial, Medicare, or Medicaid). For example, for Medicaid patients OxHP has implemented an Education and Outreach (E&O) team, composed of nonclinical staff who focus on solving social issues as well as asthma education. The team members proactively contact each Medicaid member to explain how to use primary care physicians, hospitals, and emergency departments. When members with asthma are identified during this contact, they are stratified by their level of disease severity (Mild, Moderate 1, Moderate 2, or Severe; see discussion below), and members found to be Severe or Moderate 2 are referred to the asthma disease management team for nurse case management. The E&O team tracks the members with Mild and Moderate 1 asthma to address social issues, identify potential needs for clinical management, and complete appropriate referrals.

In response to the desires of individuals served by Medicaid who have asthma and who tend to prefer face-to-face asthma education, asthma workshops have been established in hospitals in high-volume Medicaid areas. Qualified respiratory therapists or asthma-trained registered nurses conduct the workshops, adhering to the content suggested in the NIH *Guidelines for the Diagnosis and Management of Asthma*.[2] The opportunity to attend an asthma education workshop is offered to the member by the E&O team or asthma disease management team, regardless of the member's asthma severity level. Since the purpose of the workshop is to educate the member about asthma, all medical management issues are referred to the asthma nurse case managers for follow up with the member's physician.

Member education is provided in many different formats: printed materials (letters and brochures), Web sites, buddy systems (used primarily with Medicaid patients; these systems partner a nurse case manager with a specialist in solving social problems), asthma workshops, and education done in conjunction with home care. In all, it is a comprehensive education system noted for its *targeted* intervention, a consistent attempt to match the level and kind of education provided with the patient's background and level of disease severity.

Provider Education

If a disease management program is to achieve its objective of complete integration of diverse components, provider education must be in step with patient education. If the education of providers and members is coordinated, providers will be better informed about treatment guidelines and the disease management program itself. This will also improve their ability to take an active role in effectively educating their patients. In addition, the health care system can provide an educational experience to physicians about its own operations, that is, how physicians can best negotiate the system on behalf of their patients.

There are various ways in which physician education can take place. A physician packet focused on asthma, for example, could contain the program description, the criteria that patients must meet for enrollment in the program, how patients can be referred to the program, and copies of the guidelines supported by the payer. Physicians can also receive education concerning the disease management program through ongoing communication with a case manager. Continuing education classes can also be offered to keep physicians up-to-date on ongoing research, treatment, and revisions to guidelines. In fact, at OxHP we continuously distribute new information as soon as it becomes available to ensure that physicians and other providers have access to the most recent findings in asthma disease management.

In the OxHP Better Breathing program, educational materials are regularly sent to physicians who treat asthma, including primary care physicians, pulmonologists, pediatricians, and allergists. To standardize treatment according to NIH guidelines, an executive summary of the NIH *Guidelines for the Diagnosis and Management of Asthma* is provided.[6] This 44-page booklet details the key concepts in asthma diagnosis and management for adults and children. For the management of asthma during pregnancy, a brochure is provided that describes the importance of ensuring an adequate oxygen supply to the fetus while avoiding, as much as possible, drugs that pose a risk. Treatment of asthma exacerbation during labor and the effects of asthma drugs on fetal development and during lactation are also discussed. Physicians are also sent the member educational materials for adults and children as a reference.

Although it is important to standardize treatment (see the upcoming discussion of treatment guidelines) and provide access to the most recent research on asthma disease management, the most important aspect of provider—especially physician—education is comparative information in the form of statistical data. OxHP's primary emphasis in physician education is to let physicians see for themselves how their treatment plans compare with the treatment plans of other physicians in the nation, the region, and the company. OxHP remains committed to data systems, continuous quality improvement, and outcome studies, because comparative data are ultimately far more persuasive in changing physician behavior than insistence on adherence to treatment guidelines.

Treatment Guidelines

As the previous discussion begins to suggest, a disease management program's success is measured by comparing outcomes for its program participants to national statistics. However, outcome measures will be difficult to interpret if every provider uses different treatment patterns. Therefore, it is desirable that physicians comply with a set of guidelines wherever possible. Clinical guidelines provide the step-by-step method of diagnosing and guiding care by the utilization of defined treatment protocols.[5] They are based upon universal standards of clinical practice that define what needs to be accomplished during a certain period of time for a given diagnosis.[7]

At OxHP, disease management programs adopt national guidelines rather than developing new ones, unless no national guidelines or protocols have been established. While those guidelines or protocols are relied upon to reduce inappropriate variation in treatment patterns, they are used as a framework or stepping stone only. No sanctions are applied to force the adoption of guidelines; instead, OxHP prefers to rely on statistical data such as pharmacy prescribing patterns, hospital admissions, and emergency department (see Chapter 13) visits as feedback to physicians. While the guidelines do encourage similarity among treatment patterns, they are not meant to dictate what type of care the patient must receive. Instead, guidelines are put in place to give physicians a reference they can use through every step of the patient's illness and to keep them constantly apprised of the relevant literature so that they are aware of the entire range of recommendations available for managing a disease.[8]

The OxHP Better Breathing program employs NIH guidelines.[6] This executive summary includes background information, definitions, and pathophysiology of the disease and its exacerbations. It also includes algorithms for the diagnosis and management of the disease in adults, children, and infants.

Network Development

It is important that members enrolled in a disease management program feel that they are receiving the best care possible. This is feasible only if an exceptional provider network is in place. Before implementing an asthma disease management program, the quality and scope of the providers in the network must be assessed. Without a comprehensive network of quality providers, it will be difficult to implement a comprehensive program. This is especially important given that the population of members with asthma will be stratified into segments according to disease severity and coverage type. Since each segment will make different demands on the provider network, the network will require adequate "bench depth" in order to be effective. Providers in the network may include, but are not limited to, primary care physicians, specialists, hospitals, durable medical equipment providers, social workers, home care providers, and psychologists or psychiatrists.

When evaluating and developing the provider network, explicit criteria are used. Providers must be easily accessible, have varied backgrounds, and must be compliant with preestablished treatment guidelines and disease management program methods. OxHP has come to rely especially upon two resources—a list of providers who have expertise in asthma cases with special problems and a set of centers of excellence or clinics—to ensure that its provider network is offering the best care possible. These two groups help provide the best care without creating the impression that they are rivals for patients who are already well managed by OxHP physicians. Our list of providers with special expertise is not highly publicized, but it is made available to nurses managing problem cases. These special providers support both nurses and physicians; they review, prescribe for, and then return patients to their regular physician for continued care.

The OxHP case management system also employs the services of special centers of excellence for members with severe asthma and difficulty managing their condition. These centers must be headed by a director who is board certified in allergy care or pulmonology and must have a trained asthma nurse or licensed respiratory therapist on staff. The program offered must be in a dedicated outpatient facility, have a preexisting outreach program and a case management program, and provide individual counseling or group sessions on various asthma-related topics.

Case Management

The most important component in the disease management concept is case management (see also Chapter 17). Case managers (frequently nurses) collaborate with members to advocate for health care needs on an individual basis. They support and augment provider treatment and are responsible for evaluating members' health status throughout the various stages of asthma. They educate both members and providers, conduct timely discharge planning when necessary, and identify areas where care can be improved through strategic intervention. Evaluation of the status of at-risk patients includes analysis of the medical care incidents to date along with data collection regarding physical, psychosocial, environmental, and community factors that affect health care delivery and related expenditures. Case managers provide members and providers with a constant information and referral source and give continuous support to members both during and between exacerbations of their asthma.

Case managers are key players in making sure that members receive the right care at the right time during their illness. They accomplish this feat with the aid of a complex set of algorithms that are used, among other things, to intercept new patients, identify the severity of their disease, make and track referrals, and follow up on progress. The case manager is also charged with the management of data systems to track program enrollees' progress with respect to the outcome measures used to evaluate the disease management program. The OxHP asthma disease management program case management algorithms will no doubt serve as the foundation of any similar program in the organization.

Case management can be accomplished by telephone or on-site care depending on members' needs. But no matter what type of case management the member receives, it is the case manager's responsibility to remain knowledgeable about the *whole picture* of a member's care.

The case management approach, in conjunction with the physician's treatment plan, not only develops a specific plan of care but empowers the member to accomplish the plan. Because of members' close contact with the case manager, they can ask questions about medications, providers, diet, and any other concerns. This familiarity makes it more likely that members will ask questions that they may feel are too trivial to ask their physician. By probing for strengths and weaknesses in understanding, the case manager can fill in gaps in the patient's knowledge, as well as identify psychosocial problems that may require solutions. A byproduct of interaction with the case manager is long-term wellness for the patient. The interaction teaches patients about their disease and its management. In this way, the coordination of services provided by the case manager eventually leads to a reduction in utilization and an improved quality of life for the patient.

Technological Support

Asthma and other disease management relies heavily on work with an active database to track member progress and to provide data storage that can be easily mined for outcomes measures. Information systems must be able to house comprehensive patient information that enables development and refinement of treatment protocols, and to efficiently store and manipulate the asthma disease management program data. These systems enable clinical encounters to be computerized, summarized, and shared.

It would be highly difficult to conduct patient stratification and follow-up without the technical data systems that allow selective processing of patient characteristics. It would also be extremely difficult to provide valuable comparative data to physicians (showing outcomes resulting from their treatment plans versus those of other physicians) without access to pharmacy and other utilization data showing hospital admissions and emergency department visits. Complex databases will enable the future direction of patient intervention. With complex data systems, it will soon be possible to model future lapses in patient compliance by evaluating current patient behavior. With these models, and the data systems from which they are constructed, lapses in compliance will be prevented with a targeted intervention that will avoid increases in utilization and cost.

Evaluation of Outcome Measures

The movement to collect outcome information has recently escalated. Stimulated by federal initiatives to compare mortality among hospitals, by comparative outcome studies, and by payers seeking to improve quality and reduce costs, outcome measurements provide a way of evaluating the effectiveness of an asthma disease management program.

The OxHP Better Breathing program utilizes such outcome measures as the SF-12 Health Status Profile,[9] an asthma assessment questionnaire for assessing disease severity, an asthma environmental assessment, and an asthma follow-up assessment that can be used to assess progress since the last exacerbation encounter with the patient. In addition, satisfaction questionnaires are administered to both patients and physicians to improve the understanding of their level of satisfaction with the program.

The collection of outcome information remains an integral part of every disease management program, whether it is devoted to asthma or any other chronic disease. When conducted in the context of a disease management program, outcomes research enables the continuous improvement of that program, which ultimately benefits both the plan and its members.

Continuous Quality Improvement

A good asthma management program relies heavily on continuous quality improvement (CQI) strategies to investigate the program's strengths and weaknesses. These strategies mine the technical support database to statistically track asthma outcomes, pinpoint program strengths and weaknesses, and make appropriate adjustments. Early in the development of OxHP's asthma management program, program objectives were set in four areas: clinical outcomes, costs, member and physician satisfaction, and quality of life. CQI analysis is used to learn whether those objectives were met. If the objectives are not met in one area, program leaders know that part of the program needs improvement. If clear objectives are outlined at the inception of the program, those objectives can later be evaluated to assess the program's effectiveness. Analysis should be performed to compare the numbers proposed in the objectives with the actual numbers observed at the end of a specified operating period. Improvements can be made based on the results of these comparisons.

THE FOUR MOST CRITICAL STEPS

Whether you purchase the services of outside vendors or build your own program from the ground up, there are many steps involved before an asthma disease management program can begin to provide services to members: the design of an organizational structure, the development of a budget, the evaluation of vendors, and many others. In this section, we introduce what we believe are the four most critical steps in that process—the four that we think can make or break the plan.

1. identifying all the members of the organization who have asthma
2. subdividing these members into groups according to disease severity and coverage type

3. designing the right interventions for each group
4. tracking progress

In the paragraphs that follow, we will discuss each step in detail so that any health care system may implement them.

How To Locate the Members Who Should Be Targeted

At OxHP, asthmatic members who are likely candidates for the disease management program are identified through various methods depending on enrollment status and coverage type. In this section we describe those methods in some detail. They are summarized in Table 30–1.

Utilization Episode

Members who experience an asthma emergency department visit or hospital admission are referred into the program. These members are identified through authorizations, referrals from medical management teams, and member self-reporting.

Member Referral

The benefits of the Better Breathing program are communicated to asthma members through the *Healthy Mind, Healthy Body* magazine and the asthma educational member mailings. Commercial and Medicare members may self-refer into the program by telephoning the asthma disease management team. Medicaid members may self-refer by calling the Medicaid E&O team or by calling the asthma disease management team directly.

Physician Referral

Physicians may also refer members into the program by calling the asthma disease management team's 800 number. The value of the program is communicated to physicians in the *Remedies* magazine and through one-on-one education sessions with OxHP regional field staff.

Claims and Pharmacy Data

At 3-month intervals, medical claims data are reviewed for utilization of inpatient and outpatient services. Members identified via the International Classification of Diseases, Ninth Edition, Clinical Modification (ICD-9-CM) codes are referred to appropriate teams based on severity and coverage type. Pharmacy data are also regularly combed for members utilizing asthma drugs, and referrals to the appropriate teams are made.

Table 30–1 Methods for Identifying Candidates for Asthma Disease Management

	Commercial	Medicaid	Medicare
New enrollees	Member profile*	Welcome call field outreach visit	High-risk assessment
Members who are diagnosed after enrollment but have no utilization history	Claims Pharmacy utilization DME request Physician referrals Member referrals	Claims Pharmacy utilization DME request Physician referrals Member referrals	Claims Pharmacy utilization DME request Physician referrals Member referrals
Members with utilization history	Emergency department episode referral Admission referral		

*Member profile is under development.

Courtesy of Oxford Health Plan, Milford, Connecticut.

Durable Medical Equipment Request

Asthmatic members are also identified by the asthma disease management team from requests by members and physicians for asthma durable medical equipment (DME). The team may authorize DME exceptions to cover asthma equipment (spacers, nebulizers) for members who do not have a DME rider. This is an especially good time for referrals, because the member's current problem (as evidenced by the need for equipment) may have raised his or her consciousness about the need for new information regarding disease management.

Medicare High-Risk Assessment

OxHP's Medicare E&O team completes a screening survey called the High-Risk Assessment on each Medicare member after enrollment. This survey identifies asthmatics who are then referred to the asthma disease management team for appropriate intervention based on the member's asthma severity level.

Medicaid Welcome Call and Field Outreach

OxHP's Medicaid E&O team contacts each Medicaid member after enrollment by phone or home visit. During this contact, a screening survey is completed that identifies and then stratifies asthma members. Severe and Moderate 2 asthmatics are referred to the asthma disease management team for nurse case management, while the E&O team tracks Mild and Moderate 1 asthmatics (see below for a discussion of classification by disease severity).

Member Profile

This identification method for newly enrolled commercial members, still under development at this writing, requires this group of patients to complete a brief survey designed to identify individuals with various comorbidities, including asthma. Individuals identified in this way are then referred to the asthma disease management team for stratification and appropriate management.

Identifying Members' Level of Disease Severity: Patient Stratification

At OxHP, asthmatic members are stratified into one of four severity levels based on criteria consisting of the member's utilization history and the responses to three key clinical questions. Table 30–2 describes each severity level and its criteria.

While the severity levels shown in the table are closely matched to NIH severity levels published in its guidelines,[2] it should be noted that the patient stratification process can be challenging when program managers do not have access to patient charts, as in all programs not employing a full staff model. To overcome this difficulty, OxHP employs a two-stage stratification process. In stage one, claims data are sorted to preliminarily stratify members into mild, moderate, and severe categories. Mild and severe cases receive no additional stratification processing, and the intervention suitable for these cases is put into effect immediately.

Moderate cases require additional information for more precise classification. Since program managers do not have access to pulmonary function data (available only in the patients' charts, and the best method for classifying disease severity), program managers pose three questions to members by telephone. These questions act as surrogate measures to differentiate between Moderate 1 and Moderate 2 levels of severity. The questions were uncovered by polling physicians who treat asthma: (1) Is the member awakened at night by asthma symptoms? (2) Is the member currently taking systemic steroids (prednisone)? (3) Is the member using a bronchodilator more than twice a day by mouth or inhaler? A "yes" response to any of these questions places the member into the Moderate 2 severity level.

Matching the Right Intervention to the Right Stratum

Member interventions are determined by a population stratum. The strata are defined by

Table 30–2 Summary of Stratification Criteria for Placement of Program Candidates into Disease Severity Levels

Severity Level	Criteria
Mild	1. No history of asthma hospital admissions or emergency department utilization
Moderate 1	1. One episode of asthma utilization: hospital admission and/or emergency department visit 2. "No" responses to all three clinical questions
Moderate 2	1. One episode of asthma utilization: hospital admission and/or emergency department visit 2. A "yes" response to any of the three clinical questions
Severe	1. Two or more episodes of asthma utilization: hospital admissions and/or emergency department visits
Three clinical questions	1. Is the member awakened at night by asthma symptoms? 2. Is the member currently taking systemic steroids (prednisone)? 3. Is the member using a bronchodilator more than twice a day by mouth or inhaler?

Courtesy of Oxford Health Plan, Milford, Connecticut.

levels of disease severity and coverage type. In this section we describe each intervention component in detail. Table 30–3 summarizes the intervention that is appropriate for each population stratum. The discussion begins with a focus on interventions targeting commercial and Medicare members.

Asthma Case Management

Case management is reserved for individuals with Moderate 2 and Severe asthma. Nurse case managers regularly contact these members to provide telephone-based asthma assessments and education, referrals as needed to specialists and home care, and educational resources. Case managers also work closely with the member's physician to support and reinforce the physician's treatment plan, emphasizing compliance management. Also included in the asthma team are asthma coordinators who function to coordinate the nonclinical aspects of the case management process. The asthma case management processes are standardized in detailed algorithms designed to ensure consistency and adherence to program guidelines.

Co–Case Management

The co–case management process was implemented with Oxford Medical Management to improve discharge planning and coordination of care for hospitalized individuals with asthma. This process involves asthma nurse case managers proactively contacting discharge planners at admitting hospitals to determine the member's asthma care needs at home. The asthma nurses coordinate this care and follow up with the member and physician after discharge to identify an individualized care plan to improve the member's asthma management and thereby prevent readmission.

Member Education Materials

Because of the importance of education in the successful management of asthma, education materials are provided to all asthmatic members. These materials are designed to provide members with the critical information needed to understand and manage their asthma. OxHP's asthma education materials also serve as teaching tools for asthma case management interventions. These materials include the *Asthma Self-*

Table 30–3 The Customization of Asthma Interventions to Each Population Stratum

	Interventions	
Disease Severity	Commercial and Medicare	Medicaid
Mild	Asthma kit Peak flow meter	Medicaid asthma kit Peak flow meter E&O tracking Asthma workshop
Moderate 1	Asthma kit Peak flow meter Asthma coordinator tracking	Medicaid asthma kit Peak flow meter E&O tracking Asthma workshop
Moderate 2	Asthma kit Peak flow meter Asthma nurse case management	Medicaid asthma kit Peak flow meter Asthma workshop Asthma nurse case management
Severe	Asthma kit Peak flow meter Asthma nurse case management	Medicaid asthma kit Peak flow meter Asthma workshop Asthma nurse case management

Note: Member education and resources are provided to all strata; customized interventions result from the application of nurse case management and outreach tracking services and how intensely they are applied. Asthma kit contains Self-Help Series brochure (adult or child), zone chart, response card for peak flow meter, and diary grid. Medicaid asthma kit contains Medicaid asthma booklet, zone chart, response card for peak flow meter, and diary grid.

Courtesy of Oxford Health Plan, Milford, Connecticut.

Help Series: Adult, the *Asthma Self-Help Series: Childhood*, and the *Asthma Medicaid Brochure*.

Asthma Self-Management Resources for Members

This set of resources includes three items. The first is the asthma management zone system. This system utilizes the concept of red, yellow, and green zones to provide asthmatics and physicians with a method of self-adjustment of medications based on peak flow meter reading and asthma symptoms. Actions the member should take at each zone level are listed, including when to call the physician and seek emergency medical attention. This system was adopted as recommended by the NIH guidelines.[6]

The second item in the asthma kit is the peak flow meter (low and full range). This simple device uses measurements of peak expiratory flow rate to determine the degree of airflow obstruction. Regular monitoring of peak flow meter readings and asthma symptoms can predict asthma exacerbations, allowing members time to make necessary adjustments in medications to prevent or lessen the severity of the asthma attack. Peak flow meters are available in low and full ranges to accommodate both children and adults. The meters are sent directly to the members' homes.

The third item in the kit is the peak flow meter diary grid. This diary grid is used to record daily peak flow meter readings. It is sent along with peak flow meters.

As described above, a somewhat different set of interventions is provided to Medicaid patients to meet their needs. Medicaid members have historically presented unique challenges in disease management, often requiring more intensive and creative intervention than other populations to achieve desired outcomes and control inappropriate utilization. With this in mind, a special plan was implemented for Medicaid members with asthma. These interventions serve to increase the percentage of Medicaid members receiving case management and support services, as well as hands-on services such as community workshops. In combination, these specially targeted interventions tend to result in better outcomes and reduce inappropriate emergency department visits and hospital admissions.

Medicaid Education and Outreach

OxHP's Medicaid E&O team is composed of nonclinical staff who focus on solving social issues and educating members about OxHP's benefit plan policies and procedures. The E&O team proactively telephones each Medicaid member after enrollment to complete a welcome call. If phone contact is not successful, a field E&O associate visits the member at home. During the welcome call, the E&O associate explains how to use primary care physicians, hospitals, and emergency departments; confirms the member's demographic information; and ensures that the member has received identification cards and enrollment materials. Also during this contact, a screening survey is completed to identify members with asthma and then stratify them into Mild, Moderate, or Severe levels. As described above, Severe and Moderate 2 asthmatics are referred to the asthma disease management team for nurse case management. The E&O team tracks Mild and Moderate 1 asthmatics to address social issues, identify potential needs for clinical management, and complete appropriate referrals.

Buddy System

When social issues require intervention for Moderate 2 and Severe asthmatics, asthma case managers contact E&O associates for assistance. Likewise, E&O associates contact the asthma nurses for clinical support for Mild and Moderate 1 asthmatics. This process is facilitated by a buddy system that partners each asthma case manager with an E&O associate. An algorithm detailing this process has been established between Medicaid E&O and disease management to ensure consistency.

Asthma Workshops

To provide Medicaid asthmatics with face-to-face asthma education, asthma workshops were established in hospitals in high-volume Medicaid areas. Qualified respiratory therapists or asthma-trained registered nurses conduct the workshops adhering to the content suggested in the NIH guidelines.[2] The opportunity to attend an asthma education workshop is offered to the member by the E&O team or asthma disease management team, regardless of the member's asthma severity level. Since the purpose of the workshop is to educate the member about asthma, all medical management issues are referred to the asthma nurse case managers for follow up with the member's physician. The success of this initiative is evaluated by reviewing episodes of asthma-related hospitalizations and emergency department visits for those members completing an asthma education workshop.

Tracking Progress

This program is monitored using empirical data to identify its strengths and weaknesses. It is an excellent environment to employ outcomes research methods and technical support databases to evaluate program results and introduce refinements. Outcome measures suitable for this purpose should originate with the four categories of objectives outlined above. In this section, we provide an example that demonstrates how differences in emergency department utilization in two populations over a 2-year period led the OxHP asthma disease management program to revise the interventions provided to its Medicaid members.

Figures 30–1 and 30–2 compare the rates of emergency department utilization for commercial and Medicaid members over 1994 and 1995. By evaluating quarterly data over a 2-year pe-

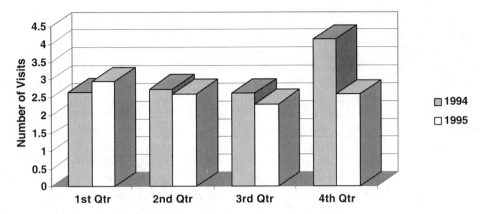

Figure 30–1 Change in Number of Visits to the Emergency Department per 1,000 Commercial Members, 1994 to 1995. Courtesy of Oxford Health Plan, Milford, Connecticut.

riod for the 2 member populations separately, a number of important differences emerge. From differences in the y-axis scales alone, it is clear that utilization among commercial members is much lower, in the vicinity of 3 visits per 1,000 members versus 25 visits per 1,000 members in the Medicaid population. Second, we can see that these data reflect the seasonality of asthma, with the fourth quarter producing the highest utilization rates, exactly as would be expected *without interventions* in the northeastern part of the country, where OxHP is located. Most important, the data show that utilization of the emergency department among commercial members did not notably increase in the fourth quarter of 1995, as would be expected by observing the pattern set in 1994, providing evidence for the effectiveness of the asthma disease management program's intervention.

A similar pattern was not observed among Medicaid members, where the fourth quarter pattern in 1995 was much the same as observed in 1994, suggesting the asthma disease management program was having little effect in the Medicaid population. This led the asthma disease management team to revise the interventions provided to Medicaid members. The new intervention relied less on mailings and phone

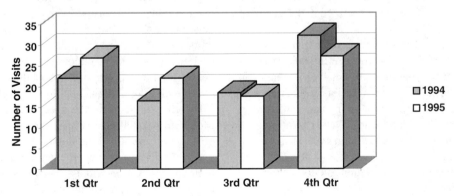

Figure 30–2 Change in Number of Visits to the Emergency Department per 1,000 Medicaid Members, 1994 to 1995. Courtesy of Oxford Health Plan, Milford, Connecticut.

calls and more on face-to-face interactions. The social support activities of E&O field representatives (see discussion above) were stepped up, and asthma workshops were put in place to enhance other educational components. This kind of self-monitoring completes an all-important feedback loop, without which the information required to improve the program remains inaccessible. The example also demonstrates the importance of data systems and statistical experience in the production and communication of such information.

INDUSTRY ALTERNATIVES TO A COMPREHENSIVE DISEASE MANAGEMENT PROGRAM

The initiation of a comprehensive program of asthma disease management is still rare in the industry, partly because there are useful alternatives to a full-blown program that may be advantageous to plans that are not yet ready to employ a wide-ranging set of targeted interventions. One such alternative is use of home-based asthma education programs, usually several visits by a nurse who also provides educational materials. Participation in the program may be limited to the time period during which the visits are occurring. Across the industry, such programs tend to average from 2 weeks to 6 months in length. Members are usually selected for this type of intervention on the basis of cost and/or utilization, and there is as yet little evidence that disease severity is also examined in the selection process.

Although all members probably receive the same intervention—no targeting of interventions is usually attempted—many members can be put through a program of this type. Additionally, while the program is in place, utilization and clinical outcomes are likely to improve. A disadvantage of this program type is that once the program period is over, and no additional outreach is attempted, patient outcomes may revert to their former status.

Another approach tends to focus on physician compliance with treatment guidelines over patient outreach and education. The advantage of this approach is that is standardizes treatment according to national guidelines. However, physicians can perceive it as punitive and reject disease management on the grounds that it is nothing more than "pushing" guidelines. The way out of this dilemma is to ensure that disease management is presented as part of a larger, more systematic program that manages asthma from many perspectives.

A third approach utilizes the assistance of pharmaceutical companies, which frequently have excellent patient and provider educational materials because they have invested heavily in their development. These institutions are also highly regarded for their sophisticated data systems and understanding of measurable outcomes. However, there are pitfalls. First, disease management done under the auspices of one pharmaceutical company tends not to include the pharmaceutical products of another company, even if the latter product (drug) is more appropriate. Second, these companies are not accustomed to the complex logistics involved in the full implementation of a disease management program. For example, they rarely have a sufficient nursing staff because nursing care is not their core competency.

A fourth approach employs asthma home care vendors to provide all aspects of disease management. These programs are well known for their "nurse power" and clinical expertise. However, they have several weaknesses. The first is technological. They usually do not have personnel trained to perform statistical monitoring of outcomes. Moreover, they may also lack the data systems upon which outcomes monitoring depends. Home care vendors also tend to focus on commercial populations and do not work for or sufficiently understand the special needs of the Medicaid population. Perhaps the most serious obstacle to use of asthma home care vendors in lieu of a disease management program is that their quality varies widely. They may play an important role in an asthma disease management program, but they will not serve well as the whole program.

Physician groups—usually pulmonologists and allergists—represent another alternative that is becoming more visible in asthma disease management. These groups promote their own clinic-based programs, which, for the most part, combine education and medical management. The great strength of this approach is that these specialists are excellent when complex medical management is required. Their weakness lies in the fact that they prefer that a plan turn patients over to them completely, an alternative that tends to offend the primary physicians of patients who are already under good management.

BARRIERS TO PROGRAM IMPLEMENTATION

While disease management is certainly becoming accepted as an efficient and cost-effective means of administering quality health care, there are still some skeptics. And their skepticism is not entirely unwarranted.

For a disease management program to be effective, patients, physicians, and other members of the health care team must make appropriate behavior changes. Redefinition and clarification of the roles of nurses, physician assistants, and other team members may be necessary to make program implementation feasible. It is often difficult to convince people to change their behavior, but if positive behavior change does not take place, disease management cannot be successful.

This observation dovetails with a second reason for skepticism. Complex and sophisticated data systems are essential if analysts are to pinpoint and then convey the wide array of information about the larger system that aggregated statistics and regional analysis can uncover. Yet the integration of the very data that is required for this effort—pharmacy, laboratory, utilization—is notoriously difficult. There are also problems in providing this information in real time. Building databases that are suitable for useful analysis takes time and planning. OxHP, has placed a high priority on providing program analysts with direct information feeds from pharmacies and laboratories, to enable comparisons between data sets.

Successful behavioral change and widely available data are related components of any disease management program. When physicians are provided with sufficient information so that they can see the need for the change themselves, they are more likely to modify their behavior. Often, data analysts can see when one region is different from another far more easily than a given region's partnerships or individual practices. The physicians just do not have access to the data. At OxHP, we have put our effort into regular face-to-face meetings with physicians in which we give them access to the same information we have: separate regions are compared with each other, to the company as a whole, and to the nation. This perspective allows physicians to draw their own conclusions and takes full advantage of the physician's empirical style. It also avoids the error of "preaching to a professional provider." It lets physicians decide on their own what behavior may need changing.

Another issue is the limited evidence to date that disease management programs actually improve health outcomes.[10] Since original implementation and refinement of a program take time, it can take several years to establish that an asthma disease management program is operating effectively. By that time, a program that did not meet its goals may end up costing company resources without providing the promised improvement and care and cost reduction.

It is also true that disease management programs may encounter difficulties as they are applied in the real world of health care delivery. Disease management programs are often initiated as a result of a clinical trial that established an effective intervention. However, it cannot be assumed that the same results that occurred in the clinical trial will happen in a real-world setting with noncompliant patients and physicians, comorbidities, a diverse population, and unexpected complications, all of which were probably missing from the experimental trial.

Moreover, the providers fear they will lose clinical decision-making power and that patient confidentiality will be compromised. Providers express the concern that decision making is moving more and more into the hands of payers. They may be hesitant to follow preestablished treatment guidelines in fear that their authority is being usurped. At the same time, both providers and patients may be skeptical of a system that tracks every aspect of a patient's care, a fear that could foster noncompliance.

CONCLUSION

Disease management is still a new idea, and asthma disease management programs will need time to become successful and effective. Certainly, attempting to fix all the problems associated with asthma at one time would be a daunting task and could lead to early failure if some caution were not exercised. OxHP has found that the best success occurred when priorities were set early and the most feasible steps targeted first. For example, once the patient population was successfully stratified, it was clear that OxHP could target the most ill patients, who consumed the most health care resources, to receive the first interventions. OxHP then set its sights on the standardization of treatment, achieved a modicum of success in that area, and moved on to the refinement and customization of intervention. Of course, there is still a long way to go. Perfecting a sound disease management philosophy throughout the company and finding the right roles and definitions for all members of the delivery team, especially patients and providers, are tasks requiring constant attention and discipline.

In spite of the effort required, OxHP team members are optimistic about asthma disease management in particular as well as disease management in general. They have adopted the philosophy that the future of disease management is consistent with the future of the information age and are now deepening their commitment to data systems, because they believe that the future of disease management lies in the use of those systems to construct models of patient behavior that can predict the level of *future compliance*. As described earlier, with these models it will be possible to predict a lapse in compliance and head off a predicted increase in utilization on a patient-by-patient basis. OxHP supports the idea that finer stratification of the patient population with such models will enable greater customization of asthma interventions and will ultimately result in even greater compliance, improved patient outcomes, and reduced cost.

As the new millennium approaches, it is now clear that disease management represents a paradigm shift in health care delivery. A philosophy of treatment based on episodic care has shifted to one based on the special needs of population segments that better understands and predicts their behavior, especially with the introduction of more sophisticated data systems and analytic methods. Recognizing the advantages of this shift will be essential as the "graying of America" is followed by an increase in the number of chronically ill patients. OxHP is aiming to meet this challenge with innovation in the hope that the objective of a new and improved health care delivery method can actually be realized.

REFERENCES

1. Weiss K, Gergen PJ, Hodgson TA. An economic evaluation of asthma in the United States. *New Engl J Med.* 1992;366:862–868.
2. National Heart, Lung and Blood Institute. *Guidelines for the Diagnosis and Management of Asthma.* National Asthma Education and Prevention Program (NAEP) Expert Panel Report II. Bethesda, MD: National Institutes of Health; 1997.
3. Plaut TF, Hershey JE, Bendich DM, Katz HP, Schoen EJ. Is asthma misdiagnosed? *J Asthma.* 1986;23(1): 23–24.
4. Ware JE, Snow KK, Kosinski M, Gandek B. *SF-36 Health Survey: Manual and Interpretation Guide.* Boston: The Health Institute, New England Medical Center; 1993.
5. Mangiofico G. Disease management: a concept in search of a definition. *Remington Rep.* September/October 1996:26–29.

6. National Heart, Lung and Blood Institute. *Guidelines for the Diagnosis and Management of Asthma.* National Asthma Education and Prevention Program (NAEP) Expert Panel Report. Bethesda, MD: National Institutes of Health; 1991.
7. Sampson E. Disease state management: new models for case management. *Remington Rep.* September/October 1996:21–24.
8. Armstrong EP. Monitoring and evaluating disease management: information requirements. *Clin Ther.* 1996; 18(6):1326–1333.
9. Ware JE, Kosinski M, Keller SD. *SF-12: How to Score the SF-12 Physical and Mental Health Summary Scales.* 2nd ed. Boston: The Health Institute, New England Medical Center; 1995.
10. Epstein RS, Sherwood LM. From outcomes research to disease management: a guide for the perplexed. *Ann Intern Med.* 1996;124(9):832–837.

BENJAMIN SAFIRSTEIN, MD, FACP, FCCP, is vice president of medical affairs for Oxford Health Plans in New York and a clinical associate professor of medicine at the Mount Sinai School of Medicine. Previously, he was chief of the pulmonary division at St. Michael's Medical Center in Newark, New Jersey, a major teaching affiliate of the College of Medicine and Dentistry of New Jersey. He was also an associate clinical professor at the New Jersey College of Medicine until 1996. In 1985, Dr. Safirstein cofounded and was founding medical director of Oxford Health Plans. He has also practiced pulmonary medicine in a multispecialty group practice in Montclair, New Jersey.

JOAN KENNEDY, MIM, is the director of disease management and behavioral health at Oxford Health Plans. She is responsible for the development, implementation, and success of 11 disease management programs and the behavioral health division. Previously, Ms. Kennedy worked for FHP Healthcare as the manager of quality/outcomes management, where she was responsible for executing company-wide clinical programs and outcomes studies.

BARBARA BARTON, RN, manages the asthma disease management program Better Breathing for Oxford Health Plans. She has over 14 years of experience in nursing, focusing on intensive care, and case management of patients with chronic diseases. She received her BS in nursing from Bowling Green University.

CHAPTER 31

Disease Management and Return on Investment

David W. Plocher and Robert S. Brody

Chapter Outline

- Introduction
- Economic Concept of Cost and Observation on Its Measurement in Disease Management
- Basic Evaluation Issues in Disease Management
- Benefits
- Costs
- Conclusion

INTRODUCTION

One of the important challenges facing those involved with making care management decisions is the growing need for economic evaluation of investment in disease management (DM) programs. DM programs have rapidly proliferated because of the widely held belief that such programs can provide solutions to ineffective care management, reflected in inappropriate and high utilization by a subset of individuals with any given diagnosis. However, the adoption of rigorous program evaluation in connection with such initiatives is surprisingly infrequent.

Recent consensus-based recommendations of an expert panel for the conduct of cost-effectiveness analyses describe methodologic approaches to improve the quality and comparability of studies where health outcomes and resource costs of health interventions are considered.[1]

This chapter focuses on methods employed to evaluate DM initiatives in which benefits are represented by savings, or diverted costs of a medical intervention, and that fall within the context of a cost benefit analysis.

ECONOMIC CONCEPT OF COST AND OBSERVATION ON ITS MEASUREMENT IN DISEASE MANAGEMENT

What we really want to measure in DM is which program components are needed and how much of admittedly limited resources is required to implement a new program for the management of patients. Economic theory suggests that the costs of such a program are not defined in terms of dollars or staff full-time equivalents. The real cost is the benefits that could be obtained by the alternative application of these resources. When resources are devoted to the development of a disease management program, then those resources are not available to produce some alternative, perhaps superior, health-enhancing capability. Because the alternatives can be broad and far reaching, they tax some of the standard methods and measurement tools upon which cost benefit analysis is based.

The small number of disease registries containing relevant longitudinal data on clinical management and outcomes over time creates difficulties in answering even the most basic questions surrounding any program. DM should be evaluated in a manner befitting an investment activity, to determine whether achievement of an anticipated or guaranteed future outcome is worth forgoing how patients with specific conditions are managed in the present. The answer to this question lies in the calculation of a program's present value, a concept defined as the current value of expected future outcome of such a program (or its return on cost).

BASIC EVALUATION ISSUES IN DISEASE MANAGEMENT

Any organization contemplating the institution of a DM initiative must estimate the costs, savings, and additional benefits to be derived from instituting a DM program. The organization should consider the program infrastructure to be created—how the DM program will be administered, including the derivation of process-based measures of the quality of the program. Because clinical detail on patient outcomes is lacking in administrative databases, it is difficult to evaluate how large an effect is to be anticipated. Estimates of the effect attributable to DM can, at times, be derived from case referent studies (also known as retrospective or case control studies), which are designed to gain insight into those independent variables, including aspects of care, that predict disease-specific outcome measures. Such data may assist organizations to predict whether anticipated benefits of a DM program will exceed its expected costs.

The basic calculation is presented in equation form at the bottom of Figure 31–1.

Several types of evaluation studies are suggested, since rarely can a single study address all of the following factors:

- patient/employee and employer satisfaction
- data on a program's administrative and clinical performance
- cost benefit or cost-effectiveness components

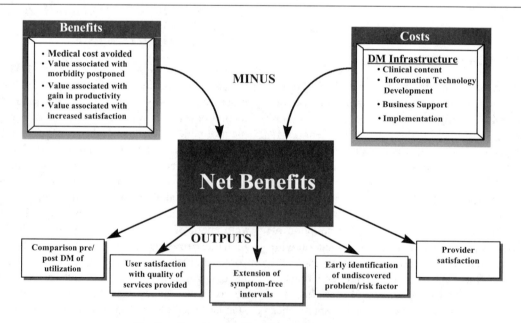

Net Benefits = Expected benefits minus Expected costs

Figure 31–1 Cost Benefit Information Flow

- changes in disease-specific functional status measures

Studies should be designed based on appropriate statistical principles, taking into consideration:

- desired analytical power
- sample size
- the number of patients that can practically be enrolled and tracked within the time allotted to demonstrate program benefits
- probability of enrolled patients subsequently electing not to "graduate" from the DM program

Internal validity concerns (eg, demonstration that the effect of the DM program exists and is not because of selection or other statistical bias) should be given greater weight than external validity concerns (eg, generalization of the effectiveness of the DM program to other persons, places, and times). Employers and health plans will require evidence of a program's effectiveness based on their own experience and are less likely to be influenced by studies performed in other populations.

The establishment of a measurement strategy can be driven by cost, impact on utilization, or quality (care management improvement). The most robust assessments consider the conditions under which care is provided in the community. A study that is naturalistic in its design would include the following elements:

- There should be a longitudinal study of all individuals meeting minimum eligibility criteria in addition to those continuously enrolled for an extended period within the health plan, whether they participate in the DM program or not (Figure 31–2). This provides a sampling frame for performing additional "nested" evaluations of the impact of the DM program that can aid in strengthening its generalization to the membership at large (Figure 31–3).
- Nested studies can be deployed simultaneously, within the longitudinal design, in order to evaluate
  - the strategy of directly measuring the impact on individuals who participate in the DM program compared to those who do not participate
  - whether there is a change in resource use and cost for members who actually use the DM service
  - other specific hypotheses related to the disease-specific practice guidelines

---

Naturalistic sampling of study subjects is preferred. Selection is performed in a way that reflects the reality of the conditions under which care is delivered.

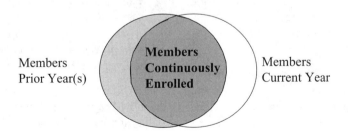

Evaluation should include those with minimum enrollment duration.
Results for continuously enrolled are one subgroup.

Figure 31–2 DM Program Evaluation Subject Selection

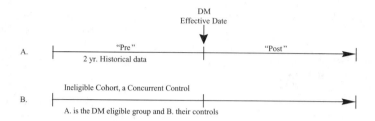

Health care resource utilization and its associated costs are evaluated in an eligible cohort and an ineligible control group. Outcome measures, including relative rates of health care utilization and their respective costs in the "Post" period, are compared with average annual outcomes in the prior 2 years, adjusted for health status.

Nested Study: Eligible DM Program Participants versus Nonparticipants

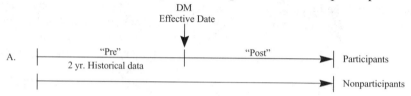

DM participants and nonparticipants are frequency matched on the basis of age (category), sex, health status in the pre-DM time frame, and plan (provider) reimbursement type. Outcomes in these groups are evaluated in a fashion similar to those described in the main longitudinal study.

Figure 31–3 Methodology: Longitudinal Studies

Indirect standardization techniques can be used to derive expected medical resource utilization based upon the assumption that specific utilization rates in the period prior to the DM program can be applied to the study population in the period after the DM program. Rates defined on the basis of independent variables that are strong predictors of health status or illness burden can be used to estimate resource use of individuals with the same level of comorbidity, permitting estimation of expenditures had the program not been implemented.

Epidemiologic studies can be designed

- to determine whether DM favorably impacts attainment of the program goals (eg, reduction in medical service utilization and costs) across populations enrolled in different plan types, in order to distinguish the effectiveness of DM, considering that many cost containment options may exist
- to evaluate the program's impact on users' level of satisfaction with the quality of patient–provider encounters, as well as ratings of overall care when DM services are used
- to establish whether the use of DM extends symptom-free intervals and facilitates the early identification of undiscovered health problems or risk factors, thereby enabling earlier intervention (the impact of the program on the occurrence and costs associated with cases that present with advanced or late stage disease or those requiring urgent care can be tracked)
- to assess providers' satisfaction with the DM process and its effect on their ability to deliver care efficiently

If a certain number of patients participate in a given DM program, if their behavior and health status improve as intended, and if their use of services and expenditures for their medical problems are found to have diminished by their participation, and behavior changes are induced, then the unbroken and consistent chain of events would support attribution of the savings to the DM program.

In evaluating outcomes performance, it is difficult to determine the exact savings. Here, too, an approach that includes a control group would be ideal, but dividing the population in half for scientific learning guarantees that the effects of the program will be only half of what the attribution of the savings to the program may be. When using historical comparison groups, savings may be estimated against the previous year's experience, though the comparison should be between the year's actual expenditures following implementation of the program and statistical adjustments to determine what expenditures would have been without the program.

Economic Study Designs

Economic evaluations seek to identify a single numerical quantity that accurately and comprehensively expresses the total amount of health improvement (both quantitative and qualitative) that could be expected from DM compared with conventional medical management. Hybrid studies that include both epidemiologic and economic evaluation components have been used to develop information to address a number of important issues, including

- support of the market position for a product or service
- pricing of the product or service
- identification of the value (and performance) of the product or service to key purchase and use decision makers

If executed properly, the study could support

- longer term business decisions regarding the development and rollout of other such programs
- pricing decisions
- service profitability objectives

In our opinion, the scope of information needs to go beyond a single study that is intended to demonstrate economic advantage. Data should be developed from naturalistic settings on the purchase and use behavior of those who opt to use the DM services, and DM's potential effect on health care utilization within the community should be appraised.

Certainly, estimates of this type can be developed based upon existing health services research data, where data reporting has been deemed to be adequate and well controlled. However, it will be important to extrapolate observed effects to different populations, circumstances of use, settings, and so on. Models that seek to extend the estimates of the DM program's effects may be of interest. Assumptions utilized in developing models and their application to the clinical setting will have to be fairly explicit and based on rigorous scientific data and methods.

A difficulty in conducting and evaluating the results of clinical economic studies is that consensus guidelines have only recently been published for conducting such work.[2] We often liken the recent state of medical economics to that period prior to the acceptance of modern accounting principles and the use of independent auditors. The Food and Drug Administration and others have formulated proposed guidelines for the conduct of these studies.[3,4] In the meantime, we refer to principles outlined by Russell et al[2] as a starting point to foster adoption of an adequate study methodology that is both rigorous and unbiased. Given the above, we would anticipate that any economic evaluation of DM would have to consider the issues presented in Exhibit 31–1.[1,2,5]

In the case of an anticipated study of DM, the analysis should focus on providing meaningful clinical and economic data to support decision making from a variety of real-world perspectives.

BENEFITS

The benefits, or diverted costs of a DM intervention, fall into four categories

1. the medical cost avoided because medical service utilization is avoided or illness complications are prevented

Exhibit 31–1 Methodologic Features of DM Program Evaluations Featuring Cost Benefit Analysis

---

1. The perspective of the analysis

   A description of the perspective of the analysis (the patient, provider, payer, employer, etc) is important to understand the context in which costs and benefits accrue.

2. Explicit hypotheses of the benefits of the DM service being studied

   In many cases, all of the benefits may not be known or are unproven. Consequently, all assumptions must be explicitly defined. In such a study, the presumed benefits will be achievement of the intended clinical result at costs that are "substantially less" than current treatment approaches. Listing specific study objectives may be preferred to listing hypotheses to be tested.

3. Cost specifications considered in the analysis

   Categories, such as the inclusion of indirect costs, should be clearly defined, and the use of actual, inferred, and/or normalized values should be indicated.

4. When costs and benefits may accrue and be realized during different periods—adjustment for differential timing using discounting

   This principle permits adjustment of cost values to a common reference point. However, if timing of costs and benefits occurs within a similar time frame (eg, a year), discounting is not required. This will be an issue only if patient outcomes are to be tracked for multiple years.

5. Sensitivity analyses testing important assumptions

   Studies typically rely on key assumptions regarding interpretation of certain findings or magnitude of outcomes. Such assumptions must be defined and a range of values tested to assess the impact of variation on the interpretation of results.

6. A summary measure of efficiency, such as a cost benefit or cost-effectiveness ratio

   The use of an index value contributes greatly to the application of the analysis and to comparison and prioritization of clinical strategies. Describing the costs saved or the utilization of resources reduced without comparison to the costs or effort required to accomplish the results is inadequate but all too common in many economic study reports.

   Source: Data from LB Russell et al, The Role of Cost-Effectiveness Analysis in Health and Medicine, *Journal of American Medical Association*, Vol 276, No 14, pp 1172–1177, © 1996, American Medical Association; NC Weinstein et al, Recommendations of the Panel on Cost-Effectiveness in Health and Medicine, *Journal of American Medical Association*, Vol 276, No 15, pp 1253–1258, © 1996, American Medical Association; and JE Siegel et al, *Journal of American Medical Associaton*, Vol 276, No 16, pp 1339–1341, © 1996, American Medical Association.

---

2. the monetary value associated with gains in an individual's productivity because morbidity and/or mortality are postponed
3. the monetary value associated with gains in an individual's productivity because a better health status is restored
4. the monetary value associated with improved satisfaction and continuation of life

The first benefit can be calculated by measuring the direct medical costs that would have been incurred had the DM program not been implemented. Using a pre-/poststudy design, medical service utilization rates for individuals of a defined health status before the implementation of a DM program can be applied using indirect standardization techniques to estimates of persons of similar health status in the population in the post-DM period to determine how estimated medical service utilization in the period following DM implementation compares to what was actually observed.

The second and third benefits include estimating the individual's income that would have been lost due to illness or, in the case of the actively employed participating in DM, the employer's salary replacement benefit and retraining costs that are avoided when the individual returns to work.

The last benefit involves estimating the monetary value of the satisfaction individuals receive from an enhanced quality and duration of life in an improved state of health. (The authors fully recognize that the monetary value of quality and duration of life may be the least important measure of this benefit. However, for purposes of this measurement, the monetary value is calculable and has been used for other purposes such as monetary rewards from insurers and the courts.) The most common method of measuring the value of a human life is the human capital approach, which discounts the value of future earnings resulting from an improvement in health or extension of life by estimating the market value of the output produced by an individual during his or her expected lifetime. An alternative method of determining the monetary value of a life is the willingness-to-pay approach, in which value is estimated based on the amount of money individuals are willing to pay for reductions in the probability of dying.

COSTS

The analysis must recognize the appropriate unit of observation, the patient/employee and his or her family. Costs, both direct and indirect, incurred by the family member must be recognized as part of the total social cost accounting framework. Account must be taken of all "informal" care provided by family members and friends.

Information about utilization for the following resource categories will need to be collected:

- physician services
- hospitalization
- nursing home stays
- home care
- homemaker services
- personal care
- meal preparation and delivery
- social/psychological counseling
- special transportation services

It is appropriate to consider the impact of the DM program on the total costs of medical care. The program evaluation should not be limited to those components that are directly influenced by the disease under investigation. For example, in studies of diabetes, costs of medical utilization for all causes, including estimates of the cost associated with diabetic care, need to be included in the analysis. Anecdotal attempts to exclude costs associated with catastrophic trauma, cancer, or organ transplantation are still controversial.

Once utilization profiles are generated, they should be costed to arrive at the required cash-flow streams. In costing utilization, a distinction should be made between costs and charges or fees. Charges (fees) represent the posted price. Costs are assumed to be less than charges, and most reimbursement programs pay reasonable costs rather than charges. From the government's perspective, cost rather than charge data reflect the expected cash flows. However, since third-party payers (and ultimately employers) pay charges or fixed fees (there may be situations where services are partially to fully capitated), one may wish to identify expected cash flows that would accrue if all parties paid charges, with or without adjustment for deductibles and copayments.

However, we recommend that cost data be used, whenever possible, in these analyses, even though charge data may be more easily obtained. Few institutions are able to isolate actual costs for individual units of service. In order to be able to exclude interinstitutional variation in charges and costs as a confounding variable in such analyses, it is suggested that normalized data be applied to represent mean values, from a source such as a well-accepted database or from similarly conducted studies, in performing cost or charge per unit of service calculations. Depending on availability of data, costs can be imputed from ratios of costs to charges (RCC). If possible, RCCs for the relevant departments of local institutions from the community should be used. Alternatively, RCCs can be used from national RCC data or from summaries of Medicare cost reports with interpretive input from experienced reimbursement consultants for the inpatient setting. In the ambulatory setting, although billed charges do not represent the expenditure in managed care plans because of negotiated discounts, customary charges for services are often applied.

As most cost benefit analyses usually span a long time period, costs and benefits accruing after the first year must be discounted to eliminate the effect of inflationary factors on the cost and benefit cash flow streams.

Some economists prefer to assess programs based on a cost-effectiveness analysis rather than a cost benefit analysis. In a cost-effectiveness analysis, efforts would be directed to quantify the medical, social, and psychological outcomes attributable to the DM program and to compare these to the costs incurred from operating the DM program. It should be determined whether data supporting the evaluation of medical, social, and mental health services (including components included in capitation arrangements with providers or where carve-outs do not permit easy availability of data) will be analyzed as part of the overall project. However, in an era of medical resource cost awareness, a cost benefit evaluation may be preferable to a cost-effectiveness evaluation that does not measure resource savings. If the DM program is worthwhile from a purely technical point of view, if alternative mechanisms for achieving comparable gains are not available, and if one is confident that the program does not harm the population at risk, then it can be argued that one need not look further at the program's advantages.

Cost-utility analysis is a form of cost-effectiveness analysis in which the measure of effectiveness combines mortality with a multidimensional perspective of morbidity. It presents a framework within which an economic evaluation can combine quality of life considerations with quantity of life considerations. Such studies are indicated when many different outcomes are possible and a common summary measure for comparison of alternatives is desired. If, for example, it were important to document the impact of the DM program on pain, performance of activities of daily living, cognitive function, social function, and emotional health, a utility approach would be needed to characterize the "best" choice, given all of the above-mentioned dimensions. However, if the outcomes can be expressed in a single variable that is readily measured in "natural units," such as symptom relief, then the economic evaluation would be better expressed as the cost per patient per level of symptom relief.

The utility approach to decision making and using quality of life measures requires definition of levels with the attributes or constructs being measured. Preferences for each level within each attribute are collected and an overall score is developed to combine all aspects of the quality of life being measured. Quality-adjusted life years (QALYs) are the preferred summary measure for the comparison of the DM with conventional health care approaches.

Studies of the Consistency of Disease Management Program Effectiveness

In order to demonstrate the consistency of the effect and economic advantages of the DM program, it will be necessary to evaluate the program's clinical efficacy and cost-effectiveness in a variety of settings. Prospective, integrated clinical and economic studies have yet to be conducted with many DM programs. In spite of multiple anecdotes proclaiming cost savings from DM programs, it is rare to see the associated start-up, implementation, and monitoring/overhead costs.

One such report[6] on congestive heart failure (CHF) patients did attempt to account for operating costs. After reviewing this study, our calculation produced a return on investment (ROI) expressed as a 9% reduction in care costs over 90 days, net of added case management expenses. This calculation was discussed with the report's chief investigator, Michael Rich (personal communication, September 1997), who confirmed the accuracy of those financial assumptions. Based on a 9% reduction in CHF care costs (total care cost from all causes was not reported), one could extrapolate to a nearly $1 billion cost reduction for CHF nationally, based on 1994 data reporting $10 billion in CHF care costs.[7]

A second example is offered by the Diabetes Treatment Centers of America (DTCA). Exhibit 31-2 shows the formula preliminarily recommended for this ROI calculation. As Exhibit 31-2 shows, care costs should decrease at least 30% in order to produce a 3.75 to 1 return on annual maintenance costs for the program. DTCA's model projects savings in excess of 30% at the end of a year of program operations. DTCA's actual experience is running ahead of the model; the program has achieved a positive ROI during its first year, a 26% reduction in care costs, according to Bob Stone, executive vice president of DTCA (personal communication, January 1998).

A third example is provided by Greineder et al. The part-time nurse operating their outreach program cost only $11,115 per year, saving approximately $87,000 in costs for asthma patients.[8]

A final example from the peer-reviewed literature provides a partial cost-of-alternative-care contrast. While not revealing all overhead costs, Chapman and Torpy[9] found that their CHF program reduced CHF admits by 30%, in an environment featuring a baseline of two to three CHF admits per CHF patient yearly, at a cost of $9,000 each. Their new outpatient clinic–based program required 15 to 20 visits per year for each CHF patient, which costs $2,000. If investing $2,000 prevents a $9,000 admission, there is the beginning of a positive ROI formula.

Exhibit 31-2 Disease Management ROI (DTCA Model as of March 1, 1997)

- Program's historic development costs
  1. $10 million
  2. Not to be included in ROI formula
- Program's *annual* maintenance ROI calculations
  1. Cell size (one site) population: 3,000 diabetics (more type II than type I diabetics)
  2. Annual cost of care for one diabetic: $5,000
  3. 3,000 diabetics × $5,000 = $15 million care cost
  4. Program implementation costs: $1 million annually
  5. Therefore, ratio of cost to operate/care costs = 1/15 = 7%
  6. Summary: If program can reduce care costs by 7%, the ROI will be 1:1 or break even
  7. Projections: Programs should be able to reduce care costs by 30%, making a (purely mathematical calculation) positive ROI of 3.75:1

Calculations courtesy of Diabetes Treatment Centers of America.

CONCLUSION

There are many reasons for a managed care organization, integrated delivery system, or organized medical group to construct and provide DM programs for certain chronic clinical conditions. One reason may be that the benefits of those DM programs exceed their costs—an important consideration in any system without infinite resources. This chapter has outlined potential approaches to performing the necessary analyses of cost benefit comparisons. It appears that for at least a few studied conditions, the benefits of DM do indeed outweigh the costs.

REFERENCES

1. Weinstein MC, Siegel JE, Gold MR, et al. Recommendations of the panel on cost-effectiveness in health and medicine. *JAMA.* 1996;276(15):1253–1258.
2. Russell LB, Gold MR, Siegel JE, et al. The role of cost-effectiveness analysis in health and medicine. *JAMA.* 1996;276(14):1172–1177.
3. Task Force on Principles for Economic Analysis of Health Care Technology. Economic analysis of health care technology: a report on principles. *Arch Int Med.* 1995;128:61–70.
4. PhRMA. Methodological and Conduct Principles for Pharmacoeconomic Research. Washington, DC:PhRMA; 1995.
5. Siegel JE, Weinstein MC, Russell LB, Gold MR. Recommendations for reporting cost-effectiveness analyses. *JAMA.* 1996;276(16):1339–1341.
6. Rich MW, Beckham V, Wittenberg C, Leven CL, Freedland, KE, Carney RM. A multidisciplinary intervention to prevent the readmission of elderly patients with congestive heart failure. *New Engl J Med.* 1995;33(18):1190–1195.
7. American Heart Association. *Heart and Stroke Facts: 1994 Statistical Supplement.* Dallas, TX: American Heart Association National Center; 1994.
8. Greineder DK, Loane KC, Parks P. Reduction in resource utilization by an asthma outreach program. *Arch Pediatr Adolesc Med.* 1995;149:415–420.
9. Chapman D, Torpy J. Development of a heart failure center: a medical center and cardiology practice join forces to improve care and reduce costs. *Am J Managed Care.* 1997;3:431–437.

ROBERT S. BRODY, MPH, is an epidemiologist with Ernst & Young's Health Care Consulting practice with responsibility for the design and conduct of studies of the cost-effectiveness of innovative medical services and therapeutics. He recently has devoted attention to enhanced performance measurement and methodologic issues in studies of return on investment of care management initiatives, such as demand and disease management programs. Previously Mr. Brody worked as a manager of research and evaluation services in the medical departments of AT&T, Motorola, and the Epidemiology Service of Memorial Sloan-Kettering Cancer Center.

Chapter 32

Managed Behavioral Health Care and Chemical Dependency Services

Donald F. Anderson, Jeffrey L. Berlant, Danna Mauch, William R. Maloney, Terri Goens, and Katherine Olberg Sternbach

Chapter Outline

- Introduction
- Key Treatment Principles
- The Ideal Continuum of Care
- Treatment Services
- Benefit Plan Design
- Utilization Management
- Channeling Mechanisms
- Behavioral Health Provider Networks
- Provider Structures for Integrated Delivery Systems To Meet Managed Care Objectives
- Quality Assurance
- Information Systems
- Public/Private Systems Integration
- Emerging Issues
- Conclusion

INTRODUCTION

Management of behavioral health (BH) treatment and costs presents special challenges. For purposes of this chapter, the term *behavioral health* includes mental health, substance abuse or chemical dependency, and serious mental illness or brain disorders. Unique factors contributing to these special challenges include the following:

- destigmatization of mental illness and chemical dependency that has made people more willing to seek help for these problems
- erosion of social support systems, including fragmentation of traditional extended and nuclear family structures
- increased complexity and stress in society, which have resulted in increased incidence and manifestation of BH symptoms
- advances in medication and psychological therapeutic techniques that have promoted more effective treatment of more disorders
- proliferation of private hospitals during the 1970s and early 1980s as a result of high profit margins, cheap capital investment, elimination of certificate-of-need laws in several large states, and exemption from reimbursement by diagnosis-related groups (DRGs)
- significant benefit restrictions for treating serious mental illnesses and addictions, which have prompted a national advocacy strategy to promote parity between mental health and physical health care benefits

---

This chapter is adapted from DF Anderson et al, Managed Behavioral Health Care Services, in *The Managed Health Care Handbook*, 3rd ed, PR Kongstvedt, ed, pp 341–366, © 1996, Aspen Publishers, Inc.

- tightening during the 1990s of public sector BH funding at the federal level, which increased pressure on local government agencies to contain costs
- increasingly vocal criticism of managed care initiatives for vulnerable populations,[1] which is contributing to intensified regulatory action

Added to these pressures is the fact that many BH problems tend to be chronic and recurring, requiring periodic treatment, sometimes intensive in nature, throughout the lifetime of the affected individual. Finally, BH diagnostic categories do not lend themselves to by-the-book utilization management with standardized length of stay and treatment protocols for specified diagnoses. The range of accepted treatment approaches for a given BH diagnosis can be broad, and severity of illness and service requirements cannot be inferred without detailed information about social context and specific symptoms.

Substantial efforts at managing BH treatment and costs first emanated from health maintenance organizations (HMOs). Early HMOs, for the most part, were wary of BH coverage. Some plans offered only diagnosis and consultation; others arranged for discounted fee-for-service care for members. The HMO Act of 1973 required only minimal BH benefits, such as crisis intervention and a maximum of 20 visits for outpatient services. No benefits for inpatient care, chronic or recurring conditions, and chemical dependency were required. Later in the 1970s and 1980s, increasing numbers of HMOs expanded BH benefits as a result of consumer demand and legislation enacted in a number of states that required enriched benefits.[2]

During the late 1970s and 1980s, when insurers and self-insured employers began instituting general utilization management techniques to help control their indemnity plan health benefit costs, it became clear that these approaches were far less effective in controlling BH costs than they were in controlling other medical benefit costs. Thus, the scene was set for development of a niche industry of specialized managed BH organizations to contract directly with HMOs, indemnity insurers, and self-insured employers and to apply specialized techniques in managing these costs. Employers traditionally have been the ultimate payers for most BH treatment managed by specialty BH entities (whether in-house HMO, insurance-carrier based, or freestanding). Increasingly in recent years, government BH agencies have become purveyors and/or purchasers of managed BH services as budgets have constricted, federal regulations have been administered more flexibly, and accountability has migrated to local government levels.

There has been a progressive homogenization of specialized carve-out BH managed care organizations (MCOs). Competitive pressures to provide managed care services at lower prices have made it increasingly difficult to engage in more than narrow utilization review activity. Yet the larger strategic need is to promote more effective care and generate more clinical value for every BH care dollar. Increasingly, limited MCO dollars also curtail investment in clinical information systems (infrastructure) and in processes for data aggregation and analysis necessary for the development of outcomes tracking systems.

The following pages describe managed BH care as it undergoes transformation and reinvention during an era of ferment and change.

KEY TREATMENT PRINCIPLES

Special Issues and Common Problems

Any MCO venturing into management of BH care faces the dilemma of how to address potentially large unmet treatment needs that place demands on scarce resources and may compete for resources from other medical care specialties. Several factors limit BH resources: a pattern of poor insurance benefits for BH care, particularly stemming from benefit reductions put into place during the late 1980s; a legacy of underinvestment and avoidance of treatment of BH disorders left by pioneering general medical-surgical HMOs; biases underestimating the prevalence, morbidity, and mortality of BH disorders; and apprehension over assuming the moral hazard of coverage for a large and poorly delineated pool of service needs.

On an operational level, it has been difficult to establish the boundaries of BH service obligations. The concept of "medical necessity" begins to blur when the causes of the disorder encompass social, personality, and biological factors, and when necessary services often must address stabilization of social supports; these factors are not universally recognized as medical needs.

When an organization is designing a delivery system, this need for social stability as a critical prerequisite for clinical stability requires a broader, more diverse continuum of programs and services than is seen in the general medical/surgical realm.

Due to recent advances in diagnostics, psychopharmacology, and psychotherapeutic techniques, there is a growing demand for powerful new treatment options during a time of shrinking resources. All these factors enhance the need for incisive management of BH care.

Goals of Treatment

Ideally, the goal of treatment for the health plan should be to *improve the BH status of a defined population*. A well-managed system should aim to reduce suicide and homicide rates, substance abuse–related impairments, and mortality and morbidity from accidents related to substance abuse or mental disorders. A well-managed system should improve the clinical status of a population in terms of symptomatic distress levels and improve life functioning in several areas.

Another central goal of managed BH care should be *conservation* and *rational allocation of resources to optimize return on expenditures*. Finding the correct balance between conservation of resources and provision of the appropriate mixture of effective services is the fundamental task for managed care.

Objectives of Treatment

There are a number of important clinical objectives for a managed care system to pursue.

- rapid symptomatic relief
- protection of the physical safety of the patient and others
- satisfaction of the patient/client and family
- improved life functioning

To conserve resources, managed care systems need to invest in cost-effective treatments and high-return therapeutic activities and maximize medical cost offsets (decreased costs for general medical and surgical care).

Strategic Approaches

Historically, MCOs have considered BH care services very cautiously. Coming down strongly on the side of conservation of resources, at least in terms of short-term, direct costs of care, they have pursued two general strategies: controlling demand and controlling supply.

Typical strategies for controlling demand make use of the established fact that demand for mental health services is very price sensitive. Techniques based on this price sensitivity include setting higher copayments and deductibles, delaying access to treatment, and limiting benefits, including imposing lifetime ceilings on BH benefits. Typical strategies for controlling supply have included benefit restrictions, program limitations, gatekeepers, triage systems, and waiting lists.

Benefit and program restrictions have at times been profound, severely limiting or excluding BH services entirely from the benefit package, excluding certain diagnostic-specific disorders or chronic illness, and providing few or no psychiatric inpatient services and little or no long-term outpatient treatment. Some contracts have excluded certain member groups from coverage, such as people with mental retardation, organic psychoses, alcoholism, and/or intractable personality disorders. Others have limited or refused to provide court-ordered services, thereby reducing liability for uncooperative clients. Some contracts have excluded geriatric patients, violent or assaultive patients, primary substance abusers, heroin-dependent persons, and people with sexual dysfunction, severe learning disabilities, or attention deficit hyperactivity disorder. Virtually all managed care plans use some form of utilization review. Although many use primary care practitioner case managers (ie, gatekeepers), large HMOs (over 200,000 enrollees) usually allow self-referral. Large case management or catastrophic management is also used.

Beyond a certain point, however, limitations on services can result in underservice of legitimate needs. To better meet the BH care needs of a population, MCOs are exploring strategies for improving the clinical value received for each BH dollar.

From a clinical perspective, managed care should favor

- use of multiple clinical pathways, providing simpler treatment plans for uncomplicated cases and more intensive treatment plans for more intensive cases
- development of a network of effective, efficient providers selected and retained on the basis of demonstrated superior clinical performance
- comprehensive assessment of the types and intensity of services needed
- matching the treatment problem with the optimal provider(s)
- selection of treatment innovations and clinical best practices to optimize effective and efficient patient response
- minimal disruption of everyday social role obligations
- treatment at the least restrictive but most effective level of care, favoring community-based over facility-based services
- coordination of all the patient's BH services
- measurement and tracking of clinical performance, focusing on clinical outcomes, management of resources, and efficiency of response
- systematic methods for assisting treatment of refractory patients to gain access to highly skilled, specialized services, including the use of centers of excellence for specific problems
- reducing relapse through identifying and planning for ongoing support for therapeutic and social needs

Finally, there is a need for the collective management of aggregate clinical expenditures in comparison to budgeted resources, concurrently identifying reasons for unexpected excessive expenditures and incisively constructing corrective action plans. Managed care should try to tie useful clinical information to financial information so that changes in clinical practices can target high-risk areas.

Emerging Strategic Approaches

From Carve-Out to Carve-In

To reduce costs and produce better outcomes, BH care services are being reincorporated into capitated medical-surgical systems. This newer paradigm counters the historic tendency of general medical-surgical HMOs to distance themselves from BH care and to use specialized carve-out utilization review organizations for BH issues. Although pioneering efforts over several decades in using brief behavioral interventions to reduce medical utilization suggested potential savings, little has been done to refine and develop this approach. The advent of automated clinical tracking in more sophisticated systems may facilitate targeting of BH care interventions in a manner previously unfeasible.

In Search of Medical Cost Offsets

Recent epidemiological research finds two types of relevant linkages:

- high prevalence rates of comorbid depressive and anxiety disorders among several major medical disorders, particularly neurological disorders, certain cancers, diabetes mellitus, and autoimmune disorders
- depression in particular as an adverse, rapidly modifiable prognostic factor for outcomes of certain medical disorders (eg, post–myocardial infarction)

In general, depression is more prevalent in the presence of more severe medical illness. Independently, however, depression as a comorbid factor is associated with lower survival rates, longer and more frequent hospital stays, lower compliance with treatment, diminished ability to care for self, and a lower quality of life.

In the case of major depression associated with myocardial infarction, prospective studies have found a doubling of mortality rates 12 years postinfarction and a quadrupling of mortality at 6 months[3] (and nearly as much at 18 months). The presence of depressive symptoms, in these studies, has been found to be an adverse prognostic factor, with a sevenfold increased risk of mortality at 18 months exceeding that of intrinsic cardiac risk factors such as frequent premature ventricular contractions (PVCs), low left ventricular ejection fraction, history of previous infarction,[4] and need for angiotensin-converting enzyme inhibitors. Certain clinical subgroups, such as those with depressive symptoms and frequent PVCs, have a very high mortality rate at 18 months.[5] Studies currently in progress will provide data on the capacity of newer antidepressant agents with low cardiotoxicity to lower these risk rates.

The potential for modifying service burdens of medical-surgical illness through attending to behavioral disorders is diverse and extensive, so much so that managed care systems need effective mechanisms to identify site-relevant problems and systematically develop intervention programs. Broad-based efforts to detect and treat mood and anxiety disorders in primary practice, however well intentioned, face the difficult challenge of training primary care practitioners to refocus on behavioral disorders and to incorporate diagnostic screenings into already tightly time-limited clinical encounters. Other strategies to supplement broad-based efforts may include targeted surveillance and detection of high resource utilizers and behavioral interventions with high probability for return on resource investment. Such strategies take the following general form:

- identification of high-cost, high-prevalence medical-surgical care problems as target groups
- identification of behavioral problems causing difficulties or adverse prognosis in the target group
- profiling the distribution of behavioral problems within the target group
- devising therapeutic interventions likely to have low-cost, high-return effects
- identification of specific individuals for targeted intervention
- location and treatment of targeted individuals

The reintegration of BH care with medical-surgical care requires an understanding of and special attention to BH treatment methods.

Methods of Treatment

Specialized managed BH care is rooted in four key principles of clinical treatment: alternatives to psychiatric hospitalization, alternatives to restrictive treatment for substance abuse, goal-directed psychotherapy, and crisis intervention.

Alternatives to Psychiatric Hospitalization

Partial hospitalization (day, evening, and/or weekend nonresidential) programs have been proven to be effective alternatives to hospital inpatient treatment in many outcome studies.[6,7] In a plan with adequate coverage for alternatives to inpatient services, and with informed decision making about which patients can benefit from these alternatives, economical and effective treatment can be provided to acutely ill patients in a partial hospital setting.

Alternatives to Restrictive Treatment for Substance Abuse

Research does not provide evidence that inpatient or residential substance abuse treatment is superior to outpatient or partial hospitalization approaches.[8,9] The central question of which patients truly need inpatient treatment and which can benefit equally well from outpatient or partial hospitalization has yet to be answered definitively. In the absence of support for the superiority of inpatient programs for the general treatment population, specialized managed BH systems tend to emphasize the more economical alternatives.

Goal-Directed Psychotherapy

The research literature supports the effectiveness of brief, goal-directed psychotherapeutic approaches for a number of problems.[10,11] Specialized managed BH care systems generally emphasize an interpersonal rather than an intrapsychic focus of therapy. These systems also place emphasis on therapy that is designed to be brief and time limited and not just a truncated version of long-term therapy.

Crisis Intervention

Successful managed BH systems are designed to make use of crisis intervention as a key service in the overall constellation of services. Research has demonstrated that short-term, intensive support of individuals during life crises or periodic acute episodes of psychiatric illness is an effective way to diminish the incidence of future crises and can substantially reduce the inappropriate use of psychiatric care.[12]

Additional clinical methods, utilized especially when applying managed care principles to the care of severely ill persons, include

- accurate behavioral diagnosis and attention to potential medical and neurological diagnostic issues
- detection and management of substance abuse
- prompt access to services for high-risk clients
- effective management of safety issues
- coordination of services from other agencies and multiple providers
- prevention of relapse through specialized clinical and case management services and adoption of a longitudinal treatment perspective for chronic disorders
- integrated use of multidisciplinary providers for exceptional cases, driven by a coherent, comprehensive treatment plan
- intensive community treatment of high-risk patients
- use of social stabilization measures to reduce relapse

THE IDEAL CONTINUUM OF CARE

Despite historical separation of substance abuse and mental health treatment programs, effective systems integrate treatment programs that tailor the appropriate mix of services to each individual's treatment needs.

Entry into the system requires an intake function, not necessarily geographically centralized, to triage cases, gather initial data, establish the presence of a BH disorder requiring treatment, determine the clinically appropriate level of care and mix of service types, and refer the patient to appropriate services. Immediate access to emergency evaluation services is also essential.

Mobile emergency services should also be available on a 24-hour basis for on-site evaluations of the need for acute inpatient services and to provide stabilization services as an alternative to hospitalization. Other important emergency services include the capacity to schedule next-day outpatient appointments and to provide psychiatric nursing backup for problems that might arise after hours.

Patients not stabilized despite on-site interventions may require 24-hour observation and assessment by a multidisciplinary team in a short-term behavioral crisis unit providing 1 to 5 days of 24-hour voluntary or involuntary observation, containment of assaultive or self-destructive behavior, and treatment of acute psychiatric emergencies.

Because of the high prevalence of dual diagnoses, chemical dependency detection and treatment protocols as well as staff with specialized training in both chemical dependency and mental disorders should be standard components for all basic services, as well as for inpatient and residential programs.

TREATMENT SERVICES

Substance Abuse Services

Few patients with substance abuse problems require inpatient treatment. Patients with mild to moderate withdrawal symptoms who need more than social support to maintain abstinence can be referred for ambulatory detoxification with daily medical management and monitoring by a physician–nurse practitioner team, including administration of medications as needed.

Patients with more severe problems need at least three types of alternative treatment levels:

- social detoxification centers for those who require removal from their usual living environment due to an inadequate support system
- residential rehabilitation for medically supervised detoxification when moderate withdrawal symptoms are present or there is a problem with compliance with instructions
- inpatient medical detoxification, usually in a general hospital setting, for patients with severe withdrawal syndromes of an imminently life-threatening nature, such as delirium tremens or withdrawal seizures

A full spectrum of nonintensive outpatient chemical dependency treatment services should be available, including brief alcohol and substance abuse treatment, maintenance counseling for individuals who need long-term support, and medication services for those requiring longer-term chemical stabilization.

Most patients unable to control substance use despite outpatient efforts can benefit from a partial hospital or intensive outpatient program, including standardized, systematic group education and therapy, core information about chemical dependency, and development of peer supports. Standard treatment packages may include an initial intensive phase with at least 20 evenings of treatment, followed by progressively less intensive treatment for the remainder of at least a year. Drug counselors in the intensive outpatient program discourage dropout by contacting patients who fail to attend meetings to determine whether relapse is occurring and to encourage return to treatment.

For those patients who relapse despite best therapeutic efforts and completion of treatment in the intensive phase of an intensive outpatient program, the continuum of care needs to provide several levels of care and therapeutic programs.

- There should be residential chemical dependency rehabilitation with 24-hour supervision during initial rehabilitation treatment in order to identify and correct factors interfering with the ability to receive successful treatment at an outpatient level. Once these factors have been removed, discharge to an intensive outpatient program can proceed.
- There should be relapse prevention programs providing specialized, more individualized techniques to address unmet treatment needs and specialized aftercare for those for whom standard methods are ineffective.
- There should be therapeutic halfway houses, linked to participation in a relapse prevention program, for those who repeatedly fail outpatient efforts.

Basic Mental Health Services

The vast majority of patients with mental health problems need only outpatient therapy services, including brief (less than 12 sessions) individual, group, and family psychotherapy; medication management services; and, for those at risk of relapse and deterioration, long-term maintenance therapy. Complicated cases need a designated primary therapist who is responsible for formulating and implementing a master treatment plan and for coordinating referrals to other outpatient services. Very complicated cases may require individualized services, such as on-site clinical case management assistance, social service interventions, and home-based support services.

Patients unable to succeed by using only outpatient therapy services need access to intensive outpatient services. These may consist of crisis services such as daily intensive individual, group, or family therapy sessions or outpatient medication visits; home-based or school-based therapeutic services, including in-home family therapy; or modular outpatient programs with an array of psychoeducational modules combined with specialized individual outpatient services and interdisciplinary treatment team involvement.

For more severely ill patients who cannot be adequately served by outpatient or intensive outpatient services, multidisciplinary partial hospital programs (PHPs) provide several hours per day of structured, integrated, modular treatment and psychoeducational services throughout the week and weekend. PHP replaces the range and intensity of services, except for 24-hour supervision and security, previously found in inpatient psychiatric programs.

Some patients require brief removal from troubled environments for stabilization of potentially life-threatening situations or situations that may cause family disintegration. As an alternative to acute hospital services or a behavioral crisis unit, crisis/respite house services may avert the need for a more restrictive and intensive facility placement. Such settings provide brief removal from a destructive or dangerous social situation or from an excessively strained family system for periods up to 2 weeks to allow stabilization of the living environment, placement in a more suitable living arrangement, or investigation by protective service agencies. This level of care would be ideal for runaway adolescents with oppositional behavior and limited substance abuse problems, battered spouses with highly disruptive adjustment disorders, self-mutilating nonpsychotic patients, and chronically mentally ill patients with families needing respite from excessive care needs or unremitting levels of conflict.

Despite intensive efforts, return home is unfeasible in some situations due to excessive long-term danger related to family violence or conflict, risk of violence by the patient, or predatory sexual behavior on the part of the patient. For such patients, community-based residential treatment services, such as a range of residential alternatives for out-of-home placement, need to be available, including therapeutic homes under the care of a family with parenting training and therapeutic group homes for small groups of adolescents and chronically ill adults with frequent disruptive behavior or without the skills to live independently or semi-independently.

Some children or adults may require placement in conventional large residential treatment centers for modification of subacute dangerous behaviors that exceed the skills capacity and security of community-based therapeutic services. Such centers provide 24-hour, tightly coordinated behavioral modification and medication treatment services, preferably with programs designed to prepare patients as rapidly as possible for placement in less-restrictive therapeutic settings.

Psychiatric acute care facilities remain essential for patients requiring high-security and very intensive treatment for imminently life-threatening conditions.

Dual Diagnosis

The combination of substance use disorders with major mental disorders, usually referred to as "dual diagnosis," has emerged as a central clinical focus for managed care approaches to public sector BH care. Systems for treating each type of disorder have evolved along separate lines in the past, resulting in limited competencies for treating individuals who have both disorders. Dual diagnosis, often a marker for poor treatment compliance, resistance to medication interventions, and multiple social problems, represents a disproportionate burden on resource utilization. The introduction of managed care into public sector psychiatry has prompted attention to the long-standing system failures for treating these difficult cases—resulting in the creation of specialized integrated dual diagnosis treatment programs and even the reorganization of separate agencies responsible for different types of disorder. In addition to having specialty units for the integrated treatment of individuals with primary mental and substance use disorders, there is growing interest in integrating well-targeted BH services into mainstream managed health care.

To address the treatment needs of the large population of patients with both mental disorders and substance abuse disorders, the continuum of care should include two general types of program elements: routine surveillance and cross-training in both disciplines at all levels of care, and specialized dual diagnosis programs to facilitate simultaneous treatment of both types of disorders when simpler treatment methods fail.

For more severely ill patients with a dual diagnosis, outpatient programs need to address abuse of a wide range of substances, because polysubstance abuse is highly prevalent among dual diagnosis patients. Intensive day and evening programs are needed for motivated patients with dual diagnoses, including psychotic mental disorders without severe residual symptoms, personality disorders without severe behavioral disturbance, and moderately severe coexisting anxiety, mood, and post-traumatic stress disorders. In these specialized dual diagnosis treatment programs, abstinence may be a goal rather than a prerequisite for entry. An ideal system will make provision for programs integrating interventions from both psychiatric and substance abuse treatment camps: continuous treatment teams, monitored medication compliance, behavioral skills training to prevent both psychiatric relapse and lapses into substance abuse, close monitoring of drug abuse, modified 12-step groups, behavioral reinforcement programs (such as a token economy) to reward abstinence and healthier behaviors, and assertive case management to reengage poorly compliant participants.

Specialized dual diagnosis treatment programs may exist at the level of crisis houses, social detoxification houses, behavioral crisis units, partial hospitals, community therapeutic residential programs, large-scale residential treatment centers, and acute inpatient services.

Paradigmatic Shifts in Progress

During the 1990s, expansion of managed care into public sector BH care systems challenges the applicability of earlier strategies and methods. Government mandates to meet the BH care needs of a more seriously ill population require modification of clinical methods and planning techniques. Brief, cognitive interventions requiring high levels of patient motivation and compliance do not meet the needs of individuals with severe mental illness or chemical dependency who, due to the seriousness of their symptoms, may lack motivation and/or the ability to comply. Rather, managed care systems serving the public sector must encompass a wide range of treatment options, including social support, outreach, and intensive case management programs. Without appropriate treatment, persons with severe illnesses can incur poor clinical outcomes, including higher mortality rates; higher nonelective, inpatient utilization rates; and higher medical morbidity and associated costs.

Modifications in medical management approaches to persons with severe mental illness and/or chemical dependency represent more than technical adaptations to special populations. These changes reflect a maturing trend in managed clinical care to refocus systems planning and care management onto the problems of a defined population, rather than solely on the care of individual patients. Two initiatives promote the shift toward population-based case management: the growth of capitated and subcapitated reimbursement systems, and the increase in population-defined service mandates of public sector systems. The pressure of capping health care expenditures while expanding managed care technologies to (historically underserved) vulnerable populations requires careful consideration of the systemic consequences of managed care technologies.

The most distinctive feature of the shift toward systems planning is the emphasis on examining the consequences, especially the unintended consequences, of changing clinical practices and strategies. For example, studies comparing the unintended consequences of different pharmacy cost containment strategies find that lower unit costs of apparently similar medications may result in higher system costs. Because there are comparable rates of efficacy for all classes of antidepressants, the least expensive agent would seem to be the rational choice for treatment. Although the direct unit cost of tricyclic antidepressants is considerably lower than for newer agents such as selective serotonin reuptake inhibitors, the overall costs of the use of tricyclics is at least as great and perhaps greater, if additional costs (laboratory, psychiatric and medical office visits, psychiatric and medical hospitalizations) are included.[13–17] Particularly important, negative effects of tricyclic use may include higher costs related to intensive medical care for tricyclic overdoses, care for falls due to orthostatic hypotension, and accidents due to diminished cognitive clarity.

Another example is the lower overall costs of care associated with the use of the more expensive, newer atypical neuroleptic agents recently marketed for the treatment of schizophrenia.[18] Due to fewer adverse effects, favorable effects on negative schizophrenic symptoms, and the capacity to treat patients who are unreceptive to conventional neuroleptics, these medications result in higher patient acceptance and compliance and better symptomatic improvement. The cost savings result from fewer treatment failures and hospital admissions.

The system effects of using newer psychotropic agents parallel similar findings in primary care medicine in which newer agents, although more expensive on a unit-cost basis, do not result in cost containment for several common disorders. Even the restricted formulary use of generic medications in place of newer single source agents, a commonly used cost savings method (see Chapter 26), may unexpectedly result in higher overall costs due to higher aggregate drug costs and an increase in the number of drugs dispensed. Cost containment strategies other than drug formulary restriction (eg, strict gatekeeping and visit copayments) may achieve their purpose better.[19]

The emerging shift to a systems paradigm promotes several other modifications of conventional managed care practice. In the older paradigm, the emphasis was on cost containment through minimizing unit costs of individual care, standardizing care methods, and decreasing access to services by controlling the supply of services. In the newer paradigm, there is an emerging emphasis on determining the lowest cost of effective care for a population, promoting and comparing competing clinical care methods, and proactively reducing the need for more costly services. As an example, in the older managed care paradigm and prior to legislation curbing the practice, services for alcohol-related disorders such as delirium tremens were often not covered under HMO benefits. In the newer paradigm, trauma-prone persons with alcohol problems are sought out for treatment in order to reduce more costly large-case trauma related to alcohol use, such as automobile or motorcycle accidents, falls, or physical battery.

Previously, the focus was on the service needs of an individual, the selection of efficient techniques for expediting episodes of care, and the avoidance of high-risk patients. In the new paradigm, the emphasis is on determining the service needs of groups within the service population and developing systems for the tightly coordinated management of care on a longitudinal basis, targeting the highest risk individuals within the population.

Past emphasis was on cost reduction, primarily through reduction of direct, point of service costs and of service utilization in general. In the newer paradigm, there is an emerging emphasis on enhancing the clinical value of resources invested in services, maximizing cost offsets of services to defray direct costs, and shaping utilization to lower the overall cost of care by enriching care in specific areas.

In the emerging, population-based paradigm for cost containment, several strategies for enhancing clinical value are prominent.

- Accelerate the onset of response.
- Develop systems to ensure follow-up and continuity of care to avoid waste of high-quality, intensive care.

- Eliminate counterproductive, low-quality interventions.
- Prevent illness, especially trauma-related illness, through treatment of predisposing behavioral disorders.
- Enhance medical cost offsets.
- Lower complication rates.
- Lower recidivism rates.
- Improve prognosis for medical disorders and surgical procedures.

BENEFIT PLAN DESIGN

Benefits design for services, including BH services, is beyond the scope of this chapter and this book. However, until passage of the 1996 Mental Health Parity Act,[20] the design of BH services almost always involved a substantial difference between benefits for basic medical-surgical services and those for BH. The parity legislation, effective January 1998, requires group health plans that have annual or lifetime dollar limits for medical or surgical benefits to also have the same dollar limits on mental health benefits, thereby promoting parity between physical and mental health care; it must be borne in mind that this applies only to dollar limits, not necessarily to other nondollar limitations on coverage. In addition to extending mental health coverage (substance abuse treatment is not covered by the Mental Health Parity Act), the law provides a venue to accurately document the financial impact of mental health treatment and to identify cost savings attributable to medical cost offset by managed mental health programs. If mental health parity causes premium costs to rise greater than 1%, the plan may be able to appeal the requirement for parity (though at this time, calculating this cost escalation looks as if it will be difficult). Within this context, BH benefit design, like all health benefit design, needs to address two key issues: coverage limits and incentives.

Coverage Limits

Given this new mental health parity law, coverage limits are essentially a method to limit or control benefit cost in the setting of dollar parity. Coverage limits can include maximum days, visits, or copayment/coinsurance amounts (eg, 50% coinsurance) and can be based on levels of care (eg, inpatient, partial hospitalization, structured outpatient), types of disorder (eg, acute psychiatric, chronic, custodial, specific diagnoses), types of treatment (eg, psychosurgery, psychoanalysis, nutritionally based therapies), and/or types of providers (eg, physician; psychologist; social worker; marriage, family, and child counselor [MFCC]). The optimal benefit design for a managed BH program will provide adequate coverage for inpatient treatment and its alternatives as well as for treatment providers from various professional disciplines.

Levels of Care

Traditional indemnity plans and many HMO plans have limited coverage to inpatient hospital care and minimal outpatient care for mental health problems and inpatient detoxification. To support a comprehensive managed BH program, the benefit should cover a number of levels of care (Exhibit 32–1).

Exhibit 32–1 Managed Mental Health Benefits: Covered Levels of Care

Mental Health
- Hospital inpatient services
- Nonhospital residential treatment
- PHP/day treatment
- Individual/group outpatient treatment
- Crisis intervention
- Outreach services

Substance Abuse
- Detoxification (inpatient, noninpatient residential, and outpatient)
- Hospital rehabilitation
- Nonhospital residential rehabilitation
- Intensive outpatient rehabilitation
- Individual/group outpatient rehabilitation

Source: Reprinted from DF Anderson et al, Managed Behavioral Health Care Services, in *The Managed Health Care Handbook,* 3rd ed, PR Kongstvedt, ed, p 348, © 1996, Aspen Publishers, Inc.

Table 32–1 Typical Coverage of Disorders in Plans with Specialized Mental Health/Substance Abuse Management

Category of Disorder	Percentage of Plans Offering Coverage
DSM diagnoses	100
Chronic mental disorders	71
Sexual addiction	21
DSM V codes	7
Codependency	7
Nicotine addiction	7
Custodial care	0

Courtesy of William M. Mercer, Inc, San Francisco, California.

Types of Disorders

Another way that some managed BH plans limit plan liability is through limiting covered disorders. Respondents to a survey indicated considerable variation in the types of disorders covered by plans featuring BH management (Table 32–1).

Some plans also exclude coverage for specific *Diagnostic and Statistical Manual IV (DSM IV)* diagnostic categories such as learning disorders and autism, as well as medical diagnoses with potential psychiatric treatment regimens, such as obesity.

Types of Treatment

Many plans built around specialized BH management limit specific treatments covered. Table 32–2 indicates variation among respondents as to coverage of selected types of treatment. Many plans also exclude from coverage such treatments as biofeedback and electroconvulsive therapy.

Types of Providers

Many traditional indemnity plans have covered only the services of MDs and PhDs for outpatient BH psychotherapy. HMOs and managed indemnity BH plans have expanded coverage to a broader range of mental health professionals. Table 32–3 indicates patterns of provider coverage for plans with specialized BH management. Some plans also cover pastoral counselors and family practitioners for BH services. For public sector managed care initiatives, an even broader range of providers is necessary. These networks usually include community mental health centers, substance abuse treatment agencies, and other specialty organizations that typically receive funding through state and local initiatives.

Table 32–2 Typical Coverage of Treatment Types in Plans with Specialized Mental Health/Substance Abuse Management

Category of Treatment	Percentage of Plans Offering Coverage
Brief problem-focused therapy	93
Long-term psychodynamically oriented therapy	64
Psychosurgery	15
Nutritionally based therapies	7

Courtesy of William M. Mercer, Inc, San Francisco, California.

Table 32–3 Typical Coverage of Provider Types in Plans with Specialized Mental Health/Substance Abuse Management

Category of Provider	Percentage of Plans Offering Coverage
MD	100
PhD psychologist	93
MA social worker	87
MA psychiatric nurse	87
MFCC	83
MA psychologist	73
Certified alcoholism counselor	57

Courtesy of William M. Mercer, Inc, San Francisco, California.

Incentives

The greater the incentives to access and comply with the managed BH system, the greater the effect. Most employers are not comfortable with a plan that offers no BH coverage outside the managed system. For this reason, most managed BH plans tend to offer point of service choice where patients can select a network or an out-of-network provider. Point-of-service coverage usually has a higher deductible and coinsurance. The typical managed indemnity plan offers a $0 deductible in-network benefit with a coinsurance of 20%. Out-of-network coverage typically will feature a deductible of $250 with 50% coinsurance.

An optimal coinsurance differential may be 40% (eg, 10% in network and 50% out of network). Managed BH plans typically do not publish a preferred provider list. For practical purposes, then, coverage differentials actually apply to the plan member accessing a gatekeeper and accepting channeling to a network provider rather than accessing a provider directly without going through the gatekeeper.

UTILIZATION MANAGEMENT

Utilization management in specialized BH programs falls into two general categories: utilization review (UR) and case management. In practice, distinctions between the two functions often become blurred, but it will be instructive to discuss them separately.

Utilization Review

In the mid-1980s, when an increasing number of employers had installed UR systems to help contain costs of indemnity plans, it became clear that UR conducted by nonspecialized staff with general medical backgrounds was ineffective when applied to BH cases. As a response, specialized BH UR developed that employed specialized staff applying BH-specific utilization criteria. Specialized UR typically includes preadmission certification of inpatient BH cases and concurrent review of inpatient and residential cases (and sometimes of outpatient cases) to determine the presence or absence of medical necessity of treatment. Operational characteristics of effective specialized UR programs are as follows:

- Telephone-based treatment review is conducted by credentialed BH professional reviewers, usually MA-level psychiatric nurses, MA-level social workers, and PhD- or MA-level psychologists.
- Reviewers as a group are trained and experienced in inpatient and outpatient treatment for BH for adults, adolescents, and children.
- Initial and concurrent review episodes involve direct contact with the primary clinician instead of, or in addition to, the facility UR nurse.
- There is readily available high-level, back-up clinical supervisory staff for front-line reviewers. Such back-up staff includes, at a minimum, board-certified adult and child/adolescent psychiatrists and a certified addictionologist.
- Medical necessity/level of care criteria employed by reviewers are age and diagnosis specific and behaviorally descriptive and encompass all levels of care, including, for example, nonhospital residential programs and partial hospitalization. Criteria are tested and retested continually and modified as needed.

UR construed narrowly as determination of medical necessity is typically installed to prevent abuses in a traditional fee-for-service plan. Although specialized BH UR has proved to be somewhat more effective in containing costs than nonspecialized UR, utilization management has been far more effective in conjunction with a specialized BH network with point of service choice.[21] This comprehensive approach to managing BH care generally invokes case management as the utilization management tool of choice.

Case Management

As comprehensive managed BH programs have evolved during the late 1980s and early

1990s, the case management function has crystallized as a focal point for promoting cost-effective, quality BH care. BH case management encompasses traditional UR but extends beyond into a broader form of patient advocacy, addressing the longitudinal course of care as well as discrete episodes of intensive treatment. Comprehensive case management includes four overlapping components.

- *Promoting correct diagnosis and effective treatment.* Assisting plan members to access the best level, type, and mix of treatment; keeping alert to opportunities for enhancing the quality and efficacy of care; acting to make provider and patient aware of these opportunities (UR strives to exclude payment for unnecessarily intensive treatment, whereas case management strives to direct patients into effective forms of treatment at appropriate levels of intensity).
- *Promoting efficient use of resources.* Helping the patient/family access the most effective resources with the minimum depletion of family finances and finite available insurance dollars (directing patients into effective care may be the most potent cost-saving method of all).
- *Preventing recidivism.* Monitoring progress subsequent to intensive treatment episodes; encouraging and, if necessary, helping arrange for inter-episode care to prevent recidivism.
- *Monitoring for and containing substandard care.* Identifying potential quality of care defects during treatment; investigating and, when needed, intervening to ensure remediation.

Comprehensive case management goes beyond determination of medical necessity and seeks to promote enhancement of the quality, efficacy, and continuity of care. As such, it is a more demanding discipline than simple UR. It is practiced optimally by qualified front-line case management staff with a minimum of 5 to 10 years of relevant clinical experience who are thoroughly trained in case management techniques, backed up by readily available doctoral-level advisors with relevant clinical experience (including managed care experience), and supported by well-articulated systems to assist with the case management task. Examples of such systems include the following:

- *Triage systems.* Every managed BH system must devise a mechanism for directing cases to the proper case manager. This includes, for example, ensuring that cases with medical issues are directed to a psychiatric nurse rather than to a social worker and that substance abuse cases are directed to case managers specifically qualified and experienced in this area.
- *Quality screens.* Diagnosis-based criteria for the use of case managers, delineating typical best practice patterns of high-quality care for specific problems as well as screens for common quality of care defects, should be employed routinely as cases are reviewed. Such screens assist in early identification of mismatches between treatment plans and diagnosis as well as pinpoint more subtle opportunities to enhance quality and efficacy of care (eg, when providers may be unaware of or unwilling to use superior treatment methods).

CHANNELING MECHANISMS

A key aspect of any managed BH system is a channeling mechanism to assess initially and direct an individual to the appropriate type and intensity of treatment. This gatekeeper function is crucial to the effectiveness of the managed BH program and is fraught with potential implementation problems. Who should conduct the initial assessment to determine whether there is a BH problem for which an evaluation and treatment plan are in order? Who should conduct a thorough clinical evaluation and formulate a treatment plan? Who should carry out the treatment plan? The candidates for some role in the gatekeeper function may include an employee assistance program (EAP), a primary care physician (PCP) in a general managed medical system, and/or a specialized BH case manager and designated assessor clinician belonging to a contracted BH provider network.

In practice, the gatekeeper role in a managed BH system is often divided among a number of system participants. EAP counselors may be credentialed to make direct treatment referrals for certain types of cases but may be required to review decisions with a case manager before making other types of referrals. PCPs may have full authority to treat mental health problems, may have authority to refer cases directly for BH treatment with notification to the BH managed care system, or may yield all authority for BH treatment to the BH manager. Protocols detailing roles and responsibilities of all concerned must be carefully worked out, understood, and agreed to.

The EAP as Gatekeeper

EAPs play a unique role in corporate America, serving as a wide-open point of access for employees and dependents with various problems and concerns. Before the advent of specialized BH systems, EAPs were often the only reliable source of information and guidance for individuals needing BH services. In this role, the EAP assesses an individual's BH status and, if necessary, makes a referral for treatment.

The positive aspect of having EAP counselors serve as gatekeepers for the managed BH benefit is that they are numerous, are generally knowledgeable, and cast a wide net. They are likely to come in contact with people early, when problems of living have not necessarily grown to become major BH problems. Drawbacks of assigning gatekeeper responsibilities to EAP counselors include the fact that not all are clinically credentialed and qualified, virtually none has the medical background to enable identification of medical and medication problems that may mimic or underlie BH problems, and some may not be philosophically in tune with the goals of the managed BH program.

The PCP as Gatekeeper

Many managed medical care programs (including many HMOs) restrict direct access to mental health practitioners and require the approval of the PCP before mental health specialists may be consulted. In some managed care programs, the PCP is expected to diagnose and treat common, uncomplicated mental disorders.

The advantage of investing gatekeeping responsibility in the PCP is that it encourages continuity of care and concentrates authority for preventing unnecessary use of all specialty services in the hands of one person. A major disadvantage of using PCPs as gatekeepers for BH services is that medical clinicians have been shown to be dramatically less likely to detect or treat mental disorders than mental health specialists.[22] Historically, HMOs have gradually acknowledged the value of allowing direct access to mental health services.

The Mental Health/Substance Abuse Case Manager and Assessor as Gatekeepers

Most specialized managed BH systems are organized to utilize some combination of case managers and designated assessor-clinicians within the contracted provider network as gatekeepers/channelers to appropriate treatment. Some systems rely on case managers to conduct a fairly detailed initial assessment over the telephone and to make referrals for treatment on that basis for all but the most complex cases (which are referred to a field clinician for further evaluation). Other systems routinely channel virtually every case to one of a group of specially designated assessors for detailed face-to-face evaluation and treatment planning.

In either instance, important triaging occurs at the outset. Many systems are able to case match referrals to assessors or treatment clinicians on the basis of the therapist's specialty interests, gender, language, ethnicity, and so forth. Among systems that encompass a broad spectrum of mental health providers (eg, MD, PhD, MSW, RN), few have developed a practical theory or usable criteria for matching cases to specific provider disciplines.

BEHAVIORAL HEALTH PROVIDER NETWORKS

Assembling and administering a specialized BH provider network involves a more labor-intensive selection and monitoring process than is usually required for a general medical provider network. Some of the criteria could apply to any network: geographic accessibility, inclusion of a full continuum of care, willingness to negotiate favorable rates in exchange for channeling of patients, willingness to cooperate with utilization management procedures and standards, and structural evidence of quality, such as appropriate credentials, current licensure, certification, and the like. Some other issues related to continuum of services, practice patterns, and practice philosophy are uniquely relevant to specialized BH networks. Therefore, although network formation is not the subject of this book, a brief discussion on pertinent aspects of a BH provider network is warranted. Generally, managed BH organizations adhere to a network development process that is similar to other network development processes but has a few unique aspects.

Size and Scope of the Network

To pinpoint the size and scope of the network, the organization must take into account the benefit design to be administered (ie, the array of services and the range of provider types covered), the demographic characteristics of the population to be served, area geographic characteristics (eg, physical or psychological barriers to provider access), and any specific payer requirements related to the size and composition of the network.

The above factors influence the characteristics of a network in any particular area, but certain general rules of thumb apply across most specialized BH networks.

1. No plan member has driving time of more than
   - 1 hour to a full-service hospital
   - 30 minutes to an emergency room
   - 30 minutes to an outpatient substance abuse program
   - 30 minutes to an individual provider or program
   - 30 minutes to an assessor
2. Network coverage ratios should be at least
   - individual provider per 1,000 covered members
   - assessor per 3,000 covered members
3. The distribution of network providers by discipline generally falls within the following ranges:
   - up to 30% psychiatrists
   - 0% to 30% PhD psychologists
   - 40% to 60% MA-level providers (psychologists, social workers, nurses, MFCCs)

Selection Criteria

Many providers completing the application typically are eliminated as a result of failure to pass the screening process (most BH organizations have a formalized set of screens that are applied to applications to narrow the field of eligible network participants). Virtually all organizations conduct an in-person site visit to facility-based programs before approving them for network membership. With individual providers, there is considerably more variation. Many organizations rely completely on written applications, some include a telephone interview, some conduct face-to-face site visits/interviews for selected providers, and a few require site visits/interviews for all individual providers admitted to the network. Some common selection criteria for facilities and individual providers are listed in Exhibit 32–2.

For public sector–oriented agencies such as community mental health centers (CMHCs), chemical dependency organizations, and other specialty services organizations, network admission criteria are variable. Virtually all MCOs

Exhibit 32–2 Common Selection Criteria for Providers

Facilities
- Must provide a continuum of levels of care (not only acute inpatient)
- Average length of stay for acute inpatient cases <10 days

Psychiatrists
- Accustomed to filling medication management role in conjunction with other therapists handling individual therapy
- Usual practice pattern involves referring patients to psychologists and social workers for individual therapy
- Work primarily with serious, complicated conditions

Psychologists
- Usual practice pattern involves referring to physician for medication evaluation when appropriate
- Do not routinely test all patients unless specifically indicated

Social workers
- Demonstrated experience in treating sociofamilial issues
- Experienced with assessment, especially in community mental health center settings

Nurses
- Some general medical nursing experience
- Demonstrated current knowledge of psychopharmacology

All practitioners
- Knowledge, experience, and training in goal-focused, brief therapy techniques
- Experienced in multidisciplinary treatment approaches
- Routinely use peer support system to discuss difficult cases
- Demonstrated familiarity with community resources

Courtesy of William M. Mercer, Inc, San Francisco, California.

---

require state licensure of specialty service *programs* and professional staff, as well as documented qualifications of nonlicensed staff who may provide valuable support services for which a professional license is not required. Beyond that, state and local governments usually promulgate regulations and standards for public sector managed care networks.

PROVIDER STRUCTURES FOR INTEGRATED DELIVERY SYSTEMS TO MEET MANAGED CARE OBJECTIVES

The preceding section focused on aspects of network formation from the perspective of MCOs. Market changes are rapidly moving the BH delivery system toward mergers of providers into vertically or horizontally integrated systems and toward the integration of providers and MCOs. Therefore, this section will focus on aspects of network formation from the point of view of such emerging systems.

Importance of Planned Integrated Delivery Systems

The nature of psychiatric and addiction disorders and the secondary disabilities that manifest as a result of the severity and persistence of these disorders underscore the importance of integrated delivery systems. A range of treatment interventions must be simultaneously available to address numerous and discrete demands for crisis intervention, stabilization and relief of acute symptoms, and continuing treatment and psychoeducational support for recovery and relapse prevention.

Historic Structures: Public and Private

Integrated service delivery systems can offer better access and accountability while guarding against clinical risk and cost shifting. In the past, BH delivery structures in the private sector were one dimensional (a hospital) or two dimensional (a hospital and outpatient clinic). These limited structures were inadequate to address the heterogeneity of the client population and its needs. Interventions more intensive than an outpatient visit were either carried out in expensive hospital settings or not available. Public care systems began to develop a broader range of services in the 1960s under the umbrella of comprehensive CMHCs.

Until the advent of managed care, CMHCs represented the majority of comprehensive and integrated care systems. Managed BH care organizations adopted community mental health approaches and became leaders in creating integrated service delivery networks, initially for the private sector and more recently for Medicaid and Medicare recipients.

Move to Provider Networks

Integrated service delivery systems have a comprehensive array of services organized to meet the needs of a defined population and geographic base. Fully integrated systems in BH care comprise acute and intensive care services, continuing care and relapse prevention, and community support and long-term care. Integrated care systems provide a single point of clinical and fiscal accountability to patients and payers, promoting access, managing utilization, and ensuring quality.

Integration has been achieved through consolidation and/or affiliation of providers into defined delivery networks. The model of a physician–hospital organization (PHO), familiar to health practitioners, is less common in BH care. More common are preferred provider organizations (PPOs), designed to link individual and small group practitioners and established by hospitals, insurers, and MCOs. Horizontal networks, comprising provider organizations in similar lines of business (ie, hospitals *or* CMHCs *or* residential providers) are most often formed to consolidate a broader geographic and client base, to achieve management efficiencies, and to position the combined organizations to compete for managed care business. Vertical networks incorporate hospitals with ambulatory service providers. In the BH arena, this may include acute care services or a combination of acute, continuing, and long-term care services (ie, hospitals *and* CMHCs *and* residential providers).

Factors in and Constraints on Carve-in and Carve-out Strategies Varying by Eligibility Population

In order to succeed in the current reimbursement environment, BH networks require the capacity to integrate internally across programs and facilities, and externally to primary health care providers. Carve-out approaches, where both reimbursement and management of BH benefits are administered separately from broader health benefits, persist where payers believe that separate administration strengthens accountability, lowers cost, and/or improves access to care. Carve-outs are most common in the private sector in areas where benefits were historically generous, utilization was high, and the provider community was well developed. In the public sector, the strategy has been focused most often on the population with disabilities, which represents the greatest risk, clinically and financially.

Carve-in approaches are most frequently found in HMOs that provide all health and BH services for a single capitated rate and limit even specialty service utilization to providers within the organization or network. Carve-in strategies are viewed as useful in controlling inappropriate health utilization driven by behavioral disorders and in promoting more integrated care. BH delivery systems must organize to accept payment on a carve-out basis as well as on a carve-in basis if volume is to be maintained and growth achieved. This capacity is particularly important in the short term to preserve continuity with clients whose insurance coverage may shift and to mitigate the financial impact of low HMO expenditures and subcapitated payments for BH.

The capacity to play on both terms is considered essential to positioning for the long term, for which the forecast is greater integration between physical health and BH.

QUALITY ASSURANCE

Quality management (QM) refers to activities designed to prevent and/or correct quality problems. QM in basic medical-surgical care is discussed in Chapter 15. In managed BH systems, core QM activities are focused on the qualifications and behavior of case managers and providers and (to some extent) on the treatment results achieved by providers. The following is a delineation of common elements of internal QM programs for managed BH organizations.

Utilization Review/Case Management

Internal QM programs should include the following elements designed to ensure quality in the UR/case management process:

- *Credentialing/recredentialing.* Typical requirements are that case managers have at least MA-level BH clinical credentials, have a minimum of 3 to 5 years of clinical experience, and maintain current licensure and certification to practice. Many organizations consistently exceed these standards in practice; for example, it is not uncommon for case managers in a given setting to average 10 to 15 years of clinical experience at various levels of care.
- *Clinical rounds.* Staff must participate in educationally oriented interdisciplinary conferences that include senior clinical staff.
- *Formal supervision.* Provision must be made for regular direct supervision and coaching of case managers by clinically qualified supervisors.
- *Clinical audits.* Routine internal audits of case management notes must be performed with attention to administrative and clinical performance, routine feedback to case managers, and individualized remedial activities when standards are not met.
- *Analysis of patient complaints/grievances.* An ongoing process to review complaints and grievances must be available with focus on clustering complaint categories, analysis of implications for policy/procedural modifications, and feedback to clinical and administrative personnel.
- *Patient/consumer satisfaction surveys.* Written tools for obtaining recommendations and measuring patient satisfaction with both the process and outcomes of care must be distributed to a sample of patients and analyzed at least annually.
- *Data tracking.* Staff-specific, diagnosis-specific outcome data must be tracked (eg, average length of stay) with comparison to norms, analysis of implications for case management technique, and feedback to case managers.
- *Inservice training.* Inservice training programs for case managers must be shaped and driven by the findings of the internal QM monitoring system.

Network Providers

Internal QM systems in BH programs should include the following elements to ensure quality in the provider network:

- *Credentialing/recredentialing.* Minimum requirements usually include academic credentialing, licensure, certification, confirmation of criterion-level malpractice insurance, and clearing of malpractice history. Some organizations independently check licensure directly with state licensing boards and perform direct checks on legal actions concerning malpractice. Recredentialing should be done on a continual basis (eg, every 2 years), including systematic reminders to providers when current licensure or insurance is about to expire.
- *Case manager ratings.* Routine global ratings of providers by case managers per contact episode must be based on cost-effectiveness, quality of care, and degree of cooperation with the managed care system.

- *Provider profiling.* Diagnosis-based provider profiling must be based on measures of cost and utilization with feedback to providers on network norms. This topic is also addressed in Chapter 38.
- *Treatment chart audits.* There must be routine audits of provider treatment charts, often focused on profile outliers, with feedback to providers.
- *Provider communications.* These include bulletins, newsletters, memoranda, and so forth given to network providers. The materials address administrative and clinical issues; choices of issues to be addressed are driven by findings of the internal QM system.
- *Provider education.* Providers must attend formal education programs driven by findings of the internal QM system.
- *Provider satisfaction surveys.* The plan must conduct routine monitoring of network provider satisfaction with clinical and administrative requirements of the managed care system and provide the opportunity for constructive suggestions for system changes.
- *Outcome monitoring.* There must be diagnosis-specific, provider-specific tracking of outcome measures including patient satisfaction, recidivism/relapse, mental and/or physical health status change, mental and/or physical claims costs, and functional change (through employer-based data such as absenteeism rates and productivity measures).

External Quality Assurance Monitoring

It has been suggested that the incentives and conflicts of interest inherent in a managed BH program are too great to be overcome entirely by internal self-regulation. In recognition of this problem, some state and federal regulatory agencies and employer/payers have instituted routine external quality monitoring of managed BH systems.

The results of such external auditing activities reveal considerable variation in performance among managed BH organizations and within organizations over time and at different service delivery locations.

Routine monitoring of the quality of patient care services may be a useful check and balance mechanism. Audits of treatment and case management records can reveal significant areas for improvement in the service delivery system not otherwise detected by internal quality assurance methods. Determining these areas may help improve the MCO's quality of care and its competitive position. Following are some examples of variation and common weaknesses in systems.

Utilization Criteria

Most organizations have criteria that specify clear behavioral criteria for various levels of care. Some organizations, however, have adopted criteria that do not provide clear guidance to case managers. General, nonbehavioral criteria are difficult to apply with any precision. In some other instances, criteria are clear but inefficient. For example, some organizations use published 50th percentile norms to assign initial lengths of stay, thus missing the opportunity to influence cases for which earlier discharge would be reasonable and achievable.

As specialized BH MCOs have matured, there has been a growing consensus among organizations concerning the essential criteria for inpatient care. There has also been serious attention paid to indications for outpatient care and elaboration of UR criteria for intermediate levels of care in the continuum of care.

Staff Qualifications

Some organizations lack case managers or even supervisory personnel with relevant BH background and experience. Some lack doctoral-level advisors who can engage in matched peer review with doctoral-level providers. Some programs have MDs without psychiatric or substance abuse background functioning as psychiatric medical directors. This is inappropriate, at best.

Inservice Training

Some organizations select inservice training programs on the basis of apparently random or arbitrary topic selection rather than needs identified through an internal QM system. Many have no inservice training, orientation, or QM oversight applied to doctoral-level advisors. Some have no discernible inservice training program at all.

Quality of Care Problem Identification

The incidence of quality of care problems such as misdiagnosis, subtherapeutic or toxic medication dosages, unexplored medical complications, mismatch of diagnosis and treatment plan, and mismanagement of dangerous behavior has not diminished over time, and specialized MCOs have yet to devise effective methods for improving care at the point of UR. In general, review programs document detection of and action on these problems in only a small minority of cases, although informal activity is believed to occur in some programs. When problems are identified by case managers in these programs, action by doctoral-level advisors can also be too rare. The potential for conserving resources through methodical improvement of the quality of care has hardly been explored.

Provider Credentialing

In the most minimal level of QM for a provider network, the BH system requires that all network providers meet certain baseline credentialing standards. Some programs fail to thoroughly document and independently to confirm credentialing when providers are admitted to the network, and many programs fail to recredential consistently to ensure that network members continue to meet basic requirements.

Progress in Outcomes Measurement, Tracking, and Assessment

The ultimate gateway to true continuous quality improvement is the reliable measurement of treatment outcomes and analysis of the relationship among treatment approach, provider type, case management technique, and treatment outcome. Some BH programs have begun to track treatment outcomes in a number of ways, and joint meetings between MCOs and large provider entities have been held to stimulate consensus on proposed tentative conceptual schemes and data measurement tools. There remains, however, great variation among programs and providers in the degree of conceptual development of these approaches, in the sophistication of information systems available to put data to use, and in the extent of agreement about appropriate measures and methods.

INFORMATION SYSTEMS

BH care information systems are a subset of general health care informatics. Consequently, many of the issues facing the automation of BH care processes mirror those facing health care generally. This section focuses on the balance that BH systems must reach between the necessarily unique BH features and those features that both types of systems have in common. The use of data and profiling in the medical-surgical environment is discussed in Chapters 37 and 38.

Unique Features of BH Systems

An information system designed specifically for BH diverges functionally in several ways from similar medical-surgical systems. Good BH systems include, for example, *DSM IV* diagnosis codes (including all axes). They allow for residential and partial care settings, nontraditional treatment alternatives, and BH testing. Many important methods for delivering BH services under managed care involve the use of intensive, noninpatient, alternative care settings. These alternatives are incompatible with the basic inpatient/outpatient structure and coding schemes of typical medical-surgical systems.

The best BH management information systems developers recognize the more chronic/long-term nature of BH problems and have structured system functions to accommodate this reality. These systems smoothly handle issues of multiple and extended authorizations for all levels of care, review, and approval of treatment plans, and episodes of care that are routinely longer than those in medical-surgical systems. Contracting and provider modules have well-developed BH credentialing and profiling systems and allow for provider searches on the full range of provider experience, treatment preferences, and education. A wide range of contracting options should be accommodated, and utilization against these contracts should be tracked.

Level of Integration

While good BH information systems have many features that distinguish them from typical medical-surgical systems, there are many functions that can be shared. More important, there are many functions that must be the same. One example is eligibility information. In most cases, the BH benefit is part of a larger medical benefit and, therefore, the eligibility information for the two benefits must be the same.

Typically, the BH system relies on the corresponding medical-surgical or employer system for eligibility information. The level of integration between these corresponding systems determines the eligibility file access alternatives. The level of integration can be represented as a continuum, with the highest level being a single system for both medical-surgical and BH and the lowest level being two independent systems with incompatible eligibility file structures.

At the high integration end of the continuum, BH processing is accomplished on the medical-surgical information system. Historically, this has led to significant functional compromises in the quality and specificity of the BH data, but it does have the positive effect of making access to the eligibility file simple. Since the BH staff is using the same system as the medical-surgical staff, they have access to the same eligibility functions and the same eligibility file. No transfer of eligibility information between systems is required.

At the other end of the integration continuum, there are many independent BH systems that have varying degrees of compatibility with the employer systems or medical-surgical systems from which they must obtain their eligibility data. In the worst case, the BH staff must either access the medical-surgical system themselves for the eligibility data, or rely on paper printouts or phone calls to the medical-surgical staff.

At the midpoint of the integration continuum, duplicate eligibility files are maintained on each system. This requires transferring the data from one system to the other over a leased line or by tape. Duplicating the files leads to new issues, including scheduling the replication process, reconciling the files, and accessing the original file between replications when eligibility questions arise.

The best integration options utilize client/server approaches. In these cases, there is only one eligibility file, which is maintained on its own eligibility server. When either a user of the medical-surgical system or a user of the BH system checks the eligibility of a client, the system sends a message or remote procedure call to the eligibility server, which returns with the appropriate eligibility and demographic data. The user is unaware that the system has accessed an external resource to answer the query.

This last approach allows the BH system the independence required to preserve its unique BH functions without requiring the duplication of files that need to be accessible to all systems. It also makes it easy to develop BH-specific data files that contain information not required by medical systems. These files can be accessed by the BH client application at the same time as the shared eligibility file. The BH system user receives an answer that contains information from both the unique BH file and the systemwide eligibility file.

Key Issues

The key to a successful BH information system is found in the balance between unique system functions and data and those functions and data that must be integrated with the remainder of the benefit plan. The eligibility function, for example, must be well integrated. So should accumulators against benefit plan maximums, integrated claims files, member service systems, and contracting.

Many other system functions and data, as indicated above, must be developed independently. The quality of the service provided is compromised when these functions are combined; the medical-surgical information systems do not support the unique needs of BH care. Treatment planning provides a good example. Medical-surgical applications have not been designed to accommodate treatment plans prior to the delivery of the service. There is much less variability in the possible treatments, and they are typically not delivered over the longer time spans that BH care requires. Consequently, medical-surgical systems do not analyze treatment plans and progress against treatment plans in determining the appropriateness of service delivered. However, in BH this is the main method of precertification and concurrent review. It is much more efficient and effective to develop this function as a separate mental health module or as an entirely independent system.

PUBLIC/PRIVATE SYSTEMS INTEGRATION

BH is unique in the health care world for the dominant role the public sector has played in the financing and delivery of care. Approximately two public dollars are spent for every private dollar in the financing of psychiatric and addiction treatment services. Moreover, publicly financed and operated systems historically cared for individuals with the most serious forms of illness, contrary to tertiary care practices in the medical-surgical arena, where the sickest people more often accessed care in the best-staffed teaching hospitals.

The BH field moved from a medical to a psychosocial model of care in the last 30 years to support the decongregation of public psychiatric hospitals and the development of community-based care. Considerable technology was developed in community mental health and addiction services for the management of care in alternative and less costly settings. Adoption of these practices was key to the success of the early managed BH care organizations.

Managed BH care was formally established in response to private sector demand for an alternative to unregulated and growing use of inpatient and outpatient care. Emergence of managed care in the public sector has primarily been driven by a desire to manage the cost of the benefit, combined with aspirations to improve access, quality, and outcomes of the care provided. Despite the fact that first-generation behavioral managed care developed from public sector approaches, the advent of managed care in the public sector has been accompanied by the notion that the private sector is more consistent and considered in its approach, which can therefore benefit the public sector.

Managed care has also been accompanied by a government privatization effort that has (more than managed care techniques) promoted public/private systems integration. Opportunities for a positive fusion of public and private sector technologies and competence are a great benefit accrued to patients at a time when the amount and cost of service benefits are being reduced. Through privatization and managed care initiatives, those with the most serious disorders now have access to the best hospitals at more affordable rates. At the same time, privately insured persons now have access to less restrictive and broader types of care. The interactive effects of public sector community treatment technology and private sector quality improvement and information management hold great promise for consumers of care.

The promise of public/private systems integration can be realized through a deliberate and planned approach to implementation of a reformed system. Steps to be taken include

- understanding the shifting roles of government players in the local environment as the

Departments of Mental Health, Public Health and Medical Assistance reframe their policy, regulatory, financing, and provider roles
- analyzing the case-mix characteristics and utilization patterns of publicly insured persons to identify client risk groups and project utilization and cost associated with their care
- assessing political and regulatory challenges to implementing new provider arrangements, service models, and reimbursement rates
- evaluating the potential for integration of publicly and privately insured persons at the provider level to reduce segregation, maximize resources, and improve access
- establishing a process and standards for quality assurance and improvement of all care programs
- incorporating the voice and interests of consumers in the planning, delivery, and evaluation of accountable services
- developing benchmarks to guide monitoring of client utilization and professional practice patterns as a safeguard against underservice
- framing agreements and a plan for allocation of savings as a return on public investments

EMERGING ISSUES

As with managed health care in general, the BH care field remains highly dynamic, with new issues emerging every year. The most important emerging issues in BH care today are discussed below.

The paradigm shift toward population-based care management challenges the limits of earlier generations of BH managed care. Prompted by poor BH care outcomes and vocal patient/family advocacy, government and employer requirements to address the needs of individuals with more severe mental illnesses are increasing. MCOs must refocus systems planning and care management onto the problems of defined and often vulnerable populations.

Involvement of a large advocacy community in the past and the more recent involvement of primary consumers in the public sector advisory process requires accommodation by the private sector as more public services are privatized. As noted earlier, the Mental Health Parity Act, effective January 1998, requires that group health plans with annual or lifetime dollar limits for medical or surgical benefits have the same dollar limits on mental health benefits. This national effort to promote parity between physical and mental health care is prompting renewed discussion on the health benefits of integrating physical and behavioral care management and the potential for medical cost offset through BH treatment.

The potential for medical cost offset as a result of timely and targeted psychiatric and addiction treatment is recognized but infrequently measured. As data emerge and full risk capitation arrangements grow, the demand for behavioral treatment in primary and tertiary care settings grows. A substantial proportion of the highest cost tertiary care patients have psychiatric and substance abuse disorders that increase morbidity and mortality if left untreated. The implications for redistribution of resources to BH are dependent upon the ability of the BH field to produce data and educate payers and practitioners.

BH providers are challenged to integrate horizontally to achieve comprehensiveness of service continuum, geographic base, and covered lives. They are also challenged to integrate vertically to complete continuums with primary health and tertiary care providers. BH providers/networks require the capacity to operate as, and accept varying payments on, both carve-in and carve-out bases.

Legal, ethical, cultural, and accountability challenges common in public care systems are emerging in managed BH care systems.

- *Legal:* Legally mandated civil commitment produces uncontrolled expenses in length of stay and legal representation, driving financial risk to capitated systems.
- *Ethical:* Providers are challenged to ration care under managed and capitated arrange-

ments where fiscal incentives may promote underservice.
- *Cultural:* As managed care penetration increases, particularly among publicly insured clients, demands increase for providers to be culturally competent, for treatments to be culturally fit, and for programs to be culturally accessible.
- *Accountability:* Patient and family member advocacy groups are organizing and demanding greater accountability from insurers, employers, and governments.

CONCLUSION

This chapter outlines some of the key components of, and issues and recent developments in, specialized managed care programs addressing BH treatment. BH care efforts present unique management problems that are increasingly being addressed through specialized managed care systems with specific and separate operational guidelines, managed care personnel, provider networks, and QM approaches.

REFERENCES

1. National Alliance for the Mentally Ill (NAMI). *Stand and Deliver: Action Call to a Failing Industry.* Washington, DC; 1997.
2. Bennett MJ. The greening of the HMO: implications for prepaid psychiatry. *Am J Psychiatr.* 1988;145:1544–1549.
3. Frasure-Smith N, Lesperance F, Talajic M. Depression following myocardial infarction. *JAMA.* 1993;270:1819.
4. Frasure-Smith N, Lesperance F, Talajic M. Depression and 18-month prognosis after myocardial infarction. *Circ.* 1995;91:999.
5. Schene AH, Gersons VP. Effectiveness and application of partial hospitalization. *Acta Psychiatr Scand.* 1986;74:335–340.
6. Rosie JS. Partial hospitalization: a review of recent literature. *Hosp Community Psychiatr.* 1987;38:1291–1299.
7. Mosher LR. Alternatives to psychiatric hospitalization. *N Engl J Med.* 1983;309:1579–1580.
8. Annis HM. Is inpatient rehabilitation of the alcoholic cost effective? *Adv Alcohol Substance Abuse.* 1986;5:175–190.
9. Saxe L, Goodman L. *The Effectiveness of Outpatient vs Inpatient Treatment: Updating the OTA Report.* Hartford, CT: Prudential Insurance Company; 1988.
10. Husby R, Dahl AA, Dahl CI, Heiberg AN, Olafsen OM, Weisaeth L. Short-term dynamic psychotherapy: prognostic value of characteristics of patient studies by a two-year follow-up of 39 neurotic patients. *Psychother Psychosom.* 1985;43:8–16.
11. Horowitz M, Marmar CR, Weiss DS, Kaltreider NB, Wilner NR. Comprehensive analysis of change after brief dynamic psychotherapy. *Am J Psychiatr.* 1986;143:582–589.
12. Whittington HG. Managed mental health: clinical myths and imperatives. In: Feldman S, ed. *Managed Mental Health Services.* Springfield, IL: Thomas; 1992:223–243.
13. Sclar DA, Robison LM, Skaer TL, et al. Antidepressant pharmacotherapy: economic outcomes in a health maintenance organization. *Clin Ther.* 1994;16(4):715–730.
14. Melton ST, Kirkwood CK, Farrar TW, Brink DD, Carroll NV. Economic evaluation of paroxetine and imipramine in depressed outpatients. *Psychopharmacol Bull.* 1997;33(1):93–100.
15. Simon GE, Von Korff M, Heiligenstein JH, et al. Initial antidepressant choice in primary care: effectiveness and cost of fluoxetine vs tricyclic antidepressants. *JAMA.* 1996;275(24):1897–1902.
16. Lapierre Y, Bentkover J, Schainbaum S, Manners S. Direct cost of depression: analysis of treatment costs of paroxetine versus imipramine in Canada. *Can J Psychiatry.* 1995;40(7):370–377.
17. Keck PE Jr, Nabulsi AA, Taylor JL, et al. A pharmacoeconomic model of divalproex vs. lithium in the acute and prophylactic treatment of bipolar I disorder. *J Clin Psychiatry.* 1996;57:213–222.
18. Meltzer HY, Cola PA. The pharmacoeconomics of clozapine: a review. *J Clin Psychiatry.* 1994;55(suppl B):161–165.
19. Barefoot JC, Helms MJ, Mark DB, et al. Depression and long-term mortality risk in patients with coronary artery disease. *Am J Cardiol.* 1996;78:613–617.
20. Anderson D. How effective is managed mental health care? *Business Health.* November 1989:34–35.
21. Wells KB, Hays RD, Burnam MA, et al. Detection of depressive disorder for patients receiving prepaid or fee-for-service care. *JAMA.* 1989;262:3298–3302.
22. Shadle M, Christianson JB. The organization of mental health care delivery in HMOs. *Admin Ment Health.* 1988;15:201–225.

DONALD F. ANDERSON, PHD, founded, and for 10 years directed, the behavioral health care consulting practice at William M. Mercer, a human resources consulting organization. He is now responsible for the supervision of several national specialty health care consulting practices at Mercer, including the behavioral health care practice. He is a clinical psychologist with extensive experience in the evaluation and design of managed mental health and chemical dependency programs.

JEFFREY L. BERLANT, MD, PHD, is an assistant clinical professor in the department of psychiatry at the University of Washington School of Medicine. He also has been a consultant for mental health and substance abuse services. He has broad experience in evaluation of both public and private sector managed mental health and substance abuse programs.

DANNA MAUCH, PHD, is the president of Magellan Public Solutions, a managed behavioral health care organization. She has extensive experience in strategic planning, operations management, systems evaluation, and the development and implementation of innovative managed care programs.

WILLIAM R. MALONEY, MBA, is a principal in the Phoenix office of William M. Mercer. He serves as national practice leader for the Health Care Information Practice. His focus is on health care information systems. Assignments have included information systems planning, vendor selection, and information systems and operations evaluations in both public and private sector health care organizations.

TERRI GOENS is a William M. Mercer consultant for mental health and substance abuse prevention and treatment services. Her consulting specialty is in designing and evaluating managed care substance abuse programs.

KATHERINE OLBERG STERNBACH, MED, MBA, is a principal with William M. Mercer's Behavioral Health Care Practice. Her consulting specialty is in the design, delivery, and implementation of managed behavioral health systems of care.

Part XI

Clinical Quality and Outcomes Measurement and Management

Best practices in medical management must by definition attend heavily to issues of quality and outcomes. Quality management has evolved as have all other medical management activities, but it has evolved in a somewhat different way. The earlier paradigms have not been replaced but have been supplemented with models that draw from more industrial models of quality management.

The measurement of outcomes is no easy task. Crafting definitions that apply to actually measuring quality and outcomes is potentially complicated, especially if there is insufficient information available. The incorporation of outcomes measurement into medical practice is increasing, but it needs to take on an even greater role as managed health care continues to achieve cost savings. Although this incorporation is potentially complicated, it can and should be done.

Chapter 33

Quality Management in Managed Care

Pamela B. Siren and Glenn L. Laffel

Chapter Outline

- Traditional Quality Assurance
- Components of a Quality Management Program: Building on Tradition
- A Process Model for a Modern Quality Management Program
- Setting the Improvement Agenda
- Conclusion

There are a variety of approaches to quality management in the managed care setting. These approaches are complementary and employ the principles of measurement, customer focus, and statistically based decision making. This chapter provides an overview of quality management in managed care, from traditional quality assurance to modern performance assessment and continuous improvement. It is hoped that readers will be able to utilize both methods once they have completed this chapter.

This chapter is adapted from PB Siren and GL Laffel, Quality Management in Managed Care, in *The Managed Health Care Handbook*, 3rd ed, PR Kongstvedt, ed, pp 402–426, © 1996, Aspen Publishers, Inc.

TRADITIONAL QUALITY ASSURANCE

Advocacy for performance assessment in health care can be traced to EA Codman, a surgeon who practiced at Massachusetts General Hospital in the early 1900s. He was among the first advocates of systematic performance assessment in health care. His efforts included evaluation of the care provided to his own patients.

In the 1960s and 1970s, the introduction of computers and large administrative data sets (used initially to support Medicare claims processing) permitted investigators to use powerful epidemiological methods in their analyses of practice variations and related phenomena. In this period, Avedias Donabedian developed three criteria for the assessment of quality that are still used today: structure, process, and outcome.[1] His approach to quality assessment of care has stood the test of time and remains useful in managed care settings.

Structure Criteria

Structural measures of health care performance focus on the context in which care and services are provided. These measures provide inferences about the managed care organization's (MCO's) capability to provide the services it proposes to offer. Structural measures include board certification of physicians, licensure of facilities, compliance with safety codes, recordkeeping, and physician network appointments. Many such requirements are delineated in federal, state, and local regulations that govern licensing or accreditation and mandate periodic review and reporting mechanisms.

Accreditation and regulatory bodies have traditionally emphasized structural criteria because of their ease of documentation. Purchasers support this tradition by requesting such information in their contract negotiations with MCOs. The role of the MCO's leadership in improving performance is increasing and is evaluated by accrediting agencies through assessment of committee function. The MCO needs a complete understanding of its leadership's role in performance improvement.

As MCOs form into integrated delivery systems, the structural criterion of performance assessment becomes more complex. The regulations and standards that may govern MCOs, such as those of the National Committee for Quality Assurance (NCQA), may be different from the standards to which member hospitals are held accountable, such as those of the Joint Commission on Accreditation of Healthcare Organizations. Reconciliation of at least the minimal and widely accepted standards within the MCO and across an integrated delivery system is the first step to developing structural measures and evaluating structural performance and its impact on the quality and cost of health care delivery.

Structural measures generally do not offer adequate specificity to differentiate the capabilities of providers or organizations beyond meeting minimum standards. In addition, the relationship between structure and other measures of performance, such as outcomes, must be clarified to ensure that enforcing structural standards leads to better results.[2]

Process Criteria

The second traditional criterion for health care quality assessment is process. Process of care measures evaluate the way in which care is provided. Examples of care process measures for MCOs include the number of referrals made out of network, health screening rates (eg, cholesterol), follow-up rates for abnormal diagnostic results, and clinical algorithms for different conditions. Such measures are frequently evaluated against national criteria or benchmarks. Process of service measures are also frequently used. These include appointment waiting times and membership application processing times.

As with structural measures, it is important to link process measures to outcomes. Although the field of outcomes research is growing, the link between many health care processes and key outcomes has not always been clearly defined.

Outcome Criteria

The third traditional category of quality assessment is the outcome of care or service. Traditional outcomes measurements include infection rates, morbidity, and mortality. Relatively poor outcomes performance generally mandates careful review. Exhibits 33–1 and 33–2 illustrate common outcome criteria used to assess quality of inpatient and outpatient care. Unfortunately, although outcomes measures are purported to reflect the performance of the entire system of care and service processes, they often offer little insight into the causes of poor performance.

Despite the limitations of current outcomes assessment, most MCOs have systems in place to assess for adverse events. These screening criteria are often evaluated during the utilization review process to detect sentinel events. Some of these same measures are being applied to the peer review process within the MCO.

Peer Review and Appropriateness Evaluation

In addition to Donabedian's three quality criteria, peer review and appropriateness review have been key components of the traditional quality assurance model. Because of their applicability to managed care, they are discussed here.

Exhibit 33–1 Examples of Events among Hospitalized Patients That May Indicate Inadequate Quality of Care

Adequacy of discharge planning
- No documented plan for appropriate follow-up care or discharge planning as necessary, with consideration of physical, emotional, and mental status/needs at the time of discharge

Medical stability of the patient at discharge
- Blood pressure on day before or day of discharge: systolic, < 85 mm Hg or > 180 mm Hg; diastolic, < 50 mm Hg or > 110 mm Hg
- Oral temperature on day before or day of discharge $> 101°F$ (rectal $> 102°F$)
- Pulse < 50 beats/min (or < 45 beats/min if patient is on a beta blocker) or > 120 beats/min within 24 hours of discharge
- Abnormal results of diagnostic services not addressed or explained in the medical record
- Intravenous fluids or drugs given on the day of discharge (excludes the ones that keep veins open, antibiotics, chemotherapy, or total parenteral nutrition)
- Purulent or bloody drainage of postoperative wound within 24 hours before discharge

Deaths
- During or after elective surgery
- After return to intensive care unit, coronary care, or special care unit within 24 hours of being transferred out
- Other unexpected death

Nosocomial infections
- Temperature increase of more than $2°F$ more than 72 hours from admission
- Indication of infection after an invasive procedure (eg, suctioning, catheter insertion, tube feedings, surgery)

Unscheduled return to surgery within same admission for same condition as previous surgery or to correct operative problem (excludes staged procedures)

Trauma suffered in the hospital
- Unplanned removal or repair of a normal organ (ie, removal or repair not addressed in operative consent)
- Fall with injury or untoward effect (including but not limited to fracture, dislocation, concussion, laceration)
- Life-threatening complications of anesthesia
- Life-threatening transfusion error or reaction
- Hospital-acquired decubitus ulcer
- Care resulting in serious or life-threatening complications not related to admitting signs and symptoms, including but not limited to neurological, endocrine, cardiovascular, renal, or respiratory body systems (eg, resulting in dialysis, unplanned transfer to special care unit, lengthened hospital stay)
- Major adverse drug reaction or medication error with serious potential for harm or resulting in special measures to correct (eg, intubation, cardiopulmonary resuscitation, gastric lavage), including but not limited to the following:
  1. Incorrect antibiotic ordered by physician (eg, inconsistent with diagnostic studies or patient's history of drug allergy)
  2. No diagnostic study to confirm which drug is correct to administer (eg, culture and sensitivity)
  3. Serum drug levels not measured as needed
  4. Diagnostic studies or other measures for side effects not performed as needed (eg, blood urea nitrogen, creatinine, intake and output)

Source: Reprinted from Health Care Financing Administration, 1986.

Peer Review

Peer review involves a comparison of an individual provider's practice either by the provider's peers or against an acceptable standard of care. These standards may be developed within the MCO (eg, practice guidelines), described by national professional associations, or required by a regulatory or legislative agency. Cases for peer review are identified either as outliers to specific indicators or through audits of medical records. Peer review has traditionally been used as an informal educational tool. It is typified by morbidity and mortality conferences currently in existence in hospital systems.

Peer review has its limitations. First, opportunities for improvement may be missed by a paradigm that rests on conformance with standards. Deming emphasized that meeting specifi-

Exhibit 33–2 Examples of Inpatient Diagnoses That May Indicate Inadequate or Improper Outpatient Care

- Cellulitis (extremities)
- Dehydration of child younger than 2 years who has severe diarrhea
- Diabetic coma—ketoacidosis
- Essential hypertension
- Gangrene (angiosclerotic, extremities)
- Hemorrhage secondary to anticoagulant therapy
- Hypokalemia secondary to potassium-depleting diuretic
- Low-birthweight infant (premature, <2,500 g)
- Malunion or nonunion of fracture (extremities)
- Perforated or hemorrhaging ulcer (duodenal, gastric)
- Pregnancy-induced hypertension (preeclampsia, eclampsia, toxemia)
- Pulmonary embolism (admitting diagnosis)
- Readmission of same condition within 14 days
- Ruptured appendix
- Septicemia (admitting diagnosis)
- Status asthmaticus
- Urinary tract infection (bacturia, pyuria)

Courtesy of Blue Cross and Blue Shield Association, Chicago, Illinois.

cations does not result in constant improvement but rather ensures the status quo.[3] Second, studies have shown that there is poor inter-reviewer reliability among panels of physician reviewers and that the level of physician agreement regarding the quality of care is only slightly higher than the level expected by chance alone.[4] Third, peer review is limited by the scope of the indicators or processes under review. Despite these limitations, peer review continues to serve an important role in MCOs' quality management programs.

Appropriateness Evaluation

Appropriateness evaluation reviews the extent to which the MCO provides necessary care and does not provide unnecessary care. Appropriateness review frequently occurs before an elective clinical event (admission or procedure). Procedures or admissions most frequently selected for appropriateness review include those for which there is a wide variation of opinion as to their usefulness or effectiveness and those that have been notably expensive. Examples of procedures frequently selected for appropriateness review include hysterectomy, coronary artery bypass surgery, and laminectomy. The proposed indication for the event is compared with a list of approved indications obtained from a professional society or a specialty vendor or designed by the MCO itself. Appropriateness review is intended to identify and minimize areas of overutilization.

Appropriateness review provides a snapshot of a care decision and does not lend itself to an understanding of the events that may have preceded the admission or procedure in question. In addition, this review does not evaluate the effectiveness of the procedure once it has been authorized.

COMPONENTS OF A QUALITY MANAGEMENT PROGRAM: BUILDING ON TRADITION

The traditional quality assurance model provides a sound foundation for a modern quality management program. The quality assurance model can be improved, however, with an infusion of systems thinking, customer focus, and knowledge for improvement.

First, systems thinking offers a method for assessment and management of performance with a clear aim or purpose. The traditional quality assurance model does not incorporate this important concept. Lacking a shared aim, payers and providers risk forming a disconnected, inefficient network. This disconnected network will eventually engage in contradictory and inefficient behaviors. Organizational goals can be achieved first by identifying customer needs of an organization, unifying the purpose within the organization, and expanding the shared purpose across the integrated delivery system. For further information about systems thinking and organizational goal setting, the reader is referred to the work of Peter Senge (listed in the Suggested Readings).

Second, the cornerstone of a modern quality management program is customer focus. The traditional quality assurance model was driven, in part, by regulations and accreditors without explicit knowledge of what the customer (member, purchaser, provider) needed. The modern quality management program identifies key customers, measures customer needs, and improves processes to meet those needs.

Finally, an enhancement of the traditional quality assurance model is knowledge for improvement. According to Moen and Nolan, three fundamental questions can be used as guides for improvement efforts.[5]

1. What are you trying to accomplish? Information gained from understanding customer needs, the current process and outcome performance, and expected performance will assist the MCO in answering this question.
2. How will you know that a change is an improvement? Establishing performance expectations before implementing an improvement activity assists the MCO in understanding whether a change is an improvement and minimizes any potential confusion between measures of utilization and indicators of quality.
3. What changes can be made that will result in an improvement?

To develop tests and implement changes, the plan-do-study-act cycle is used as a framework for an efficient trial and learning model. The term *study* is used in the third cycle to emphasize this phase's primary purpose: to gain knowledge. Increased knowledge leads to a better prediction of whether a change in a current process will result in an improvement.[6]

A PROCESS MODEL FOR A MODERN QUALITY MANAGEMENT PROGRAM

Figure 33–1 depicts a model for a modern quality management program that enhances the traditional quality assurance model so that it incorporates the dimensions mentioned above. The remainder of this chapter discusses the eight key steps in developing a modern quality management program.

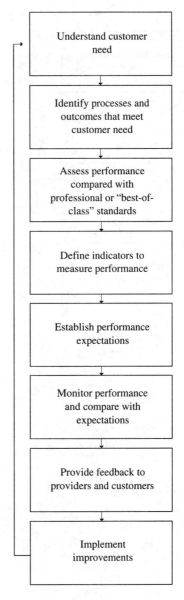

Figure 33–1 Continuous Improvement Process. *Source:* Reprinted from PB Siren and GL Laffel, Quality Management in Managed Care, in *The Managed Health Care Handbook,* 3rd ed, PR Kongstvedt, ed, p 406, © 1996, Aspen Publishers, Inc.

Understand Customer Need

Understanding customer need (Figure 33–2) is the basis of all quality management programs. Juran and Gryna described a customer as anyone who is affected by a product or process.[7] There are external customers, internal customers, and suppliers. External customers of an MCO include members or benefactors and purchasers. Internal customers include the departments and services within the MCO, such as claims processing and member education, as well as the health care professionals themselves. Customer needs may be clear or disguised, rational or less than rational. These needs must be discovered and served.[7] Negotiating and balancing the needs of these diverse and sometimes conflicting customer groups represent a challenge for MCOs, as they do for any organization.

Methods to understand customer need are as diverse as the customer groups. Customer complaints are a usual signal of a quality problem. Low levels of complaints, however, do not necessarily mean high satisfaction. Frequently, dissatisfied customers will purchase services elsewhere without ever registering a complaint. Most MCOs have a formal process to survey their membership for satisfaction with care or services (Exhibit 33–3). Yet despite the burgeoning number of satisfaction surveys, a study has shown that only 2 of 10 health care organizations conducting patient satisfaction surveys were using them as a regular feedback device to administrative and clinical departments.[8] Through marketing initiatives, MCOs are proactively determining customer needs through focus groups and interviews. These processes are designed to identify customer expectations and real (versus stated) need. The Hospital Corporation of America (now Columbia/HCA) finds it useful to identify several levels of customer expectation. At level I, a customer assumes that a basic need will be met; at level II, the customer will be satisfied; at level III, the customer will be delighted.[7] Results from member satisfaction surveys and market analyses are an integral part of strategic quality planning.

A fundamental principle of quality improvement theory is the necessity for economically meaningful partnerships between purchasers and suppliers. Purchasers, MCOs, and hospitals are negotiating contracts based on performance measurement. To illustrate this concept, US Quality Algorithms, Inc, a subsidiary of US Healthcare,

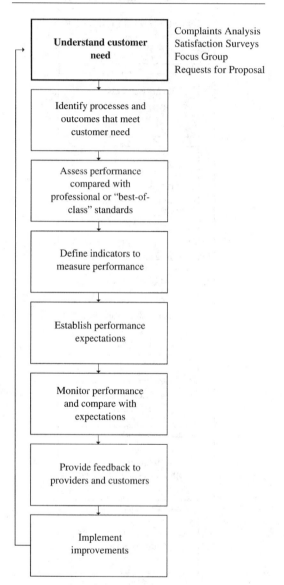

Figure 33–2 Continuous Improvement Process—Understand Customer Need. *Source:* Reprinted from PB Siren and GL Laffel, Quality Management in Managed Care, in *The Managed Health Care Handbook,* 3rd ed, PR Kongstvedt, ed, p 407, © 1996, Aspen Publishers, Inc.

Exhibit 33–3 Examples of Satisfaction Surveys

How would you rate:	Excellent	Very Good	Good	Fair	Poor
The thoroughness and technical skills of the					
Attending doctor					
Nursing staff					
Consulting doctors					
Other personnel (lab, X-ray, etc)					
The friendliness and compassion of the					
Attending doctor					
Nursing staff					
Consulting doctors					
Other personnel (lab, X-ray, etc)					
The explanations, instructions, and responses to questions by the					
Attending doctor					
Nursing staff					
Consulting doctors					
Other personnel (lab, X-ray, etc)					
Admission process (timeliness, friendliness, convenience)					
Explanation of your rights as a patient					
Discharge instructions and arrangements					
Food quality and service					
Appearance and cleanliness of the hospital					
Overall quality of care provided by the attending doctor					
Overall rating of this hospital					
Satisfaction with the outcome of your procedure (if applicable)					

Would you recommend this hospital to a friend or loved one? ☐ Yes ☐ No
Would you recommend your attending doctor to a friend or loved one?

© U.S. Quality Algorithms (USQA), 1991

How would you rate each of the following:	Excellent ◄─────► Poor 10 9 8 7 6 5 4 3 2 1	No Opinion 0
Nursing care		
Emergency room services		
Laboratory department		
Quality assurance/improvement program		
Utilization review department		
Social services/discharge planning		
Medical records		
Bed availability		
Patient satisfaction with the hospital		

continues

Exhibit 33–3 continued

Please rate the following clinical departments:	**Excellent** ◄―――――► **Poor**	**No Opinion**
	10 9 8 7 6 5 4 3 2 1	0
OB/GYN General Surgery Orthopaedics Urology Cardiology ENT Other _____ Other _____		
Would you refer a family member to this hospital? ❑ Yes ❑ No		

© U.S. Quality Algorithms (USDA), 1991

Note: This example includes selected questions from USQA's survey of members and USQA's survey of physicians.

Source: © *Journal on Quality Improvement*, Oakbrook Terrace, IL: Joint Commission on Accreditation of Healthcare Organizations, 1993, p 377. Reprinted with permission.

---

has implemented the CapTainer compensation system, which combines base payments with an annual performance-based distribution. The CapTainer system is based on a contracting process that includes the setting of performance targets, the development of a schedule for progress toward them, and the construction of a purchase/compensation schedule that translates improvement into a performance-based distribution.[9] The size of the performance-based distribution is related to progress toward goals and to the financial implications of changes in hospital or MCO operating procedures. Partnerships between MCOs and hospitals, and the positive economic relationships they imply, are only realistic and possible if the values of delivering care in a managed environment are shared.[9]

Negotiating and balancing the diverse groups of customer needs represent a challenge. Juran and Gryna stated that it is important to recognize that some customers are more important than others. It is typical that 80% of the total sales volume comes from about 20% of the customers; these are the "vital few" customers who command priority.[7] Within these key customer groups, there is a distribution of individual customers that also may have a hierarchy of importance, such as a government agency, a gold card purchaser account, or an academic teaching center. Explicit understanding of the needs of all the MCO customer groups will minimize situations in which one customer's needs are met to the exclusion of another's.

Identify Processes and Outcomes That Meet Customer Need

Identification of processes and outcomes that meet customer need is the next step of the continuous improvement process model (Figure 33–3). How do customers view the MCO's quality? To begin with, they want to know whether the MCO meets their expectations. MCOs are expected to treat members who are ill and to maintain the health and functional capabilities of those who are not. To treat sick patients, MCOs first have to make it easy for them to access services and second must provide them with appropriate care. Purchasers and members value access and appropriateness.[10] Purchasers also value assessments of disease screening activities, service quality, and encounter outcomes to the extent that they support or embellish information about access and appropriateness.[10] Similarly, purchasers know that to maintain health and functional capacity, MCOs must support prevention of illness and management of health status. Therefore, the

Quality Management in Managed Care   443

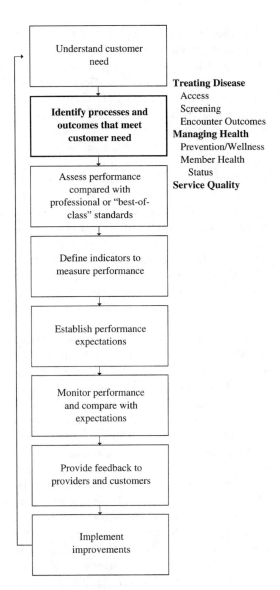

Figure 33–3 Continuous Improvement Process—Meet Customer Need. *Source:* Reprinted from PB Siren and GL Laffel, Quality Management in Managed Care, in *The Managed Health Care Handbook*, 3rd ed, PR Kongstvedt, ed, p 409, © 1996, Aspen Publishers, Inc.

two key processes in this step are treating disease and managing health.

Treating Disease

Access. The Institute of Medicine defines access as "the timely use of personal health services to achieve the best possible outcomes."[11(p4)] In an MCO, access encompasses geographical convenience and availability of providers. For purchasers and members alike, access is an absolutely critical area. For example, a 1993 study found that 93% of Americans considered access to services very important in their choice of a health system, and 76% of the same group felt that accessibility might decline given the incentive structure created by capitation.[12] Of related interest, Americans in all demographic categories consistently indicate that they will not accept the waits characteristic of other countries' health systems (up to 6 months for heart surgery in Canada, up to 4 months for a specialist appointment in Britain).[13] Finally, surveys of MCO disenrollees repeatedly show that a majority of those who left the MCO of their own volition chose to leave because they were dissatisfied with access to service.

In addition, studies have concluded that communities where people perceive poor access to medical care have higher rates of hospitalization for chronic diseases (asthma, hypertension, chronic obstructive pulmonary disease, congestive heart failure, and diabetes).[14] It has been suggested that improving access to care is more likely to reduce hospitalization rates for chronic disease than changing patients' propensity to seek health care or eliminating variation in physician practice style.[14]

Screening. Disease screening measures assess the MCO's performance in detecting the medical conditions of its membership at an asymptomatic, treatable stage. Familiar examples of disease screening include mammography, Pap smear testing, cholesterol screening, and sigmoidoscopy. Disease screening measures defined as screening rates per eligible population are easy for consumers to understand. The measures, however, are not immune to the controversies of timing of disease screening. In addition, purchasers tend to view screening activities as useful and cost-effective even though the evidence to support this is weak. Nevertheless, screening processes are likely to remain important to purchasers.

In the future, consumers and purchasers may come to value outcomes of screening more than frequency or amount of screening. After all, screening does not assess the patient's benefit from early detection. For example, an effectiveness measure in screening breast cancer may be two outcome measures—the stage of breast cancer at diagnosis and the 5-year mortality rate for breast cancer—rather than only mammography rates over time.

Encounter Outcomes. Encounter outcome measures evaluate the results of specific clinical encounters, such as a hospitalization or an office visit. Included in this category are the traditional assessments of mortality, readmission rates, adverse events, provider empathy, and satisfaction. Traditionally, encounter outcome measures have been confounded by small sample sizes, case-mix adjustment issues, and unreliable data collection methods. These problems have made it difficult to compare data across systems or even within an MCO over time. Purchasers are likely to continue asking for encounter outcomes for high-volume clinical conditions. Because of the methodological issues mentioned, however, purchasers are likely to set relatively low performance standards in these areas.

Managing Health

Prevention/Wellness. The next set of key processes comprises those associated with prevention of illness. Prevention activities are designed to keep the membership free of disease. Examples of prevention programs include smoking cessation, nutritional counseling, and stress reduction. Measures of prevention include the percentage of eligible patients enrolled in one of the above programs, immunization rates, and first trimester prenatal care visit rates. Such prevention programs assess process performance. As discussed earlier, the effectiveness of such programs is questionable without a link to outcomes. High disenrollment rates make it hard for MCOs to realize long-term benefits from prevention programs. At least in the short term, it appears that consistently poor performance in this area would dampen a purchaser's enthusiasm for an MCO.

Member Health Status. The evaluation of a member's health status may include assessment of functioning in physiological terms (eg, blood pressure or laboratory tests), physical terms (eg, activities of daily living), mental or psychological terms (eg, cognitive skill and affective interaction), social terms (eg, ability to engage in family work or school), and other health-related quality of life areas (eg, pain, energy, sleep, and sex).[15] Two purposes are served by health status evaluations. First, members at risk for need of services can be identified before a catastrophic event. Second, a member's health status assessment can serve as an outcome measure for care or treatment received. The popularity of health status assessment stems from two ideas. The first is that members' perceptions of their health are both important and easy to obtain.[16] The second is that health systems should be accountable not only for treating disease and managing health, but for enhancing members' well-being as well.

Although it is believed that purchasers will rely heavily on member health status measures in their assessments of MCO quality, the Health Care Advisory Board recently articulated a persuasive countervailing opinion.[10] According to the Advisory Board, health status data are not likely to play a prominent role in MCO selection. The Advisory Board called attention to two facts in presenting its argument. First, member health status is influenced by factors beyond the control of the MCO, including genetic predisposition to illness, sociodemographic factors, dietary and exercise habits, and so forth. Second, most systems exhibit member turnover rates of 10% or higher, and this makes it difficult to link health status to activities in any one system. According to the Advisory Board, purchasers are unlikely to hold MCOs accountable for (much less make a decisive negotiating decision in light of) the health status of its members. Only time will tell how much member health status measures will play a role in evaluations of an MCO's performance.

Service Quality

Service quality measures evaluate the timeliness, responsiveness, and courtesy with which the MCO serves its members. These attributes are of obvious importance to MCO members. The impact of managed care and the balance of cost and quality will continue to be evaluated. Although there are numerous studies showing high levels of member satisfaction with MCOs, it is worthy to note that the results were less than favorable for the MCOs in one recent survey. A total of 2,374 adults were randomly selected and interviewed over an 11-month period. Nonelderly sick persons in managed care plans reported lower out-of-pocket expenses but more problems getting the health service or treatment they or their physicians thought was necessary. The study also found that sick people in managed care plans were more likely to be unhappy with both general and specialist physician care. In addition, managed care enrollees were more likely to report difficulty getting access to specialist care and diagnostic tests and waited longer for medical care. Compared with patients in fee-for-service plans, patients in managed care plans who had illnesses or disabilities were more likely to complain that their general physician

- provided medical care that was not correct or appropriate (5% of fee-for-service patients, 12% of managed care patients)
- failed to explain what he or she was doing (6% of fee-for-service patients, 12% of managed care patients)
- neglected to explain how and when to take prescriptions at home (4% of fee-for-service patients, 10% of managed care patients)
- made them wait a long time for an appointment (7% of fee-for-service patients, 17% of managed care patients) or a long time in the waiting room (18% of fee-for-service patients, 26% of managed care patients)[17]

In addition to these service quality assessments, some MCOs are following their industry counterparts by offering service guarantees for members who are not satisfied with services received during an office visit; for example, monthly premiums may be reimbursed to members with qualified complaints.

Assess Performance Compared with Professional or "Best-of-Class" Standards

The third step of the continuous improvement process model (Figure 33–4) is assessing the MCO's performance compared with a professional or "best-of-class" standard. This concept of comparison was discussed earlier. The modern quality management program includes the components of performance assessment as described for appropriateness evaluation and peer

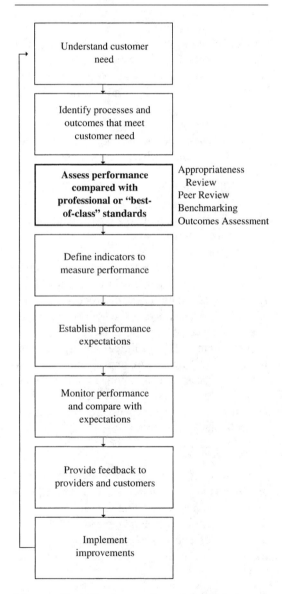

Figure 33–4 Continuous Improvement Process—Compare Performance. *Source:* Reprinted from PB Siren and GL Laffel, Quality Management in Managed Care, in *The Managed Health Care Handbook,* 3rd ed, PR Kongstvedt, ed, p 412, © 1996, Aspen Publishers, Inc.

Appropriateness Review

As discussed for the traditional quality assurance model, appropriateness indicators evaluate the extent to which the MCO provides necessary care and does not provide unnecessary care in the service location best suited for quality and cost efficiencies. Purchasers understand that they cannot obtain good value from an MCO unless it provides appropriate services, so that these indicators are as important as those for accessibility.

Unfortunately, improving the assessment of appropriateness has been dogged by methodological problems, such as adjusting the data for case mix (discussed later), and the surprising lack of data from controlled trials that would define appropriate care in the first place. This issue affects the evaluation of both overutilization and underutilization of services.

In response to these challenges, the MCO can do two things. First, the MCO can identify minimum performance standards for high-cost diagnoses and use them to select processes having excess utilization. Second, the MCO can demonstrate evidence of consistent success and/or an improvement trend in clinical appropriateness indicators. If these two approaches are employed, purchasers seem inclined to offer MCOs some flexibility in the short run even if some isolated indicators suggest that there may be quality problems.

Peer Review

As discussed previously, peer review involves a comparison of an individual provider's practice against an accepted standard of care. A key difference between peer review in a traditional quality assurance model and that in a modern quality management model is the topic of comparison.

Benchmarking

A third method of assessing and comparing an MCO's performance is benchmarking. Benchmarking was popularized by Robert Camp of Xerox over the last 20 years. Camp and Tweet define benchmarking as "the continuous process of measuring products, services and practices against the company's toughest competitors or those companies renowned as industry leaders."[18(p229)] Two types of benchmarking may be used by MCOs. First, internal benchmarking identifies internal functions to serve as pilot sites for comparison. This type of benchmarking is particularly useful in newly integrated delivery systems with multiple, diverse component entities.[18] The second type of benchmarking is external or competitive benchmarking. Competitive benchmarking is the comparison of work processes with those of the best competitor and reveals which performance measure levels can be surpassed.[18] The benchmarking process can be applied to service and clinical processes for knowledge of current performance.

Outcomes Assessment

A fourth method for an MCO to assess performance is through outcomes assessment. An outcomes assessment may be performed on the MCO's 10 highest volume or highest cost diagnoses or procedure groups. An outcomes assessment permits the MCO to assess its own performance over time and to identify variation within the MCO. Davies and others have outlined three core activities for an outcomes assessment[19]:

1. Outcomes measurements are "point-in-time" observations.
2. Outcomes monitoring includes the process of repeated measurements over time, which permits causal inferences to be drawn about the observed outcomes.
3. Outcomes management is the application of the information and knowledge gained from outcome assessment to achieve optimal outcomes through improved decision making and delivery.

The purpose of an outcomes assessment is to provide a quantitative comparison among treatment programs, to map the typical course of a chronic disease across a continuum, or to identify variations in the outcome of care as potential markers of process variation.[19]

Define Indicators To Measure Performance

Defining indicators to measure performance is the fourth step of the continuous improvement process model (Figure 33–5). The MCO may apply the quality criteria (structure, process, and outcome) as discussed for the traditional quality assurance model. In addition, it is useful for MCOs to evaluate their process and outcomes by populations of customers served. The MCO quality management matrix (Figure 33–6) is a diagram of how this may occur. A key issue faced by MCOs in indicator definition and analysis is case-mix adjustment.

Case-mix adjustment is the process to correct data for variations in illness or wellness in patient populations. It is a statistical model that takes into account specific attributes of a patient population (eg, age, sex, severity of illness, chronic health status, etc) that are beyond the control of the MCO or health care provider.[20] This adjustment is particularly important in comparative analyses between providers or among MCOs.

Case-mix adjustment permits fair comparisons among same-population groups because it accounts for preexisting phenomena that may affect the outcome of care. Potentially required variables in a broadly useful risk adjustment system include the following[21]:

- demographic factors
- diagnostic information
- patient-derived health status
- claims-derived health status
- prior use of all services
- prior use of nonelective hospitalization
- prior use of medical procedures

Issues of case mix affect the analysis of both inpatient and outpatient care. The problem, however, is more serious for some performance measures than for others. Case mix is important for clinically oriented indicators such as appropriateness and encounter outcomes. It also has a significant impact on assessments of health status, resource use, and member satisfaction. Case mix is not nearly as important for measures of access and prevention, and thus these measures should be considered for physician profiles and report cards.

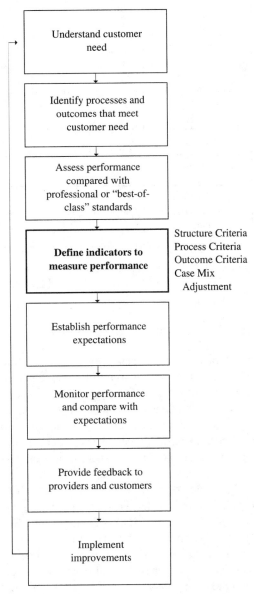

Figure 33–5 Continuous Improvement Process—Measures of Performance. *Source:* Reprinted from PB Siren and GL Laffel, Quality Management in Managed Care, in *The Managed Health Care Handbook,* 3rd ed, PR Kongstvedt, ed, p 414, © 1996, Aspen Publishers, Inc.

	Treatment of Disease				Managing Health		
Population \ Key Function	Access	Appropriateness	Screening	Encounter Outcomes	Prevention	Health Status	Service Quality
Primary Care	# of PCPs with open panels # days for routine physical		Mammography Cholesterol		Childhood immunization Adult immunization		Member satisfaction
Senior Care		% seniors with > 7 prescriptions					
Specialty Care							
High Risk Obstetrics Care							
Other High-Volume or Special Need Population							

Figure 33–6 Quality Management Matrix. *Source:* Adapted from N Goldfield, Case Mix, Risk Adjustment, Reinsurance, and Health Reform. *Managed Care Quarterly,* Vol 2, No 3, p iv, © 1994, Aspen Publishers, Inc.

Establish Performance Expectations

Establishing performance expectations is the fifth step of the continuous improvement process model for an MCO (Figure 33–7). Performance expectations are defined by understanding customer needs (step 1), evaluating the performance of the processes and outcomes designed to meet those needs (step 2), and comparing performance against "best-of-class" standards either internal or external to the MCO (step 3). Purchasers have had an influence on establishing performance expectations. In 1990, Digital Corporation identified priority areas where quality improvement efforts might promote better outcomes. Digital began this effort with the development of health maintenance organization (HMO) standards and by setting expectations in the areas of utilization management, access, quality assurance, mental health services, data capabilities, and financial performance.[22] Digital examined its health care costs and used weightings that drew on multiple data sources to identify priority areas to be considered by the participating plans. Clinical indicators selected for performance measurement and improvement included mental health inpatient readmissions and inpatient days per patient, Caesarean section rates, prenatal care in the first trimester, screening mammography rates, asthma inpatient admissions, and blood pressure screenings. The results from these measurements were not meant to be used punitively but rather enabled Digital to gauge the participating managed care plans in terms of their success in managing specific aspects of health care.

Monitor Performance and Compare with Expectations

Following established expectations, the sixth step is the actual monitoring of performance and comparison with expectations. The frequency of monitoring is determined by the indicators the

Provide Feedback to Providers and Customers

The seventh step of the continuous improvement process model (Figure 33–8) is providing feedback. Two methods of feedback are discussed here: profiling assesses the performance of individual providers, and report cards assess overall MCO performance.

Profiling

Profiling focuses on the patterns of an individual provider's care rather than that provider's specific clinical decisions. The practice pattern of an individual provider—hospital or physician—is expressed as a rate or a measure of resource use during a defined period and for a defined population.[23] The resulting profile can then be compared against a peer group or a standard. MCOs are using profiling to measure providers' performance, to guide quality improvement efforts, and to select providers for managed care networks.[24]

The Physician Payment Review Commission (PPRC) has suggested several guidelines for effective physician profiling.[25] According to the PPRC, profiles first must be analyzed for a well-defined population. Second, they must include a sufficient number of observations to ensure that differences are not due to chance. Third, they should include adjustments for case mix. Finally, profiles must be analyzed for a small enough organizational unit that the parties involved can be responsible for the results and take the necessary courses of action for improvement. A successful profiling system defines an episode of care, accounts for severity of illness and comorbidities, and identifies all the resources used per episode of care.[24] Most profiling systems rely heavily on standard billing information, such as diagnosis-related groups, categories in the tenth revision of the International Classification of Diseases, and current procedural terminology codes.

Examples of measures used in provider profiling include average wait time to schedule a routine physical, number of hospital admis-

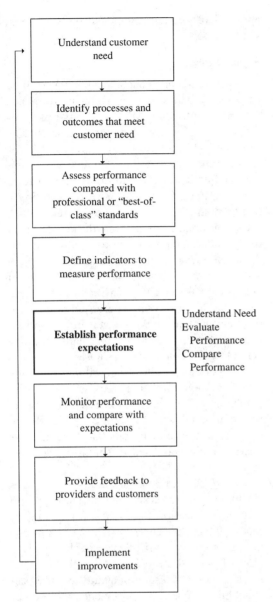

Figure 33–7 Continuous Improvement Process—Establish Expectations. *Source:* Reprinted from PB Siren and GL Laffel, Quality Management in Managed Care, in *The Managed Health Care Handbook,* 3rd ed, PR Kongstvedt, ed, p 416, © 1996, Aspen Publishers, Inc.

MCO has selected to measure performance. An MCO can compare its performance against its own over time and against other MCOs if the same indicator definitions are used.

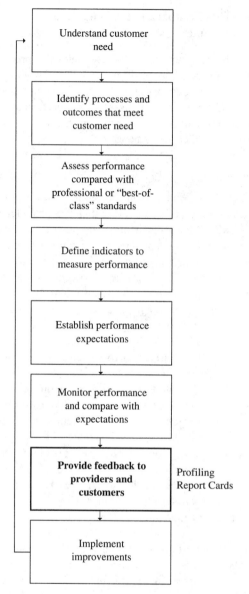

Figure 33–8 Continuous Improvement Process—Feedback. *Source:* Reprinted from PB Siren and GL Laffel, Quality Management in Managed Care, in *The Managed Health Care Handbook,* 3rd ed, PR Kongstvedt, ed, p 416, © 1996, Aspen Publishers, Inc.

sions, number of referrals out of network, number of emergency department visits, member satisfaction, percentage compliance with the MCO's clinical practice guidelines, and, if applicable, the percentage of children receiving appropriate immunizations and the Caesarean section rate.

Report Cards

Report cards have become a popular method of conveying information about performance within an individual MCO with multiple geographic sites or across many diverse MCOs. The purpose of a report card is to provide customers (purchasers and consumers) with comparable quality and cost information in a common language for the purpose of selecting a health plan. Purchasers have formed groups across the country to facilitate the development of a standardized approach to health plan performance measurement. For example, in 1993, 27 corporate and government purchasers of health care formed the Massachusetts Health Care Purchaser Group. The group challenged the health plans in Massachusetts to submit data on six clinical indicators: mammography screening, prenatal care, Caesarean section rate, hypertension screening, asthma admission rate, and mental health admissions after an inpatient stay[26] (Exhibit 33–4). Each health plan was compared with the clinically significant average range, and a consumer-friendly pie chart graphic was used to summarize performance (Figure 33–9).

The NCQA, a nonprofit group that accredits HMOs, organized a national test pilot report card demonstration for 21 health plans representing 9.6 million enrollees. The NCQA judged the plans on a subset of the Health Plan Employer Data and Information Set (HEDIS) measures: standard measures of quality, member satisfaction, membership enrollment, and resource utilization measures.

The report card concept is equally valuable when applied to internal customers of the MCO. Key quality measures can be tracked, trended, and utilized for strategic quality planning and to assess the effectiveness of improvement efforts. For example, in 1993, the Northern California region of Kaiser Permanente released a self-assessment that it referred to as its report card.[27] This report card is organized into seven categories: childhood health, maternal care, cardio-

Exhibit 33–4 Massachusetts Health Care Purchaser Group Clinical Indicators

Mammography Screening Rate:	Percentage of members aged 52–64 who were continuously enrolled in the plan during 1991 and 1992 who received mammograms.
Hypertension Screening Rate:	Percentage of members aged 52–64 who were continuously enrolled in the plan in 1991 and 1992 who were screened for high blood pressure.
Asthma Admission Rate:	The number of hospital admissions for asthmatics of both sexes between the ages of 1 and 19 and ages 20 and 64 divided by the number of enrollees in the plan of the same age cohorts over a 1-year period.
Prenatal Care Rate:	The percentage of pregnancies among women who delivered babies and who were continuously enrolled for 7 months in 1992 for which prenatal care was received during the first trimester of pregnancy.
Caesarean Section Rate:	The percentage of all deliveries in 1992 that were performed by Caesarean section.
Mental Health Readmission Rate:	Males and females aged 18–64 years continuously enrolled in a given health plan for the previous 2 years, and hospitalized with a discharge date in the second year for psychiatric care. There were two measures: the average number of individual hospital admissions per patient, and the average number of mental health hospital days per patient for all hospital admissions.

Source: © *Journal on Quality Improvement*, Oakbrook Terrace, IL: Joint Commission on Accreditation of Healthcare Organizations, 1995, p 169. Reprinted with permission.

vascular disease, cancer, common surgical procedures, other adult health, and mental health/substance abuse. In designing categories, developers selected areas that affected many enrollees and tried to depict care from the patient's perspective (ie, what would the patient need during the course of his or her illness?). The report card assessed enrollee satisfaction as a separate entity.

The benefits of the report card movement include the stimulus for MCOs to build the capacity to produce performance information and strengthen data quality. Public disclosure of performance information also lends itself to plan, provider, and hospital accountability. The main limitation of the report card movement continues to be measurement. Although the NCQA and HEDIS have made moves to standardize measurement, there continues to be variation in measurement, coding, and clinical classification. Additionally, there is variation in the administrative source data sets that plans use to obtain their measurements. Risk adjustment and a broader clinical focus are opportunities for improvement. Finally, no conclusion can be drawn about processes or outcomes that are not assessed by the report card measurements.

Implement Improvements

The eighth step of the continuous improvement process model (Figure 33–10) is implementation of improvements. Current strategies employed by MCOs as tools to improve health care delivery processes and outcomes are practice guidelines, case management, quality improvement (QI) teams, and consumer education.

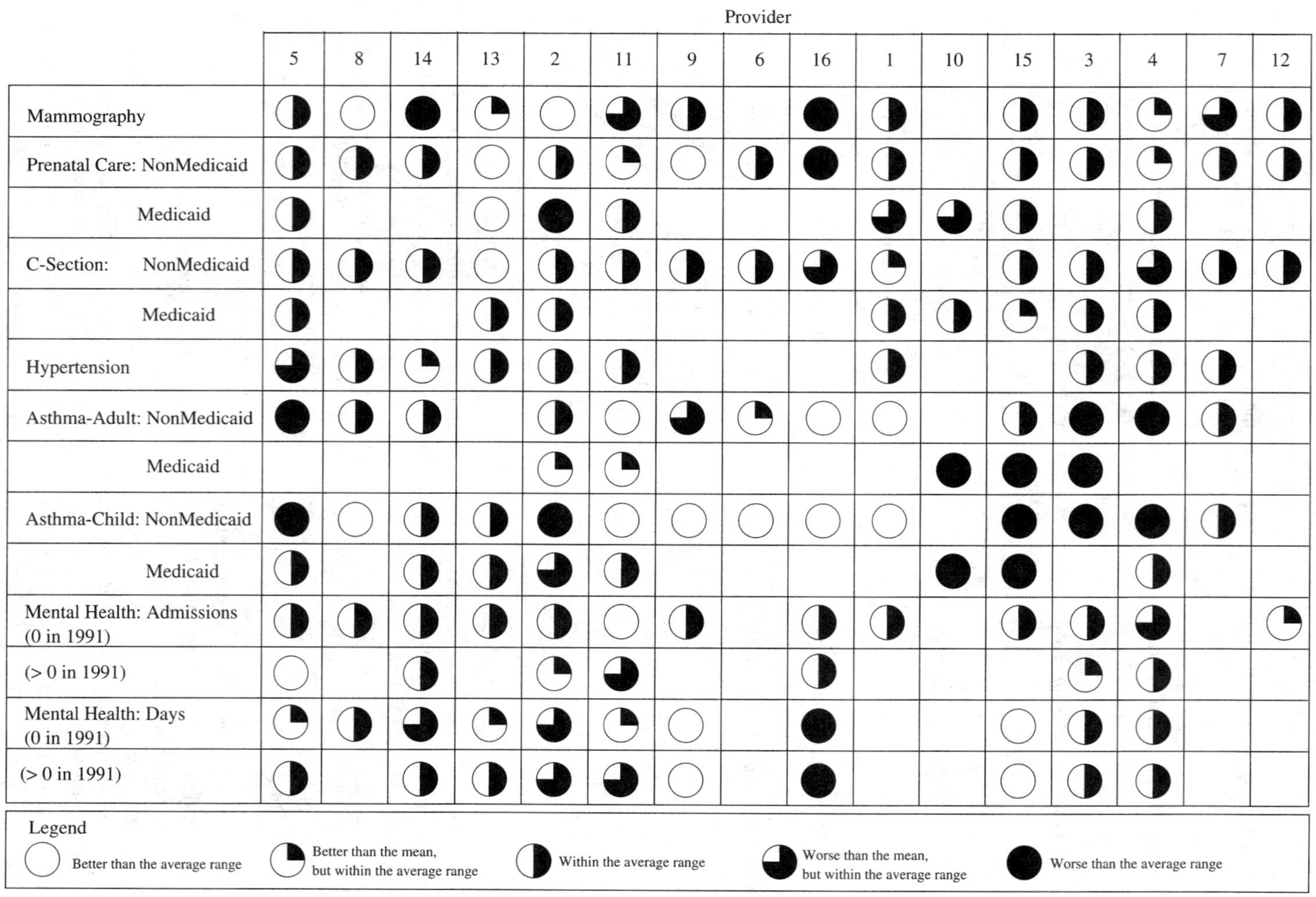

Figure 33–9 Massachusetts Health Care Purchaser Group 1992 Summary Table. *Source:* © *Journal on Quality Improvement*, Oakbrook Terrace, IL: Joint Commission on Accreditation of Healthcare Organizations, 1995, p 171. Reprinted with permission.

Quality Management in Managed Care 453

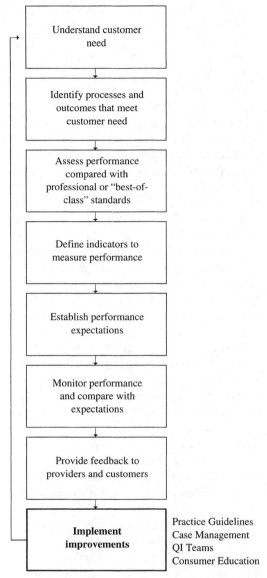

Figure 33–10 Continuous Improvement Process—Implement Improvements. *Source:* Reprinted from PB Siren and GL Laffel, Quality Management in Managed Care, in *The Managed Health Care Handbook,* 3rd ed, PR Kongstvedt, ed, p 420, © 1996, Aspen Publishers, Inc.

Practice Guidelines

Clinical practice guidelines are systematically developed statements to assist practitioners and patients in making decisions about appropriate health care for specific clinical circumstances. Guidelines offer an opportunity to improve health care delivery processes by reducing unwanted variation. An appointed committee of the Institute of Medicine recommended the following attributes of guideline design[28]:

- Validity: Practice guidelines are deemed valid if they lead to the health and cost outcomes projected for them.
- Reliability/reproducibility: If given the same evidence and development methods, another set of experts would come up with the same recommendations. The guidelines are interpreted and applied consistently across providers.
- Clinical applicability: Guidelines should apply to a clearly defined patient population.
- Clinical flexibility: Guidelines should recognize the generally anticipated exceptions to the recommendations proposed.
- Multidisciplinary process: Representatives of key disciplines involved in the process of care should participate in the guideline development process.
- Scheduled review: Guideline evaluation should be planned in advance and occur at a frequency that reflects the evolution of clinical evidence for the guideline topic.
- Documentation: Detailed summaries of the guideline development process should be maintained that reflect the procedures followed, the participants involved, the evidence and analytical methods employed, and the assumptions and rationales accepted.

In addition to a development process, guideline programs also have an implementation process. The first step in designing an implementation strategy for clinical guidelines is to identify the forces driving and restraining clinical practice change.[29] Thus, an MCO may want to convene a group of local content experts along with its own medical leadership to initiate guideline planning and adoption. An effective implementation team strengthens the driving forces for the guideline and weakens the restraining forces for a given clinical practice change. Performance assessment is measured on two levels. First, the gap between prior and optimal practice is measured to assess the degree of implementation. Second, feedback is given to providers to reinforce the change in clinical practice. As an example, the following is a summary of United HealthCare's guideline implementation process[30]:

1. Prioritize your objectives. Select guidelines that
   - are likely to be accepted by physicians
   - have a cost impact for the health plan
   - affect a quality issue for patients
   - affect a large population
   - fulfill a regulatory issue
2. Document the need to change.
3. Look for guideline credibility.
4. Get the word out.
5. Use timely feedback to physicians.
6. Remember, you are dealing with a system.

Practice guidelines are not without limitations. Studies have shown that traditional methods of guideline dissemination have not resulted in significant changes in practice.[31,32] Frequently, guidelines are not designed to be implemented directly into practice. This has a particular impact in preferred provider organizations (PPOs) and independent practice associations (IPAs), where there are multiple and varied processes. An MCO can facilitate the implementation of guidelines through the corresponding development of algorithms, summaries, laminated cards, medical record tools, and reminder systems. Second, as mentioned earlier in this chapter, meeting specifications does not necessarily result in constant improvement but rather may maintain the status quo.[3] Guidelines should be designed with flexibility to encourage improvement and innovation.

Case Management

Case management is a model of patient care delivery that restructures and streamlines the clinical production process so that it is outcome based.[33] Case management, like practice guidelines, can reduce unwanted variation. As a model, case management mobilizes, monitors, and rationalizes the resources a patient uses over the course of an illness. In doing so, case management aims at a controlled balance between quality and cost.[34]

Case management plays an integral part in an MCO's quality management program. First, a case manager is an integral part of the health care team and participates in establishing an individualized treatment plan with the member, physician, and MCO. Second, case management can be applied to the identification of members at risk for high-cost, catastrophic illness. After identification of these members, case managers monitor their care on an ongoing basis to assess whether quality care is being provided in an appropriate setting. The case manager plays an important role as a resource manager for the MCO. Third, case managers can evaluate the implementation and effectiveness of practice guidelines.

To date, little evidence exists regarding the long-term effectiveness of case management in MCOs or integrated delivery systems. The effectiveness of case management, however, has been studied in preventive services and community mental health. A number of studies have shown that maternity care coordination and preventive services improve child health and are cost-effective but are under-used.[35-42] Replicated findings suggest that case management during pregnancy increases infant birthweight.[43,44] Other studies have found that community mental health clients who received case management used more community services than those not receiving case management.[45-49] This finding has led researchers to speculate that case management of clients' vocational, educational, housing, social, recreational, and financial needs may improve their quality of life, which consequently reduces their need for rehospitalization.[45,48] These effectiveness evaluations are important to MCOs because the performance of these key functions (prenatal care and mental health care management) is a measure used for evaluation by purchasers in HEDIS.

Quality Improvement Teams

A third tool employed by MCOs to facilitate improvement of health care delivery is the quality improvement team. MCOs are complex organizations that comprise many job functions and usually cover large geographic areas. The tasks required to produce the outputs of a quality management program require diverse talents and skill sets. The variety of network configurations (eg, staff model HMO, PPO, and IPA) requires a method to incorporate provider input from different perspectives. Quality improvement teams offer an alternative in an environment where administrative expense must be controlled and minimized. Teams outperform individuals acting alone or in larger organizational groupings, especially when performance requires multiple skills, judgments, and experiences.[50]

There are several well-known phenomena that explain why teams perform well. First, the broader skill mix and know-how facilitate the team's response to multifaceted challenges, such as innovations, quality, and customer service. Second, in developing clear goals and approaches to problem solving, teams can support real-time resolution and initiative. Finally, teams provide a unique social dimension that enhances the economic and administrative aspects of work. By surmounting barriers to collective performance, team members build trust and confidence in each other's capabilities. This supports the pursuit of team purpose above and beyond individual or functional agendas.[50]

How can teams be applied to quality management in an MCO? Examples include a team consisting of MCO leaders, purchasers, members, and providers setting the evaluation and improvement agendas for the MCO by prioritizing goals. Alternately, a cross-functional team may evaluate the disease- or population-specific needs of a member group and test interventions, such as practice guidelines, for care improvement. Finally a team could form to design an MCO's strategy to meet accreditation requirements. Teams can be chartered to address most issues faced by an MCO as long as an explicit purpose and a defined time frame for completion have been identified.

Consumer Education

Many MCOs' quality management programs include evaluation of the effectiveness of consumer education. Consumer education is targeted at beneficiaries so that they can become

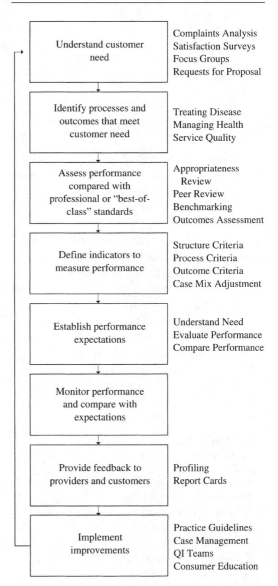

Figure 33–11 Continuous Improvement Process—Summary. *Source:* Reprinted from PB Siren and GL Laffel, Quality Management in Managed Care, in *The Managed Health Care Handbook,* 3rd ed, PR Kongstvedt, ed, p 423, © 1996, Aspen Publishers, Inc.

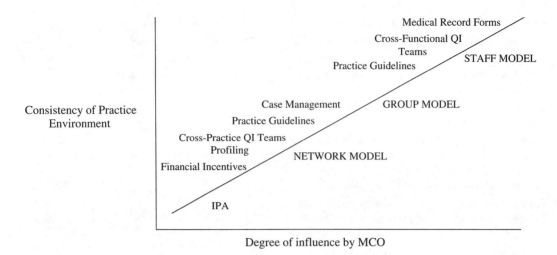

Figure 33–12 Quality Management Tools for a Variety of MCOs. *Source:* Reprinted from PB Siren and GL Laffel, Quality Management in Managed Care, in *The Managed Health Care Handbook,* 3rd ed, PR Kongstvedt, ed, p 424, © 1996, Aspen Publishers, Inc.

effective health care consumers and participate in meeting the aforementioned needs of treating disease and managing health. Examples of consumer education utilized by MCOs include telephone resource lines, health risk appraisals, work site–based consumer education programs, and consumer health education materials. Many MCOs have developed and provide members with self-care guidelines for preventing illness and treating common complaints at the time of enrollment.

SETTING THE IMPROVEMENT AGENDA

After the implementation of step 8, the MCO must evaluate whether the improvements actually made a change and met customer need. If not, the cycle begins again with step 1. If improvements did occur and customer needs were met, the cycle can begin again for new or unaddressed customer needs.

How can an MCO design such a cycle? MCOs have limited resources with which to assess and improve performance, and strategic decisions must be made to target resources effectively. An MCO's leadership group may begin the cycle of improvement by applying the following criteria:

- Identify which customer need is being addressed by the proposed project.
- Evaluate the strength of the evidence for the need to improve.
- Assess the probability that there will be a measurable impact.
- Determine the likelihood of success.
- Identify the immediacy of impact in meeting the customer's need.

CONCLUSION

Consumers and purchasers of health care are demanding quality at a reasonable price. To address this need, a quality management program in a managed care setting must be designed to reflect complex delivery systems and diverse customer groups. Success in managing cost and optimizing health outcomes begins with an understanding of customer needs, assessment of performance to meet those needs, and continuous improvement. Attention focused on the provision of appropriate care in an appropriate setting will continue to shape the quality resource programs in MCOs. The need to assess the impact of these shifts of care from one segment of the delivery system to another will continue to grow as the shifts progress.

As a part of a health delivery system, MCOs have an opportunity to affect the health status of populations through their actions and thus have a responsibility to assess and measure these effects. To achieve these goals, an MCO must have a focused aim and a process for achievement, such as that summarized in Figure 33–11. This eight-step process can be implemented on a diverse scale, such as in an IPA or network model, or at a staff model site. Improvement opportunities have different degrees of success in different organizations, as identified in Figure 33–12. A variety of methods—practice guidelines, case management, outcomes management, and others—have been introduced and, no doubt, will continue to evolve.

REFERENCES

1. Donabedian A. *Exploration in Quality Assessment and Monitoring: The Definition of Quality and Approaches to Its Assessment.* Vol 1. Ann Arbor, MI: Health Administration Press; 1980.
2. Shortell SM, LoGerfo JP. Hospital medical staff organization and quality of care: results from myocardial infarction and appendectomy. *Med Care.* 1981;19:1041–1056.
3. Walton M. Improve constantly and forever the system of production and service. In: *The Deming Management Method.* New York: Putnam; 1986:66–67.
4. Goldman RL. The reliability of peer assessments of quality of care. *JAMA.* 1992;267:958–960.
5. Moen RD, Nolan TW. Process improvement. *Qual Prog.* 1987;9:62–68.
6. Langley GL, et al. The foundation of improvement. *Qual Prog.* 1994;6:81–86.
7. Juran J, Gryna F. Understanding customer need. In: FM Gryna, ed, *Quality Planning and Analysis.* 3rd ed. New York: McGraw-Hill; 1993:240–252.
8. Nelson CW, Niederberger J. Patient satisfaction surveys: an opportunity for total quality improvement. *Hosp Health Serv Admin.* 1990;35:409–427.
9. Sennet C, Legorreta A, Zatz S. Performance-based hospital contracting for quality improvement. *Joint Commission J Qual Improvement.* 1993;9:374–383.
10. Health Care Advisory Board. *Next Generation of Outcomes Tracking.* Washington, DC: Health Care Advisory Board; 1994.
11. Millman M, ed. *Access to Health Care in America: Institute of Medicine (U.S.) Committee on Monitoring Access to Personal Health Services.* Washington, DC: National Academy Press; 1993.
12. What about Quality of Care? *PR Newswire.* September 14, 1993:3–6.
13. Alta RB. Canadian way: universal, but not immediate access. *Mod Healthcare.* 1989;6:36.
14. Bindman AB, Grumbach K, Osmond D, et al. Preventable hospitalization rates and access to health care. *JAMA.* 1995;274:305–311.
15. Batalden PB, Nelson E, Roberts J. Linking outcomes measurement to continual improvement: the serial "V" way of thinking about improving clinical care. *Joint Commission J Qual Improvement.* 1994;20:167–180.
16. Nelson EC, et al. Patient-based quality measurement systems. *Qual Manage Health Care.* 1993;2:18–30.
17. Robert Wood Johnson Foundation. *Sick People in Managed Care Have Difficulty Getting Services and Treatment.* Princeton, NJ: Robert Wood Johnson Foundation; 1995.
18. Camp RL, Tweet AG. Benchmarking applied to health care. *Joint Commission J Qual Improvement.* 1994;20:229–238.
19. Davies AR, Doyle MA, Lansky D, et al. Outcomes assessment in clinical settings: a consensus statement on principles and best practices in project management. *Joint Commission J Qual Improvement.* 1994;20:6–16.
20. Pine M, Harper DL. Designing and using case mix indices. *Managed Care Q.* 1994;2:1–11.
21. Goldfield N. Case mix, risk adjustment, reinsurance, and health reform. *Managed Care Q.* 1994;2:iv.
22. Bloomberg MA, Jordan H, Angel K, et al. Development of indicators for performance measurement and improvement: an HMO/purchaser collaborative effort. *Joint Commission J Qual Improvement.* 1993;19:586–595.
23. Lee PR, et al. Managed care: provider profiling. *J Insurance Med.* 1992;24:179–181.
24. Walker LM. Can a computer tell how good a doctor you are? *Med Econ.* 1994;71:136–147.
25. Physician Payment Review Commission (PPRC). *Conference on Profiling.* Washington, DC: PPRC; 1992.
26. Jordan H, et al. Reporting and using health plan performance information in Massachusetts. *Joint Commission J Qual Improvement.* 1995:21;167–177.

27. Executive Director's Office, Kaiser Permanente Medical Group. *Reporting on Quality KPMG Forum.* Oakland, CA: Kaiser Permanente Medical Group; 1993.
28. Institute of Medicine, Committee to Advise the Public Health Service on Clinical Practice Guidelines. *Clinical Practice Guidelines: Directions for a New Program.* Washington, DC: National Academy Press; 1990.
29. Handley MR, et al. An evidence-based approach to evaluating and improving clinical practice: implementing practice guidelines. *HMO Practice.* 1994;8:75–83.
30. Newcomber LN. Six pointers for implementing guidelines. *Healthcare Forum J.* July/August 1994:31–33.
31. Kosecoff J, Kanouse DE, Rogers WH, et al. Effects of the National Institutes of Health consensus development program on physician practice. *JAMA.* 1987;258: 2708–2713.
32. Lomas J, Anderson GM, Domnick-Pierre K, et al. Do practice guidelines guide practice? The effect of a consensus statement on the practice of physicians. *N Engl J Med.* 1989;321:1306–1311.
33. Zander K. Nursing case management: strategic management of cost and quality outcomes. *J Nurs Admin.* 1988; 18:23–30.
34. Giullano KK, Poirier CE. Nursing case management: critical pathways to desirable outcomes. *Nurs Manage.* 1991;22:52–55.
35. Gortmaker SL. The effects of prenatal care upon the health of the newborn. *Am J Publ Health.* 1979;69: 653–660.
36. Showstack JA, Budetti PP, Minkler D. Factors associated with birth weight: an exploration of the roles of prenatal care and length of gestation. *Am J Publ Health.* 1984;74:1003–1008.
37. Cohen DR, Henderson JB. *Health, Prevention, and Economics.* New York: Oxford University Press; 1988.
38. Currier R. Is early and periodic screening, diagnosis, and treatment (EPSDT) worthwhile? *Int J Rehab Res.* 1979;2:508–509.
39. Irwin PH, Conroy-Hughes R. EPSDT impact on health status: estimates based on secondary analysis of administratively generated data. *Med Care.* 1982;20: 216–234.
40. Kelle WJ. Study of selected outcomes of the early and periodic screening, diagnosis, and treatment program in Michigan. *Publ Health Rep.* 1983;98:110–119.
41. Manning WL. The EPSDT program: a progress report. *Indiana Med.* 1985;78:320–322.
42. Reis JS, Pliska SR, Hughes EF. A synopsis of federally sponsored preventive child health. *J Community Health.* 1984;9:222–239.
43. Korenbrot CC, et al. Birth weight outcomes in a teenage pregnancy case management project. *J Adolesc Health Care.* 1989;10:97–104.
44. Buescher PA, Roth MS, Williams D, Goforth CM. An evaluation of the impact of maternity care coordination on Medicaid birth outcomes in North Carolina. *Am J Publ Health.* 1991;81:1625–1629.
45. Bigelow DA, Young DJ. Effectiveness of a case management program. *Community Ment Health J.* 1991; 27:115–123.
46. Borland A, McRae J, Lycan C. Outcomes of five years of continuous intensive case management. *Hosp Community Psychiatry.* 1989;40:369–376.
47. Franklin JL, Solovitz B, Mason M, et al. An evaluation of case management. *Am J Publ Health.* 1987; 77:674–678.
48. Goering PN, Wasylenki D, Farkas M, et al. What difference does case management make? *Hosp Community Psychiatry.* 1988;39:272–276.
49. McRae J, Higgins M, Lycan C, Sherman W. What happens to patients after five years of intensive case management stops? *Hosp Community Psychiatry.* 1990; 41:175–180.
50. Katzenbach JR, Smith DK. *The Wisdom of Teams. Creating the High Performance Organization.* Boston: Harvard University Press; 1993.

SUGGESTED READINGS

Couch JB, ed. *Health Care Quality Management for the 21st Century.* Tampa, FL: American College of Medical Quality and the American College of Physician Executives; 1991.

The Deming Management Method. New York: Putnam; 1986.

Goldfield N, Pine M, Pine J. *Measuring and Managing Health Care Quality: Procedures, Techniques, and Protocols.* Gaithersburg, MD: Aspen Publishers, Inc; 1992.

Juran JM, Gryna FM. *Quality Planning and Analysis.* 3rd. ed. New York: McGraw-Hill; 1993.

Senge P. *The Fifth Discipline: The Art and Practice of the Learning Organization.* New York: Doubleday; 1993.

Senge P, Kleiner A. *The Fifth Discipline Fieldbook.* New York: Doubleday; 1994.

Youngs MT, Wingerson L. *The 1996 Medical Outcomes and Guidelines Sourcebook.* New York: Faulkner & Gray; 1995.

PAMELA B. SIREN, RN, MPH, is a senior health care consultant with ML Strategies in Boston. She helps organizations develop, implement, and evaluate medical management programs across a variety of settings. Her clients include HMOs, MSOs, PPOs, and PHOs. Previously, she was director of clinical development with Lazo, Gertman & Associates, and she was director of clinical improvement for Blue Cross and Blue Shield of Massachusetts.

GLENN L. LAFFEL, MD, PHD, is principal of Clinical Solutions in Newton Center, Massachusetts. He is recognized internationally for his work on the health care application of total quality management and is the founding editor of *Quality Management in Health Care*.

CHAPTER 34

Introduction to the Measurement of Clinical Outcomes

Michael Pine

Chapter Outline

- Introduction
- Domains of Clinical Outcomes Measurement
- Goals of Clinical Outcomes Measurement
- Six-Step Process for Measuring Comparative Risk-Adjusted Clinical Outcomes

INTRODUCTION

The success of any organization that purports to manage the delivery of health care—regardless of that organization's structure, and of which services it provides—ultimately must be determined by how often and how well its goals have been achieved.

Unfortunately, "outcomes research" has failed to provide simple answers to apparently straightforward questions about the goals of health care. Even the most basic outcomes are too complex to characterize in the absence of (1) a clearly defined input, (2) one or more processes that can transform the input to achieve the outcome of interest, and (3) a cause-and-effect relationship between at least one of the intervening processes and the outcome of interest (Figure 34–1). Measuring "outcomes" without specifying inputs and processes is a fruitless exercise that can result only in misinformation and misunderstanding.

An outcome cannot be measured until (1) an initial state is defined and (2) all factors that may influence the transformation being assessed are delineated. If these requirements are properly fulfilled, the measurement of clinical outcomes can become a powerful tool in the practical sphere of clinical management.

DOMAINS OF CLINICAL OUTCOMES MEASUREMENT

Information about clinical outcomes spans four domains of inquiry: (1) clinical status, (2) physical function, (3) social function, and (4) feelings and perceptions (Figure 34–2).

While outcomes in one domain may be related to outcomes in another, each domain provides unique, important insights into clinical performance.

Each domain is defined, in part, by a distinctive set of outcome measures. Clinical status can be characterized either by objective clinical measures or by the judgment of trained clinicians. Physical function either can be measured objectively or can be reported by patients based on objective criteria. Social function can be determined by applying objective criteria to data derived from patient reports. Finally, feelings and perceptions related to a patient's condition (eg, pain, anxiety) or to a patient's care (eg, satisfaction, perceived competence of clinical staff) are derived directly

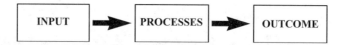

Figure 34–1 Characterization of Outcomes. Courtesy of Michael Pine and Associates, Inc, 1998, Chicago, Illinois.

from patient reports. A comprehensive assessment of clinical performance should address both desired and adverse outcomes in all four domains.

GOALS OF CLINICAL OUTCOMES MEASUREMENT

While much fanfare is attached to the transformation of data into information, information alone is no more valuable than raw data unless it can be applied. Two important applications of information about clinical outcomes are (1) the selection of individuals and organizations offering health care services and (2) the improvement of health care services, either to achieve better outcomes (ie, to improve effectiveness) or to achieve comparable outcomes while consuming fewer resources (ie, to improve efficiency). The first application requires only the assessment of performance (ie, external monitoring). The second requires not only external monitoring but also a detailed understanding of how processes of care are linked to observed outcomes (ie, internal monitoring).

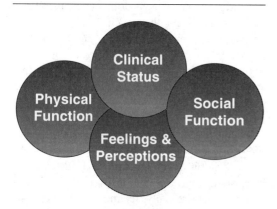

Figure 34–2 Domains of Clinical Outcomes Measurement. Courtesy of Michael Pine and Associates, Inc, 1998, Chicago, Illinois.

Both applications require that information about clinical performance be used to make informed decisions and to take appropriate actions. However, information about clinical outcomes, even if correct, will not necessarily result in truly informed decisions. Such information can be interpreted in more than one way, and each possible interpretation may support a different decision. For example, external monitoring may demonstrate conclusively that patients treated at Clinic A have uniformly better outcomes than patients treated at Clinic B, but this superiority may be due solely to Clinic A's success in treating elderly patients with cardiopulmonary diseases. In this case, it would not be advisable for a young patient with limited resources and a gastrointestinal disorder to pay a premium for "superior" care at Clinic A. Or, internal monitoring may prove that patients treated with novobiocin recover from pneumonia twice as fast as patients receiving conventional treatment—but if 10% of patients receiving novobiocin for pneumonia develop fatal dysrhythmias during therapy, clinicians would be well advised not to make decisions about whether to administer novobiocin solely on the basis of its more rapid therapeutic response.

If information about clinical outcomes is to be used in management, it must adequately support decisions by patients, purchasers, providers, practitioners, and other participants in the process of health care delivery. Decision makers must be able to draw correct conclusions that pertain directly to realistic options under consideration. Conclusions, not information, are the yardsticks by which performance monitoring ultimately must be judged.

In sum, whether for external or for internal monitoring, (1) valid data must be transformed into accurate information, (2) accurate information must be used to draw correct conclusions, (3) correct conclusions must be used to make wise decisions, (4) wise decisions must guide effective action, and (5) effective action must produce demonstrable, desired results. Any interruption in the chain of events illustrated in Figure 34–3 greatly diminishes the usefulness of all preceding steps and makes all subsequent steps extremely perilous.

SIX-STEP PROCESS FOR MEASURING COMPARATIVE RISK-ADJUSTED CLINICAL OUTCOMES

Effective health care decisions cannot be made without accurate and relevant measurements of patient outcomes. Obtaining such measurements is a challenging and often daunting task. However, this task is more manageable when divided into discrete steps. Careful completion of each step will ensure final results that reflect actual clinical performance and that are suitable for use by decision makers.

One algorithm for deriving and interpreting comparative measurements of clinical performance consists of the following six steps:

1. Clearly distinguish clinical outcomes from processes of care and select specific outcomes of interest.
2. Craft outcome measures and clinical indicators and identify potential risk factors that may influence comparative performance.
3. Define and collect data elements required to perform analyses.
4. Develop risk-adjustment models for each clinical indicator.
5. Compare risk-adjusted clinical outcomes.
6. Evaluate comparative performance based on analytic findings.

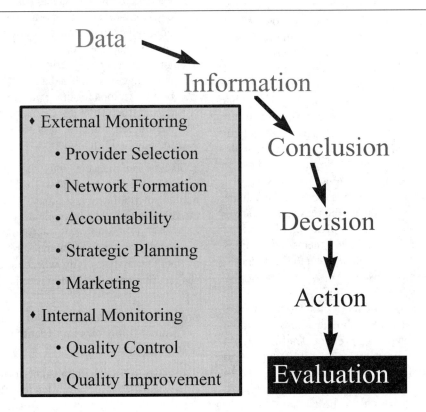

Figure 34–3 Linking Data to Action. Courtesy of Healthcare Quality Insights, Inc, 1997.

Step 1: Clearly Distinguish Clinical Outcomes from Processes of Care and Select Specific Outcomes of Interest

In theory, the distinction between *clinical outcomes* and *processes of care* is self-evident. However, in practice, outcomes and processes are easily confused. When asked to select outcomes that can be used to assess the quality of clinical care, clinicians often list actions they consider important instead of results they desire to achieve. For instance, they will propose as a measure of quality the use of angiotensin converting enzyme (ACE) inhibitors to treat patients with severe congestive heart failure, rather than focusing on the clinical (eg, reduction in objective findings of pulmonary congestion), functional (eg, increased ability to climb stairs, return to work), and cognitive (eg, reduction in dyspnea) changes associated with successful treatment of this condition. Certainly, measurement of the use of ACE inhibitors (as outlined in Chapter 28) is important, but it is a measurement of the *process* of care, not the *outcome*.

Medical practitioners can *control* processes of care but can only *influence* outcomes. For this reason, they often prefer to be judged on what they do, rather than on what they achieve. But if the objective of health care is to preserve and improve health, then achievement of clinical goals, rather than adherence to best practices, must be the ultimate measure of clinical success.

Outcomes of care always focus on the patient, not on the care. They are the reason why care is rendered in the first place. They can be derived from lists of diagnostic and therapeutic actions by asking, "What would happen to the patient if each action on the list were either omitted or performed incorrectly?"

Medical judgment about clinical outcomes is consistent and stable. Clinicians throughout the ages have desired to prevent death, to avoid complications, to reduce physical limitations, to restore social function, to relieve pain, and to comfort patients and families. On the other hand, disagreements about the best means (ie, processes) to these ends are not infrequent, and recommended practices evolve fairly rapidly. Therefore, outcomes rather than processes are the preferred yardstick for initial screening of clinical performance.

In general, it is best to begin monitoring comparative clinical performance by focusing on global rather than narrow outcomes. Global outcomes will provide a better overview of clinical quality than will their more narrowly defined equivalents. Some examples are

- occurrence of any complication that prolongs hospitalization, rather than the development of acute renal failure in particular
- admission to a hospital within 48 hours of discharge from ambulatory surgery, rather than hypotension during administration of anesthesia for such surgery
- unscheduled delivery of a premature infant in the second or third trimester, rather than the development of eclampsia
- deterioration in self-reported physical function, rather than reduction in a single measure of range of motion
- total annual cost of caring for pediatric asthmatic patients, rather than total annual cost of medications for those patients
- dissatisfaction with care provided by a health plan, rather than dissatisfaction with the plan's billing practices

The narrow measures may be very important in special studies designed to shed light on particular potential problem areas. However, cost-effective monitoring of clinical outcomes, like cost-effective monitoring of financial performance, begins with general measures and resorts to detailed analyses only when initial findings suggest that additional study is required.

Step 2: Craft Outcome Measures and Clinical Indicators and Identify Potential Risk Factors

In order to compare clinical performance, *outcome measures* must be crafted to reflect validly the actual clinical status of patients receiving care. These measures must be precisely defined and must not be unduly influenced by vagaries in data acquisition. The exact timing and method of assessment are critical because systematic differences in reporting can be mistaken easily for systematic differences in performance. For example, inpatient mortality, mortality within 30 days of admission, and mortality within 1 year of diagnosis all are reasonable measures of mortality, but information obtained using one of these measures cannot be compared directly to information obtained using another. Similarly, information about global satisfaction with care obtained using a 20-question phone survey of a random sample of clinic patients cannot be compared directly to information on the same subject obtained using a 2-question mail survey distributed to all patients leaving the clinic.

Also, observer bias must be minimized, since systematic differences in reporting may "average out" in estimates of overall results but will not "average out" when performance is compared. For example, the average rate of wound infection after abdominal surgery may be correctly estimated at 3.2%, despite systematic reporting biases by a group of surgeons who underreport their infection rate by 1.0% and by a group of surgeons who overreport their rate by 1.0%. However, if Surgeon A, from the first group, and Surgeon B, from the second group, actually have similar rates of wound infections, but Surgeon A reports his rate as 2.2% and Surgeon B reports his rate as 4.2%, a naive observer would conclude from these data that Surgeon B has almost twice the rate of wound infections as Surgeon A.

In crafting measures of clinical outcomes, clinical events that can be classified as processes rather than outcomes of care may be used as surrogates for actual clinical outcomes that cannot be measured directly in a valid, consistent fashion. For instance, hospitalization of a patient with asthma is a treatment decision (ie, part of the process of care), but it is also a marker for unsuccessful outpatient management of asthma (ie, a clinical outcome measure)—the patient's condition deteriorated seriously enough to require hospital care.

Measures of clinical outcomes may be either discrete or continuous. Discrete measures categorize an outcome either (1) as having occurred or not occurred (eg, dead or alive) or (2) as being of one of a discrete set of categories (eg, very satisfied, satisfied, indifferent, dissatisfied, very dissatisfied). Continuous measures assign one of numerous possible values to each patient (eg, alveolar-arterial oxygen gradient from 0 to 600). Discrete measures generally are reported as rates; continuous measures generally are reported as means (ie, averages) or medians (ie, the value associated with the 50th percentile).

Clinical performance can be compared only when measures are applied to well-defined populations of patients. A *clinical indicator* specifies both the measure to be applied and the population to which it is applicable. In reporting an indicator, the measure generally provides information contained in the numerator in a fraction (eg, the number of inpatient deaths, the total cost of treatment), and the population studied generally provides information contained in the denominator (eg, the number of patients hospitalized, the number of patients treated).

Single measures can be used to create multiple indicators. For instance, a specific measure of adverse outcomes can be applied to men, women, men with blue eyes, women with gray eyes, unmarried men between the ages of 40 and 65, and divorced women between the ages of 25 and 27—divisions of the patient population that may not be particularly relevant to clinical performance. Therefore, in assessing systems designed to compare clinical performance, it is best to consider individual measures rather than individual indicators.

If the population to be studied is completely homogeneous with respect to the measure being applied (ie, each patient has the same probability of achieving each possible outcome), then all data elements required for the assessment of comparative clinical performance have been defined. However, the probability that different patients in the population to be studied will achieve one or more of the outcomes being measured often varies. These differences can be related to differences in patient characteristics and conditions when care is begun (ie, to different inputs). In order to compensate for these differences, measurable potential risk factors must be identified that can be used to predict each patient's outcome given uniform care. Like outcome measures, risk factors must be clearly defined and must not be unduly influenced by vagaries in data acquisition. They must be present prior to the delivery of the care being evaluated. Together with data needed to define outcome indicators, data required to define risk factors compose the analytic data set that must be acquired to use risk-adjusted outcomes to evaluate clinical performance.

Step 3: Define and Collect Data Elements Required To Perform Analyses

The nature and quality of data used to determine comparative risk-adjusted clinical outcomes are critical to the validity and relevance of conclusions drawn from these analyses. Clear data specifications must be prepared and followed in order to obtain fair comparisons. A data element may be obtained from any one of several acceptable sources, but the comparability of data from these multiple sources must be evaluated carefully before such data are used in analyses.

Currently, billing data are readily available in electronic form, and hospital UB-92 and ambulatory Health Care Financing Administration (HCFA) 1500 formats are relatively well standardized. However, secondary diagnostic codes used in UB-92 reports do not distinguish between comorbidities present on admission (ie, potential risk factors) and complications that developed during hospitalization (ie, potential adverse outcomes of care), and HCFA 1500 reports often fail to list many important, active clinical diagnoses. More detailed hospital charge master databases also are available in electronic form and can provide a wealth of important information. However, the structure of these databases varies among facilities, and painstaking mapping must be performed in order to obtain comparable information.

Many other operational databases can be accessed to obtain information about outcomes and risk factors (eg, laboratory, pharmacy), but linking these databases and obtaining comparable data from multiple facilities are far more difficult in practice than in theory (see Chapters 37 and 38 for additional discussion about the challenges of using data from multiple sources). For all the rhetoric and hype surrounding "the electronic medical record," medical record systems remain extremely primitive and disjointed, and even when electronic linkage is achieved, incompatibly defined data often prevent valid comparisons.

The most direct method of collecting data elements required to evaluate comparative risk-adjusted clinical outcomes is to create a customized database and either to obtain required data elements directly from caregivers or to abstract them directly from medical records. Incorporating data collection for outcomes analyses into the process of documenting clinical care is appealing but has proven very difficult to implement for more than a few conditions at a limited number of institutions. On the other hand, abstraction of medical records has proven an effective but extremely costly method of obtaining data for comparative analyses of clinical outcomes.

In sum, ideal sources of data to support comparative analyses of risk-adjusted clinical outcomes currently are not available. However, some methods of reducing the cost of data collection without compromising the validity or relevance of analytic conclusions have been developed and tested. These will be discussed in Chapters 35 and 36 on practical applications.

Step 4: Develop Risk-Adjustment Models for Each Clinical Indicator

Rarely, if ever, is a population of patients so homogeneous that differences do not exist among patients in the probability of occurrence of an outcome of interest. Therefore, some adjustment must be made to compensate for these differences in "severity of illness." Without such adjustment, interpretation of analyses of "raw" outcome data may falsely attribute differences in measured performance to variation in quality of care when they really are the product of variation in patient risk (ie, differences in case mix).

Risk adjustment is the process of assigning to each patient a predicted value for each outcome indicator being measured. For discrete indicators, this value is the percentage of the time each possible result would be predicted if the patient received standard care. For example, one patient with congestive heart failure, given standard care, might have a 5% risk of dying in the hospital and, if she lived, might have a 25% probability of rating her care as excellent. On the other hand, another patient with congestive heart failure, given the same care, might have a 25% risk of dying in the hospital and, if he lived, might have a 20% probability of rating his care as excellent. For continuous indicators, predicted values are reported as the estimates of the actual result that would have occurred if the patient had received standard care. For instance, one patient receiving standard care for congestive heart failure might have a predicted length of stay of 4.2 days, and another patient receiving the care might have a predicted length of stay of 6.8 days.

It is important to note that risk is not only patient specific; it also is outcome specific. For instance, a patient undergoing emergency surgery may have a high probability of dying but a low probability of a postoperative wound infection. By contrast, another patient undergoing the same surgical procedure may have a low probability of dying but a high probability of a postoperative wound infection. And both patients may have moderate probabilities of substantial postoperative physical impairment. Therefore, severity systems that classify patients using a single score to denote differences in their burden of illness are poor risk-adjustment tools. Instead, a complete risk profile should be created for each patient by individually computing predicted values for each outcome of interest.

For instance, measurements that appear to show very different levels of care at two different hospitals may not explain that one hospital tended to treat much sicker patients or patients more frequently at risk of a particular complication. Simply put, risk-adjustment models are algorithms or equations that express the intrinsic risk (ie, severity) of a given patient or group of patients, based on specific descriptors of each patient's characteristics and condition prior to receiving care.

Complete dependence on expert judgment to classify patients according to relative probabilities of specific outcomes has proven problematic. Instead, expert judgment is best directed toward the identification of potential risk factors (see step 2) and toward review of empirically derived risk-adjustment algorithms or equations for clinical credibility. Final selection of predictive data elements and assignment of relative weights are best performed by applying statistical techniques to a large database drawn from multiple providers that serve diverse populations of patients.

While many statistical techniques can be used to develop valid risk-adjustment models, all are based on the same general approach and underlying assumptions. First, data must be evaluated carefully to ensure that it is internally consistent and relatively free of errors. Assuming that measurement errors are negligible, each patient's outcome will be dependent upon three factors (Figure 34–4): (1) those specific to each patient prior to the delivery of care (ie, patient-specific factors), (2) those specific to the quality of the care provided (ie, provider-specific factors), and (3) those due to chance alone (ie, random variation not attributable to any identifiable factor).

By limiting a risk-adjustment model to only those risk factors that have a statistically significant relationship to the outcome of interest, the influence of random variation on the model can be reduced. And since many different providers and institutions contribute to the database, the influence of differences in quality of care are greatly reduced. This permits the analyst to relate patient-specific factors directly to observed outcomes, and to use the available data to assign a relative weight to each risk factor selected for inclusion in the model. Thus, as is shown in Figure 34–5, residual random variation and provider-specific factors can be minimized, and risk factors and weights reflect mainly intrinsic patient-specific characteristics that alter the probability that a specific outcome will occur.

Unfortunately, if the effect of a potential risk factor on an outcome of interest differs for various patients in the database used to construct a risk-adjustment model, the weight assigned to that risk factor will represent an aggregate of the weights for each individual patient and will not be correct for any individual. This problem can be minimized by limiting analyses to outcome indicators that apply to relatively homogeneous populations. However, the requirement that risk-adjustment models be developed using large databases limits the precision with which a population at risk can be defined.

After a risk-adjustment model is developed, its predictive power can be assessed. For discrete indicators, this generally is done by computing a C-statistic; for continuous indicators, this generally is done by computing an R-square statistic.

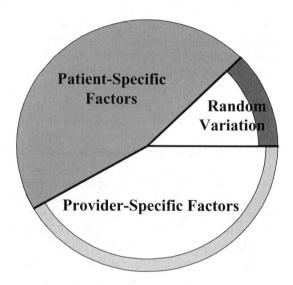

Figure 34–5 Residual Factors Affecting Risk-Adjustment Models. Courtesy of Michael Pine and Associates, Inc, 1998, Chicago, Illinois.

A C-statistic describes the area under a receiver operating characteristic (ROC) curve. This curve relates true positive and false positive rates for any rule designed to predict whether an event will or will not occur (eg, to predict that an outcome will occur if the probability of its occurrence is greater than 20%). In constructing an ROC curve, the true positive rate is computed as the number of times the rule predicts a positive event correctly divided by the number of positive events that occurred. The false positive rate is computed as the number of times that same rule predicts a positive event incorrectly, divided by the number of times the event failed to occur. A unique ROC curve can be constructed for any predictive model by computing a series of individual points, each associated with a specific rule to designate whether a finding is positive or negative. ROC curves for three risk-adjustment models are in Figure 34–6. The better the risk-adjustment model, the farther upward and to the left the curve lies in the diagram.

As is illustrated in Figure 34–6, a C-statistic of 0.5 indicates that the model is no better than simple guesswork, while a C-statistic of 1.0 in-

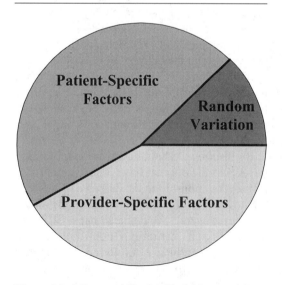

Figure 34–4 Factors Affecting Each Measured Outcome. Courtesy of Michael Pine and Associates, Inc, 1998, Chicago, Illinois.

dicates that the model predicts correctly 100% of the time.

An R-square statistic is a direct measure of the amount of variation among observed values that can be accounted for by a risk-adjustment model. An R-square of 0 indicates that the model is no better than simple guesswork, while an R-square of 1.0 indicates that the model predicts perfectly 100% of the time. Illustrations of the correlations described by other R-square statistics are shown in Figure 34–7. In these illustrations, the R-square of 0.323 indicates that 32.3% of the variation in observed values is explained by the risk-adjustment model, and the R-square of 0.785 indicates that 78.5% of the variation in observed values is explained by the risk-adjustment model.

Even if a model predicts observed outcomes reasonably well, it may be flawed because of systematic bias. For instance, for a discrete outcome of interest, low-risk patients may have systematically higher-than-predicted rates of occurrence, while high-risk patients have systematically lower-than-predicted rates of occurrence. Statistical tests can be performed to determine whether such biases exist.

Finally, every risk-adjustment model should be validated by applying it to a data set other than the one from which it was developed. If systematic biases or unusual random associations have had undue influence on the selection of risk factors, or on the weights assigned to them, evaluation of the model using the new database will reveal instability in weights and in the significance levels assigned to risk factors, as well as a marked deterioration in predictive power. If the model and its performance remain relatively stable across multiple data sets, there is a high probability that risk factors and weights accurately reflect the effect of patient-specific variation on the outcome being monitored.

Step 5: Compare Risk-Adjusted Clinical Outcomes

When combined with risk-adjustment models derived in step 4, clinical outcome measures can be converted into valid, relevant indices of clinical performance. Since observed and predicted values for a clinical measure are available for each patient to whom the measure was applied,

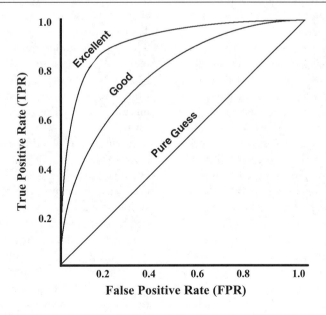

Figure 34–6 ROC Curves. Courtesy of Michael Pine and Associates, Inc, 1998, Chicago, Illinois.

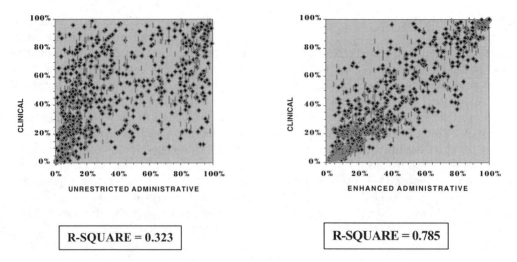

Figure 34–7 Examples of Correlations and Associated R-Squares. Courtesy of Michael Pine and Associates, Inc, 1998, Chicago, Illinois.

clinical performance can be assessed for different combinations of patients (ie, reporting categories), regardless of how these patients were assigned to risk-adjustment models (ie, to analytic categories). This flexibility permits analysts to create new clinical indicators (as opposed to measures) at will and to explore issues and concerns that were not considered when initial measurements and risk-adjustment models were designed and developed.

To prepare valid reports of comparative clinical performance from information about risk-adjusted clinical outcomes, each measured outcome must be divided into four basic components: (1) intrinsic patient-specific risk, (2) quality of care provided, (3) random variation, and (4) bias introduced by systematic errors in measurement. Figure 34–8 presents this relationship as a simple sum in which patient risk plus quality of care plus random variation plus systematic error equals measured outcome.

Because patient outcomes can be observed directly, they are far easier to measure directly than is quality of care (ie, the providers' contribution to patient outcomes). Patient risk can be calculated by measuring relevant risk factors and computing predicted values using risk-adjustment models derived in step 4. Allowance can be made for random variation using statistical computations, and systematic errors can be minimized by carefully designing and executing data acquisition and analysis. Since quality of care remains the only unknown component, it is possible to estimate its contribution to measured clinical outcome by subtracting patient risk, random variation, and systematic error from both sides of the outcomes equation described above. This yields a new equation (Figure 34–9) in which quality of care equals patients' measured outcomes minus systematic error (here assumed to be 0) minus patient-specific risk (computed using an appropriate risk-adjustment model) minus random variation (estimated using statistical formulae).

In the equation illustrated in Figure 34–9, quantities are assumed to be absolute values. However, patient risk (ie, the probability that an outcome will occur for a particular patient given standard care) is not absolute, because it depends on the arbitrary selection of one of many reasonable standards of care. When the performance of a group of organizations or providers is compared, the standard selected is often the average of all patients included in the analysis (ie, for the entire group of patients, the observed outcome is equal to the predicted outcome). Al-

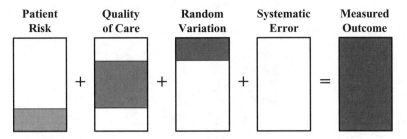

Figure 34–8 Basic Components of Measured Outcome. Courtesy of Michael Pine and Associates, Inc, 1998, Chicago, Illinois.

ternatively, a risk-adjustment model can be calibrated using a reference set of patients, and that reference then can be used to define a standard of care. The selection of a standard of care does not affect the choice of risk factors or the relative weights assigned to them, nor does it affect the relative performance of organizations or providers being evaluated. However, it does affect the designation of an organization or provider as better than, comparable to, or worse than average. If low standards are selected, everyone being evaluated may be above "average," while if high standards are used, everyone being evaluated may fail to achieve "average" levels of performance.

Once a standard of care has been selected and used to calibrate an appropriate risk-adjustment model, risk-adjusted outcomes for a group of organizations or providers can be compared. One such comparison is illustrated in Figure 34–10 for a discrete indicator (adverse outcomes in patients undergoing nonsurgical coronary revascularization), and another is illustrated in Figure 34–11 for a continuous indicator (postprocedure length of stay in patients undergoing nonsurgical coronary revascularization).

These illustrations delineate all the components in the quality equation: (1) observed rates, (2) predicted rates, and (3) ranges representing amounts of variation associated with specified levels of confidence that differences between observed and predicted rates are not merely the results of chance variation. Systematic error is assumed to be negligible. Comparisons of predicted values provide information about case mix differences (ie, the relative riskiness of patients treated by different organizations or providers). The difference between observed and predicted values reflects the degree to which actual performance was better or worse than standard care.

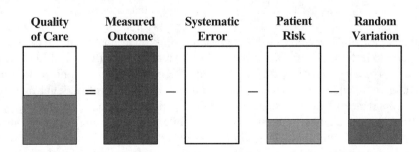

Figure 34–9 Computation To Derive Quality of Care. Courtesy of Michael Pine and Associates, Inc, 1998, Chicago, Illinois.

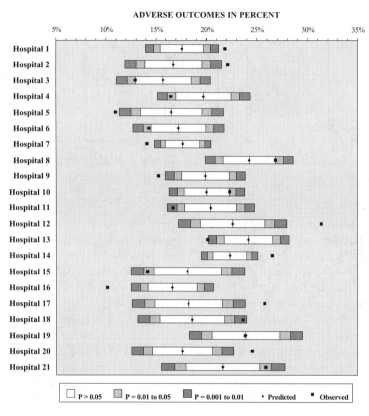

Figure 34–10 Comparison of Risk-Adjusted Adverse Outcome Rates for Patients Undergoing Nonsurgical Coronary Revascularization at 21 Hospitals in the Nationwide Cardiac Alliance. Courtesy of Healthcare Quality Insights, Inc, 1997.

Three sets of confidence limits mark the intervals within which differences between observed and predicted values should be considered statistically insignificant (ie, consistent with chance variation alone). A difference outside the smallest confidence interval will occur by chance alone less than 5% of the time; a difference outside the largest confidence interval will occur by chance alone less than 0.1% of the time. Managers can base their decisions on more or less demanding confidence limits depending on the relative importance of the decision; the larger the confidence interval, the less likely it is that a difference that is due solely to chance will be mistaken for a difference in quality of care.

The influence of random variation generally is greater for discrete than for continuous indicators. It always can be reduced by increasing the number of measurements for each organization or provider. However, sample size often can be increased only by making populations studied more heterogeneous or by increasing the time over which data are collected. Sample sizes used in reports of comparative risk-adjusted outcomes represent compromises between the desire to reduce the influence of random variation and the desire to obtain information about homogeneous groups of patients over relatively short periods of time.

While confidence limits provide information about *statistical significance* (ie, the probability that a difference between observed and predicted values is due solely to chance variation), they do not provide comparable information

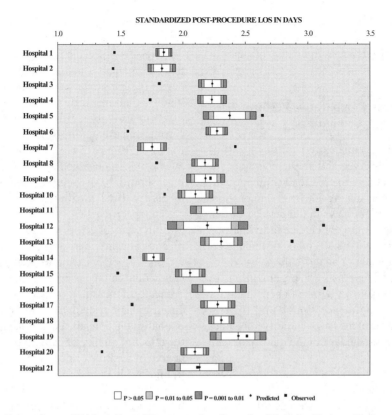

Figure 34–11 Comparison of Risk-Adjusted Postprocedure Length of Stay for Patients Undergoing Nonsurgical Coronary Revascularization at 21 Hospitals in the Nationwide Cardiac Alliance. Courtesy of Healthcare Quality Insights, Inc, 1997.

about clinical or operational *importance* (ie, whether the difference between observed and predicted values is large enough to be considered in decision making). In Figure 34–10, confidence intervals are relatively wide, and all statistically significant differences in performance also are clinically important. However, in Figure 34–11, confidence intervals are relatively narrow, and some statistically significant differences (eg, differences of less than 0.1 days) might not be considered clinically or operationally important.

When comparing large numbers of organizations or providers, it is important to remember that, as the number of comparisons increases, so does the likelihood that one or more organizations or providers will be identified as outliers (ie, as having differences between observed and predicted values that exceed the confidence interval selected for the comparison). For instance, if a confidence limit of 5% is selected, there will be less than 1 chance in 20 that a single determination will incorrectly attribute a chance difference to a difference in quality of care. However, if 20 determinations are considered, there are almost two chances in three that at least one organization or provider will be an outlier by chance alone; if 50 determinations are considered, the odds are greater than 9 to 1 that at least one organization or provider will be an outlier by chance alone. Therefore, when multiple comparisons are being considered, it is important to determine whether the distribution of differences between observed and predicted values is significantly greater than distributions that might occur by chance alone. If statistical tests indicate that this distribution is consistent with chance variation alone, care must be taken in focusing on any single difference as indicative of superior or inferior performance.

Step 6: Evaluate Comparative Performance Based on Analytic Findings

An important, statistically significant difference between observed and predicted values for a clinical indicator measured for a single organization or provider may result from one or more or the following: (1) flaws in the process of risk adjustment that reward or penalize individual organizations or providers, (2) other systematic errors in measurement or analysis that bias results in favor of or against an organization or provider, (3) random variation not accounted for by established confidence limits, and (4) real differences between the organization or provider and the reference standard in the quality of care provided.

Risk-adjustment models may not compensate completely for differences in case mix; they may either omit or underestimate the importance of one or more patient-specific risk factors (eg, poorly controlled diabetes mellitus, severe dementia). When this occurs, as illustrated in Figure 34–12, some of the difference between observed and predicted outcomes that should have been attributed to intrinsic patient-specific risk will be attributed instead to quality of care.

On the other hand, a risk-adjustment model may contain risk factors that reflect the intermediate results of the care a patient receives rather than the patient's actual status when care was begun (eg, pulmonary edema resulting from too vigorous administration of intravenous fluids, cerebrovascular accident first noted after a carotid endarterectomy). In this case, as illustrated in Figure 34–13, some of the difference between observed and predicted outcomes that should have been attributed to quality of care will be attributed instead to intrinsic patient-specific risk.

Both types of errors will result in some organizations or providers appearing to perform better, and some appearing to perform worse, than they would in the absence of these errors.

Ideally, a measured outcome will not be influenced by any systematic errors in measurement or analysis. If it is, the errors can distort some of the effect of quality of care by introducing some degree of positive or negative bias, as illustrated in Figure 34–14.

For example, one provider or organization may report minor wound infections as a complication, while another may report only wound infections that delay discharge. Or, one facility may treat every patient with hemophilia in the entire community, making it impossible to develop fair comparative standards for outcomes involving these patients. Or low-risk patients may have better risk-adjusted results than high-risk patients, thereby

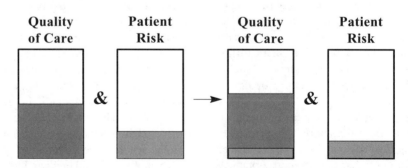

Figure 34–12 Misattribution of Patient Risk to Quality of Care. Courtesy of Michael Pine and Associates, Inc, 1998, Chicago, Illinois.

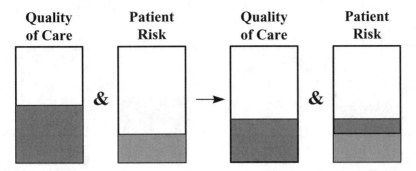

Figure 34–13 Misattribution of Quality of Care to Patient Risk. Courtesy of Michael Pine and Associates, Inc, 1998, Chicago, Illinois.

systematically favoring facilities that treat predominantly low-risk patients. Unlike the effect of random error, which can be reduced by increasing sample size, systematic errors are not affected by larger samples. Nor are there routine tests that will automatically detect the presence of all possible systematic errors. Systematic errors can be avoided only by carefully designing and critically evaluating studies of comparative risk-adjusted clinical outcomes.

Whatever confidence limits are selected, the difference between observed and predicted outcomes will be due, at least in part, to chance variation, as illustrated in Figure 34–15. The influence of chance variation on this difference can be reduced by requiring higher degrees of confidence. However, reducing the possibility of an alpha error (ie, attributing to quality of care differences that really are due to chance variation) by requiring a higher degree of confidence will increase the possibility of a beta error (ie, attributing to chance differences that really reflect quality of care).

Larger samples will reduce the relative magnitude of chance variation. However, increasing sample size generally requires that patient groups be made more heterogeneous or periods of data collection be lengthened, thereby making it more difficult to draw clinical and operational conclusions from analytic reports.

In sum, the ideal equation illustrated in Figure 34–9 must be revised to incorporate all the errors that can enter into computations of clinical performance based on risk-adjusted outcomes. As is shown in Figure 34–16, the ef-

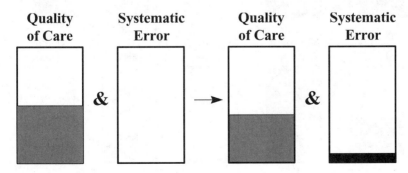

Figure 34–14 Effect of Systematic Error on Measured Quality of Care. Courtesy of Michael Pine and Associates, Inc, 1998, Chicago, Illinois.

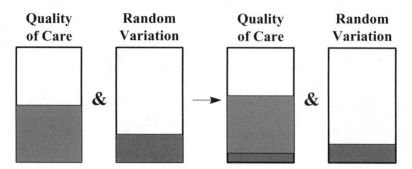

Figure 34–15 Effect of Random Variation on Measured Quality of Care. Courtesy of Michael Pine and Associates, Inc, 1998, Chicago, Illinois.

fects of intrinsic patient-specific risk and quality of care can be confused and random variation and uncorrected systematic errors can distort estimates of quality of care. These errors can never be entirely eliminated, but they can be minimized by carefully designing and executing comparative studies of risk-adjusted clinical outcomes.

If, after allowing for possible sources of error, important and statistically significant differences between observed and predicted outcomes remain, these can be attributed to differences in quality of care. However, further analysis and interpretation almost invariably are required if conclusions needed to support effective decision making are to be drawn.

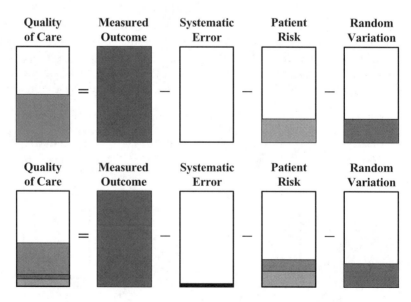

Figure 34–16 Effect of Multiple Errors on Measured Quality of Care. Courtesy of Michael Pine and Associates, Inc, 1998, Chicago, Illinois.

MICHAEL PINE, MD, MBA, is president of Michael Pine and Associates and a research associate in the section of cardiology at the University of Chicago. He is a board-certified cardiologist and has served on the medical faculties of Harvard, University of California, and University of Cincinnati. Since founding his consulting firm in 1988, he has helped purchasers, providers, coalitions, insurers, professional associations, and others to measure clinical outcomes and manage and improve the clinical quality of care.

CHAPTER 35

Crafting Valid, Relevant Measures of Clinical Performance

Michael Pine

Chapter Outline

- Introduction
- Creating Cost-Effective Databases To Monitor Risk-Adjusted Clinical Outcomes
- Using Control Charts To Obtain a Dynamic View of Performance
- Integrating Information about Health Care Services To Identify Providers of Choice
- Risk-Adjusted Functional Status
- Monitoring Clinical Outcomes of Ambulatory Care

INTRODUCTION

Clinical outcomes must be measured consistently to ensure valid comparisons of performance among providers or organizations. However, descriptive and diagnostic data are sensitive to differences in how they are observed and reported by different individuals. This is true especially when many people are involved in recording or collecting data and when they have not received consistent training and consistent evaluation of their data quality.

Objective data also may be biased if they are not obtained consistently. For instance, positive findings may be missed when tests are not performed. Or, just the fact that a test is ordered, even though results are normal, may indicate increased risk of an adverse outcome. Ideally, therefore, assessments of risk-adjusted clinical outcomes all should be based on uniformly collected objective measures such as those used in costly cooperative clinical research studies.

Because this approach would be prohibitively expensive, methods are needed to create valid measures of clinical outcomes from data that can be acquired and recorded in the course of ordinary clinical care or that can be obtained directly and affordably from patients. These measures need not correspond directly to measures used in clinical practice. However, they must (1) reflect patient outcomes accurately and (2) reflect clinical performance consistently.

One method of creating acceptable outcome measures from flawed data is as follows:

1. Screen patients using a crude indicator of an outcome of interest.
2. Based on initial findings, apply methods of statistical process control to a readily available, objective measure associated with the outcome of interest.
3. From this measure, create a new indicator that can be calibrated and applied consistently to individual providers or organizations.
4. Use the new indicator as a surrogate for the outcome of interest.

This method can be used, for example, to obtain rates of occurrence of adverse outcomes (ie, complications) that occur during hospitalization for a specific condition or procedure. Rates of reported complication are extremely unreliable for this purpose, because systematic biases in identifying, recording, and reporting complications may easily halve or double such rates. On the other hand, objective data about lengths of hospitalization and postoperative lengths of stay are readily available. Moreover, both clinical experience and research have shown that the predominant reason for an unusually long length of stay is the occurrence of a clinical complication that prolongs the need for inpatient care. Therefore, lengths of stay that are unusually long for each provider or organization can be used as a clinical indicator that accurately and consistently reflects the occurrence of an important clinical complication.

An application of this method follows. Of 393 patients with pulmonary disease treated at Sample Memorial Hospital, 19 died and 75 had reported inpatient complications. Standardized (ie, risk-adjusted) lengths of stay for all patients with pulmonary disease who were discharged alive from Sample Memorial were computed by (1) dividing observed by predicted values and (2) multiplying this ratio by the average length of stay for a reference population of patients discharged alive without reported complications. The distribution of standardized lengths of stay for patients without and with reported complications is shown in Figure 35–1. The figure shows that standardized lengths of stay for patients without reported complications rarely exceed 7.5 days. On the other hand, patients with reported complications tend to have longer lengths of stay. A substantial number of these patients still are hospitalized after 7.5 days. Similar patterns have been found consistently for numerous clinical conditions and procedures.

Next, a control chart was constructed for standardized lengths of stay for the 299 patients discharged alive without reported inpatient complications. Standardized lengths of stay that exceeded a three standard deviation upper confidence limit were removed from the data set, and confidence limits were recomputed. This process was repeated until all standardized lengths of stay in the data set were less than the upper confidence limit computed from that data set.

In the control chart for pulmonary diseases at Sample Memorial shown in Figure 35–2, the 10 lengths of stay (LOSs) removed from the data set in two successive computations are shown as squares and labeled "Prolonged LOS." Con-

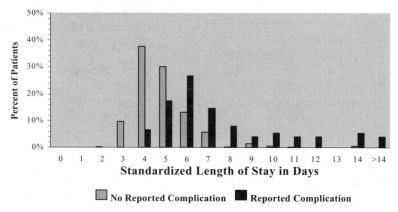

Figure 35–1 Distribution of Standardized Lengths of Stay for Patients Without and with Reported Complications During Hospitalization for Pulmonary Diseases at Sample Memorial Hospital. Courtesy of Healthcare Quality Insights, Inc, 1997.

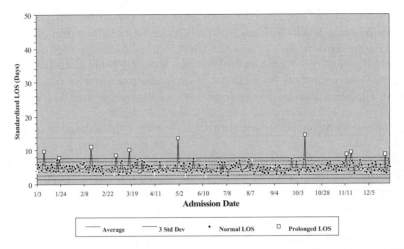

Figure 35–2 Final Control Chart of Standardized Lengths of Stay for Patients Without Reported Complications During Hospitalization for Pulmonary Diseases at Sample Memorial Hospital. Courtesy of Healthcare Quality Insights, Inc, 1997.

fidence limits are based on the 289 lengths of stay shown as diamonds and labeled "Normal LOS."

The final confidence interval derived as explained above was used to identify outliers from among the 75 patients with pulmonary diseases who were discharged alive from Sample Memorial Hospital. The results are shown in Figure 35–3. Compared with patients without reported complications, a much higher proportion of patients with reported complications had prolonged standardized lengths of stay. A few patients with reported complications had exceedingly long hospitalizations.

Finally, patients who died or who had prolonged standardized lengths of stay (as defined above) were classified as having had adverse outcomes associated with their hospitalization.

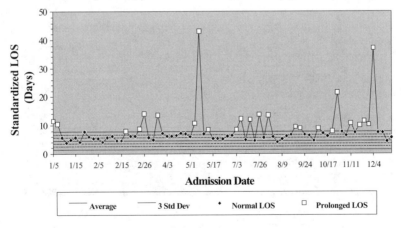

Figure 35–3 Control Chart of Standardized Lengths of Stay for Patients with Reported Complications During Hospitalization for Pulmonary Diseases at Sample Memorial Hospital. Courtesy of Healthcare Quality Insights, Inc, 1997.

Figure 35–4 shows that 10 of 299 patients without reported complications and 24 of 75 patients with reported complications had prolonged standardized lengths of stay. Thus, 53 of 393 patients with pulmonary diseases hospitalized at Sample Memorial were classified as having had adverse outcomes (ie, 19 died and 34 were discharged alive after prolonged hospitalizations).

While demonstrating how an adverse outcome rate was computed for pulmonary diseases at Sample Memorial Hospital, Figure 35–4 also indicates the quality of the hospital's data. The low rate of adverse outcomes in patients discharged alive without reported complications (ie, 3.3%) and the substantially higher rate of adverse outcomes in patients discharged alive with reported complications (ie, 32.0%) both are consistent with high standards of data integrity.

The effect that errors in reporting inpatient complications have on computed adverse outcome rates is illustrated when data reported by Sample Memorial Hospital are altered without changing any objective findings. In one facility (Meticulous Community Hospital), complications are reported for an additional 75 patients who were discharged alive; in another case (Easycount General Hospital), complications are not reported for any patient who was discharged alive. The results of analysis are shown in Figure 35–5. Reported complication rates at the three hospitals differ markedly, but adverse outcome rates remain consistent with the fact that outcomes at the three "different" facilities were identical.

Even though a measure is accurate and consistent, it may not help decision makers to draw conclusions that could lead to appropriate plans of action. For example, a report may disclose that average risk-adjusted length of stay is significantly longer than predicted for patients with a specified condition admitted to a specific hospital. However, this disclosure does not allow the purchaser, patient, clinician, or administrator to distinguish ineffective clinical care (ie, unusually high rates of hospital-acquired complications) from inefficient care. This distinction is vital in selecting providers and in quality improvement. This problem can be solved by dividing total risk-adjusted length of stay into two components. First, efficiency can be measured as the average risk adjusted length of stay for patients who had no adverse outcomes that resulted in unusually long hospitalizations. Second, average risk-adjusted length of stay for all patients discharged alive, when compared with the value predicted based on the

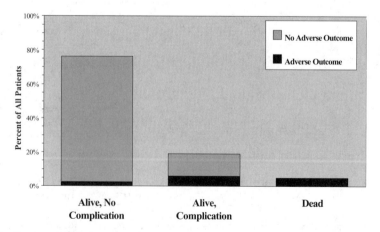

Figure 35–4 Distribution of Outcomes and Reported Complications among Patients Hospitalized for Pulmonary Diseases at Sample Memorial Hospital. Courtesy of Healthcare Quality Insights, Inc, 1997.

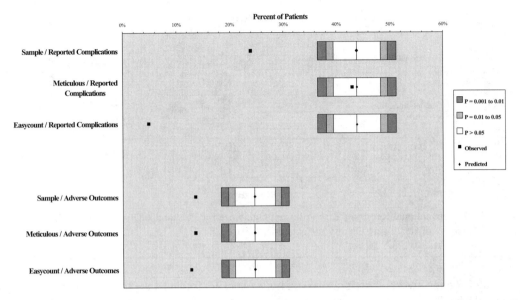

Figure 35–5 Reported Complications and Adverse Outcomes among Patients Hospitalized for Pulmonary Diseases at Three Hospitals Providing Identical Quality of Care. Courtesy of Michael Pine and Associates, Inc, 1998, Chicago, Illinois.

experience of patients without adverse outcomes, indicates how much the average length of stay could be improved by preventing serious adverse outcomes.

Figures 35–6 through 35–9 illustrate how to avoid interpretive problems associated with conventional reports of (1) risk-adjusted mortality, (2) risk-adjusted reported complications, and (3) risk-adjusted average lengths of stay for all live discharges. Figures 35–6 and 35–7 present conventional reports for patients with pulmonary diseases treated at HiComp General Hospital and SloMetic Memorial Hospital, respectively.

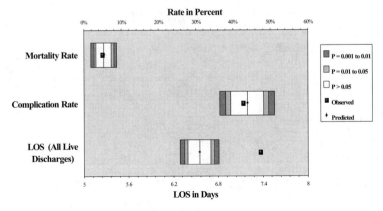

Figure 35–6 Conventional Report of Risk-Adjusted Outcomes for Pulmonary Diseases at HiComp General Hospital. Courtesy of Healthcare Quality Insights, Inc, 1997.

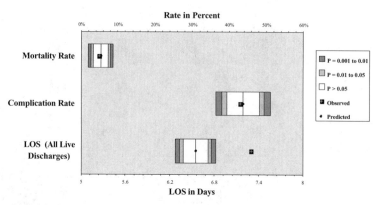

Figure 35–7 Conventional Report of Risk-Adjusted Outcomes for Pulmonary Diseases at SloMetic Memorial Hospital. Courtesy of Healthcare Quality Insights, Inc, 1997.

Results for the two hospitals are virtually identical. Both have average risk-adjusted mortality and complication rates (ie, average effectiveness) but high risk-adjusted lengths of stay (ie, poor efficiency). Based only on these findings, both hospitals might institute projects to complete routine care more expeditiously.

However, the modified reports presented in Figures 35–8 and 35–9 show that this conclusion is incorrect. In these modified reports, the relatively objective adverse outcomes measure is substituted for the more subjectively reported complication rate. Secondly, length of stay is divided into the risk-adjusted average for patients without adverse outcomes (ie, a measure reflecting efficiency of routine care) and the increase in that risk-adjusted average when it is computed for the combination of routine patients and patients with adverse outcomes who were discharged alive (ie, a measure that reflects the effect of hospital-acquired complications on average length of stay).

These graphs demonstrate clearly that HiComp General's generally long average length of stay is because of its significantly higher than predicted rate of adverse out-

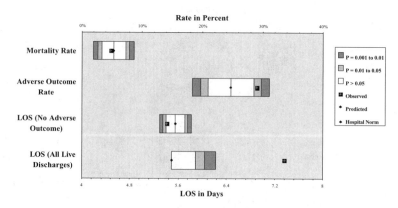

Figure 35–8 Modified Report of Risk-Adjusted Outcomes for Pulmonary Diseases at HiComp General Hospital. Courtesy of Healthcare Quality Insights, Inc, 1997.

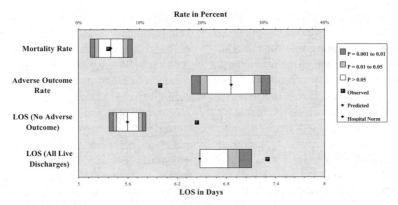

Figure 35–9 Modified Report of Risk-Adjusted Outcomes for Pulmonary Diseases at SloMetic Memorial Hospital. Courtesy of Healthcare Quality Insights, Inc, 1997.

comes, while SloMetic Memorial's generally long average length of stay is due to inefficient delivery of care to routine patients. Furthermore, reported complications were relatively low at HiComp because only fairly serious complications were reported. On the other hand, reported complications were relatively high at SloMetic because even fairly minor complications were reported. These modified reports permit decision makers to differentiate between health care organizations that consume excess resources treating serious inpatient complications (ie, organizations providing ineffective care) and organizations that consume excess resources delivering routine care (ie, organizations providing inefficient care). Knowing this distinction, decision makers can take appropriate action either to correct problems or to capitalize on superior performance.

CREATING COST-EFFECTIVE DATABASES TO MONITOR RISK-ADJUSTED CLINICAL OUTCOMES

Using methods described earlier in this chapter, reasonable risk-adjustment models can be developed using data abstracted directly from patients' medical records. However, many providers and health plans have found this method of data collection to be prohibitively expensive. Alternatively, readily available electronic billing data can be used to create risk-adjustment models. However, predicted values derived from models based on these databases correlate poorly with those derived from data abstracted from medical records of the same patients. Adding electronically available laboratory data (ie, results of chemistry, hematology, and blood gas analyses) to hospital billing data yields predictions that are very similar to those derived using data abstracted from medical records. However, linking electronic billing data and electronic laboratory data still is extremely difficult, if not impossible, for most hospitals.

The primary inadequacy of hospital billing data (with respect to adjusting for patient-specific risk) is the lack of distinction between diagnoses present when patients are admitted to the hospital (comorbidities) and diagnoses that arise after the patient is hospitalized (complications). Numerous unsuccessful attempts have been made to differentiate comorbidities from complications accurately using clinically derived algorithms. These failures are due to the inadequacy of clinical information provided in hospital billing records rather than to investigators' lack of clinical acumen or methodological rigor.

An alternative approach to distinguishing comorbidities from complications is to append to each five-digit secondary diagnostic code an additional code that specifies whether the diagnosis was present on admission or was acquired during hospitalization. This approach was first reported in 1991 by the Mayo Clinic, which found that obtaining these data consumed less than 2 minutes per record. Moreover, the rate of agreement among coders was 87%.[1] Routine submission of this information is now required both in New York State (since 1993) and in California (since 1996).

When only diagnoses documented to be present on admission are used in developing and applying risk-adjustment models, there is good correlation between patient-level predictions using these models and patient-level predictions using data abstracted directly from the same patients' medical records. For example, for patients hospitalized with pneumonia, an R-square of 0.785 was obtained, compared with an R-square of 0.323 when all secondary diagnoses were used. More widespread adoption of this new code, sometimes referred to as the sixth digit, can permit accurate

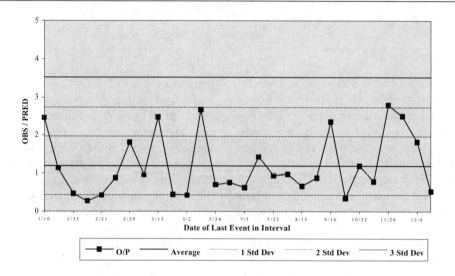

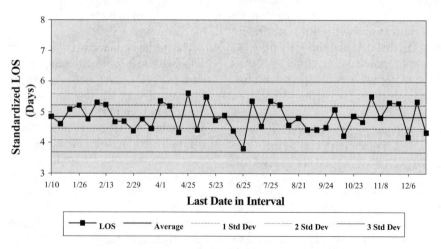

Figure 35–10 Dynamic View of Rates of Adverse Outcomes and Lengths of Stay for Pulmonary Diseases at Sample Memorial Hospital. Courtesy of Healthcare Quality Insights, Inc, 1997.

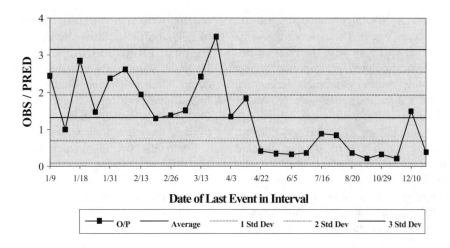

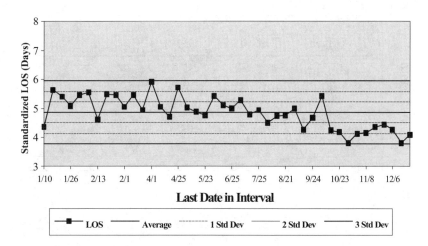

Figure 35–11 Dynamic View of Rates of Adverse Outcomes and Lengths of Stay for Pulmonary Diseases at Neway Community Hospital. Courtesy of Healthcare Quality Insights, Inc, 1997.

risk adjustment of clinical outcome indicators while avoiding both the unacceptable inaccuracies currently associated with the use of standard UB-92 billing data and the high cost currently associated with abstraction of medical records.

USING CONTROL CHARTS TO OBTAIN A DYNAMIC VIEW OF PERFORMANCE

Periodic reports of comparative risk-adjusted clinical outcomes (such as those illustrated in Figures 34–10 and 34–11) can provide useful information about performance. However, increasing the frequency of these reports will be of limited value for most practitioners or providers, because of the relatively small number of patients they treat in each diagnostic or procedural category. Small numbers increase the relative importance of random variation, which results in unacceptably large confidence limits. Therefore, it is advisable to perform comparisons to external reference standards relatively infrequently (eg, annually or semiannually) and to evaluate trends by creating control charts for standardized (ie, risk-adjusted) outcomes.

For discrete indicators such as mortality or adverse outcomes, the ratio of observed to predicted values can be charted over intervals that begin immediately after an event occurs and end with a subsequent event. The number of events in each interval will vary with the relative frequency of events and the algorithm used to terminate each interval. For continuous indicators, standardized values for successive groups of consecutive routine cases (ie, cases without adverse outcomes) can be averaged and charted. Confidence limits can be derived using standard techniques of statistical process control.

Figures 35–10 through 35–12 all were produced using the same data set as that used to study complications and adverse outcomes at Sample Memorial Hospital. Only the dates of admission were altered to create different patterns of risk-adjusted outcomes at Sample Memorial Hospital (Figure 35–10), Neway Community Hospital (Figure 35–11), and BadTime Academic Medical Center (Figure 35–12). Therefore, annual performance reports for the 393 patients with pulmonary diseases cared for at each of these three hospitals would be identical.

Figure 35–10 shows no identifiable trends and no outliers (ie, points outside of three standard deviation confidence limits) either for standardized adverse outcome rates or for standardized lengths of stay for pulmonary patients at Sample Memorial Hospital. In contrast, Figure 35–11

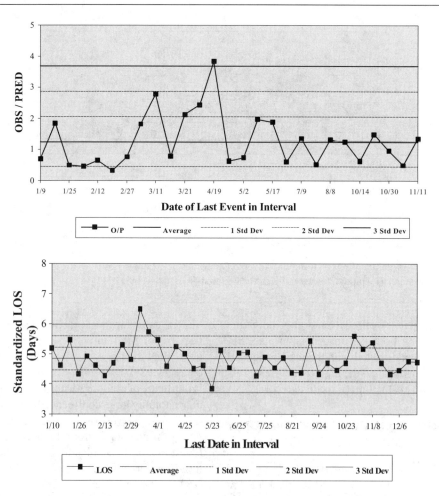

Figure 35–12 Dynamic View of Rates of Adverse Outcomes and Lengths of Stay for Pulmonary Diseases at BadTime Academic Medical Center. Courtesy of Healthcare Quality Insights, Inc, 1997.

shows a precipitous fall in standardized adverse outcome rates and a slow but unmistakable decline in standardized lengths of stay for pulmonary patients at Neway Community Hospital.

Finally, Figure 35–12 shows a single point that exceeds the upper confidence limit for standardized adverse outcome rates and a single point that exceeds the upper confidence limit for standardized lengths of stay for pulmonary patients at BadTime Academic Medical Center. These outliers are not associated with any identifiable trend. Both occurred during the months of the year when Dr. Careless was the attending physician on the pulmonary service. These findings have clear implications for the chief of pulmonary medicine.

INTEGRATING INFORMATION ABOUT HEALTH CARE SERVICES TO IDENTIFY PROVIDERS OF CHOICE

Recipients and purchasers of health care wish to obtain the best value services available. Value can be reduced to a simple equation of quality divided by cost. *Qualities* of care can be measured with reasonable precision using methods described above. However, no single equation will combine these measures to produce an aggregate indicator of overall *quality* for every purpose. Selection of "best value" requires systematic consideration of a series of questions in the light of specific patients' and payers' priorities and the realistic options available to them.

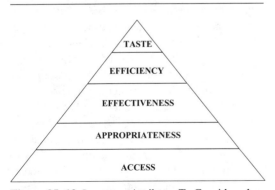

Figure 35–13 Important Attributes To Consider when Selecting Health Care Providers. Courtesy of Michael Pine and Associates, Inc, 1998, Chicago, Illinois.

These questions, in recommended order of initial consideration, are:

1. Which providers or organizations can provide adequate *access* to care?
2. Is the care offered by a provider or organization generally *appropriate*?
3. Is the care received *effective*?
4. Is the care delivered *efficiently*?
5. Are there *other considerations* that make a provider or organization more or less desirable?

This hierarchy of considerations, illustrated in Figure 35–13, systematically identifies providers or organizations that (1) can provide needed health care, (2) provide only health care that is needed, (3) achieve established clinical goals, (4) achieve these goals without consuming excessive resources, and (5) do not offend the tastes or sensibilities of patients and payers. In practice, final decisions may require simultaneous consideration of some or all of these attributes. However, by reviewing each consideration systematically and individually, decision makers can avoid losing discrete but important concerns within the morass of more compelling global impressions.

Issues related to access include geographic location, services provided and difficulties encountered in obtaining them, and willingness and ability to meet special requirements imposed by patients or payers (eg, Saturday office hours, acceptance of global fees). External monitors of clinical performance provide little assistance in dealing with these issues.

Issues related to appropriateness are extremely complex and are best discussed after effectiveness and efficiency have been considered.

Effective health care is care that results in better clinical outcomes than would be obtained in the absence of such care. External monitoring of risk-adjusted clinical outcomes can identify providers and organizations that provide health care more effectively than their competitors in one or more dimensions for one or more clinical conditions or procedures. However, it is rare that a single provider or organization excels in every dimension for every condition or procedure. Therefore, global assessments of performance will depend upon the priorities of the patients or payers involved in the process of selection. For any decision maker, the clinical performance of multiple health care providers or organizations can be summarized with a single measure based on a spectrum of risk-adjusted outcome indicators that have been weighted according to that decision maker's explicitly stated priorities.

Efficiency relates effectiveness to resources consumed in providing care. Measures of resource consumption can be developed in much the same way as the measures of clinical outcomes that were described above. Risk-adjustment models can be constructed and analyses performed using detailed charge master data, but careful mapping of cost centers across organizations is required if reports of comparative risk-adjusted resource consumption are to provide valid, relevant reflections of resource consumption. Billed charges are totally inappropriate for comparisons of resource consumption, and cost-to-charge ratios provide only crude estimates of comparative efficiency.

If quality is equated to clinical performance and cost is equated to resource consumption, then value can be equated to clinical performance divided by resource consumption. This equation is valid from the perspective of organizations that provide care, but from the perspective of a payer, value is equal to clinical performance divided by the price paid for clinical outcomes obtained. Figure 35–14 shows that cost, from a purchaser's perspective, encompasses not only resource consumption but also financial efficiency and the health care provider's operating margin.

Financial efficiency incorporates such items as the cost of bad debt, the types of financing employed, the cost of capital, the prices paid for labor and supplies, and the cost of administration and other overhead. Superior financial efficiency can permit clinically inefficient providers to offer extremely competitive

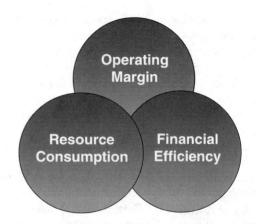

Figure 35–14 Components of Cost to Purchaser. Courtesy of Michael Pine and Associates, Inc, 1998, Chicago, Illinois.

prices; poor financial efficiency can force clinically efficient providers to charge uncompetitively high prices.

Finally, operating margins can be raised or lowered almost at will to maintain short-term competitive prices. However, purchasers must be wary of entering into long-term arrangements with clinically inefficient providers that have poor or average financial efficiency. Competitive prices sometimes are offered solely on the basis of negative operating margins that cannot be sustained over prolonged periods of time.

Appropriate health care now can be defined as care that, over time, is more effective or more efficient than alternative care. By this definition, inappropriate care is care that either is ineffective or is less effective and efficient than alternatives for any reasonable combination of patient or payer interests. Unfortunately, the information required to identify inappropriate care using this definition currently is, for the most part, unavailable.

In the absence of relevant data about long-term clinical effectiveness, appropriateness generally is assessed using algorithms that delineate acceptable and unacceptable practices. These algorithms are usually developed by panels of experts, and they often rely on published research that may or may not replicate clinical situations to which the algorithms are applied. On occasion, last year's best practice will become this year's questionable practice and next year's malpractice. Therefore, such algorithms should be used conservatively to identify markedly aberrant patterns of care, rather than normatively as a marker for superior care.

After all objective measurements are completed, subjective factors can play an important role in the selection of health care providers. Satisfaction with health care services is an important clinical indicator, and satisfaction does not correlate completely with any clinical measure or combination of clinical measures. While it is wise to postpone subjective considerations until all objective data have been weighed carefully, it is foolish to ignore individual tastes and preferences in dealing with so personal a service as health care.

The following description of the creation of a hospital network will illustrate the proper integration of information obtained from external monitoring of risk-adjusted clinical outcomes into the process of selecting health care providers or organizations. The example is based on an actual case study, but the procedure followed has been expanded to illustrate the entire process outlined above.

Of 35 hospitals that are geographically accessible to employees of the Firm, 29 agreed to meet the Firm's service requirements and expressed an interest in being considered for inclusion in the Firm's new network.

Rates of conformance to a conservative set of appropriateness algorithms were compared for these 29 facilities. Three were found to have rates of inappropriate care that were greater than 25% higher than average for all 29 facilities. In each of the three cases, the difference between the observed rate of inappropriate care and the average rate for all facilities was far beyond the 0.1% confidence limit (ie, there was less than 1 chance in 1,000 that the difference was due to chance alone). Therefore, the Firm decided to eliminate these three facilities from further consideration.

Next, the Firm selected outcomes monitoring systems that covered all four domains (Figure 34–2) of clinical effectiveness. It obtained performance reports on risk-adjusted clinical outcomes of interest. At the same time, the Firm convened a task force that assigned relative weights to specific conditions and procedures based on the perceived importance of these conditions and procedures to the Firm and its employees. For each condition and procedure considered, the task force assigned relative weights to each outcome measure based on the perceived importance of available measures to the Firm and its employees. Finally, an algorithm was used to produce a report (Figure 35–15) that combined measured results and priorities established by the task force.

In this report, hospitals were divided into seven categories, each represented by a different shade in Figure 35–15. Higher scores indicated better performance; placement in nonadjacent categories indicated important differences in overall performance. The seven hospitals in Groups 6 and 7 (the bottom two sets in Figure 35–15) were eliminated from further consideration.

Final bids and evidence of financial viability were reviewed for the 19 hospitals still being considered. One hospital was eliminated because financial analysts at the Firm believed that the hospital's negative operating margin precluded long-term maintenance of services without substantial increases in price. The Firm convened a second task force to project annual utilization of specific hospital services and to explicitly classify the Firm's sensitivity to differences in price. Based on these determinations, an algorithm was used to produce a report (Figure 35–16) that combined clinical performance and projected cost of service.

In this report, hospitals were divided into six categories, each represented by a different shade in Figure 35–16. Higher scores indicated better value (eg, better performance at the same cost, similar performance at a lower cost); placement in nonadjacent categories indicated important differences in value. The four hospitals in Groups 5 and 6 (the bottom two sets in

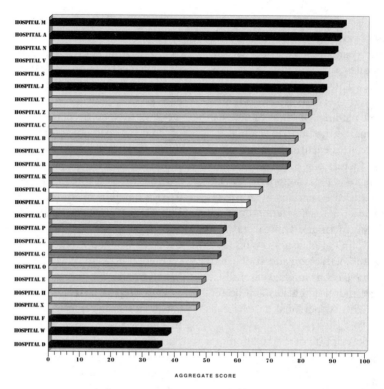

Figure 35–15 Ratings of Overall Clinical Effectiveness Derived by Applying Utilities Established by the Firm to Measures of Risk-Adjusted Clinical Outcomes at 26 Hospitals. Courtesy of Michael Pine and Associates, Inc, 1998, Chicago, Illinois.

Figure 35–16) were eliminated from further consideration.

Two of the remaining 14 hospitals (ie, Hospital Y and Hospital Q) were eliminated from further consideration based on subjective considerations. One hospital's physical facilities were considered unacceptably distasteful by a small but influential group of the Firm's senior management. The other hospital was owned by a multinational corporation that recently had been convicted of waste, fraud, and abuse.

The Firm entered into negotiations with the five hospitals of highest value and concluded contracts with four. After reviewing these four facilities' locations and the array of services they provided, the Firm entered into negotiations with two hospitals from Group 2 (ie, Hospital C and Hospital R) and one hospital from Group 3 (ie, Hospital T). These hospitals (unlike others in their group) were selected because the Firm believed their inclusion in the network would improve both access to important specialized services and access in general. Hospital S, for instance, was not approached because it was only two blocks away from Hospital N and did not offer any specialty services beyond those already provided by Hospital N. Of 35 original candidates, 7 hospitals (ie, Hospitals M, N, A, J, C, R, and T) were included in the Firm's health care network.

The Firm currently is considering using a similar process to designate Centers of Excellence in several specialty areas. All interested hospitals will be considered, but preference will be given to hospitals that already are included in the Firm's health care network.

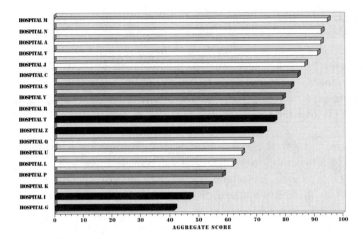

Figure 35–16 Ratings of Relative Value Offered to the Firm by 18 Hospitals Based on Ratings of Overall Clinical Effectiveness, Projected Costs of Hospital Care, and the Firm's Price Sensitivity. Courtesy of Michael Pine and Associates, Inc, 1998, Chicago, Illinois.

RISK-ADJUSTED FUNCTIONAL STATUS

Measures of functional status promise to add an important dimension to monitoring and managing clinical outcomes. Traditional measures of clinical performance have emphasized the early effects of care for acute conditions or interventions (eg, death in patients hospitalized for acute pneumococcal pneumonia, wound infection after partial colectomy). Many of these measures document the occurrence (or avoidance) of adverse events (eg, death, complications) rather than the achievement of therapeutic objectives (eg, alleviation of symptoms, or recovery). To paint a complete picture of the value of health care services, an outcomes monitoring system also must provide information about the positive contribution of health care services to long-term well-being.

Three complementary approaches to monitoring functional outcomes over time are

1. periodic disease-specific objective functional assessment, performed by trained clinicians
2. periodic condition-specific patient surveys, designed to measure functional capacity in areas related to each patient's underlying pathology
3. periodic surveys of patients' or beneficiaries' general functional capacity

The medical profession traditionally has employed disease-specific objective functional assessment to document and monitor the progression or regression of disease-related functional impairment. Often such assessments include patient-derived information obtained and edited by clinicians, who interpret and modify patients' responses to direct questions. Standardized objective functional assessments, performed on a fixed time schedule, are an integral part of many clinical research studies. However, both standardization and adherence to schedules are difficult, if not impossible, to achieve in ordinary health care settings. Despite the appeal to health care professionals of clinician-derived functional measures, the usefulness of such measures is limited severely by the following factors:

1. failure of clinicians to collect comparable data about patient function
2. systematic biases introduced by collection of data on samples of patients that are not random (eg, only on patients who return for 6-month follow-up appointments)

3. problems with comparison of data collected at different times after an acute episode (eg, follow-ups performed on Surgeon A's patients 3 months and 1 year after hip replacement, compared with follow-ups performed on Surgeon B's patients 6 months after hip replacement)

Until these problems are solved, either by creating more uniform patterns of follow-up assessment or by developing analytic techniques to compensate for diversity in clinical practice, disease-specific objective functional assessment will provide little useful information for comparative monitoring of clinical performance.

In lieu of clinician-derived information about functional status, periodic surveys of patients treated for a given condition can be used to assess patient functional capacity in areas related directly to underlying pathology. When well designed, these surveys can parallel historical information traditionally used by health care professionals. Data collection, selection of patients, and timing of assessments all can be controlled more rigorously than is possible when data collection is dependent upon routine clinical follow-up. However, surveys designed to assess functions affected by a single clinical condition or intervention may provide misleading information about (1) patients who have several coexisting conditions (eg, patients with diabetes, coronary artery disease, and arthritis), and (2) patients whose function is affected by processes not normally associated with the condition or intervention for which the survey was designed (eg, patients with chronic obstructive pulmonary disease who have an acute myocardial infarction with resulting chronic congestive heart failure). Despite these limitations, condition-specific surveys designed to monitor patients' functional status can provide important information about clinical performance, particularly when these surveys are administered by trained interviewers.

As an alternative to condition-specific surveys, surveys of patients' or beneficiaries' general functional capacity (eg, the SF-36 or SF-12 surveys) can provide valuable, valid information about changes in functional status over time. This information is particularly useful in monitoring (1) general health status, as opposed to the functional sequelae of specific diseases or interventions, and (2) the results of clinical interventions intended to produce major alterations in functional status over a short period (eg, a 3-month outpatient rehabilitation program). However, general surveys may fail to detect important changes in function that result directly from disease-specific clinical interventions, or may confuse such changes with other changes in function so that valid interpretation of findings becomes impossible.

Considerable attention has been devoted to the relative merits of disease-specific measures and general measures of functional status, but little notice has been given to the difficulties of drawing conclusions about comparative clinical performance from information about patients' functional status. Purchasers and providers of health care who would never think of using raw mortality data to evaluate clinical performance appear ready to accept raw data about functional status for the same purpose. The following case study illustrates the dangers inherent in uncritically using information about functional status to identify superior or substandard health care providers.

In this hypothetical situation, 15 hospitals provide inpatient and follow-up care for patients admitted with signs and symptoms of acute myocardial infarction. Functional status prior to the onset of the symptoms that prompted admission and functional status 6 months after admission both are assessed. Reliable, valid measures yield scores from 100 (no functional impairment) to 0 (no function whatsoever). Information is obtained on 1,000 consecutive discharges from each hospital. Superior performance (ie, average score 3 points or more above average) is rewarded by full return of a 40% withhold to participating clinicians. Average performance (ie, average score from 3 points below to 3 points above average) recoups 75% of the withhold, while the remaining 25% is distributed equally among clinicians at facilities with superior performance. (If no facilities demonstrate superior performance, average performance results in full return of the withhold.) Below-average performance (ie, average score more than 3 points below average to average score 9 points below average) recoups only 50% of the withhold, while the remaining 50% is used to support focused quality improvement and remediation. Poor performance (ie, average score more than 9 points below average) results in all withheld funds being used to support focused quality improvement and remediation.

Functional status 6 months after admission varies among facilities, from 14.1 points below average for all patients to 9.2 points above average (Figure 35–17). When comparisons are based on the difference between postdischarge functional status and preadmission functional status (Figure 35–18), variation remains substantial: from 9.1 points below average to 16.0 points above average. However, case-mix differences detected by considering functional status prior to admission are significant enough to change the ranking of 4 out of 15 fa-

cilities. This demonstrates clearly that single measurements of function cannot be used to evaluate clinical performance, even if these measurements are both accurate and important.

Before-and-after assessments also are inadequate for detecting real differences in performance and for avoiding erroneous conclusions that differences in performance are present. In this illustration, different distributions of 35 case types were treated by the 15 hospitals. In some cases, important preexisting functional limitations were reversible; in others, they were either minimal or irreversible. In some cases, myocardial damage was minimal; in others, it was substantial and irreversible on arrival at the hospital; and in others, it was potentially substantial but could be reversed by prompt, appropriate treatment after arrival. In some cases, there was a high risk of subsequent infarction if critical lesions were not corrected in a timely fashion; in other cases, no additional critical lesions were present. Finally, some patients were candidates for car-

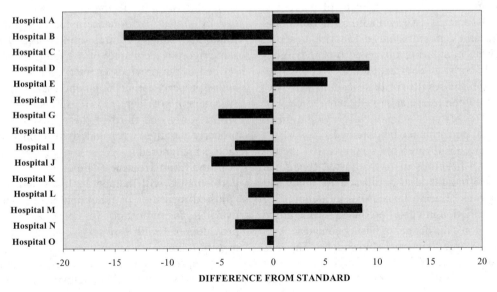

Figure 35–17 Reported Functional Status 6 Months after Acute Myocardial Infarction. Courtesy of Michael Pine and Associates, Inc, 1998, Chicago, Illinois.

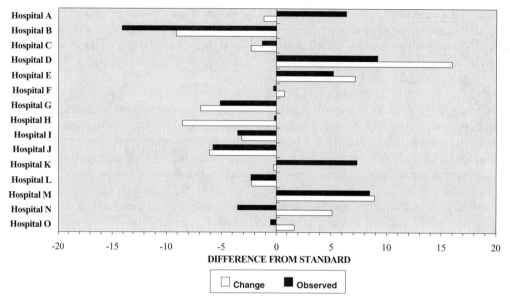

Figure 35–18 Reported Functional Status 6 Months after Acute Myocardial Infarction: Comparison of Status and Change in Status. Courtesy of Michael Pine and Associates, Inc, 1998, Chicago, Illinois.

---

diac rehabilitation that, if properly administered, would improve their functional status. Effective and ineffective care of the 35 case types resulted in 158 sequences of outcomes, each associated with a preadmission functional score and a postdischarge functional score. Only by comparing observed 6-month functional scores at each hospital to predicted results (ie, the results for that hospital when average outcomes are achieved there for each of the 35 case types) can a valid evaluation of hospital performance be obtained.

Figure 35–19 presents a comparison among these 15 hospitals of risk-adjusted functional status 6 months after admission for signs and symptoms of acute myocardial infarction. The wide variation in values predicted for the group underscores the danger of basing conclusions on postdischarge functional status alone. The lack of correspondence between the gray and white bars in Figure 35–20 demonstrates that differences between observed and predicted values cannot be estimated using measures of preadmission functional status, because these differences are largely the product of how each patient's underlying clinical condition evolves with effective or ineffective care. Proper evaluation of clinical performance using measures of functional status requires application of the same rigorous techniques of risk adjustment described in the previous chapter. Failure to risk adjust properly can result in wholesale misclassification of providers, as is illustrated in Figure 35–21: only one third of these hospitals are properly classified when underlying clinical risk factors are ignored.

In the future, routine evaluations of clinical performance will include sophisticated, risk-adjusted measures of functional status. However, it is important for purchasers and providers of health care services to avoid premature reliance on techniques that may accurately represent clinical outcomes but are not yet able to support valid conclusions about the relative quality or value of health care services.

Crafting Valid, Relevant Measures of Clinical Performance 497

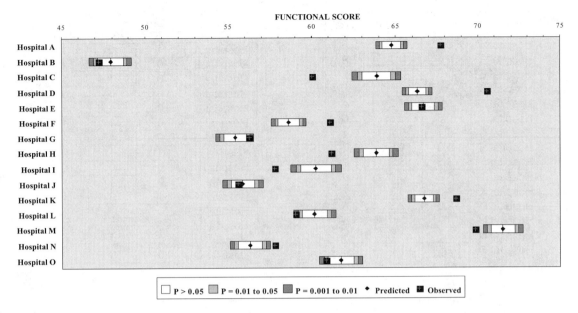

Figure 35–19 Risk-Adjusted Functional Score 6 Months after Acute Myocardial Infarction. Courtesy of Michael Pine and Associates, Inc, 1998, Chicago, Illinois.

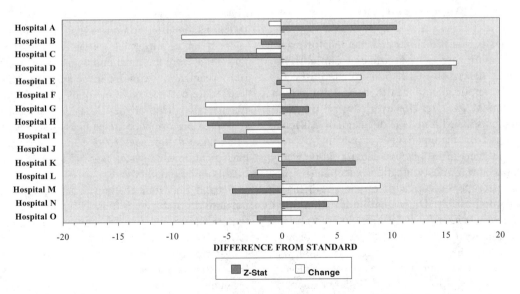

Figure 35–20 Reported Functional Status 6 Months after Acute Myocardial Infarction: Comparison of Change in Status and Risk-Adjusted Status. Courtesy of Michael Pine and Associates, Inc, 1998, Chicago, Illinois.

	SCORE	CHANGE	Z-STAT
Hospital A	6.4	-1.1	10.5
Hospital B	-14.1	-9.1	-1.8
Hospital C	-1.3	-2.3	-8.7
Hospital D	9.2	16.0	15.5
Hospital E	5.2	7.2	-0.4
Hospital F	-0.3	0.8	7.6
Hospital G	-5.1	6.9	2.4
Hospital H	-0.2	-8.5	-6.7
Hospital I	-3.5	-3.2	-5.3
Hospital J	-5.8	-6.1	-0.8
Hospital K	7.3	-0.2	6.7
Hospital L	-2.3	-2.3	-3.0
Hospital M	8.5	8.9	-4.5
Hospital N	-3.5	5.1	4.1
Hospital O	-0.5	1.7	-2.3

Superior
Average
Below Avg
Poor

From To	SCORE CHANGE	SCORE Z-STAT	CHANGE Z-STAT
Hospital A	-1	0	1
Hospital B	0	2	2
Hospital C	0	-1	-1
Hospital D	0	0	0
Hospital E	0	-1	-1
Hospital F	0	1	1
Hospital G	0	1	1
Hospital H	-1	-1	0
Hospital I	0	0	0
Hospital J	0	1	1
Hospital K	-1	0	1
Hospital L	0	-1	-1
Hospital M	0	-2	-2
Hospital N	2	2	0
Hospital O	0	0	0

Delta = 1
Delta = 2

Figure 35–21 Classification of 15 Hospitals According to Functional Status, Change in Functional Status, and Risk-Adjusted Functional Status 6 Months after Acute Myocardial Infarction. Courtesy of Michael Pine and Associates, Inc, 1998, Chicago, Illinois.

MONITORING CLINICAL OUTCOMES OF AMBULATORY CARE

Ideally, the principles and methods of external monitoring of risk-adjusted clinical outcomes described in Chapter 36 should be directly applicable to health care delivered in outpatient settings. However, several practical problems have limited the diffusion of this technology from the inpatient environment.

First, very little objective data is routinely collected during most outpatient encounters. This makes proper classification of patients difficult, if not impossible. Diagnostic information often is incomplete, and it is far more likely to be inaccurate than is diagnostic information for hospitalized patients. Important chronic conditions may pass unnoticed or unnoted during relatively brief, poorly documented ambulatory encounters for self-limited acute medical problems. When a chronic condition is noted, little information may be provided about its duration, extent, or progression. Current ambulatory care classification systems either gloss over these problems, creating groupings that are clinically suspect, or require such extensive documentation that only the most enthusiastic, resource-rich organizations can use these systems. Thus, until more cost-effective methods of accurately classifying patients are developed, differences in measured performance are as likely to be due to systematic differences in documentation and classification as to systematic differences in the quality of ambulatory care.

Second, important changes in health status often unfold slowly, while dramatic, rapid changes that precipitate many ambulatory encounters often are self-limited and transient. Incomplete long-term follow-up can introduce systematic biases that invalidate comparisons of alternative providers or patterns of care. Unfocused measures of general health status may fail to uncover important differences in condition-specific outcomes or may reveal differences without providing any insight into their underlying cause. On the other hand, condition-specific measures can be misapplied when diagnoses are incomplete or incorrect, and these measures are problematic in numerous cases in which multiple chronic conditions coexist. Thus, problems with interpreting apparent differences in performance and properly relating these differences to actionable alternatives remain important barriers to the widespread adoption of outcomes monitoring in ambulatory settings.

Finally, multiple sources of data generally are required to track outcomes related to ambulatory care and to create and apply appropriate risk-adjustment models. Numerous technical difficulties and considerable expense are associated with collecting, integrating, managing, and analyzing a vast array of data from multiple sources. In a cost-conscious environment that focuses on the provision, rather than the assessment, of health care services, there is a strong tendency to accept sloppy, misleading evaluations rather than to commit the resources needed to develop cost-effective systems that ensure the accuracy and relevance of analytic findings.

If monitoring risk-adjusted clinical outcomes in acute care settings is in its infancy, monitoring risk-adjusted clinical outcomes in outpatient settings has yet to be born. However, patient-derived information about functional status is applicable to the ambulatory environment, and several areas of outpatient care that are well suited to developmental work can provide useful information for both purchasers and providers of care.

First, important chronic conditions can be identified and tracked using objective markers rather than inconstant diagnostic assignment. For instance, in HEDIS 3.0 (see Chapter 37), treatment with insulin or oral hypoglycemic agents is used as a marker for diabetes mellitus. This technique parallels the use of prolonged risk-adjusted length of stay as a marker for important hospital-acquired complications. It will not identify all patients in a category (eg, with diabetes), but it will identify a relatively uniform subset of such patients. Similarly, alterations in patterns of care can be identified and used to mark important outcomes of ambulatory care. To successfully use such alterations as a proxy for ambulatory outcomes, actual baseline patterns must be characterized for individual practitioners. The use of universal external standards is inappropriate for proxy measurement.

Second, patients can be selected for study based on the occurrence of particular adverse outcomes, rather than on diagnoses or findings at the onset of an episode or course of ambulatory care. Care must be taken when interpreting evaluations of care in these instances, because analytic techniques required to draw useful conclusions from these patients differ markedly from standard methods described in the preceding chapter.

Third, measures of adherence to well-substantiated standards of care can substitute for measures of outcomes in situations in which scientific evidence linking processes to outcomes is extremely strong, and the benefits of adherence to standards occur only after considerable time has elapsed. A compendium of such practice standards is available in the *Guide to Clinical Preventive Services* (2nd edition, 1996) prepared by the US Preventive Services Task Force. Recommendations rated "A" (for good evidence supporting intervention) are the best candidates for incorporation in process-based performance measures. When relying on process-based measures, it is important to acknowledge circumstances in which processes must be altered (eg, failure to perform periodic Pap smears after total hysterectomy for benign disease), or where adherence to standards is more difficult due to factors beyond the control of providers of care (eg, administration of vaccines to patients who may be allergic to eggs). This can be accomplished either by excluding these cases from analyses, thereby limiting the applicability of findings, or by risk adjusting for these factors.

Finally, ambulatory care following acute episodes or interventions can be evaluated using methods described in the preceding chapter. For instance, care following discharge from a hospital or following ambulatory surgical procedures can be evaluated by risk adjusting using patient characteristics at the conclusion of the acute care intervention. Similarly, patients entering formal rehabilitation programs are good candidates for external monitoring of risk-adjusted clinical outcomes. In these situations, data for risk adjustment are more readily available because data collection is linked to an acute intervention that requires more intensive clinical monitoring than is generally needed in routine ambulatory settings.

Because of growing concerns with the quality of ambulatory care, tremendous demand exists for plausible systems to monitor outcomes attributable to outpatient management. However, it is important to remember that plausible information may be neither accurate nor valid. To ignore methodological barriers and limitations is to court disaster, since invalid conclusions can result in poor policy, poor management, and poor practice and can ultimately undermine the credibility of outcomes monitoring in general. Only by carefully investing in limited solutions that can serve as prototypes for expanded development and applications can comprehensive monitoring of risk-adjusted outcomes of ambulatory care be achieved.

REFERENCE

1. Naessens JM, Brennan MD, Boberg CJ, et al. Acquired conditions: an improvement to hospital discharge abstracts. *Quality Assurance in Health Care.* 1991; 3(4):259.

MICHAEL PINE, MD, MBA, is president of Michael Pine and Associates and a research associate in the section of cardiology at the University of Chicago. He is a board-certified cardiologist and has served on the medical faculties of Harvard, University of California, and University of Cincinnati. Since founding his consulting firm in 1988, he has helped purchasers, providers, coalitions, insurers, professional associations, and others to measure clinical outcomes and manage and improve the clinical quality of care.

Chapter 36

Introduction to the Management of Clinical Outcomes

Michael Pine

Chapter Outline

- Introduction
- Components of Clinical Processes
- Characterization of Clinical Processes
- Relating Clinical Outcomes to Processes of Care
- Conclusion

INTRODUCTION

Clinical outcomes cannot be managed directly. Attempts to do so will involve doctoring data, which, in contrast to doctoring patients, is not acceptable to most people. Therefore, the management of clinical outcomes must consist of linking these outcomes to processes of care and then managing these processes in order to maintain or improve resulting outcomes.

Any contribution to or component of clinical care can be described as one or more processes. Most health care involves complex combinations of processes that produce a broad array of interrelated outcomes. When a patient must wait to be treated, all the activities (or lack of activity) that contribute to waiting time are processes, including scheduling, testing to arrive at or confirm a diagnosis, and obtaining consent for treatment. On the other hand, outcomes related to these processes include the time the patient actually has to wait for treatment and changes in the patient's mood or clinical condition during the waiting period. The time the patient actually has to wait for treatment also may be considered a surrogate measure that helps characterize the combination of processes involved in patients' seeking and receiving treatment.

COMPONENTS OF CLINICAL PROCESSES

Attempts to manage clinical outcomes often center on creating and implementing algorithms or on describing best clinical practices. Such clinical pathways can be extremely useful for

1. obtaining consensus on appropriate clinical management
2. clarifying current practices
3. monitoring and improving the consistency of health care delivery
4. redesigning clinical care plans to improve effectiveness or efficiency

However, clinical pathways are often either too general or too detailed to provide much assistance in explaining or correcting unsatisfactory clinical outcomes.

To link clinical outcomes and processes successfully, it is useful to begin by dividing processes of care into three distinct components as illustrated in Figure 36–1. These components are (1) judgment, (2) technique, and (3) style.

Judgment includes all clinical decisions that have a consistent, measurable effect on one or more clinical outcomes. *Technique* describes the manner in which judgments are implemented. Good technique often cannot compensate for bad judgment, and bad technique may produce poor outcomes even when initial judgments were correct. Good judgment makes optimum use of resources available. For instance, the most efficacious procedure overall (ie, the procedure that, in the best hands, produces the best results) may not be the best choice in a specific setting. If a patient cannot be referred to another setting for care, good judgment will select, not the most efficacious procedure, but the procedure that will give the best results in the setting in which the patient is receiving care. Risk-adjusted clinical outcomes are the product of the interaction of judgment and technique in discrete clinical settings.

Style describes differences in clinical practice that do not have consistent, measurable effects on clinical outcomes. Stylistic differences may be very obvious and may incite controversy. However, confusing stylistic issues with judgment or technique issues will guarantee the failure of a quality improvement initiative.

Clinical pathways (see Chapter 18 for additional discussion of critical pathways in clinical care) often address judgment, technique, and style simultaneously. However, serious efforts to link clinical outcomes to processes of care must focus on critical points of judgment or technique within the scope of a clinical pathway. There are many reasons for selecting a particular style of practice, and consistency in style can help ensure uniformly high-quality care. But clinical outcomes are managed best by concentrating on a limited number of critical points; then, analysts and decision makers can better identify actionable links between outcomes and processes. Clinicians and managers can use the insights gained to effect changes that have a high probability of altering the substance, rather than just the form, of health care delivery.

CHARACTERIZATION OF CLINICAL PROCESSES

Measures of clinical processes, like measures of clinical outcomes, may be discrete or continuous. Discrete measures generally address specific judgmental issues (eg, Should the patient receive Drug A, Drug B, or Drug C? Should cardiac catheterization be performed? Should the patient be hospitalized? Should a Caesarean section be performed? Should the patient be referred to a specialist?).

Continuous measures generally characterize a combination of judgment and technique (eg, How long did a procedure last? How many prenatal visits preceded a term delivery? How long did a patient remain in the intensive care unit? How long after an operation was a patient extubated?).

Often, critical points in care can be highlighted by tracking the occurrence of clinical milestones. These milestones are important points on the road to a clinical outcome (eg, resumption of ambulation after orthopaedic surgery, extubation after general anesthesia, dis-

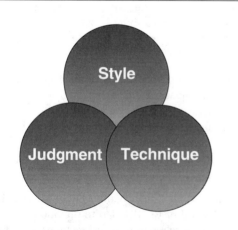

Figure 36–1 Components of Processes of Care. Courtesy of Michael Pine and Associates, Inc, 1998, Chicago, Illinois.

continuation of antibiotics after treatment for acute bronchitis, transfer to a step-down unit after acute myocardial infarction, discontinuation of steroids after an exacerbation of asthma). Clinical milestones can be monitored as continuous process measures.

The creation of process indicators parallels the creation of outcome indicators described above. Since clinical judgment is not absolute and since technique may vary depending upon a patient's intrinsic characteristics and condition, risk adjustment of process indicators often is as appropriate as risk adjustment of outcome indicators. Methods for developing risk-adjustment models are similar for process indicators and outcome indicators (described above).

Characterization of discrete process indicators is identical to characterization of discrete outcome indicators. Observed and predicted rates are computed and compared for a discrete outcome indicator. Characterization of continuous process indicators parallels characterization of continuous outcome indicators, but additional characterization is needed to facilitate later analyses. Three comparative measures are recommended, as illustrated in Figures 36–2 through 36–4, for risk-adjusted extubation time after coronary artery bypass graft (CABG) surgery for nine hospitals in the HealthyHeart Cardiac Alliance.

The first measure, as illustrated in Figure 36–2, compares average observed and predicted values for the indicator in routine patients (ie, patients without adverse outcomes) after removal of unusual values (ie, those that are outside of confidence limits derived from a control chart of standardized values). This indicator measures the average risk-adjusted value ordinarily achieved in routine patients for the process being characterized.

A second measure, illustrated in Figure 36–3, compares short-term variations in standardized (ie, risk-adjusted) values for the indicator. To derive this measure, standard deviations are calculated for successive groups of standardized values for a predetermined number of consecutive routine cases (ie, cases without adverse outcomes or unusual standardized values of the measure). These standard deviations are used to create a control chart. Confidence limits are derived using standard techniques of statistical process control. The size of these confidence limits is used as a measure of the degree of short-term variation. Measures of short-term variation are not risk adjusted; hence, all predicted values in Figure 36–3 are identical. This indicator measures the ordinary amount of variability in the process being characterized.

Finally, as illustrated in Figure 36–4, the percentage of routine patients (ie, patients without

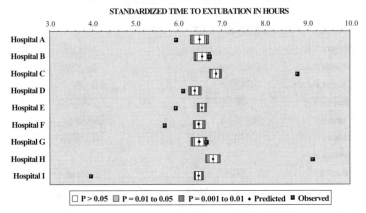

Figure 36–2 Routine Risk-Adjusted Average Extubation Times after CABG Surgery in Patients Without Adverse Outcomes. Courtesy of Michael Pine and Associates, Inc, 1998, Chicago, Illinois.

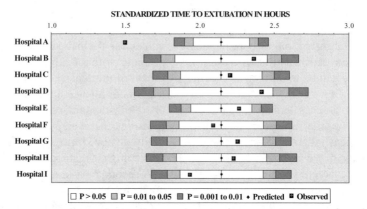

Figure 36–3 Variations in Standardized Routine Extubation Times after CABG Surgery in Patients Without Adverse Outcomes. Courtesy of Michael Pine and Associates, Inc, 1998, Chicago, Illinois.

adverse outcomes) that had unusual (eg, prolonged) standardized values for the indicator is computed and compared to the value predicted based on an external standard. This indicator measures how often the ordinary process is not achieved in routine patients.

Each of the three measures described above applies to routine patients who do not have confounding adverse outcomes. Changes in these measures for patients with adverse outcomes can provide clues about how adverse clinical outcomes may be linked to critical processes of care.

RELATING CLINICAL OUTCOMES TO PROCESSES OF CARE

Methods associated with process improvement and clinical research generally concentrate on investigating how specific processes of care affect clinical outcomes. This section introduces several methods to identify processes of care that are responsible for differences in measured risk-adjusted outcomes.

The first method focuses on the distribution and timing of initial complications associated with adverse outcomes of clinical care. By lim-

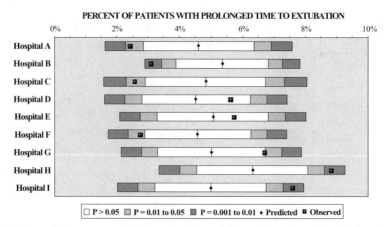

Figure 36–4 Risk-Adjusted Percentages of Patients Without Adverse Outcomes Who Had Prolonged Extubation Times after CABG Surgery. Courtesy of Michael Pine and Associates, Inc, 1998, Chicago, Illinois.

iting this investigation to patients who have experienced important adverse outcomes, the effect of reporting biases on analytic findings can be reduced. By focusing on initial events rather than on later sequelae, the analysis can focus on potential root causes rather than on complicating factors. By comparing findings for an individual provider or organization with findings for a reference population and by adjusting for the individual provider's or organization's rate of adverse outcomes, decision makers can gain valuable insights into underlying causes of superior or unsatisfactory performance. They also can identify (1) isolated problem areas when overall performance is average or above average and (2) isolated areas of excellence when overall performance is average or below average.

Findings using this method are illustrated in Figures 36–5 and 36–6. In these illustrations, the mortality associated with CABG surgery is the adverse outcome being evaluated. Cutemup Regional Medical Center's observed mortality rate is more than one third higher than predicted. Figure 36–5 demonstrates that this excess mortality is associated with initial cardiopulmonary complications, many of which can be attributed to problems associated with the surgical procedure itself. Consistent with this observation, Figure 36–6 demonstrates that excess mortality is associated almost entirely with initial complications that occur within a day of operation. With these findings, attention can be directed to potential problems in judgment and technique associated with operative and early postoperative clinical management.

A second method evaluates the effect of ordinary variation in process on risk-adjusted clinical outcomes. These analyses focus on general performance rather than on performance by individual providers or organizations. Therefore, measurements of process are standardized to obliterate the effect of both intrinsic patient risk and differences in clinical practice. Findings are applicable to all settings from which data have been obtained.

This method is illustrated in Figures 36–7 through 36–9. Using data from the HealthyHeart Cardiac Alliance, the analyses evaluate the association between standardized extubation times

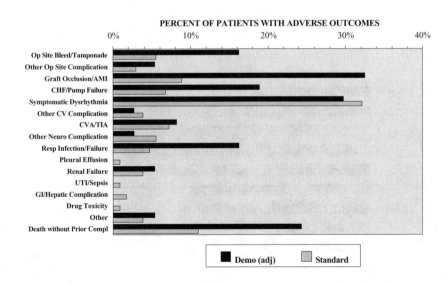

Figure 36–5 Comparison of Adjusted Proportions of Specific Initial Complications among Inpatients Who Died During or after CABG Surgery at Cutemup Regional Medical Center and at All Hospitals in the HealthyHeart Cardiac Alliance. Courtesy of Michael Pine and Associates, Inc, 1998, Chicago, Illinois.

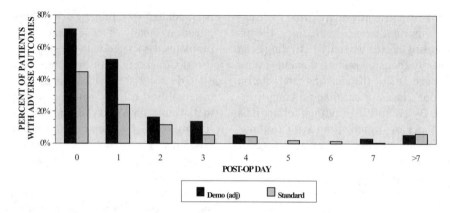

Figure 36–6 Comparison of Times of Occurrence of Initial Complications among Inpatients Who Died During or after CABG Surgery at Cutemup Regional Medical Center and at All Hospitals in the HealthyHeart Cardiac Alliance. Courtesy of Michael Pine and Associates, Inc, 1998, Chicago, Illinois.

after CABG surgery and both risk-adjusted adverse outcomes and risk-adjusted postoperative lengths of stay.

Figure 36–7 shows the distribution of standardized extubation times after CABG surgery for all hospitals in the HealthyHeart Cardiac Alliance. Slightly more than 5% of these patients have standardized extubation times that exceeded by more than three standard deviations the average value for routine patients at the hospital at which they were treated.

Figure 36–8 shows a steady rise in adverse outcome rates as standardized extubation times increase above 5 hours, even when these times are not extraordinary for individual providers or organizations. This finding suggests that more consistent early extubation may reduce risk-adjusted adverse outcome rates across the entire Alliance. The marked increase in risk-adjusted adverse outcome rate with prolonged extubation time is consistent with the general occurrence of complications that result both in

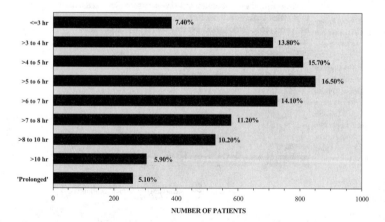

Figure 36–7 Distribution of Standardized Extubation Times after CABG Surgery. Courtesy of Michael Pine and Associates, Inc, 1998, Chicago, Illinois.

Introduction to the Management of Clinical Outcomes 507

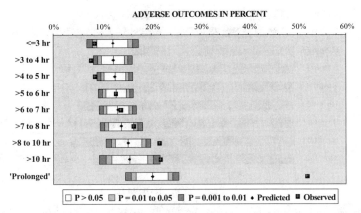

Figure 36–8 Relation of Risk-Adjusted Adverse Outcome Rates to Standardized Extubation Times after CABG Surgery. Courtesy of Michael Pine and Associates, Inc, 1998, Chicago, Illinois.

prolonged extubation times and in adverse outcomes.

Figure 36–9 shows a sudden rise in adverse outcome rates as standardized extubation times increase above 8 hours, even when these times are not extraordinary for individual providers or organizations. This finding suggests that, at all hospitals in the Alliance, even late extubation that does not qualify as prolonged may be associated with longer risk-adjusted postoperative lengths of stay in patients who do not experience adverse outcomes. On the other hand, average extubation times are not associated with any increase in routine risk-adjusted postoperative lengths of stay.

A third method evaluates potential provider-specific effects of extraordinary variation in processes on risk-adjusted clinical outcomes. For individual providers, patients who had extraordinary variation in a process of care are evaluated by comparing observed clinical outcomes to outcomes predicted after adjusting for the following:

1. intrinsic patient-specific risk of the clinical outcome

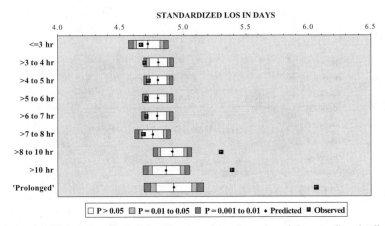

Figure 36–9 Relation of Risk-Adjusted Routine Postoperative Lengths of Stay to Standardized Extubation Times after CABG Surgery. Courtesy of Michael Pine and Associates, Inc, 1998, Chicago, Illinois.

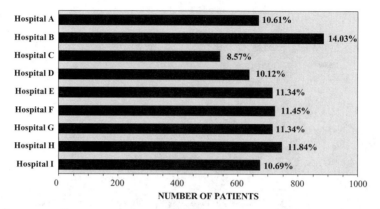

Figure 36–10 Distribution of Patients Undergoing CABG Surgery in 1 Year. Courtesy of Michael Pine and Associates, Inc, 1998, Chicago, Illinois.

2. the overall association of the clinical outcome and extraordinary variation in the process of care
3. the provider-specific relation between observed and predicted clinical outcomes among patients for whom the process of care being studied was ordinary (ie, standardized values for the process were within provider-specific confidence limits)

Important and statistically significant differences between observed and predicted clinical outcomes in patients with extraordinary variation in a process of care suggest that, for the provider or organization being studied, the process has a direct relation to the clinical outcome beyond the aggregate relationship for providers or organizations as a group. Identification of such a relationship enables decision makers to concentrate on reinforcing or altering processes that are likely to be having direct effects on clinical outcomes of interest to them.

This method is illustrated in Figures 36–10 through 36–12, which evaluate the association between prolonged standardized (ie, risk-adjusted) extubation times after CABG surgery and risk-adjusted adverse outcome rates for nine hospitals in the HealthyHeart Cardiac Alliance.

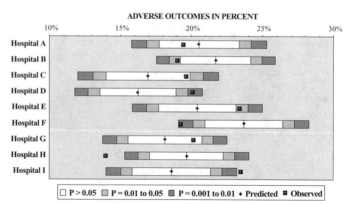

Figure 36–11 Risk-Adjusted Adverse Outcome Rates after CABG Surgery. Courtesy of Michael Pine and Associates, Inc, 1998, Chicago, Illinois.

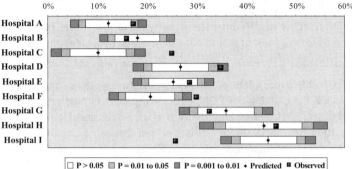

Figure 36–12 Risk-Adjusted Percentages of Patients with Adverse Outcomes Who Had Prolonged Extubation Times after CABG Surgery. Courtesy of Michael Pine and Associates, Inc, 1998, Chicago, Illinois.

Figure 36–10 shows the number of patients undergoing CABG surgery in 1 year at each hospital. Figure 36–11 shows risk-adjusted adverse outcome rates for patients undergoing CABG surgery at each hospital. Rates at Hospitals B, F, and H are significantly lower than predicted; rates at Hospitals D, E, and I are significantly higher than predicted. Figure 36–12 shows risk-adjusted adverse outcome rates for patients who had prolonged standardized extubation times after undergoing CABG surgery at each hospital. Risk adjustment was performed to account for (1) intrinsic patient-specific risk of an adverse outcome after CABG surgery, (2) the overall association of adverse outcomes after CABG surgery and prolongation of standardized extubation times, and (3) the provider-specific relation between observed and predicted adverse outcome rates in patients who had ordinary standardized extubation times after CABG surgery. Important and significantly higher than predicted rates of adverse outcomes in Hospitals A, C, D, and F suggest that, in patients undergoing CABG surgery, the process of extubation and associated respiratory issues are of particular interest at these facilities. The important, significantly lower than predicted rate of adverse outcomes in Hospital I suggests that the high risk-adjusted rate of adverse outcomes observed at that hospital (Figure 36–11) is not directly related to the process of extubation and associated respiratory issues.

In combination, the three methods described in this section can suggest and support hypotheses about how clinical outcomes can be improved by altering specific processes of care. They provide a powerful supplement to clinical and managerial insight and judgment, to standard methods of statistical quality control and process improvement, and to more familiar methods of clinical investigation.

CONCLUSION

Clinical outcomes measurement (ie, external monitoring) can provide valuable guidance to patients, purchasers, and providers of health care. Internal monitoring in conjunction with clinical process control and improvement can be combined into programs of clinical outcomes management that can improve the effectiveness and efficiency of clinical care and can provide a competitive edge for providers and organizations that utilize them successfully. However, as in many highly technical areas, casual approaches to clinical outcomes measurement and management can be disastrous. Poorly designed and executed programs can demonstrate quickly the wisdom behind the old adage: it isn't what you don't know that hurts you; it's what you know that isn't so.

On the other hand, well-designed and executed programs of outcomes measurement and management can provide insights that would otherwise be unobtainable. The have a special authority to inform and educate, because they describe an organization's performance accurately, without distortion. Properly used, they embody the true spirit and purpose of managed care.

MICHAEL PINE, MD, MBA, is president of Michael Pine and Associates and a research associate in the section of cardiology at the University of Chicago. He is a board-certified cardiologist and has served on the medical faculties of Harvard, University of California, and University of Cincinnati. Since founding his consulting firm in 1988, he has helped purchasers, providers, coalitions, insurers, professional associations, and others to measure clinical outcomes and manage and improve the clinical quality of care.

PART XII

Use of Information in Care Management

Best practices in medical management are data and information driven. Data and information show medical managers where to focus their attention and what happens when they do. The use of information generally (but never exclusively) is focused on one of two broad categories: provider profiling and everything else. That is exactly how the information is presented in Part XII.

CHAPTER 37

Using Data in Medical Management

Peter R. Kongstvedt

Chapter Outline

- Introduction
- General Requirements for Using Data To Manage the Health Care Delivery System
- Focus
- Hospital Utilization Reports
- Outpatient Utilization
- Provider Profiling
- Conclusion

INTRODUCTION

Using data and information is rapidly becoming one of the most important components of managing health care. A medical manager's ability to use data and information intelligently to improve health care delivery systems will ultimately separate excellent plans from only adequate ones. This is not to say that other medical management activities are unimportant; just the opposite, it is the use of data that allows those other activities to be carried out more effectively. It is important to bear in mind, however, that information is not magic. Data and information are merely powerful tools to help the medical manager carry out necessary functions.

This chapter should be read in the context of a managed care plan's specific needs and in conjunction with the information presented in other chapters. The chapter will not review all reports that may be produced by a plan's management information system (MIS or IS) but rather concentrate on those reports specific to utilization and medical management that will help medical directors carry out their jobs. Clearly, the need for reports will be influenced by a plan's configuration and its controls and incentives. Administrators may find that not all the reports discussed in this chapter are helpful, or that other utilization reports they need to use are not discussed here. It is up to the medical director to decide what reports are necessary, and it is up to the director of MIS to provide them.

GENERAL REQUIREMENTS FOR USING DATA TO MANAGE THE HEALTH CARE DELIVERY SYSTEM

Data Characteristics

To use data for managing health care costs, certain basic requirements must be met. First, the data must have integrity. Errors are common, especially in data that require manual entry (ie,

---

This chapter is adapted from PR Kongstvedt, Using Data in Medical Management, in *The Managed Health Care Handbook*, 3rd ed, PR Kongstvedt, ed, pp 440–452, © 1996, Aspen Publishers, Inc.

data entered via keystrokes); such errors must be prevented when possible, and identified and corrected when present. In some plans, especially large insurance companies, the database may not even use all the available information; for example, in order to hold down personnel costs, the plan may only key in the first three digits of the diagnostic code (each keystroke costs money!) and thus may not be able to refine diagnostic data.

It is not unusual for data to come from multiple sources. For example, a health plan may use more than one system to administer different activities (eg, enrollment and billing on one system, general ledger on another, utilization management on another, claims on still another). It is also possible that multiple plans, or a combination of a plan and a provider system such as an integrated delivery system (IDS), will want to combine data to improve the robustness of the database. In such cases, the data must be integrated into a common database. To integrate data successfully, there must be a standardized format for use in data analyses.

Data must be made consistent among providers. Providers may code differently for the same procedure, or a hospital may code an event differently than the attending physician does. Diagnostic coding is particularly problematic when one is analyzing data from physician outpatient reports. Because diagnostic coding is not important in determining what a physician is paid (except for those claims systems that match diagnostic code to procedure code), there is great laxity in diagnostic coding for office visits. Procedure coding tends to be more accurate because there is a direct relationship between what a provider codes as having been performed and what the provider gets paid (except in capitated systems). Accuracy, however, does not rule out creative coding, common upcoding, or even fraud, resulting in deliberate coding inconsistencies. For example, one surgeon may bill for a hysterectomy while another surgeon in the same situation may bill for an exploratory laparotomy, removal of the uterus, removal of the ovaries, and lysis of adhesions, all of which generate a fee. The need for consistency may mean having to change or otherwise modify data to force conformance of meaning.

Data must also be valid: They must actually mean what you think they mean. Even when there is great attention to diagnostic coding, the reason for the visit may not be related to everything done during the visit (eg, a patient is seen with the diagnosis of hypertension but also gets a hearing test), or the diagnostic code may not be the same as the underlying disease (eg, a patient is seen for an upper respiratory infection but the relevant diagnosis is emphysema). In addition to coding validity, it is important to validate data against other potential sources of the same data; for example, physician identification data may be kept in two separate databases that may not match.

The measures must be meaningful. It is of no value (other than academic) to measure things that have no real impact on the plan's ability to manage the system or a physician's ability to practice effectively. Even worse, there is potential harm in producing reports that purport to mean one thing but really mean another.

The sample size must be adequate. Measuring encounters or referral statistics by physician is of little value if a physician has only 20 members in the panel. Even large databases may fall prey to this problem if the claims and clinical data are spread over too large a provider base, so that there are insufficient data for any given provider. Even when there are sufficient outpatient data for participating primary care physicians (PCPs), there frequently are insufficient data regarding inpatient admissions to be meaningful, even in large insurance claims databases.[1,2]

The data must encompass an adequate time period. Simple snapshots in time do not reveal the true picture. This is particularly important when one is looking at total health care resource consumption of patients. This is even more important when one is trying to determine whether a provider's behavior is consistent. Analyses that encompass very long periods of time need to be viewed with the knowledge that practice patterns and behavior do indeed change over time, and that must be taken into account when comparing long time periods to short ones for the same types of episodes.

General User Needs

End users working with data must find the data useful and accessible. Raw data, for instance, has no immediate value to the typical manager. Users must be able to access usable data as directly as possible. If a manager must stand in line to supplicate the priests of MIS in order to get critical information, opportunities will be lost. Access must also be as timely as possible, and the system should be as easy to use as possible.

Systems should also allow managers to have considerable flexibility when working with data. If a manager must accept a hard-coded report and cannot cut the data in another fashion without a lot of wasted time and coding expense, then that manager will be trapped into managing only with whatever information the programmers have allowed for.

Ability To Use System Data with Other Tools

It is important that managers be able to obtain data from the system and use that data with other analytic tools. Advanced statistical analysis programs can be very useful to the medical department when managers are performing practice profiling (discussed below) or other trend analysis. The ability to export or download data into other plan programs such as spreadsheets or database programs in personal computers is also desirable. The ability to transmit analyzed data to physicians' offices is a feature that will become important over time.

Format

How reports are formatted depends on taste and the MIS department's abilities. The easiest type of report for MIS to produce is one that tabulates columns of numbers. That is also usually the type most deadly to a busy manager. An already overburdened medical director has better things to do than sift through 20 pages of printout looking at raw numbers of referrals for each physician to get an idea of the referral rate.

The best report formats usually fit onto one or two sheets of paper. Those reports should summarize the important data, indicate the outliers and deviations from the norm (or from preset standards), and indicate whether the manager will need to seek more detail. If managers need the raw data, they can always ask for them. For example, a two-page report giving the overall referral rate for the plan and the annualized referral rate per 1,000 members per year for each PCP for the month and the year to date may be sufficient. If there are PCPs who are grossly over the norm, the medical director can then ask for the detail behind the report.

Graphic reports (especially color graphics) are highly useful for conveying large amounts of information quickly to busy managers and providers, especially ones who are not used to looking at reports. Unfortunately, most mainframe computer systems are not set up to produce graphic reports, so data must be entered (or downloaded and then imported) into a personal computer before the graphs can be produced. This cumbersome process limits the production of these reports. As computers and software become more sophisticated and interlinked through client/server systems, production of graphic reports will become more common.

Routine and Ad Hoc Reports

To manage information wisely, managers need to decide which reports they want on a routine basis and which reports they want on an ad hoc basis. For example, in a stable open panel plan, it is unnecessary for the medical director to receive a monthly report listing the recruiting activity or membership for each participating physician. That information, if it is needed, could be provided once per quarter. On the other hand, the medical director or associate medical director will usually want a hospital report on a daily basis.

The basic rule of thumb is to ask for routine reports for those functions that require constant management and will provide sufficient data to spot trends and aberrations. Routine reports should allow administrators to decide when to focus on specific areas for further investigation. For example, watching the trend in referral costs could reveal an upswing that would result in an administrator requesting detail about utilization by specialty. That in turn could lead to a need to look at utilization by individual providers in a single specialty. Managers should save the highly detailed reports for infrequent intervals or ad hoc requests. Time spent deciphering cryptic reports is time spent not managing.

Further discussion of useful summary reports follows. The message here is that reports for busy managers should be concise, readable, and easily interpreted and allow the manager to request further detail as needed. One common problem is too much detail. Judging by the stacks of computer printouts that are seen holding up the ceiling in many offices, reports in some plans must be valued by weight. It is easy to believe that the more data and detail the better. Too much detail, and the manager might miss seeing the forest for the trees, and spend more time grinding through reports than managing. Computers are wonderful tools, but they can smother you with data. Know what to ask for and when to ask for it.

FOCUS

Reports may be focused in a variety of ways to reveal useful information. For example, the overall admission rate for the plan may be normal, but a report focusing on where the patients are admitted may reveal that most of the admissions are to high-cost or even to nonparticipating hospitals. What follows is a general guide to the different ways in which data can be focused.

Plan Average

Plan average simply looks at the average performance for the entire plan. It is useful in that it will relate closely to the plan's financial performance. For example, if the plan is over budget in medical expense, a plan average report that reveals hospital admissions to be greatly over budget will give management its initial focus. Plan average also allows for comparative data between plans that may have somewhat different care delivery arrangements.

Plan average is limited because it is relatively insensitive to specific causes of problems. That can be an advantage in some circumstances, however. Some plans manage by trying to keep performance clustered around a norm, but that norm can sometimes be mediocre. If the plan average reports and the provider-specific reports are similar (ie, there are no real outliers in performance), and if the plan is not doing as well as it should, then it is clear that there is a general problem of attitude or skills in the managers themselves and not a problem with a few recalcitrant providers or hospitals.

Plan average reports are frequently required by regulatory agencies and are also useful for reporting the overall performance of the plan to participating physicians and corporate parents. Plan average reports also function as the backdrop against which other reports are viewed. A plan with multiple lines of business such as commercial, Medicare, and Medicaid will likely create additional plan average reports that focus on each line of business.

Health Center, Individual Practice Association, Provider Organization, or Geographically Related Center

The purpose of this focus is to provide midlevel managers with data for their own areas of responsibility. In many plans, especially large or geographically diverse ones, it is common to divide up responsibility into manageable units. The problem of span of control in large or diverse plans can be very real. In closed panels, units often encompass a health center or a small number of geographically related health centers. In open panels, units may be discrete multiple individual practice associations (IPAs), subunits within the overall health plan such as pools of doctors (PODs), or geographically divided territories. In plans that contract with IDSs that are vertically integrated, physician-hospital organizations (PHOs), or management services organizations (MSOs), it will be important to develop reports focused on each IDS.

Individual Physician

Most managed care plans produce reports that focus on individual physicians. This may refer to PCPs who are functioning as gatekeepers or care coordinators but may apply equally to open access health maintenance organizations (HMOs) or preferred provider organizations (PPOs). Virtually all the types of utilization reports discussed later in this chapter can be oriented to focus on individual physicians.

Physicians become understandably paranoid about the plethora of reports that are produced about them. They feel that they are being judged by machines or by standards that fail to take into account any extenuating circumstances and that their fate will be decided on the basis of sterile reports. In truth, it is the ability to report the behavior of individual physicians that provides managed care plans with their most powerful tool and physicians with their greatest source of both concern and potential help.

Care must be taken when one is using physician-specific reports. The medical director must look behind the data of the report for the reasons for the reported performance. This is not to say that any behavior should be rationalized. Rather, this is to say that individual physician performance reports need to be used intelligently and properly.

Service or Vendor Type

This type of report refers to the entity delivering the service (eg, a hospital or a type of referral specialist). Focusing reports on those delivering the service (sometimes referred to as vendors) will be of great value when one is negotiating contracts and will allow for improved utilization control. These types of reports also help focus on areas where attention should be paid. Remember Sutton's Law: Go where the money is!

Premium Source Group

The premium source group focus tracks utilization and other data by enrolled group. This focus most frequently applies to individual commercial groups (eg, Wendy's Widget Corp), but it can also apply to any group of enrollees whose premiums come from a common source (eg, Medicare or Medicaid). For those plans that are allowed group benefits premiums, it will be necessary to develop the actual cost experience; even for those plans that must accept governmental (and nonnegotiable) rates, these data will tell you whether there is a problem with a group that may need to be addressed. Also, some large employers are demanding such data as a requisite for offering plans to their employees. Medicare risk plans must provide Health Plan Employer Data and Information Set (HEDIS) 3.0 reports, but there are plenty of non-HEDIS reports to produce as well. Exhibit 37–1 illustrates the HEDIS 3.0 data set.

HOSPITAL UTILIZATION REPORTS

Routine hospital utilization management reports may be divided into two categories: the daily log and monthly summaries. Many plans now automate their utilization management systems. In addition to producing reports as discussed below, these systems allow for on-line access to far more information than would be practical on a printed report. Nevertheless, printed reports regarding hospital utilization may remain useful to medical managers, who often need to review reports in a manner better done and for a length of time better spent away from the computer.

Daily Log

It is almost a requirement for a managed care plan to produce a daily hospital log. This docu-

Exhibit 37-1 HEDIS 3.0/1998 Reporting and Testing Set Measures

I. Effectiveness of Care
Reporting Set Measures
  Advising smokers to quit
  Beta blocker treatment after a heart attack
  The health of seniors
  Eye exams for people with diabetes
  Flu shots for older adults
  Cervical cancer screening
  Breast cancer screening
  Childhood immunization status
  Adolescent immunization status
  Prenatal care in the first trimester
  Low birthweight babies
  Check-ups after delivery
  Follow up after hospitalization for mental illness
Testing Set Measures
  Number of people in the plan who smoke
  Smokers who quit
  Flu shots for high-risk adults
  Cholesterol management of patients hospitalized after coronary artery disease
  Aspirin treatment after a heart attack
  Outpatient care of patients hospitalized for heart failure
  Controlling high blood pressure
  Prevention of stroke in people with atrial fibrillation
  Colorectal cancer screening
  Follow up after an abnormal Pap smear
  Follow up after an abnormal mammogram
  Assessment of how breast cancer therapy affects the patient's ability to function
  Substance counseling for adolescents
  Availability of medication management and psychotherapy for patients with schizophrenia
  Patient satisfaction with mental health care
  Screening for chemical dependency
  Appropriate use of psychotherapeutic medications
  Continuation of depression treatment
  Treating children's ear infections
  Family visits for children undergoing mental health treatment
  Monitoring diabetes patients
  Chlamydia screening
  Prescription of antibiotics for the prevention of HIV-related pneumonia
  Use of appropriate medications for people with asthma

II. Access/Availability of Care
Reporting Set Measures
  Availability of primary care providers
  Children's access to primary care providers
  Availability of behavioral health providers
  Annual dental visit
  Availability of dentists
  Adults' access to preventive/ambulatory health services
  Initiation of prenatal care
  Availability of obstetrical/prenatal care providers
  Low birthweight deliveries at facilities for high-risk deliveries and neonates
  Availability of language interpretation services
Testing Set Measures
  Problems with obtaining care
III. Satisfaction with the Experience of Care
Reporting Set
  Satisfaction survey
Testing Set
  Consumer Assessments of Health Plans Study (CAHPS)
  Disenrollment survey
  Satisfaction with breast cancer treatment
IV. Health Plan Stability
Reporting Set
  Disenrollment
  Provider turnover
  Indicators of financial stability
  Years in business/total membership
V. Use of Services
Reporting Set
  Well-child visits in the first 15 months of life
  Well-child visits in the third, fourth, fifth, and sixth year of life
  Adolescent well-care visit
  Frequency of selected procedures
  Inpatient utilization—nonacute care
  Inpatient utilization—general hospital/acute care
  Ambulatory care
  Caesarean section and vaginal birth after Caesarean rate (VBAC rate)
  Discharge and average length of stay for females in maternity care
  Births and average length of stay, newborns
  Frequency of ongoing prenatal care

continues

Exhibit 37–1 continued

> Mental health utilization—percentage of members receiving inpatient, day/night, and ambulatory services
> Readmission for specified mental health disorders
> Chemical dependency utilization—percentage of members receiving inpatient, day/night care, and ambulatory services
> Mental health utilization—inpatient discharges and average length of stay
> Readmission for chemical dependency
> Outpatient drug utilization
> Testing Set
>   Use of behavioral services
> VI. Cost of Care
> Reporting Set
>   High-occurrence/high-cost DRGs
>   Rate trends
>
> Testing Set
>   Health plan costs per member per month
> VII. Informed Health Care Choices
> Testing Set
>   Counseling women about hormone replacement therapy
> VIII. Health Plan Descriptive Information
> Reporting Set
>   Board certification/residency completion
>   Provider compensation
>   Arrangements with public health, educational, and social service organizations
>   Weeks of pregnancy at time of enrollment
>   Diversity of Medicaid membership
>   Unduplicated count of Medicaid members
>   Enrollment by payer (member years/months)
>   Total enrollment
>
> *Note:* HEDIS 3.0/1998 is a registered trademark of the National Committee for Quality Assurance.
>
> *Source:* Reprinted with permission from the National Committee for Quality Assurance; *HEDIS 3.0/1998, Volume I: Narrative, What's in It and Why It Matters*, pp 34–37, © 1997 by National Committee for Quality Assurance.

ment serves as a working tool for the utilization management nurse and the medical director in controlling institutional utilization. It should be designed to provide the necessary information to manage current or prospective cases actively. Data should be sorted and printed by whatever management criteria make sense. For example, you may wish to print each hospital's census separately so that the utilization review nurse can take it when making hospital rounds. In plans where associate medical directors will have primary responsibility, you may want to print the log so that it sorts by geographic region, IPA, IDS, or health center.

Any daily log should include at least the elements listed in Exhibit 37–2. Additional daily log information that is useful in most health plans is listed in Exhibit 37–3.

Monthly Summary

A monthly summary report of hospital utilization should also be produced. This differs somewhat from the daily log because it is used to identify patterns for overall management rather than to serve as a mechanism for performing concurrent utilization review. A monthly report might include the data illustrated in Exhibit 37–4 for both the month ended and the year to date.

Exhibit 37–2 Minimum Data Elements for a Daily Hospital Log

> Current census
> - Name of patient
> - Hospital
> - Diagnosis and procedures
> - PCP
> - Admitting physician
> - Consultants or specialists
> - Admission date
> - Length of stay to date
> - Free-text narrative with clinical information
> - In-network compared to out-of-network status
>
> Hospital statistics
> - Bed days per 1,000 members today
> - Bed days per 1,000 members month to date
>
> Prospective admits and outpatient surgeries

Exhibit 37–3 Additional Useful Data Elements for a Daily Hospital Log

> Service type (as part of current census)
> - Medicine
> - Surgery
> - Pediatrics
> - Gynecologic surgery
> - Obstetrics
> - Mental health
> - Chemical dependency
> - Intensive care unit/cardiac care unit
> - Neonatal intensive care unit
> - Rehabilitation
> - Outpatient surgery
>
> Estimated length of stay or maximum length of stay
>
> Admissions and discharges today and month to date
>
> Authorization or denial status
>
> Catastrophic case report
>
> Line of business code
> - Commercial
> - Medicare
> - Medicaid
> - Self-insured vs. fully insured
> - Special accounts

Exhibit 37–4 Sample Data Elements for a Monthly Summary of Hospital Utilization

> Plan statistics
> - Bed days per 1,000 members
> - Admissions per 1,000 members
> - Average length of stay
> - Average per diem cost
> - Average per case (per admission) cost
> - Emergency department visits and average cost
>
> Hospital- and provider-specific statistics
> - Bed days per 1,000 members
> - Admissions per 1,000 members
> - Average length of stay
> - Average per diem cost
> - Average per case (per admission) cost
> - Emergency department visits and average cost
>
> Statistics by service type (eg, intensive care unit, med/surg, rehab)
> - Bed days per 1,000 members
> - Admissions per 1,000 members
> - Average length of stay
> - Average per diem cost
> - Average per case (per admission) cost
>
> Retrospective authorizations
>
> Pended cases for review
>
> In-network compared to out-of-network statistics
>
> Number and percentage of denied days
>
> *Note:* The plan will want to produce these statistics not only for the entire plan, but for major lines of business as well (ie, commercial, Medicare, Medicaid, self-insured vs. fully insured, and so forth).

OUTPATIENT UTILIZATION

Although daily reports are necessary for controlling hospital utilization, in only the most tightly managed health plans will they be necessary for controlling outpatient utilization. In general, outpatient utilization control is usually best done by using monthly reports, both routine and ad hoc. Reports should include data both for the month ended and for the year to date. Data may also be reported by month on a 12-month rolling basis. Data for such reports might include elements as illustrated in Exhibit 37–5, depending on the needs of medical management.

Categories of outpatient or ambulatory care may be divided into several components, each with unique characteristics. Office visits for primary care, including any testing or procedures, is one such category, as is the related category of office visits for specialty care. Ambulatory procedures are a different matter, however, as is the setting for the procedure. The identical procedure may be performed in a physician's office, an ambulatory care center, or the outpatient department of a hospital.

Some plans have addressed the issue of ambulatory care, especially outpatient procedures, by using statistical groupings. One method is ambulatory patient groups (APGs), a method developed under contract by 3M Systems for the Health Care Financing Adminis-

Exhibit 37–5 Sample Data for a Monthly Summary of Outpatient Utilization

Primary care encounter rates
- Visits per day (closed panels only)
- Visits per member per year (annualized)
- Percentage of new visits
- Revisit interval rates (to look for churning)

Preventive care
- Immunization rates
- Mammography
- Pap smears
- Other

Laboratory/pathology utilization per visit

Radiology utilization per visit
- Total
- Focused (eg, magnetic resonance imaging)

Prescriptions
- Prescriptions per visit or prescriptions per member per year
- Average cost per prescription
- Percentage generic

Referral utilization
- Referral rate per 100 primary care visits or per 1,000 members per year
- Comparison of PCP referral rate to peer group

- Initial referrals compared only to total referral visits
- Cost per referral by PCP, plan average, and specialty
- Number of visits and cost by specialty
  - Top specialty referrals for each PCP
  - Average cost per visit
  - Per member per month cost by specialty

Out-of-network specialty care in point of service plans
- Percentage of total specialty care
- Cost
- Specialty and utilization categories

Ambulatory procedures
- By ambulatory patient groups (APGs)
- By ambulatory care groups (ACGs) and ambulatory diagnosis groups (ADGs)
- By diagnostic or procedure code

Ancillary care
- Physical therapy and other rehabilitation therapies
- Podiatry
- Eye care
- Oral surgery
- Other

Note: The plan will want to produce these statistics not only for the entire plan, but for major lines of business as well (ie, commercial, Medicare, Medicaid, self-insured vs. fully insured, and so forth).

---

tration (HCFA) for use in Medicare (Medicare plans to introduce them in the next several years), but a number of private health plans have adopted them for reimbursement purposes. APGs are to outpatient services what diagnosis-related groups (DRGs) are to inpatient ones, although APGs are based on procedures rather than simply on diagnoses and are considerably more complex. Under APGs, all the services associated with a given outpatient procedure or visit are bundled into the APG reimbursement. More than one APG may be billed if more than one procedure is performed, but there is significant discounting for additional APGs. There are 297 APGs. If the number of events is quite high, a plan may analyze them all; most plans, however, will probably need to cluster the APGs into sets in order to achieve statistical validity.

Another statistical approach is to use ambulatory care groups (ACGs), a methodology that focuses on a resource-based measure of burden of illness.[3] Ambulatory patients are monitored for all encounters, and each encounter is classified as one of 34 ambulatory diagnosis groups (ADGs) based on medical resource used over a 1-year period and based on the expectation of recurrence of that diagnosis over time. The set of ADGs for each patient is then combined with measures of age and sex to assign the patient to one of 51 mutually exclusive ACGs. ADGs and ACGs may also be looked at independently.[4] ACG and ADG methodology requires a high level of statistical sophistication, and the programming cannot always be handled by the plan's MIS.

As has been mentioned earlier, once a plan decides on the routine reports, it can use those to decide what additional reports to request. For example, if total expenses for cardiology appear to be high, a manager could investigate further by requesting reports that show who is ordering the referrals, what ancillary testing is being done, what specialists are seeing the patients and how much they are charging, and so forth.

Open access systems, or systems that do not use a primary care gatekeeper model, present special problems in monitoring utilization. In a PPO or managed indemnity plan, there will be no physician-specific membership base to use as a denominator. In HMOs that allow open access to specialists or allow specialists to self-authorize revisits or secondarily to authorize referrals to other specialists, there will be no way to measure specialist utilization against a fixed membership base (the base is for only the PCPs, not the specialists).

In these situations, plans must be willing to accept less precise methods of measuring utilization of referral services and specialist utilization. Reports should focus on those areas under control of the specialist as well as primary care. Examples of such data elements are illustrated in Exhibit 37–6.

PROVIDER PROFILING

Closely related to all the issues discussed in this chapter is provider profiling. Profiling means the collection, collation, and analysis of data to develop provider-specific profiles. Such profiles have a variety of uses, but the most important ones are producing provider feedback reports to help the providers modify their own behavior, recruiting providers into the network, and choosing which providers may not be (or are not) the right fit with the plan's managed care philosophy and goals. Other uses include determining specialists to whom the plan will send certain types of cases, detecting fraud and abuse, determining how to focus the utilization management program, supporting performance-based reimbursement systems, and performing economic modeling. This important topic is discussed in Chapter 38.

Exhibit 37–6 Sample Data for an Open Access Model Plan

Outpatient Services
- Average number of visits per member per year
- Average number of visits per member per year to each specialty
- Diagnostic utilization per visit
  –Laboratory
  –Radiology and imaging
  –Other
- Average cost per visit
- Procedures per 1,000 visits per year (annualized)
  –Aggregate
  –By procedure for top 10 by specialty type
  –By individual specialist
- Average cost per episode (as defined for each sentinel diagnosis) over a defined time period, including charges not directly billed by provider

Inpatient Services
- Average total cost per case, including charges not billed by provider, for hospitalized cases
- Average length of stay for defined procedures
- Average rate of performance of a procedure, such as:
  –Caesarean section rate
  –Hysterectomy rate
  –Transurethral prostatectomy rate
  –Cardiac procedures
- Readmission rate or complication rate
  –Use of resources before and after the hospitalization

Incorporation of Other Data

Many plans incorporate other data into a provider profile analysis. Claims and encounter data are enormously useful, as are data from hospital episodes, but there are additional sources of data as well. Credentialing data may be automated and referenced. Member services data such as complaints, transfer rates, or administrative problems may be incorporated. Advanced MCOs incorporate data from the quality management program (see Part XI) and member satisfaction data into their profiling reports and compensation programs.

Feedback

Medical management reports should not be confined to plan managers. As mentioned in several chapters in this book, feedback to providers is a useful adjunct to other medical management activities. Feedback to providers must be clear, easy to understand, and accurate.

Feedback should be meaningful and useful to both parties, not just the plan or the provider. When feedback reports are clearly linked with performance expectations, and when such reports can help a provider alter a behavior in a positive way (which will in turn benefit that provider), then feedback may be successful. This is especially true when feedback is linked to the financial incentive system.

Providers will alter their behavior in response to feedback for a variety of reasons. Natural competitiveness and peer pressure may exert influence. More important, the opportunity to increase market share and to improve their revenue will be a powerful reason for physicians to respond to feedback. Fear of possible adverse actions by the plan may also play a role if a provider is a clear outlier and if feedback provides a concrete measure of expectation by the plan.

Hospitals may benefit from feedback reports as well. Hospitals are providers in their own right, even though the physicians on staff give the orders. Nevertheless, hospitals have their own policies and procedures that influence how care is rendered, and hospitals certainly have their own billing practices. Hospitals can also have a strong role in influencing the practice behavior of the physicians on staff and can work effectively with managed care plans to effect changes.

Feedback is not always effective in changing behavior, however. The topic of changing physician behavior, including the use of data and feedback, is discussed in Chapter 39.

Focused Utilization Management

As noted earlier, profiling provides medical managers with the ability to focus utilization management more efficiently. Some providers may perform at such a high level of cost-effectiveness that the plan can essentially rely on feedback and case management support rather than more traditional methods of managing utilization; in other words, those providers would need little oversight or intervention by the plan. In other cases, the plan may determine that heightened levels of utilization review and precertification are required for some providers who are clear outliers.

Profiling and data management may also reveal systemwide issues of utilization that require a broad approach. For example, it may be found that emergency department usage is uniformly high, not due to a small number of outlier physicians. In that case, a focused approach to demand management (see Part IV) would have greater utility than focusing on individual physician behavior.

Lastly, profiling will enable the medical director to determine which specialists should receive more referrals and preferential business and which specialists are less cost-effective, provide a lower quality of care, or simply manage too low a volume for a competitive market.

CONCLUSION

Medical management reports are powerful and absolutely necessary tools for managers of health plans. Routine reports must be simple to read and compact, providing only those data needed to manage the plan. They should provide managers with sufficient information to order other, more detailed reports required to solve specific problems that surfaced in the routine reports. Provider profiling is taking on an ever greater role in managed care, but it remains complex. Data overload is a frequent and troubling problem, but intelligent use of reports should prevent data overload from occurring. As systems evolve, managers' ability to directly access useful information and manipulate it as needed will provide a clear competitive edge.

REFERENCES

1. Lasker RD, Shapiro DW, Tucker AM. Realizing the potential of practice pattern profiling. *Inquiry*. 1992;29:287–297.
2. Nathanson R, Noether M, Ozminkowski RJ. Using claims data to select primary care physicians for a managed care network. *Managed Care Q*. 1994;2(4):50–59.
3. Starfield B, Weiner J, Mumford L, Steinwachs D. Ambulatory care groups: a categorization of diagnoses for research and management. *Health Serv Res*. 1991;26:53–74.
4. Weiner J, Starfield B, Steinwachs D, Mumford L. Development and application of a population-oriented measure of ambulatory care case-mix. *Med Care*. 1991;29:452–472.

SUGGESTED READINGS

Betty WR, Hendricks HK, Ruchlin HS, Braham RL. Physician practice profiles: a valuable information system for HMOs. *Med Group Manage*. 1990;37:68–75.

Braham RL, Ruchlin HS. Physician practice profiles: a case study of the use of audit and feedback in an ambulatory care group practice. *Health Care Manage Rev*. 1987;12:11–16.

Doubilet P, Weinstein MC, McNeil BJ. Use and misuse of the term "cost effective" in medicine. *N Engl J Med*. 1986;314:253–256.

Eisenberg JM. Clinical economics: a guide to the economic analysis of clinical practices. *JAMA*. 1989;262:2879–2886.

Gotowka TD, Jackson M, Aquilina D. Health data analysis and reporting: organization and system strategies. *Managed Care Q*. 1993;1(3):26–34.

Harris JS. Watching the numbers: basic data for health care management. *J Occup Med*. 1991;33:275–278.

Hughes RG, Lee DE. Using data describing physician inpatient practice patterns: issues and opportunities. *Health Care Manage Rev*. 1991;16:33–40.

Nathanson R, Noether M, Ozminkowski RJ. Using claims data to select primary care physicians for a managed care network. *Managed Care Q*. 1994;2(4):50–59.

Physician Payment Review Commission. *Physician Payment Review Commission Conference on Profiling*. Washington, DC: Physician Payment Review Commission; 1992.

Chapter 38

Provider Profiling

Peter R. Kongstvedt and David W. Plocher

Chapter Outline

- Introduction
- What To Measure?
- Episodes of Care
- Adjusting for Severity and Case Mix
- What Specialty *Is* the Physician?
- What Constitutes the Group? What Linkages Exist?
- Incorporation of Other Data
- Comparing the Results of Profiling
- Selection of a Profiling Vendor
- Conclusion

INTRODUCTION

Closely related to the issues of using data in medical management (discussed in Chapter 37) is provider (or practice) profiling—the collection, collation, and analysis of data to develop provider-specific profiles. Providers in this chapter are assumed to be physicians, though the more generic term is used because the same concepts may be applied to profiling nonphysician providers (including hospitals) as well.

Practice profiles have a variety of uses, but the most important ones are producing feedback reports to help the providers modify their behavior, recruiting providers into the network, and choosing which providers may not be (or are not) the right fit with the organization's managed care philosophy and goals, whether the organization is a managed care organization (MCO), an organized medical group, an integrated delivery system (IDS), a pool of doctors (POD), or an independent practice association (IPA) (for this chapter, MCO will be used to refer to all these types of organizations, which are defined in the Glossary). Other uses include supporting performance-based reimbursement systems, selecting specialists to whom the MCO will send certain types of cases, detecting fraud and abuse, determining how to focus the utilization management program, and performing financial modeling.

The initial focus of many profiling activities has historically been inpatient care, partially because inpatient care is so costly. Also, a hospital case is usually easily definable (except for cases that are transferred or readmitted), and the physicians delivering care are usually identifiable. Basic hospital care profiling (adjusted for case mix and severity—see below) combined with feedback to physicians and active intervention has been shown to effectively reduce length of stay.[1] Recent activity has shifted to consider outpatient procedural and office-based care as well, recognizing that care occurs across a continuum rather than in isolated episodes and that most physicians will have more data from the ambulatory environment.

Some provider profiling systems simply look at the behavior of the provider against certain norms. Comparison against norms is certainly necessary, but it is fraught with potential difficulties. How do you define the norm? What aspects of provider care do you choose to look at? Most profiling activities focus solely on the actions of the provider. It is better, however, to attempt to examine provider behavior from the standpoint of total health care resource consumption and outcome, including resources not directly delivered or billed by the provider, and to look at true episodes of care and outcomes as opposed to constellations of single visits. Exhibit 38–1 lists many key items to consider when constructing practice profiling reports; Chapter 37 provides a more detailed listing. It is as easy to collect data that produce bad results as it is to collect data that produce good results. Exhibit 38–2 provides a partial listing of reasons that data can produce bad results. Below are some issues to bear in mind in order to avoid these pitfalls.

Exhibit 38–1 Design Issues for Profiling Reports

1. *Compare* your results with published performance.
2. *Report* performance using a uniform clinical data set.
3. *Determine* levels of comparison (eg, averages versus gold standards).
4. When possible, *employ* an external data source for independent validation of the provider's data.
5. *Consider* on-site verification of data from the provider's information system.
6. *Present* comparative performance using clinically relevant risk stratification.
7. *Require* measures of statistical significance.
8. *Revise* performance measurements using formal severity adjustment instruments.

Exhibit 38–2 Potential Problems with Integrity of Cost and Quality Data

- Bad data (ie, incorrect or grossly inaccurate data) are used.
- Managing physician is not correctly identified.
- Specialist category is not consistently identified.
- Practice does not match specialist category.
- Parameter is not practical to measure.
- There is no adjustment for illness severity.
- There is no statistical significance testing.
- There is no agreement on episode limits.

WHAT TO MEASURE?

Deciding what to measure is not always obvious. There are certain requirements that must be met in order for a measurement to be useful. The first general requirement is to start with high-volume outpatient measures such as the use of laboratory and imaging, office visits, referral rates, and so forth. As the frequency diminishes, so does the ability to capture meaningful data. Even then, as has been noted above and as we shall see below, if the data are not understood in the context of episodes of care, outcomes, and overall use of resources, the data will be of limited value.

Even if correct or useful data are collected, it is easily possible that there will be insufficient data to achieve statistical significance. While some plans are willing to use statistically insignificant results in their profiling activities, we do not endorse that approach.

Another key component to address is what end result(s) you want to measure. We have used terms such as cost-effectiveness, cost and quality, and outcomes. It is beyond the scope of this chapter to discuss what these are (see Part XI for thorough reviews of outcomes and quality measures). For our purposes, it is important to stress that it is best to examine all these components simultaneously, not just one at a time. For the MCO to succeed or thrive, managing cost is crucial; if quality is not maintained or improved, then cost reduction efforts are worse than fool's work. Therefore, as discussed below, attention to the outcomes of care within defined episodes is as important as understanding the total use of resources to achieve those outcomes.

EPISODES OF CARE

Episodes of care are defined as time-related intervals that have meaning to the behavior you are trying to measure. Episodes may vary considerably both by clinical condition and by the provider type that is being measured. In the case of obstetrics, obvious measures such as Caesarean section rate and average length of stay are important but will not reveal the full picture. Looking at the entire prenatal and postnatal episode may reveal significant differences in the use of ultrasound and other diagnostics, differences in early detection and prevention of complications, or perhaps a great deal of unbundled claims during the prenatal period. In the case of some medical conditions, the episode may extend for years or have no endpoint short of the patient's death (or in the case of a payer organization, disenrollment, at which point data are no longer available). Furthermore, patients with multiple medical conditions may have overlapping episodes of care, making it more difficult to sort out what resources are being used for what episode.

A related difficulty is determining which provider is actually responsible for care. As an example, an internist or a diabetologist may be responsible for the care of a patient with diabetes but may have little responsibility for managing that patient's broken leg other than to refer the patient to a good orthopaedist (see Chapter 29). Identification of the responsible physician is also difficult when patients are hospitalized; it is common for the admitting physician and the attending physician to be different people, especially when surgery is involved.

The hallmark of episode definition is the ability to link up all the health care resources into a defined event. This may mean diagnostic services (eg, laboratory or imaging), therapeutic services (eg, physical therapy), consultations, outpatient visits, and inpatient visits. In other words, it must be a patient-based analysis rather than a provider-based one; the analysis of the behavior of providers hinges on what happens to their patients. Various vendors have constructed proprietary groupers for the purpose of simplifying episode development.

ADJUSTING FOR SEVERITY AND CASE MIX

Practices have differences in the age and sex make-up of their patient panel that must be accounted for. These variables have been the traditional methods that served as a proxy for severity and case-mix adjustments. Age and sex are intuitively useful, and capitation payments are routinely modified based on these two parameters. The basic argument, which has validity, is that utilization is predictable based on age and sex, using actuarial tables. While this is true for any large population of individuals (such as a large insurance company would use to set rates), it provides little real value to any individual physician's expected utilization profile, because when the numbers are small, chance has more of an influence than do population-based statistics. (This is sometimes referred to as the "Law of Small Numbers": when there are few events to measure, then chance is more influential than are predictions based on large numbers of events.) Yet it is both common and necessary to include adjustments for age and sex when looking at any type of practice profile, because even if the influence of those factors is lessened, that influence does not disappear. Besides, providers, MCOs, and purchasers have come to expect these adjustments.

Geographic differences may also account for some differences in utilization. This certainly occurs when comparing the West Coast of the United States to the East Coast (as discussed in Chapter 15). It is likewise common to see differences between rural and urban levels of utilization. As noted above, these trends, whether or not they make empirical sense, are useful when observing population-based numbers but retain little relevance when looking at small numbers of events (eg, covered lives, surgical procedures, and so forth). Unlike age and sex, geographic location may or may not be a legitimate adjustment when crafting profiles. It is more likely to be useful when looking at large numbers of providers or patients that share the same geographic location; it is less likely to be useful if applied to individual providers based on single ZIP codes.

Case mix and severity are always issues of contention when one is profiling providers: Providers with costly profiles will always complain that they have the sickest patients. Whether or not these complaints seem valid, the issue of severity *must* be accounted for in profiling. Statistical manipulation such as trimming in outlier cases is commonly employed (ie, if only a few cases are outliers, one brings those cases back to the mean). Another technique for doing so is to use severity of illness indicators. Severity of illness is most often used in hospital cases (for example, 3M's All-Patient diagnosis-related groups [AP-DRGs], which assign patients to DRGs and adjust that assignment based on four levels of severity), and most recently, diagnostic care groups (DCGs). Severity adjustment methodologies also may be applied to outpatient care as well; examples include ambulatory care groups (ACGs, recently adapted to include the entire continuum), ambulatory patient groups (APGs), and ambulatory diagnostic groups (ADGs).

Adjusting for severity and case mix is important and cannot be bypassed. However, it is interesting to note that these factors probably account for only a small amount of the variation noted in practice behavior. At least one study has reported that adjusting for severity and case mix significantly reduced the number of physicians that appeared to be outliers,[2] although there was a good counterargument that what the methodology actually did was to make genuine outliers look normal.[3] Other studies have reported that these adjustments accounted for little of the variation in practice that was found.[1,4,5] Furthermore, the population-based utility of ACGs must be contrasted with narrower, episode-based measures described above.

WHAT SPECIALTY *IS* THE PHYSICIAN?

It is not always clear what specialty a physician really is. Most MCOs have provider files that indicate what specialty type a physician has self-indicated, but it is surprising how often that information does not match up with specialty indicators in the claims file. Of course, MCOs that perform comprehensive verification of board specialty status will have more accurate data than MCOs that depend on self-reporting by physicians. Even when the specialty designation is accurate, there is no guarantee that the provider actually makes a living at that specialty.

The problem of provider specialty definition is particularly acute when one is looking at primary care. Many board-certified medical specialists actually spend a considerable amount of time performing primary care, whereas others spend the majority of their time practicing true specialty medicine. This has great implications for how an MCO will evaluate performance of specialists as well as primary care physicians when comparisons to peers are used (a common practice). A related issue is in determining which physicians will be considered specialists; the MCO may not want to refer members to specialists who are not active in their designated specialties.

Even within a single specialty there will be differences in how "specialized" a specialist is. For example, a specialist may have a larger percentage of primary care or may not care for patients in the intensive care unit. The MCO therefore will want to look at the degree to which a physician is truly a specialist in his or her mix of routine and complex cases.

Even when the issue of specialty definition is resolved, there remains another problem: no two practices are exactly alike. For example, general internists either perform flexible sigmoidoscopies or they do not. If one looks only at charge patterns, the internist who performs the procedure will look more expensive compared to the internist who does not, but that analysis will fail to pick up the fact that the internist who does not perform flexible sigmoidoscopies instead refers them all to a gastroenterologist who charges more than the first internist (of course the first internist could be overutilizing the procedure, or the second internist could be failing to provide this common preventive care activity, but that is a separate type of analysis).

WHAT CONSTITUTES THE GROUP? WHAT LINKAGES EXIST?

The next issue is the problem of providers who behave as though they are in a group but are not legally connected and do not appear as a group in the MCO's provider file. An example would be two physicians who share an office, share calls, and see each other's patients but who have different tax numbers and billing services. This is important in managed care because if the MCO contracts with one provider but not the other, the member may wind up seeing the nonparticipating physician and be subject to balance billing. Even if the physicians agree not to balance bill, the MCO still may not want the other physician in the network, even occasionally.

Related to the above dilemma is the ability to detect linkages between practices and ancillary services. Examples include orthopaedists who own physical therapy practices and neurologists who have a proprietary interest in a magnetic resonance imaging center.

INCORPORATION OF OTHER DATA

Many MCOs incorporate other data into a provider profile analysis. Claims and encounter data are enormously useful, as are data from hospital episodes, but there are additional sources of data as well. Credentialing data may be automated and referenced. Data from member services such as complaints, transfer rates, or administrative problems may be incorpo-

Exhibit 38–3 Examples of Additional Data To Add to Profiling Reports

---

Clinical measures or data, such as
- Condition-specific functional status measures
- Laboratory or imaging results; that is, not only the blood sugar or hemoglobin A1c CPT-4 code but the numeric result of the lab test compared to a desired level
- Measures specific to Medicare and Medicaid

Nonclinical measures or data, such as
- designation of the imputed primary care physician; that is, for networks in which primary care physician assignment is not required, advanced profilers deduce by resource consumption pattern which provider is the primary care physician
- compliance with administrative priorities (eg, being able to communicate electronically with the MCO)

---

rated. Data from the quality management program (see Part XI) and member satisfaction reports are now included in the profiling reports and even compensation programs of advanced MCOs (see *The Managed Health Care Handbook*, 3rd Edition, for a description of several of these types of physician reimbursement systems). Examples of supplemental data incorporation include (but are not limited to) those listed in Exhibit 38–3.

COMPARING THE RESULTS OF PROFILING

Practice profiles are of no use unless the results are compared to some type of standard. Yet there are certain problems inherent to comparisons in provider profiling. All these problems are resolvable, but medical managers need to be aware of them before embarking on profiling. The usual ways of comparing profiling results are to provide data for each individual practice in comparison to one or more of the following:

- *MCO average results.* This standard is simply the average for the entire MCO. It is the crudest method of comparison.
- *IPA, POD, or IDS.* A variation of MCO average, this compares the practice only to other practices within a set of providers smaller than the entire network. This approach may be combined with multiple other approaches when an MCO contracts through organized provider systems. In the absence of organized provider groups, providers within certain geographic areas may be compared.
- *Specialty-specific or peer group.* This compares providers in each practice only to other providers within the same specialty. For example, internists are compared only to other internists.
- *Peer group, adjusted for age, sex, and case mix/severity of illness.* This is the most complicated approach (as noted earlier), but it provides the most meaningful comparative data.
- *Budget.* This compares the profile to budgeted utilization and cost, a necessary activity when providers are accepting full or substantial risk for medical expenses.
- *Advanced and statistically based comparisons.* These comparisons should be coupled with confidence intervals so that a provider will know whether the difference from the peer group is statistically significant (see Chapters 34 and 35 for greater discussion about this issue).

In the near future, profiles may rely less on administrative databases, to the great relief of many who lament claim coding inaccuracies. Instead, the computerized patient record promises eventually to enrich the information used to populate these profilers.

SELECTION OF A PROFILING VENDOR

Unless an MCO has an extraordinary information system, it will have to purchase or license services from an outside vendor of profiling systems. There are several distinguishing features that one looks at to aid in the selection of a system.

- multiple products for HMO, point of service, Medicare, Medicaid
- comprehensible by average PC user
- independently validated risk adjustment methodology
- carve-out accommodated
- prioritization of services for focused review
- Health Plan Employer Data and Information Set (HEDIS) 3.0 production

Multiple Products for HMO, Point of Service, Medicare, Medicaid

While profiling in the "lock-in" or 100:zero plan HMO environment is usually straightforward, point of service products add new complexity. Whether referred by the primary care physician with or without the MCO's approval or if self-referred by the member, resource consumption out of network and in-service area or out-of-service area strains the information collection completeness and timeliness. Metrics for Medicare must include influenza vaccination adherence rates, pneumonia and congestive heart failure readmissions, and additional items beyond HEDIS 3.0 requirements. Medicaid populations must build profiles that address maternities with high risk, asthma, human immunodeficiency virus (HIV) and acquired immune deficiency syndrome (AIDS), care for substance abuse, and care for the elderly, blind, and disabled.

Comprehensible by Average PC User

Customers for profiling software and services may settle for shipping a claim tape to the vendor and waiting for a report. However, the recent users are asking for the option to have a terminal on their own bench and training to design ad hoc reports for customized circumstances in real time. They prefer the visual relief provided by a graphical user interface and deplore tabular data. They want to be self-managing.

Independently Validated Risk Adjustment Methodology

Vendors have decided either to license an established risk adjustment program or grow their own. Watch out for the latter. It is challenging enough for the former to demonstrate the predictive validity of their instrument (ability to explain differences in resource use) through the peer-reviewed literature.

Carve-Out Accommodated

As MCOs have separate agreements with subcapitated programs (managed behavioral health, chiropractic, pharmaceuticals, lab, etc), the better profilers are equilibrating their report packages to ensure apples-to-apples comparisons. Although important, profiling from within any capitated entity (especially physician group) will not be possible if encounter CPT-4 data are not submitted, and MCOs have had to develop reward programs for the completeness-of-capture of encounter information. In addition, pharmaceutical information *can* get to the level of drug name, dose, and route of administration.

Prioritization of Services for Focused Review

Briefly mentioned earlier in this chapter, this capability represents an essential management tool for MCO utilization management departments. They don't want to hassle righteous physicians. They want to reduce the overhead attached to operating these oversight activities. They would prefer not having to do old-fashioned "utilization review" at all. The better profilers arm them with information to perform this targeting.

HEDIS 3.0 Production

Profiling vendors vary in their willingness to produce the administrative data portion of HEDIS 3.0 reports (see Chapter 37 for a table of HEDIS data requirements). Conservative vendors argue that claim data integrity is unknown, so the electronic production of such a report is unreliable. Other vendors dedicate energy to claim tape edits and "cleansing" processes, whereby a level of confidence is achieved. Users can investigate a vendor's track record by examining an external audit of a HEDIS 3.0 report created by that vendor.

CONCLUSION

Profiling has become a necessary tool for any medical manager or provider in order to compare performance and results against both peers and expected results. While profiling is often seen as threatening (and it has sometimes been used that way), it can also provide highly useful data to allow a physician (or other provider) to improve performance. Profiling is far more complex than simply taking snapshots of individual activities of a provider; in fact, that type of profiling has little value. Profiling must be performed from the perspective of what happens to the patient, it must incorporate adjustments for severity and case mix (as well as age and sex), and it must be meaningful and useful to the medical managers and the providers themselves. Profiling is a continually evolving tool that will become more useful over time.

REFERENCES

1. Bennett G, McKee W, Kilberg L. Case study in physician profiling. *Managed Care Q*. 1994;2(4):60–70.
2. Salem-Schatz S, Moore G, Rucker M, Pearson SD. The case for case-mix adjustment in practice profiling: when good apples look bad. *JAMA*. 1994;272(11):871–874.
3. Welch HG, Black WC, Fisher ES. Case-mix adjustment: making bad apples look good. *JAMA*. 1995;273(10):772–773.
4. Nathanson R, Noether M, Ozminkowski RJ. Using claims data to select primary care physicians for a managed care network. *Managed Care Q*. 1994;2(4):50–59.
5. Welch HG, Miller ME, Welch WP. Physician profiling: an analysis of inpatient practice patterns in Florida and Oregon. *N Engl J Med*. 1994;330(9):607–612.

SUGGESTED READINGS

Betty WR, Hendricks HK, Ruchlin HS, Braham RL. Physician practice profiles: a valuable information system for HMOs. *Med Group Manage.* 1990;37:68–75.

Braham RL, Ruchlin HS. Physician practice profiles: a case study of the use of audit and feedback in an ambulatory care group practice. *Health Care Manage Rev.* 1987;12:11–16.

Doubilet P, Weinstein MC, McNeil BJ. Use and misuse of the term "cost effective" in medicine. *N Engl J Med.* 1986;314:253–256.

Eisenberg JM. Clinical economics: a guide to the economic analysis of clinical practices. *JAMA.* 1989;262:2879–2886.

Goldfield N, Boland P. *Physician Profiling and Risk Adjustment.* Gaithersburg, MD: Aspen Publishers, Inc; 1996.

Gotowka TD, Jackson M, Aquilina D. Health data analysis and reporting: organization and system strategies. *Managed Care Q.* 1993;1(3):26–34.

Harris JS. Watching the numbers: basic data for health care management. *J Occup Med.* 1991;33:275–278.

Hughes RG, Lee DE. Using data describing physician inpatient practice patterns: issues and opportunities. *Health Care Manage Rev.* 1991;16:33–40.

Iezzoni L, Shwartz M, Ash AS, Hughes JS, Daley J, Mackierman YD. Severity measurement methods and judging hospital death rates for pneumonia. *Med Care.* 1996;34(1):11–28.

Physician Payment Review Commission. *Physician Payment Review Commission Conference on Profiling.* Washington, DC: Physician Payment Review Commission; 1992.

Thomas JW, Ashcraft MLF. Measuring severity of illness: six severity systems and their ability to explain cost variations. *Inquiry.* 1991;28:39–55.

Part XIII

Changing Behavior in Managed Care

We are all creatures of habit. We are also all prone to doing things that may not contribute to our welfare or may actively work against it. Physicians are also subject to habits and biases. As a practical matter, if behavior does not change, then positive results are difficult to achieve. The focus on change has been mostly on providers, primarily physicians in the managed care arena, but efforts to achieve behavioral change in the members or patients are also taking place and hold real promise for long-term positive results.

CHAPTER 39

Physician Behavior Change in Managed Care Plans

Peter R. Kongstvedt

Chapter Outline

- Introduction
- Inherent Difficulties in Modifying Physician Behavior
- General Approaches to Changing Behavior
- Programmatic Approaches to Changing Physician Behavior
- Changing the Behavior of Individual Physicians
- Conclusion

INTRODUCTION

The practice behavior of physicians in a managed care organization (MCO) is the most important element in controlling cost and quality. Attending to physician practice behavior begins when physicians are selected and goes beyond the issue of basic credentialing. Selecting physicians who already practice high-quality, cost-effective medicine is the best way to achieve success, although profiling physicians, as discussed in Chapter 38, is no easy task. Even in the best of worlds, one cannot be assured that every physician participating in the plan will be solid gold, and marketing and delivery system needs dictate that geographic areas be adequately covered, even when that means accepting some B players rather than all A players.

The best contractual arrangements in the world will be of little value if there are poor utilization patterns or a lack of cooperation with plan policies and procedures. There will be some physicians in the medical community who will not modify their practice behavior. There will also be some physicians who are frankly hostile and some who, for various reasons, plans will not want, regardless of how friendly or cooperative they are. The majority of physicians, however, will want to cooperate and to be valued participants.

Given these realities, the purpose of this chapter is to present some of the issues involved in modifying the practice behavior of those participating physicians who can and will work with the plan. Financial incentives are clearly a useful method of influencing behavior,[1,2] but they are not the subject of this book. (An in-depth discussion of reimbursement methodologies may be found in *The Managed Health Care Handbook,* 3rd Edition.)

This chapter is adapted from PR Kongstvedt, Changing Provider Behavior in Managed Care Plans, in *The Managed Health Care Handbook*, 3rd ed, PR Kongstvedt, ed, pp 427–439, © 1996.

INHERENT DIFFICULTIES IN MODIFYING PHYSICIAN BEHAVIOR

Physicians are professionals with an inordinately large set of built-in biases because of their training, the current environment of medical practice, and the pressures they are now feeling. There is also great heterogeneity in attitudes and prior training in cost containment.[3] None of these issues are unique to the medical profession, but the combination and depth of the issues make for a number of inherent difficulties in changing the behavior of physicians.

What follows is a brief discussion of some of the more important issues. It is wise for managers to be sensitive to these issues, although that does not mean that they should fail to apply proper management methods.

Strong Autonomy and Control Needs

There is perhaps no more emotionally charged issue than autonomy and control. Physicians are trained to function in an autonomous way, to stand up for themselves, and to be authorities. It is difficult for them to accept a role in which another entity, whether it is managed care, peer review, or practice guidelines, has control over their professional activities.[4,5] Because of that, physicians participating in MCOs often feel antagonistic when they perceive that their control has been lost or lessened. By definition, managed care introduces elements of management control into the arena of health care delivery, management that clearly reduces the physician's autonomy. In one large study, physicians who entered into contracts with health maintenance organizations (HMOs) expected lower earnings, lower quality of care, and lessened autonomy; neither earnings nor quality declined, but there remained a general perception that physician autonomy did decline.[6] In a different study, physicians maintained a mildly negative attitude toward practicing medicine in an open panel HMO setting, and yet their perceived negative attitudes regarding autonomy and income were not supported by actual facts about their practice when asked specific questions on these issues.[7] At least one other study, however, has shown that practicing under managed care does not produce a uniformly lower level of satisfaction.[8]

There has been an increase in the amount of external control over the years. HMOs, preferred provider organizations (PPOs), indemnity plans with managed care elements (eg, preadmission authorization requirements), Medicare, and Medicaid are all programs that have been increasing their control over medical practice as health care costs have risen. The degree of control will vary considerably depending on the type of program involved, but managed health care, particularly in tightly managed HMOs, currently exerts the greatest degree of external control other than medical residency training. The greater the degree of external control, the greater the danger of overt or covert resistance to achieving the goals of the plan.

This chapter discusses many issues pertinent to ameliorating some of the anxieties that arise in dealing with control issues. It is important to point out that if the private sector and the physician community fail to control medical costs, there are likely to be even greater interventions by nonphysicians charged with bringing medical costs under control. Enlisting the physician's help in achieving the plan's goals is possible by empowering the physicians within the system. The following are suggestions for some specific approaches to working with control issues.

Control of Where Care Is Received

Virtually all managed care plans will have some controls over where members receive their care. In a simple PPO, that control will be confined to a differential in benefits that is based on whether a member uses participating hospitals and physicians. In a tightly managed HMO, the plan will allow only the use of participating providers, and even then only for certain services. For example, the HMO may have an exclusive contract for mammography; even though all the participating hospitals have the ability to perform mammography, only one provider will be allowed to do it and get paid.

If a plan intends to have a highly restricted panel of participating providers, it is sometimes helpful to elicit the opinions of those physicians already in the panel, even though the final decision will still rest with the plan. For example, if the decision has been made to use only two or three orthopaedic groups to provide services, the primary care physicians could be canvassed for nominations of groups to approach. The plan should clearly state that it is not having a majority rule vote but is looking for people to approach; the final selection will be based on a combination of the plan's regular credentialing process, the group's willingness to cooperate with plan policies and procedures, and cost.

Control of Patient Care

Much more volatile than controlling where care is given, controlling patient care is a hot button with most physicians. This control can range from the retrospective review of claims that is found in most plans to the mandatory preauthorization of all non–primary care services that is found in most HMOs. The greater the degree of plan involvement in clinical decision making, the greater the chances of antagonism between physicians and plan managers, but also the greater the degree of medical cost control.

Because this management of medical services is the hallmark of managed care, it is neither possible nor desirable to eliminate it. How that control is exercised will have a great effect on its acceptance and success, however. If the plan intervenes in an arbitrary and heavy-handed manner, there will be problems. If interventions are done with an element of understanding and respect, there should be greater cooperation.

The techniques described in a later section of this chapter are particularly important here. Frequent and regular contact, both positive and negative, with physicians will help a great deal. Discussing cases and suggesting and soliciting alternatives for case management will yield better results than arbitrary demands for improvement.

Control of Quality

The most common objection that physicians will voice about managed care is that it reduces the quality of care. That argument may sometimes be a smoke screen for complaints about economics, yet the issue of quality is valid. Any system that requires the use of a restricted network of providers and has an authorization system has the potential of reducing the quality of care delivered. There is no real evidence that managed care systematically results in inferior care. Despite the lack of evidence that managed care is inferior, concerns about quality persist in most physicians' minds.

The best approach here is to place responsibility for participating with the plan's quality management (QM) program squarely with the physicians themselves. It is vital to have a properly constructed QM program so that participation is meaningful. A solid QM program will allow the physicians to feel that the plan genuinely does have an interest in quality and should allow for some pride in participation. A more detailed discussion of QM programs is found in Chapter 33.

Role Conflict

It is often stated that physicians are trained to be the patient's advocate. This is partially true, but that notion presupposes a system whereby a patient, like a plaintiff or defendant in a lawsuit, needs an advocate. In fact, physicians are trained to be the patient's caregiver, that is, the coordinator and deliverer of medical care.

The issue of advocacy arises when a physician feels that the needs of the plan and the needs of the patient are in conflict.[9] When that happens, the physician feels genuinely torn between being the patient's advocate and the plan's advocate. This conflict most frequently arises when patients request or demand a service that is not really necessary or is of marginal clinical benefit. Physicians feel uncomfortable if they must deny the service; they feel as if they are in conflict with their patients, and that patients may be wondering, "Just whose side are you on, anyway?" This is a difficult situation that is handled better by some physicians than others.[10]

Plan managers need to acknowledge this conflict, even though there may be less conflict in reality than in perception. Because of poor provider understanding of the insurance function (discussed below), the conflict may come up when the physician feels a service is medically necessary but the service is not a covered benefit. In some cases, there is poor understanding of the difference between what is medically necessary and what is essentially a convenience. The health plan is not in the business of denying truly needed services, assuming that they are covered under the schedule of benefits; denial of such services would be ethically and financially foolish.

But the health plan does intend to cut the fat out of the system. The physician is charged with conserving the resources, primarily economic, of the plan to ensure availability of those resources to those who truly need them. It is the physician who will best be able to determine what is really needed and what is really not, and that will help provide more appropriate allocation of those resources. The plan's utilization management efforts are (or should be) aimed at aiding the physician in carrying out that function.

Poor Understanding of the Insurance Function of the Plan

As mentioned above, some of the problems of role conflict stem from a poor understanding of the insurance aspect of the plan. HMOs in particular are marketed as offering comprehensive benefits, even though there are clearly certain exclusions and limitations, just as there are for any form of health care coverage. Physicians often do not differentiate between what is medically necessary and what is a covered benefit.

Every plan has certain exclusions and limitations of coverage. For example, a member may require 3 months of inpatient psychiatric care, but the plan only covers 30 days. Another example is an experimental transplant procedure. In each case, an argument can be made that the treatment is necessary, but it is not a covered benefit under the plan's schedule of benefits.

Plan management may make exceptions to the exclusions and limitations policy, but that should only be done rarely and after much thought. In some cases, it will be clearly cost-effective to do so (eg, providing 30 days of home durable medical equipment to avoid a hospitalization). In other cases, it will not be. If frequent exceptions are made, it can lead to an open-ended commitment to provide lifetime noncovered services, a commitment that the plan cannot afford if it is to remain in business.

Helping a physician understand the coverage provided by the plan, including its limitations, will be a wise investment for plan managers to make. It is often helpful for a plan manager to contact a member to explain that a decision was made based on contract (ie, schedule of benefits) issues, and that the physician was not being callous.

Bad Habits

All of us have habits and patterns in our lives. Most physicians have habits and patterns in their practices that are not cost-effective but are difficult to change. One example is a practice of not seeing patients or making rounds on Wednesdays; the physician's partner may not feel comfortable discharging another physician's patient, so the stay is lengthened by an extra day. Another example is a physician who keeps a routine, uncomplicated surgical case in for 5 days, stating "That's the way I've always done it, and it's worked just fine for me!"

This problem is a touchy one. It is usually poor form to accuse a physician of bad practice habits. The frontal assault is generally met with the indignant question, "Are you questioning my judgment?" You are not, of course; you are questioning a bad habit.

It is preferable to lead physicians to the appropriate conclusion themselves. If you discuss the issue objectively, present supporting information, and ask physicians to examine critically the difference in practice behavior, a number of physicians will arrive at the conclusion that their old habits must change. By allowing physicians gracefully and quietly to make the change, you run less risk of creating the need for a rigid defensive posture on their part.

If calm and rational discussions fail to effect a change, firmer action is needed; physicians may cooperate but may tell the patient that the health plan is forcing them to take certain actions. In most cases, that type of grumbling will go away after a short while. If it does not, the medical director must counsel these physicians about appropriate behavior, especially in this litigious era. If there is an adverse outcome, even though it had nothing to do with the changed practice pattern, the chances of a lawsuit are probably heightened if those types of comments have been made. Despite recent laws passed in some states that encourage plaintiffs to sue MCOs for malpractice, physicians should realize that they may still be dragged through that same lawsuit. If genuine malpractice has occurred, then appropriate management and legal steps should be taken and the patient's problems attended to. If, however, malpractice has not occurred, it is not in the interest of either the physician or the plan to engage in the types of communications that would encourage baseless legal action.

Poor Understanding of Economics

Even though physicians and their business managers are becoming more sophisticated about managed care, there is still a surprising lack of understanding of managed care economics, especially in capitated or other performance-based reimbursement systems. There may be little understanding of the withholds and incentive pools, or physicians may feel so distant from those pools that there is little or no effect on behavior.

It is worthwhile to have continual re-education about the economics of the plan as it relates to the physician's income. Related to this is the need for accurate and timely feedback to the physicians about their economic status on the basis of payments and utilization. Inaccurate feedback is far worse than no feedback at all.

The hoary old cliché that money talks is absolutely true. Because of that, plan management should always be aware of the whole dollars involved in compensating physicians. A small number, such as an $11.25 per member per month capitation payment, may seem like funny money to a physician, but if that $11.25 per member per month really means $40,000 per year, that has a considerable impact on the financial health of a practice. Helping physicians realize the contribution that managed care is making to their bottom line can be eye opening.

Poor Differentiation among Competing Plans

Considerable difficulty arises when there is little or no differentiation among competing plans; this is essentially a problem in open panels. In many HMOs, particularly when the state or federal government sets standards, the benefits may be the same and the provider network may be similar or the same; the only difference among plans is the rates (then, the market takes on the ominous characteristics of a commodity market).

This lack of clear differentiation becomes a problem when each plan has different internal policies and procedures with which the physicians and their office staff must comply. If a physician is contracting with three or more plans, the frustration involved with trying to remember which one wants what can be quite high. This problem is exacerbated when the same patient changes to a different managed care plan. For example, on Friday Mr. Jones was with the ABC Health Plan, but when he came in for his return appointment on Monday he had switched to the XYZ Health Plan; the office staff did not take notice, which resulted in claims or authorization denials. This can be a real morale problem with the physician's office staff. When frustration rises, compliance falls.

This frustration is best addressed by increased attention and service to the physicians and their office staff. Frequent and timely communications will help, especially when they are handled in person, because newsletters have a way of getting to the bottom of the parakeet cage without being read. Some physicians have ready access to e-mail, but that is inconsistent; the physician may access e-mail at home rather than at the office and not transmit the information to the office staff.

In this area, nonmonetary issues can have as much impact as monetary ones. Examples include difficult-to-use forms that require a lot of unnecessary writing, frequent busy signals on service lines, and inconsistencies in responses to questions. Prompt and courteous responsiveness to questions and concerns is *required*. You do not have to give the answer that you think physicians will want to hear; you do have to give an answer or response that is consistent, clear, and fair.

GENERAL APPROACHES TO CHANGING BEHAVIOR

Translating Goals and Objectives

A useful way of looking at communications between plan management and physicians is to consider the concept of translation. It is easy to overlook the fact that managers and physicians may have radically different ways of viewing matters relating to the delivery of health care services to plan members.

For example, the area of cost containment is rife with possibilities for opposing views. Physicians frequently look upon cost containment measures as unnecessary intrusions into their domain, whereas nonphysician managers view the same measures as the only way to control headstrong physicians. Translating the goal of cost containment into terms that are understandable and acceptable to both parties will take you far toward obtaining cooperation and acceptance. To ensure that the economic resources will be available to compensate providers and to make services available (at all) to patients, cost containment must take place.

Rewards Are More Effective Than Sanctions

A tenet of behavior modification theory is that positive interactions or rewards are more effective than negative interactions or sanctions at achieving long-term changes in behavior. Furthermore, it is rarely good policy for managers to impose their will on others in an arbitrary manner. In some cases it is necessary, but if it is done as a matter of course, cooperation will not be enthusiastic. In the worst case, it can lead to widespread dissatisfaction and defection from the plan. Even without such attrition, overt cooperation can occur, but covert sabotage undoes any progress made. This can be especially true with physicians. Unlike regular employees, physicians (even in closed panel operations) behave with a great deal of autonomy and have much power.

In the context of this discussion, rewards refer primarily to forms of positive feedback and communication about good performance. Clearly, good case management should yield economic rewards as well, but positive feedback from plan management will be a reward system all its own. Other rewards could include continuing education seminars about managed care, small gifts, acknowledgments for good work, and so forth.

Although it is unrealistic to expect that every physician will embrace every policy and procedure the plan has, the odds of cooperation will increase when the interactions between the physician and the plan are more positive than negative. This is not to be confused with capitulation on necessary policies and procedures: There were once plenty of physician-friendly health plans that are now little more than smoking rubble. Rather, this is to emphasize that too heavy a hand will eventually cause problems.

Be Involved

It is shocking how often managers of health plans fail to maintain an active involvement with the participating physicians. Frequently, the only communications with the physicians are occasional newsletters or memos, claims denials, and calls from the utilization management department harassing the physicians about hospital cases. Those types of interactions will not add to the luster of plan management in the physicians' eyes.

Frequent and regular contact, either through scheduled meetings, personal visits, or telephone calls, will help create an environment for positive change. If the only time physicians hear from the plan is when there is a problem, they will try to avoid contact in the future and will tend to have decreased responsiveness to the plan's needs.

Offer advice, suggestions, and alternatives, not just demands to change something. Ask intelligent questions about the clinical issues at hand, and solicit advice about alternative ways to provide the care. Work to get to the point where physicians will be asking themselves the same questions you would ask, without your having to ask them.

Involvement is a two-way proposition. It is fair and reasonable to expect practicing physicians to participate in plan committees to help set medical policy, monitor quality, and so forth. Soliciting active participation in such functions helps promote a sense of ownership on the part of the involved physicians and will clearly give the plan some valuable input. In fact, for those MCOs that are members of the American Association of Health Plans, such physician participation is required. Whether the plan compensates the physicians for the time spent on such activities is a local decision, but an honorarium is common and recommended.

PROGRAMMATIC APPROACHES TO CHANGING PHYSICIAN BEHAVIOR

Formal Continuing Medical Education

Formal continuing medical education (CME) is the provision of additional clinical training through seminars, conferences, home study, and so forth. The hallmark of CME is that it provides CME credits by virtue of the accreditation of the sponsoring body. This method of information dissemination, while traditionally the most prevalent, has a mixed effectiveness when it comes to changing behavior. One large review found little evidence that traditional CME changed patient outcomes or changed behavior.[11] However, another study found that changes in behavior will occur when the curriculum is *designed* to change specific types of behavior.[12] A more recent and extensive review of CME (which specifically excluded programs that were tied to financial incentives) supports the conclusion that traditional CME can have a small effect on behavior, with a somewhat greater effect on behavior when the techniques of academic detailing (ie, one-on-one education focused on specific issues), reminders (ie, specific reminders at the time of a patient visit), and possibly the additional influence of opinion leaders is brought into play.[13]

Based on this evidence, formal CME will remain a useful tool for disseminating clinical information and will be a useful adjunct of changing physician behavior in general. Formal CME is not currently a very useful tool for a managed care plan to use to change specific physician behavior when compared to other available methodologies.

Data and Feedback

As has been mentioned in other chapters, particularly Chapter 37, data regarding utilization and cost are an integral part of a managed care plan. The value of data is not restricted to plan managers; data are equally important to individual physicians. If the only data physicians get are letters at the end of the year informing them that all their withhold is used up, they can credibly argue that they have been blindsided.

Providing regular and accurate data about an individual physician's performance, from both a utilization and (for risk/bonus models) an economic standpoint, is vital to changing behavior. Most physicians will want to perform well, but they can do so only when they can judge their own performance against that of their peers or against plan norms.

The research literature is actually a bit mixed in its support for feedback as a means of changing behavior, although a modest majority of the research data is positive. There are numerous studies showing significant reductions in utilization and costs in response to feedback about individual physician behavior.[14–22] There are, however, some studies that are more ambiguous regarding the role of feedback, or that report that feedback has little lasting effect unless it is continuously reinforced.[23–29]

When reviewing the possible reasons why feedback may be ineffective (at least in the long run), it is possible to make conjectures about conditions that improve the effectiveness of feedback. First, the physicians must believe that their behavior needs to change, whether for clinical reasons, for economic reasons, or simply in order to remain part of the participating panel in the plan; if physicians do not believe that they need to change, then feedback provides nothing of value. Feedback must also be consistent and usable; in other words, physicians must clearly understand the data in the report, be able to use that information in a concrete way, and be able to keep using it to measure their own performance. Feedback needs to be closely related to what a physician is doing right at that time; in other words, feedback about behavior that is remote in time or infrequent is less likely to be acted upon. Feedback must be regular to sustain the changed behavior; when feedback is sporadic, physician behavior is likely to regress, to return to the behavior before the feedback had generated an improvement. Lastly, feedback that is linked to economic performance is more likely to produce substantial change than is feedback that is not so linked.

Practice Guidelines and Clinical Protocols

Practice guidelines and clinical protocols refer to codified approaches to medical care. Guidelines may be for both diagnostic and therapeutic modalities, and they may be used to guide physicians in the care of patients with defined diseases or symptoms or as surveillance tools to monitor practice on a retrospective basis. Clinical pathways or protocols are discussed in great detail in Chapter 18 and in Part X, and the reader is urged to review those chapters.

Some physicians have an initial negative reaction to practice guidelines; they feel that guidelines make for cookbook medicine and do not allow for judgment or that guidelines represent a high risk in the case of a malpractice suit (because guidelines provide a template against which all actions will be judged). Nevertheless, practice guidelines have been gaining in popularity, at least among medical managers.

Implementing practice guidelines is not always easy, particularly in an open panel setting. There is frequent lack of enthusiasm on the part of the physicians, and the plan's ability to monitor the guidelines is limited. Generally, the plan's QM process is best able to monitor the use of guidelines (see Chapter 33), although the claims system may be able to help do so as well.

Attempting to put comprehensive practice guidelines into place in a managed care plan is a daunting task. In an open panel, it will be exponentially more difficult. There is some evidence that simple publication of practice guidelines alone may predispose physicians to consider changing their behavior but that such guidelines by themselves are unlikely to effect rapid change.[30,31] When such protocols are accompanied by direct presentations by opinion leaders, so-called academic detailing, then changes are more sustained.[32] Lastly, as discussed in Chapter 18, clinical pathways developed by the physicians who will use those pathways, especially in the inpatient setting, are most likely to have significant effects, at least for the type of care that the pathway addresses, and there are multiple interventions that can improve compliance with the guidelines.[33]

CHANGING THE BEHAVIOR OF INDIVIDUAL PHYSICIANS

Stepwise Approach to Changing Behavior Patterns

Changing provider behavior involves a stepwise approach. The first and most common step is collegial discussion. Discussing cases and utilization patterns in a nonthreatening way, colleague to colleague, is generally an effective method of bringing about change.

Far less common is positive feedback. (The use of the term "positive feedback" here is different than when using the term "feedback" regarding data. While both forms of feedback provide information to the provider regarding performance, data feedback is objective, while positive feedback in the context of this section refers to subjective information from plan managers.) Positive feedback is an even more effective tool for change, but most managers fail to use it to any great degree. Positive feedback does not refer to mindless or misleading praise but to letting a physician know when things are done well. Most managers get so involved in firefighting that they tend to neglect sending positive messages to those providers who are managing well. In the absence of such messages, providers have to figure out for themselves what they are doing right (the plan will usually tell them what they are doing wrong), and that may not be optimal.

Persuasion is also commonly used. Somewhat stronger than collegial discussion, this tactic involves plan managers persuading providers to act in ways that the providers may not initially choose themselves. For example, if a patient requires intravenous antibiotics for osteomyelitis but is otherwise doing well, that patient is a candidate for home intravenous therapy. Some physicians will resist discharging the patient to home therapy because it is inconvenient to follow the case; keeping the patient in the hospital is a lot easier. The physician must then be persuaded to discharge the patient because of the cost-effectiveness of home therapy.

Firm direction of plan policies, procedures, and requirements is the next step after persuasion. If a physician refuses to cooperate with the plan to deliver care cost-effectively and discussions and persuasion have failed, a medical director may be required to give a physician firm direction, reminding him or her of the contractual agreement to cooperate with plan policies and procedures. Behind firm direction is the implied threat of refusal to pay for services or even more severe sanctions. It is clearly a display of power and should not be done with a heavy hand. When giving firm direction, it is best to not allow oneself to be drawn into long and unresolvable arguments. Presumably the discussions and even the arguments have already occurred, so it is pointless to keep rehashing them. This is sometimes called a broken record type of response because, rather than respond to old arguments, the medical director always gives the same response: firm direction.

The last steps are sanctions and termination. Sanctioning should rarely be required, and termination is very serious. These topics are discussed below.

One last thought in this section: Avoid global responses to individual problems. When managers are uncomfortable confronting individual physicians about problems in behavior, a dysfunctional response is to make a global change in policy or procedure because of the actions of one or two physicians. That type of response frequently alienates all the other physicians who have been cooperating and fails to change the behavior of the problem providers. If a policy change is required, make it. If the problem is really just with a few individuals, however, deal with them and do not harass the rest of the panel.

Discipline and Sanctions

This section discusses the most serious form of behavior modification. Sanctions or threats of sanctions are applied only when the problem is so serious that action must be taken and the provider fails to cooperate to improve the situation. In some cases, the provider may be willing to cooperate, but the offense is so serious that sanctions must be taken anyway. An example of this is a serious problem in quality of care, such as malpractice resulting in death or serious morbidity. In any event, the sanctioning process has legal overtones that must be kept in mind.

Plan management may initiate disciplinary actions short of a formal sanctioning process. In most cases, such discipline is helpful in creating documentation of chronic problems or failure to cooperate. Discipline may involve verbal warnings or letters; in either case, the thrust of the action is to document the offensive behavior and to describe the consequences of failure to cooperate.

One example of discipline is sometimes called ticketing, so named because it is similar to getting a ticket from a traffic cop. This is a verbal reprimand about a specific behavior; the behavior and corrective action are described, as are the consequences of failure to carry out the corrective action. The manager refuses to get into an argument at that time and requires the offending provider to make an appointment at a future date to discuss the issue (similar to a court date). This allows tempers to cool off a bit and ensures that the disciplinary message does not get muddied up with other issues. When a manager issues a ticket, there should be a document placed in a file that describes what transpired.

A more formal approach is an actual disciplinary letter. Like a ticket, the letter describes the offending behavior and the required corrective action and invites the provider to make an appointment to discuss the issue. In the case of a verbal ticket or a disciplinary letter, the consequence of failure to change errant ways is initiation of the formal sanctioning process.

Formal sanctioning has potentially serious legal overtones. Due process, or a policy regarding rights and responsibilities of both parties, is a requirement for an effective sanctioning procedure, at least when one is sanctioning for reasons of quality. The Health Care Quality Improvement Act of 1986 has formalized due process in the sanctioning procedure as it relates to quality and must be adhered to in order to maintain protection from antitrust action. Although this act was primarily aimed at hospital peer review activities, HMOs are specifically mentioned, and other forms of managed care may be implied in the future.

The Health Care Quality Improvement Act of 1986 describes the requirements of due process as follows:

(a) a professional review action must be taken
   (1) in the reasonable belief that the action was in the furtherance of quality health care,
   (2) after a reasonable effort to obtain the facts of the matter,
   (3) after adequate notice and hearing procedures are afforded to the physician involved and after such other procedures as are fair to the physician under the circumstances, and
   (4) in the reasonable belief that the action was warranted by the facts known after such reasonable effort to obtain facts and after meeting the requirements of paragraph (3)
(b) A health care entity is deemed to have met the adequate notice and hearing requirement of subsection (a)(3) with respect to a physician if the following conditions are met (or are waived voluntarily by the physician):
   (1) Notice of Proposed Action—The physician has been given notice stating—
      (A) (i) that a professional review action has been proposed to be taken against the physician,
          (ii) reasons for the proposed action,
      (B) (i) that the physician has the right to request a hearing on the proposed action,

(ii) any time limit (of not less than 30 days) within which to request such a hearing, and
(C) a summary of the rights in the hearing under paragraph (3).
(2) Notice of Hearing—If a hearing is requested on a timely basis under paragraph (1)(B), the physician involved must be given notice stating—
(A) the place, time, and date of the hearing, which date shall not be less than 30 days after the date of the notice, and
(B) a list of the witnesses (if any) expected to testify at the hearing on behalf of the profession review body.
(3) Conduct of Hearing and Notice—
(A) the hearing shall be held (as determined by the health care entity)—
(i) before an arbitrator mutually acceptable to the physician and the health care entity,
(ii) before a hearing officer who is appointed by the entity and who is not in direct economic competition with the physician involved, or
(iii) before a panel of individuals who are appointed by the entity and are not in direct economic competition with the physician involved;
(B) the right to the hearing may be forfeited if the physician fails, without good cause, to appear;
(C) in the hearing the physician involved has the right—
(i) to representation by an attorney or other person of the physician's choice,
(ii) to have a record made of the proceedings, copies of which may be obtained by the physician upon payment of any reasonable charges associated with the preparation thereof,
(iii) to call, examine, and cross-examine witnesses,
(iv) to present evidence determined to be relevant by the hearing officer, regardless of its admissibility in a court of law, and
(v) to submit a written statement at the close of the hearing; and
(D) upon completion of the hearing, the physician has the right—
(i) to receive the written recommendation of the arbitrator, officer, or panel, including a statement of the basis for the recommendations, and
(ii) to receive a written decision of the health care entity, including a statement of the basis for the decision.[34]

Following the requirements of the Act regarding due process is cumbersome and is obviously the final step before removing a physician from the panel for reasons of poor quality care. Because it is such a drastic step, compliance with the Act, including the reporting requirements, is the best protection the plan has against a legal action.

It should be emphasized that the Act is in regard to peer review activities resulting in actions against physicians for quality problems. If a physician fails to cooperate with contractually agreed-to plan policies and procedures, the plan may have reason to terminate the contract with the physician for cause. Even in that case, it may be wise to have a due process policy that allows for formal steps to be taken in the event that the plan contemplates termination. Presentation of facts to a medical advisory committee made up of physicians who are not in direct economic competition with the involved physician provides a backup to plan management. Such a committee may be able to effect changes by the physician where the medical director may not. Finally, the backing of a committee underscores that severe sanctions are not arbitrary but the result of failure on the part of the physician, not plan management.

There may arise situations where a physician's utilization performance is such that there is a clear mismatch with managed care practice philosophy. The quality of the physician's medical care may be adequate, and there even may have been no gross lack of cooperation with plan policies and procedures, but the physician simply practices medicine in a style that results in medical resources being heavily and inappropriately overutilized. In such cases, the medical director must assess whether the physician can change his or her behavior. Assuming that the medical director concludes that the provider in question cannot change (or change sufficiently) or has failed to change despite warnings and feedback, the plan may choose to terminate the relationship solely on the basis of contractual terms that allow either party to terminate without cause when adequate notice is given (see *The Managed Health Care Handbook,* 3rd Edition, for a discussion of contracting).

When the plan takes a physician off its list of participating providers in this way, it is often not subject to a due process type of review. The reason is that the separation is based on practice style and fit, not accusations of rule breaking or poor quality. Although this may not seem fair at first blush, in point of fact most contracts certainly allow physicians to terminate if they feel the fit is poor; plans have the same right, even if they do not exercise it frequently. Terminating physicians in this manner has the potential for creating adverse relations in the network if there is the perception that the plan is acting arbitrarily and without reason. On the other hand, assuming that the terminated physician does indeed practice profligately, the other physicians in the network are probably aware of it, so that there may not be that much shock and surprise.

Even so, such steps are drastic and should not be done frequently or taken lightly. It should also be noted that in some states, legislative efforts to prevent health plans from terminating physicians without "due cause" have been undertaken and remain the subject of heated debate.

CONCLUSION

Changing physician behavior is crucial to the success of any managed care plan, but it is not always easy. Physicians tend to have a strong need for autonomy and control, potential for role conflicts, uneven understanding of the economics or insurance functions of managed care, and ingrained practice habits. Plan managers can exacerbate the difficulties in changing physician behavior by failing to be responsive and consistent, failing to differentiate their plan from other plans, failing to provide positive feedback, failing to address specific problems with providers early, and failing to take a stepwise approach to managing change.

Systematic approaches to changing physician behavior can be successfully used for many aspects of practice. Continuing education, creation and dissemination of practice protocols, and data feedback are all useful techniques, especially when combined with financial incentives.

When reasonable efforts to improve physician behavior are unsuccessful and the problems are serious, discipline and sanctions must be applied. Due process must be followed before termination for poor quality, and it may be useful in other settings as well. In the final analysis, it is the plan's responsibility to effect changes in provider behavior that will benefit all the parties concerned and to take action when necessary.

REFERENCES

1. Hillman AL, Pauly MV, Kerman K, Martinek CR. HMO managers' views on financial incentives and quality. *Health Aff.* Winter 1991:207–219.
2. Hillman AL, Pauly MV, Kersten JJ. How do financial incentives affect physicians' clinical decisions and the financial performance of health maintenance organizations? *N Engl J Med.* 1989;321:86–92.
3. Greene HL, Goldberg RJ, Beattie H, et al. Physician

attitudes toward cost containment: the missing piece of the puzzle. *Arch Intern Med.* 1989;149:1966–1968.
4. O'Connor SJ, Lanning JA. The end of autonomy? Reflections on the postprofessional physician. *Health Care Manage Rev.* 1992;17(1):63–72.
5. Salmon JW, White W, Feinglass J. The futures of physicians: agency and autonomy reconsidered. *Theor Med.* 1990;11:261–274.
6. Schulz R, Scheckler WE, Girard C, Barker K. Physician adaptation to health maintenance organizations and implications for management. *Health Serv Res.* 1990;25:43–64.
7. Deckard GJ. Physician responses to a managed environment: a perceptual paradox. *Health Care Manage Rev.* 1995;20(1):40–46.
8. Baker LC, Cantor JC. Physician satisfaction under managed care. *Health Aff.* 1993(suppl):258–270.
9. Emanuel EJ, Dubler NN. Preserving the physician-patient relationship in the era of managed care. *JAMA.* 1995;273(4):323–329.
10. Anderson RO. How do you manage the demanding (difficult) patient? *HMO Pract.* 1990;4:15–16.
11. Davis DA, Thomson MA, Oxman AD, Haynes RB. Evidence for the effectiveness of CME: a review of 50 randomized controlled trials. *JAMA.* 1992;268:1111–1117.
12. White CW, Albanese MA, Brown DD, Caplan RM. The effectiveness of continuing medical education in changing the behavior of physicians caring for patients with acute myocardial infarction: a controlled randomized trial. *Ann Intern Med.* 1985;102:686–692.
13. Davis DA, Thomson MA, Oxman AD, Haynes RB. Changing physician performance: a systematic review of the effect of continuing medical education strategies. *JAMA.* 1995;274(9):700–706.
14. Myers SA, Gleicher N. A successful program to lower Cesarean section rates. *N Engl J Med.* 1989;319:1511–1516.
15. Wennberg JE, Blowers L, Parker R, Gittelsohn AM. Changes in tonsillectomy rates associated with feedback and review. *Pediatrics.* 1977;59:821–826.
16. Frazier LM, Brown JT, Divine GW, et al. Academia and clinic: can physician education lower the cost of prescription drugs? A prospective, controlled trial. *Ann Intern Med.* 1991;15:116–121.
17. Marton KI, Tul V, Sox HC. Modifying test-ordering behavior in the outpatient medical clinic. *Arch Intern Med.* 1985;145:816–821.
18. Berwick DM, Coltin KL. Feedback reduces test use in a health maintenance organization. *JAMA.* 1986;255:1450–1454.
19. Billi JE, Hejna GF, Wolf FM, et al. The effects of a cost-education program on hospital charges. *J Gen Intern Med.* 1987;2:306–311.
20. Billi JE, Duran-Arenas L, Wise CE, et al. The effects of a low-cost intervention program on hospital costs. *J Gen Intern Med.* 1992;7:411–416.
21. Manheim LM, Feinglass J, Hughs R, et al. Training house officers to be cost conscious: effects of an educational intervention on charges and length of stay. *Med Care.* 1990;28:29–42.
22. Zablocki E. Sharing data with physicians. In: Zablocki E, ed. *Changing Physician Practice Patterns: Strategies for Success in a Capitated Health Care System.* Gaithersburg, MD: Aspen Publishers, Inc; 1995.
23. Dyck FJ, Murphy FA, Murphy JK, et al. Effect of surveillance on the number of hysterectomies in the province of Saskatchewan. *N Engl J Med.* 1977;296:1326–1328.
24. Lomas J, Enkin M, Anderson GM, et al. Opinion leaders vs. audits and feedback to implement practice guidelines: delivery after previous Cesarean section. *JAMA.* 1991;265:2202–2207.
25. Lee TH, Pearson SD, Johnson PA, et al. Failure of information as an intervention to modify clinical management: a time-series trial in patients with acute chest pain. *Ann Intern Med.* 1995;122:434–437.
26. Axt-Adam P, van der Wouden JC, van der Does E. Influencing behavior of physicians ordering laboratory tests: a literature study. *Med Care.* 1993;31(9):784–794.
27. Parrino TA. The nonvalue of retrospective peer comparison feedback in containing hospital antibiotic costs. *Am J Med.* 1989;86:442–448.
28. Soumerai SB, McLaughlin TJ, Avorn J. Improving drug prescribing in primary care: a critical analysis of the experimental literature. *Milbank Q.* 1989;67: 268–317.
29. Martin AR, Wolf MA, Thibodeau LA, et al. A trial of two strategies to modify the test-ordering behavior of medical residents. *N Engl J Med.* 1980;303:1330–1336.
30. Kosecoff J, Kanouse DE, Rogers WH, et al. Effects of the National Institutes of Health Consensus Development Program on Physician Practice. *JAMA.* 1987;258:2708–2713.
31. Lomas J, Anderson GM, Domnik-Pierre K, et al. Do practice guidelines guide practice? The effect of a consensus statement on the practice of physicians. *N Engl J Med.* 1989;321:1306–1311.
32. Soumersai SB, Avorn J. Principles of educational outreach ("academic detailing") to improve clinical decision making. *JAMA.* 1990;263:549–556.
33. Ellrodt AG, Conner L, Riedinger M, Weingarten S. Measuring and improving physician compliance with clinical practice guidelines: a controlled intervention trial. *Ann Intern Med.* 1995;122:277–282.
34. Health Care Quality Improvement Act of 1986. 45 USC §11101–11152. Sec 412, Standards for Professional Review Actions.

SUGGESTED READINGS

Berenson RA. Commentary: a physician's view of managed care. *Health Aff.* 1991;10(4):106–119.

Chernov AJ. Managed care and the doctor-patient relationship. *Med Interface.* February 1993:30–32.

Greco PJ, Eisenberg JM. Changing physicians' practices. *N Engl J Med.* 1993;329(17):1271–1274.

Eisenberg JM. *Doctors' Decisions and the Cost of Medical Care.* Ann Arbor, MI: Health Administration Press; 1986.

Mittman BS, Siu AL. Changing provider behavior: applying research on outcomes and effectiveness in health care. In: Shortell SM, Reinhardt UE, eds. *Improving Health Policy Management: Nine Critical Research Issues for the 1990s.* Ann Arbor, MI: Health Administration Press; 1992.

Nash DB, ed. *The Physician's Guide to Managed Care.* Gaithersburg, MD: Aspen Publishers, Inc; 1994.

Zablocki E, ed. *Changing Physician Practice Patterns: Strategies for Success in a Capitated Health Care System.* Gaithersburg, MD: Aspen Publishers, Inc; 1995.

Chapter 40

Member Behavior Change

Nancy W. Spangler

Chapter Outline

- Introduction
- They Know Better, So Why Don't They Just Stop?
- Models for Affecting Patient Behaviors
- Tools for Enhancing Change
- From Theory into Practice: Humana's CHIP Program
- Conclusion

INTRODUCTION

In recent decades, most people in the United States have blindly placed their trust in the miracles of the medical system. They have been content to be taken care of and have "followed doctor's orders" obediently. With the advent of managed care, however, patients are now being asked to

- Be proactive in preventing disease and disability.
- Become involved in health care decision making.
- Take part in actively managing chronic conditions.
- Interact effectively with providers.

All of these expectations require a significant change in attitudes about health. Achieving greater active participation from and assigning greater responsibility to people previously conditioned to be passive recipients of care is no easy task. This chapter explores some of the major constructs and theories of behavior change and adult learning and how they apply to such areas as health risk reduction, demand management, disease management, compliance, and community health initiatives. Examples of and rationales for some of the strategies being used by managed care organizations (MCOs) to affect patient behavior will be provided.

THEY KNOW BETTER, SO WHY DON'T THEY JUST STOP?

Just watch any old movie from the 1940s and notice the amount of cigarette smoking. While intending to appear sophisticated and refined, the actors (probably) did not know at the time the negative effect of all that smoking on their health. In today's movies, characters light up much less often. When they do, it is more likely to indicate shadiness than to indicate refinement. With today's knowledge about the hazards of smoking, large numbers of people attempt to quit. Smoking has declined since the 1960s, yet a large portion of the United States' population continues to smoke. If they consciously acknowledge that they would be better off if they didn't smoke, overeat, abuse alcohol, or drive without seat belts, why do they continue these self-defeating behaviors? Why not just stop? This is a question asked by many professionals in fields from adult education to health psychology, primary care to health promotion. The answer appears far from simple. Attempting to change the behavior of human beings can be complex and problematic.

Readiness To Change

According to Prochaska and DiClemente, originators of the transtheoretical theory (also known as the stages of change model), simple knowledge that one *should* change a certain behavior will not necessarily cause a person to initiate or sustain a change.[1,2] The following example is familiar to many. After nagging your smoking patient (or loved one) to stop, and providing yet more information on nicotine patches and other quitting strategies, you are met not with the typical disinterested stare and nod, but with outright belligerence and anger. Your response? A mental note to yourself not to bring up the subject again. After all, you don't want the patient to stop coming to you all together. (In the case of a loved one, you opt for harmony rather than another argument.) Unfortunately, the message your patient hears in your silence about the behavior in succeeding visits is "Smoking must not be all that important. My doctor doesn't even mention it any more."

Prochaska and DiClemente point out that efforts to change patient behaviors focus most of their resources in techniques appropriate for those in an active state of change, though fewer than 20% of people in a target population are prepared for action at any given time. The remainder are in one of several other stages of readiness to change. Figure 40–1 depicts an adaptation of Prochaska's model to illustrate the cyclical nature of change and the type of support that will be most effective in moving people toward action. Table 40–1 provides additional description of these phases or events.

Cycling between the stages is common, and successful termination (ending the cycle of change in permanent maintenance) typically requires numerous attempts to change. Tailoring the health professional's response to individuals based on their stage may be helpful in moving patients through the change cycle. As in the previous example with the smoking patient, a threatening approach or suggestion of tools and techniques will likely elicit resistance and defensiveness from a person who is not yet con-

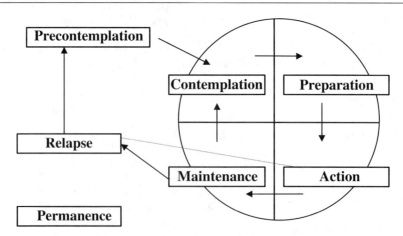

Figure 40–1 Stages of Change Model. *Source:* J Prochaska and C DiClemente, Stages and Processes of Self-Change of Smoking: Toward an Integrative Model of Change, *Journal of Consulting and Clinical Psychology,* Vol 51, pp 390–395, Copyright © 1983 by the American Psychological Association. Adapted with permission.

Table 40–1 Patient Approaches Based on Stage of Readiness To Change

Stage	Patient Characteristics	Tailored Response Needed
Precontemplation	Unaware of the need to change; unwilling or too discouraged to try, at least within the next 6 months; may be defensive.	Consciousness raising to increase patients' awareness of the negative consequences of the behavior and the inaccuracy of their denial or other defenses; nonjudgmental information.
Contemplation	Self-reflection; open to information; asking more questions; evaluating options for change, and weighing the pros and cons; ambivalence about next steps. Seriously considering change in next 6 months.	Emotional arousal; assistance in evaluating the pros and cons of change and ways to reduce the cons; provision of information; identification of supportive tools and resources.
Preparation	Determined to take action within next 30 days; sense of confidence and commitment.	Gain commitment to action; assist in setting attainable goals and dates for achieving them; praise incremental efforts; help with skill development; encourage support seeking.
Action	Overt change in behavior; attempts at reaching new goals; skill development.	Encourage rewards for achieving goals; assist in thinking through potential relapse situations and how to avoid; explore irrational self-talk ("I can't, I must") and encourage counterthinking; continue to reinforce social support.
Maintenance	Action sustained for 6 months or more; potential overconfidence may lead to slips in behavior if patients let up their guard.	Reinforce likelihood of slips and erosion of resolve; reduce self-blame for lapses and encourage sticking with plan; remind of achievements.

templating change in that behavior, while a matter of fact, nonjudgmental approach, advising the patient to quit and repeating the consequences of the behavior at *each* visit, may invoke a less emotional response and, over time, move the patient toward contemplating life as a nonsmoker. Thus, the health professionals' "success" (both in terms of patient health and the professionals' abilities to help) must be measured not only by the end behavior, but by incremental movements toward the goal.

For many health professionals, working with patients who are in the precontemplation stage can be frustrating. Some patients are simply unaware of the value of changing their behaviors. A discussion of social marketing to increase knowledge and motivation will follow later in this chapter. For many others, however, one can often sense an attitude of resignation, a "Why bother?" mindset. What are some factors that could contribute to lingering in this stage of precontemplation?

Effect of Beliefs

Bandura's theory of self-efficacy suggests that a person's goal-directed behavior toward changing a health habit is based on two expectancies held by the individual:

- *Outcome expectancy*—a belief that a particular behavior will result in a desired outcome (eg, that exercise could help one lose weight)
- *Efficacy expectancy*—a belief that the individual is capable of performing the behavior (eg, that he or she could learn the necessary skills and overcome whatever barriers might get in the way)

Thus, self-efficacy can be said to be based on a sense of control over one's abilities and one's environment. Without a sense of self-efficacy, a person is unlikely to contemplate changes that require risking failure.[3]

Additional Theories

Seligman's work has examined how our early experiences may play a part in how we develop a sense of control and ability to cope. Seligman's theory of learned helplessness was established through experiments by his student, Madelon Visintainer, where rats were placed in highly stressful situations with no means of escape. Initial goal-directed escape behaviors of the active, aroused rats included multiple attempts at problem-solving behaviors to gain access to an escape route. As these attempts failed, the rats grew angry, agitated, and vocal. With repeated attempts at unsuccessfully controlling their circumstances, however, the rats reduced their attempts at escape and fell into a passive state of helplessness, comparable to human depression. This learned helplessness, due to the blockage of goal-directed behavior, also was found to compromise immune system function. The comparison rats who were allowed to experience success over their circumstances were better able to reject tumor growth than those who experienced early helplessness. The rat's "childhood" mastery experience served as an immunization against cancer.[4]

Seligman's subsequent work has been directed toward factors that modulate a sense of learned helplessness in people's lives. He has postulated that a sense of optimism can also be learned and that this optimism can positively affect health outcomes as described. According to Seligman, optimistic people can develop

- a stronger immune system
- a belief in their abilities to stick with health regimens and seek medical care
- an ability to cope with change and negative life events
- stronger systems of social support

Much of the direction of Seligman and his colleagues was inspired by the work of Ellen Langer and Judith Rodin, whose research looked at issues of personal control.[5,6] In their studies, individuals in nursing homes were given greater control over decisions about their day-to-day lives (meals, activities, room arrangement, etc) and some responsibility (plants that they were assigned to care for). After 18 months, levels of activity, alertness, and general well-being improved in the group with greater control and got worse in those who were not similarly empowered. In addition, lower levels of mortality were found in the group with enhanced control. This body of work suggests that as we age, control becomes of special significance, because older people may be viewed as less competent and may be assisted with tasks that they had previously accomplished independently. The resulting sense of limited self-efficacy, perceived lack of control, and helplessness may hasten a decline in physical and emotional functioning.

In applying such work to human children, we can see that exposure to traumatic life circumstances they are unable to control, such as divorce, alcoholic or abusive parents, and danger in inner cities, could create a pervasive sense of helplessness. In fact, Wallerstein postulates that this resulting generalized powerlessness, or lack of control over living conditions, employment opportunities, social status, and so on, should receive greater attention as a risk factor for many diseases. Interventions that build up community empowerment may, thus, result in an improved collective sense of control and ability that contributes to improved population health status, as shown in Figure 40–2.[7]

MODELS FOR AFFECTING PATIENT BEHAVIORS

If poor health results from the factors described above, what accounts for the fact that some people *do* make changes in their lives, do become optimistic, do begin to take charge of their health? Prochaska and colleagues suggest that in moving from precontemplation to action an individual comes to perceive that the "pros" of changing outweigh the "cons," or the benefits outweigh the barriers.[2] As summarized in Figure 40–1, the processes used in moving toward change may include consciousness raising, emotional arousal, self-evaluation, commitment, rewards, and helping relationships. What intervention models can be used by organizations to support this change?

System-Based Models

MCOs (and organized medical care delivery systems, a subset of MCOs) are ideally positioned to have an effect on health attitudes and behaviors because of their access to patient populations and their ability to systematically measure improvement in health status. In addition, unique approaches to communicating with patients in a controlled fashion may be attempted by MCOs with adequate contact database systems. Health promotion, demand management, and disease management can reach new heights with "social marketing," an approach currently uncommon in health care, to raise health consciousness and create conditions for self-evaluation and decision making in targeted populations. Kotler and Roberto define social marketing as "a strategy for changing behavior. It combines the best elements of the traditional approaches to social change in an integrated planning and action framework and utilizes advances in communication technology and marketing skills. . . . The goal is to advance a social cause, idea, or behavior."[8(p24)]

While most MCOs have used public relations campaigns to promote issues such as immunizations and healthy lifestyles, few have become highly sophisticated in the marketing techniques used by many businesses. Corporations such as Nike or Philip Morris have not affected buying behaviors of the American public by mailing out photocopied fliers to interested consumers who call for information, a primary promotional technique for many health education departments on a shoestring budget. On the other extreme, many

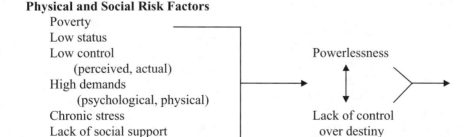

Figure 40–2 Disease as Related to Powerlessness. *Source:* Reprinted with permission from N Wallerstein, Powerlessness, Empowerment, and Health: Implications for Health Promotion Programs, *American Journal of Health Promotion*, Vol 6, pp 197–205, © 1992.

MCOs are currently bombarding their members indiscriminately; the overwhelmed members tire of searching for what might be meaningful in the sea of printed information.

Techniques that will increase effect on behavior include

- segmenting the target audience according to geographic, demographic, or psychographic variables
- "product" and brand name testing
- positioning research to determine perceptions of target audiences
- "product packaging," communications testing, and postcommunication recall testing
- test marketing for adoption behavior, and research on and selection of distribution channels

Use of computer-tailored communications has great promise for affecting behavior. Strecher et al found that using patients' perceived benefits of and barriers to quitting smoking in creating a highly personal letter recommending that they quit had a significantly greater effect on quit rates than a generic letter.[9] Such techniques can better target the individual's personal beliefs and attitudes and improve persuasiveness.

Community Systems

To reach improved levels of population health, health professionals must become better at viewing member care from a systems view. In this view, one part of a system rarely changes in isolation. A family member will be more successful in changing eating habits if the whole family changes. One family will be more successful if the entire community begins adopting healthier habits of exercising, relating positively to one another, reducing smoking, and so on. A common, or at least perceived to be common (not having been studied systematically), rationale among MCOs is to invest in programs that will produce an effect within 2 years. "Why invest in patients who will likely be in someone else's plan before there is a return on our investment?" some executives have been heard to ask (or imputed to be thinking, based on their actions). This is not systems thinking.

With a systems view, *all* MCOs in a community work collaboratively in issues of health improvement. Media campaigns are created with sufficient power and persuasion to raise the population's consciousness on targeted issues, and larger numbers of people are moved toward action. MCOs can contribute jointly to analyses of cultural incentives for particular behaviors, such as teen pregnancy, alcohol use, or high-risk behaviors, and in strategies to address those issues. Community programs to improve personal safety, transportation, job availability, and neighborhood pride and social support should be supported politically, financially, and through broad involvement by major health organizations serving the community. People *do* change when their attitudes and opinions are influenced. In fact, people will do amazing things, both positive and negative, when they *believe* they can and should. Just as the rudder of a ship is powerful in changing the ship's direction, so can MCOs become powerful in positively changing the behavior of a community and reap the rewards over the long term.

Patient–Provider Models

Direct interaction between the patient and physician or other clinician can also be very effective in encouraging changes in health behaviors. According to Greenfield, DiMatteo, and others, efforts at improving patient–physician communication and enhancing the patient's sense of control through participation in treatment decisions can result in

- improved *adherence* to medication and other treatment regimens[10]
- improved *health outcomes*, such as blood pressure and blood sugar control[10]
- enhanced *patient satisfaction*[11]

When written information about the patient's medical condition was provided and patients were coached in behavioral strategies (such as asking questions of the provider, negotiating treatment options, and decreasing anxiety and feelings of intimidation), the group's functional status and other health measures were improved.

Most patients respect their physician's knowledge and value information they receive from him or her highly. Therefore, the role of the physician in changing behavior cannot be overemphasized. Unfortunately, increased pressures for providers to help cut costs by seeing more patients in less time have made many providers feel reluctant or unable to educate or counsel patients as they might have done in the past. Few physicians are well prepared in counseling techniques during medical training, and many report feeling ill equipped for these tasks. Furthermore, most physicians tend to be pessimistic about their patients' ability to change even when they do discuss lifestyle issues with patients. Numerous studies, however, document the effectiveness of repeated advice and brief behavior counseling in such areas as alcohol abuse, smoking, obesity, and lack of physical activity.

The physician recommendation or brief intervention is more likely to *motivate* the patient toward greater readiness to change, gaining their *commitment* and offering them *hope* that others just like them have made similar changes, than in teaching them the actual *skills* for change. Teaching skills demands more time than an office visit could allow, but motivating, gaining commitments, and offering hope can be brief, but powerful, considering that an estimated 70% of adults visit their physician yearly. And, while a limited number of people actually enroll in formal behavior change programs, many will attempt a change on their own. (It is estimated that 95% of smokers who quit do so on their own without participating in a group program. Most people will make several, if not many, attempts at quitting before they finally quit for good.)[12] Fiore recommends assessment of smoking status as the "fifth vital sign."[13] In other words, by asking every patient about their smoking status and documenting it at every visit (as is standard practice for vital signs such as blood pressure and weight), physicians can ensure that all smokers are identified and routinely advised to quit. Exhibit 40–1 lists ways in which physicians can personalize reasons to quit smoking.

The "4 A's" method was developed by the National Cancer Institute[14] for physicians to fol-

Exhibit 40–1 Personalizing the Reasons To Quit Smoking

New smokers
- Easier to quit now

Long-term smokers
- Reduce risks for cancer and heart disease
- Be able to enjoy retirement and grandchildren

Smokers with a positive family history
- Reduce risks for cancer or heart disease

Asymptomatic adults
- Reduce risks for heart disease, cancer, emphysema
- Cost
- Wrinkles
- Inconvenience
- Bad breath
- Socially unacceptable

Pregnant women
- Miscarriage
- Low-birthweight infant
- Fetal death

Symptomatic adults
- Respiratory infections, cough
- Dyspnea
- Claudication
- Esophagitis
- Sore throats
- Ulcers
- Osteoporosis
- Gum disease

Teenagers
- Bad breath
- Cost
- Cough
- Respiratory infections
- Sore throats
- Effect on sports
- Life controlled by cigarettes

All smokers
- Cost
- Ability to exercise
- Sense of well-being
- Health

Source: Adapted with permission from CG Husten and MW Manley, How To Help Your Patients Stop Smoking, *American Family Physician,* © 1990, American Academy of Family Physicians.

low for enhancing smoking cessation, but it can be applied to other issues in health promotion and disease management as well. It consists of these tasks:

1. *Ask* about smoking status at every visit. If patients smoke, ask how much, how soon after waking, if they have ever tried to stop before, and if they are currently interested in stopping.
2. *Advise* all smoking patients to quit. Personalize reasons according to the individual.
3. *Assist* patients in stopping. If patients express interest, help them set a quit date, provide self-help materials, and discuss nicotine replacement therapies. If patients resist, simply let them know that when they eventually become ready, support will be available.
4. *Arrange* follow-up visits. Since relapse (for any behavior change) is common in the first 2 weeks, a follow-up visit within 1 to 2 weeks of the selected quit date is recommended. If the patient has lapsed, circumstances for the lapse should be discussed and strategies for the next attempt determined.

Stepped Model

To reach optimal effect of behavior change interventions, the stepped care and matching model advanced by Abrams et al[15] also serves as an excellent guide for delivering the appropriate level of intervention. The authors acknowledge that intensive clinician intervention can be highly effective, yet may not be necessary for all patients and can be costly and difficult to access for many. While health education approaches of self-help pamphlets and posters have a wider reach, their effectiveness is lower. Even so, following this stepped model, by tailoring interventions according to such factors as the patient's motivational level, level of nicotine dependence, comorbidities, and number of previous attempts to change, a larger total effect can be achieved. For example, smokers who are ready to quit, are not heavily addicted, and have made no previous attempts to quit would first be given low-cost self-help materials and encouragement to attempt to quit on their own.

If these smokers' attempts to quit are unsuccessful independently, the approach would move to brief counseling with follow up (eg, by telephone). If smokers are still unsuccessful, intensive clinical treatment with a specialist highly experienced in behavior change would take place. This stepped-up approach protects individuals from a sense of failure by assuring them that there is another novel approach "if at first they don't succeed"; the approach does not recycle through the same old approaches. It also reserves the time of highly trained specialists for those who truly need it while broadening the effect of the total intervention.

Dealing with Relapse

Success in sustaining change may be predicted in the way the individual reacts to a momentary lapse, or return to a previous unhealthy behavior. As Marlatt and Gordon describe, if individuals attribute lapses to a global failure of their personal and moral character (observed through such statements as "I'm just basically weak, no wonder I blew it."), this negative emotional state can create a mindset that makes it likely for the individual to relapse completely.[16] If, however, the individual can be assisted to view the lapse as an isolated mistake and not a *pattern* of failure, to learn from the lapse, to prepare cognitively for similar situations in the future, and to set a new date, the person is much more likely to try again and stay on track. The encouragement of the physician here again cannot be understated. These thinking styles begin early and contribute to many patterns of life behaviors.

Relapse can also be looked at through concepts in cognitive neuroscience. When a person is learning any new motor pattern, a multitude of cortical pathways in the brain are used initially. After many repetitions, however, the movements become automatic and are managed by brain centers other than the initial cortical connections. For example, when first learning to drive, people consciously think about where to place their feet, how quickly to press the gas pedal when entering traffic, and so on. Years later, drivers can reach their destinations without giving much thought to how they got there. Operating an automobile has become a "no brainer."

Similarly, when first consciously attempting to change a health behavior, people are highly vigilant and attentive to their task. Many cortical subsystems are activated, and multiple synaptic connections are utilized. Memory traces, or engrams, are encoded and become strengthened with each repetition of the new behavior. This analogy from Kosslyn and Koenig is illustrative of this concept:

> During the initial phases of memory encoding, it is as if one is preserving the shape of a letter by walking a particular route on a lawn. The pattern is dynamic, and is only evident in the way one moves. After a period of time, however, the grass will wear through, creating a dirt pathway. At that point, one can stop walking; the information is preserved structurally.[17(p351)]

The analogy suggests that as one performs a new behavior, over time, and with many repetitions, the memory traces and neural pathways become stronger, as in wearing down a path. Yet if one stops the behavior before the grass has worn through, so to speak, the likelihood of relapse remains higher. If people try to "get back on the right path," the traces of their former steps remain, making it easier to stay on track with each successive attempt.[17] These authors also offer a neurological rationale for using imagery for relapse prevention. Brain scans of patients asked to simply imagine they are moving objects have documented the same neural activity in the motor cortex of the frontal and parietal lobes as patients who actually moved the objects. Thus, patients' mental preparations for situations that could be tempting are likely to involve the same neural subsystems that patients would use if they were in that situation; memory traces for positive coping skills can begin developing in advance.

Worksite Models

Progressive MCOs work in partnership with their purchasers when they realize the advantages inherent in offering health promotion and rehabilitation programs at the work site. These include

1. Policies, such as limitations on smoking, and environmental support, such as availability of healthy foods, flextime, and adequate work spaces, create opportunities for healthy practices.
2. Support from peers to help increase readiness to change and reinforce maintenance.
3. Incentives, whether direct financial incentives, tangibles (T-shirts, fitness equipment, gift certificates, etc), reward days off, or social recognition.
4. Employee assistance programs to help employees deal with the emotional issues that frequently affect health.
5. Early return to work programs and on-site rehabilitation following injuries, which promote a sense of ability rather than disability and keep workers accustomed to their work routine and connected to vital social support systems.
6. On-site support staff for individual coaching, periodic tracking of health status, and group education.

Providing programs at employer sites enables MCOs to use the employer's internal marketing approaches to advertise programs and reach a more "captive" audience. While the US workplace is a melting pot of cultures, workplace programs can reduce some of the variables that make teaching group programs at clinics very difficult, such as vast differences in age, language, and health status. In addition, workplace programs eliminate problems in taking time off work and obtaining transportation. Access to corporate training departments will frequently allow use of advanced teaching approaches ideal for adult learning.

According to Knowles, adult learning differs vastly from learning of children.[18] Adults learn best when

- They feel respected.
- New learning is related to their own life experiences.
- New learning has immediate usefulness to them.
- They are allowed to *do*, or discover concepts actively (we remember 20% of what we hear, 40% of what we hear and see, and 80% of what we hear, see, and do).

Knowles also addresses readiness to learn, suggesting that movement from one stage of life to another—getting married, having children, losing a loved one—can trigger a "need-to-know" situation. For example, until one has children, there is little motivation to learn about parenting skills, discipline methods, or childhood immunizations. Engaging employees in "diagnostic experiences" where they can assess where they are now (as through the use of health risk appraisals; see Part I) and receive support to determine where they want to go (through worksite health promotion staff or telephone "coaches"; see Chapter 6) can provide opportunities for valuable learning.

TOOLS FOR ENHANCING CHANGE

With patients in various stages of readiness and with many types of health behaviors, developing strategies to support change can be challenging. The following are some examples of approaches that are in use. As the high interest in behavior change generates research over the next decade, health professionals' level of sophistication and the effectiveness of tools will increase significantly.

Communications

As mentioned in previous sections, communication techniques employed to help patients understand the consequences of their current behavior and to see the possibilities of changing it can be very helpful in moving people from "just thinking about it" to "doing something about it." Broad, highly visible campaigns around targeted health topics can be implemented for this purpose. Table 40–2 shows various uses of media for communicating information, contrasting the qualities and abilities of each.

In addition to selecting media carefully, targeting information to critical life stages is recommended (for example, a birthday card to women on their 40th birthday to encourage a mammogram or information given to parents of 4-year-olds to encourage continued immunization).

Reinforcers

For individuals who are in a preparation or action stage of change, there are a number of ways to support and reinforce desired behaviors.

Tracking Methods

Tools that assist the patient in tracking behaviors (such as number of cigarettes smoked and time of day, amount and perceived level of exertion when exercising, types and amounts of foods consumed and feelings of satisfaction after eating) are effective ways to increase awareness about behaviors. They assist in setting goals and identifying barriers, actively involve the patient in the change process, and reinforce progress. In many cases, it is best to track the *behavior* (eating pattern), rather than the *result* (actual daily weight), because the behavior is more in the control of the patient and is easier to reinforce. Such tools as blood pressure wallet cards and personal medical records for referring to during interactions with providers can also stim-

Table 40–2 Comparative Value of Media for Health Communication and Education

Type	High Emotional Appeal, Persuasive	Able To Convey Detailed or Complicated Information	Easy To Personalize	Low Cost	Life-long
Print materials					
• Newspaper advertisements	xxx	x		xx	
• Newsletters	x	xx	x	xx	x
• Magazine articles	xx	xxx			xx
• Pamphlets	x	xx	x	xxx	xxx
• Postcards	xx		xxx	xxx	x
• Books	x	xxx		xx	xxx
Billboards	xxxx				
Television advertisements or programs	xxxx				
Radio advertisements	xxx	x			
Audiotapes	xx	xx	x	x	xx
Videotapes	xxx	x			x
Telephone contacts	xx	xx	xxx	xx	x
Interactive CDs	xx	xx	x		x

Key: (blank indicates minimal application)
x = low suitability
xx = medium to low suitability
xxx = medium to high suitability
xxxx = high suitability

ulate a greater sense of individual responsibility, particularly if the patient is encouraged by the provider to use the materials.

Action Plans and Contracts

Written plans and contracts serve several purposes (an example is provided in Exhibit 40–2). By thinking through goals, patients personalize the approach, planning the series of steps needed. Preparing ahead equips them for inevitable barriers and solutions. Signing the plan with another person (physician, medical assistant, program facilitator, family member) serves as a public announcement, a declaration of the intention to change, and an expectation that the cosigner will follow up with patients on their progress. In addition, the physical act of writing the goals, rather than just thinking about them, uses additional neural subsystems and develops a visual memory trace, possibly reinforcing success, as mentioned earlier.

Reminder Systems

Tools for reminding patients of desired behaviors can take many forms. Pill boxes allowing patients to separate their various pills for the day in small compartments are helpful, as are pill containers that can be clipped to the toothbrush, serving as a reminder for adherence to medications. Written reminders for exercise sessions recorded in the patient's weekly calendar can help reduce the perceived barrier of "not enough time."

Exhibit 40–2 Sample Action Plan

Name _____

Member ID# _____

Your Action Plan for _____
(Insert goal you chose on enrollment form)

Specific objectives and dates for achieving them:

_____

_____

Success strategies for reaching goal:

_____

_____

Roadblocks that might get in my way and how I will deal with them:

_____

_____

Additional information or support I need:

_____

_____

My reward and when I will give it to myself:

_____

_____

Return original with enrollment form. Keep copy for your records.

Courtesy of Humana, Inc, 1996, Kansas City, Missouri.

Incentives and Rewards

Patients should be encouraged to establish personal rewards for achieving goals as part of the action plan/contract process. Rewards should be set for each progressive step toward the goal to reinforce a perception of momentum. As with tracking, the reward should be based on completing specific behaviors rather than achieving specific physiologic outcomes. Rewards may be tangible items the patient might be preparing to buy but can postpone the purchase of, or they can be gifts of time to be spent in a unique way, such as browsing in a museum or attending a sporting event. Work sites have successfully used rewards and recognition to reinforce behaviors. This setting is ideal for promoting good-natured competitions and lotteries for targeted behaviors (eg, all participants who record the type and amount of physical activity engaged in over a period of weeks may receive a chance to win a gift certificate toward exercise clothing or equipment).

Social Support

Coaching

Whether completed face-to-face or by phone, coaching to assist patients in setting progressive goals, identifying barriers, recovering quickly from lapses, and preparing cognitively for future problems has been used successfully in areas of lifestyle change and medication adherence. This type of intervention has been effective both with patients who have expressed an interest in changing, as well as with "nonvolunteer" smokers. Just setting up the expectation that the coach will be following up with them can be reinforcing for some patients. Coaches should be well trained in motivational counseling techniques that enhance empathy and support self-efficacy. These include exploring resistance in a nonthreatening way, asking open-ended questions, reflective listening (responding to the speaker with a clarification of what you heard), and eliciting concerns and fears. Coaches should also be trained in sensitivity to cultural and emotional issues that may be at the root of many behaviors.

Enlisting Support

Family members can be enlisted to actively support patients' revised behavior. Their inclusion is especially important when the changes will affect them as well (such as changes in diet or in ways of communicating to better manage stress). Support groups abound for many conditions and interests. Most are directed by lay leaders, and many have been highly successful in helping patients maintain changed behavior.

FROM THEORY INTO PRACTICE: HUMANA'S CHIP PROGRAM

This section presents an example of a program that turned these concepts into action. Discussions between Kansas City administrators of the MCO Humana and the pharmaceutical company Hoechst Marion Roussel about improving care for patients with cardiovascular health problems led to a partnership in patient education between the two organizations. The program, called the Cardiovascular Health Improvement Process, or CHIP, was developed in 1995 and implemented in 1996. Patients with hypertension were selected for the CHIP intervention due to the prevalence of hypertension within the Humana population and the potential reduction in cardiovascular complications that could be achieved with hypertensive management through lifestyle change and medication compliance.

With Prochaska and DiClemente's stages of change model in mind (refer to "Readiness To Change" above), hypertensive members were subdivided according to their response to an initial mailing (Figure 40–3). The level of intervention was determined by the member's expressed commitment to change. The groups were labeled as follows:

1. *Participants* showed they were *contemplating* change by participating in the cardiac risk check (CRC), a computerized assessment of risks for cardiovascular disease. They received encouragement, first through a reminder postcard, then through a video, to commit to change by enrolling in the CHIP program.
2. *Enrollees*, or patients who indicated *active* readiness for a lifestyle change by completing the CRC *and* enrolling (ie, selecting a particular area of lifestyle change or medication compliance and setting specific goals to work on), were provided intervention. The intervention consisted of printed booklets specific to the lifestyle area selected and a customized CHIP newsletter providing information on behavior change, lifestyle, and medications.

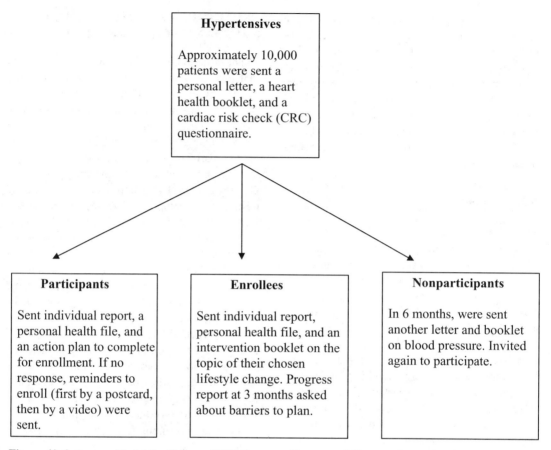

Figure 40–3 Process Model for Humana CHIP Program. Courtesy of Humana, Inc, 1996, Kansas City, Missouri.

Other interventions, including telephone support, were also explored but print interventions were selected as the focus for the first phase. Materials were developed for all participants and enrollees to encourage self-monitoring of blood pressure, medications, and health status and to enhance effective interaction with providers.

3. *Nonresponders* were those members who did not respond after several invitation reminders to participate. This group was thought to include many "precontemplators" who were not ready to begin a change process. Nonresponders were contacted in 6 months, provided information on the benefits of hypertension management, and invited again to participate.

In addition to the printed mailings to patients, meetings were held with Humana's Kansas City area physicians to describe the program and to discuss newly developed guidelines for treating hypertensive patients. The guidelines, based on recommendations in the Fifth Report of the Joint National Committee on Prevention, Detection, Evaluation, and Treatment of High Blood Pressure (JNC V), placed a heavy emphasis on lifestyle modifications both prior to and in conjunction with drug therapy for hypertension management.[19]

Program Effect

Telephone interview research provided by Hoechst Marion Roussel in October 1997 elicited valuable information regarding patients' opinions of the CHIP program, process, and materials. One hundred patients from each of the three groups were contacted.

Patient Changes

Overall, 56% of patients reported making positive lifestyle changes after receiving the CHIP information, with the largest response being from those who made a formal commitment to change and developed a written plan of action (84% of enrollees, 60% of participants, 24% of nonparticipants). Of those who made changes, 70% maintained them for 6 months or more, a time period considered significant for behavior maintenance.

Changes included

- Chose more healthful foods (78%)
- Increased activity levels (53%)
- Looked more at food labels (36%)
- Read more about high blood pressure (30%)
- Became more aware of triggers (eg, for smoking/stress/eating) (26%)
- Made more attempts to manage stress (24%)
- Used reminders for medications (23%)
- Asked physician more questions (21%)
- Reduced or quit smoking (8%)

While hypertension is generally considered to be an "older person's disease," younger patients were more likely to make a behavior change.

- 20–39 year olds (67%)
- 40–59 year olds (74%)
- 60–79 year olds (57%)
- 80+ year olds (43%)

Participation Information

The main reasons given for *not participating* in CHIP included

- Patient didn't recall receiving the information (56%)
- Patient thought he or she *did* return the questionnaire (11%)
- Forgot (7%)
- Just not a priority right now (7%)

Main reasons for not *enrolling* included

- Didn't recall the enrollment information (29%)
- Didn't want to commit to a "program" (24%)
- Not a priority (16%)
- Didn't want to complete the action plan required for enrolling (14%)

Of all those who did enroll, 58% reported that the goal setting process was very helpful. Interestingly, a large percent (92%) of African-American enrollees found this process very helpful.

Materials

Responses to all of the CHIP materials were favorable, and most patients (64%) said they would like to continue to receive information about high blood pressure, medications, and healthy lifestyles (59% of nonparticipants, 60% of participants, 73% of enrollees, 76% of African Americans, 60% of Caucasians).

Favored formats for intervention include

- mailed materials (85%) (This strong response supports the decision to use print intervention as the primary vehicle for patient education in projects like CHIP.)
- videotapes (26%)
- appointments with health professional (15%)
- telephone support (12%)
- group classes (6%)
- Internet programs (6%)

Effect on Opinion

Many patients (72%) reported that programs like CHIP affect their opinion of Humana in a very favorable way. Clearly, patients have valued CHIP and are eager for the health information and support the plan provides through such programs.

CONCLUSION

Patient behavior change may well be the next frontier in modern medicine. While not an easy task, improving patient adherence to lifestyle modifications, drug therapy regimens, and other treatment goals can enable managed care organizations to reduce costs and improve the quality of care. Efforts at applying current theories of behavior change as well as support of research to expand our body of knowledge in this area will become increasingly important in the near future.

REFERENCES

1. Prochaska J, DiClemente C. Stages and processes of self-change of smoking: toward an integrative model of change. *J Consult Clin Psychol.* 1983;51:390–395.
2. Prochaska J, DiClemente C. Towards a comprehensive model of change. In: Miller WR, Heather N, eds. *Treating Addictive Disorders: Processes of Change.* New York: Plenum Press; 1986:3–27.
3. Bandura A. *Principles of Behavior Modification.* New York: Holt, Rinehart, and Winston; 1969.
4. Seligman M, Visintainer M. Tumor rejection and early experience of uncontrollable shock in the rat. In: Brush FR, Overmier JB, eds. *Affect, Conditioning, and Cognition: Essays on the Determinants of Behavior.* Hillsdale, NJ: Erlbaum; 1985:203–210.
5. Langer EJ, Rodin J. Effects of choice and enhanced personal responsibility for the aged: a field experiment in an institutional setting. *J Personality Soc Psychol.* 1982;34:437–439.
6. Rodin J. Effects of the sense of control. *Science.* 1986;233:1271–1276.
7. Wallerstein N. Powerlessness, empowerment, and health: implications for health promotion programs. *Am J Health Promotion.* 1992;6:197–205.
8. Kotler P, Roberto E. *Social Marketing: Strategies for Changing Public Behavior.* New York: Free Press; 1989.
9. Strecher V, Kreuter M, Den Boer D, et al. The effects of computer-tailored smoking cessation messages in family practice settings. *J Fam Pract.* 1994;39:262–270.
10. Greenfield S, Kaplan S, Ware J, et al. Patient's participation in medical care: effects on blood sugar and quality of life in diabetes. *J Gen Int Med.* 1988;3:448–457.
11. DiMatteo R, et al. The significance of patients' perceptions of physician conduct: a study of patient satisfaction in a family practice center. *Community Health.* 1980;6:18–34.
12. Orleans CT. Understanding and promoting smoking cessation: overview and guidelines for physician intervention. *Ann Rev Med.* 1985;142(1):52–57.
13. Fiore M. The new vital sign: assessing and documenting smoking status. *JAMA.* 1991;266(22):3183–3184.
14. Glynn TJ, Manley MW. *How To Help Your Patients Stop Smoking: A National Cancer Institute Manual for Physicians.* National Institutes of Health Publication no. 90-3064. Bethesda, MD: US Department of Health and Human Services, Public Health Service, National Institutes of Health, National Cancer Institute; 1990.
15. Abrams DB, Orleans CT, Niaura RS, et al. Integrating individual and public health perspectives for treatment of tobacco dependence under managed health care: a combined stepped-care and matching model. *Ann Behav Med.* 1996;18(4):290–304.
16. Marlatt GA, Gordon JR, eds. *Relapse Prevention.* New York: Guilford Press; 1985.
17. Kosslyn SM, Koenig O. *Wet Mind: The New Cognitive Neuroscience.* New York: Free Press; 1992.
18. Knowles M. *The Adult Learner: A Neglected Species.* Houston, TX: Gulf; 1978.
19. Joint National Committee on Detection, Evaluation, and Treatment of High Blood Pressure. The Fifth Report on the Joint National Committee on Detection, Evaluation, and Treatment of High Blood Pressure. *Arch Intern Med.* 1993;153:153–183.

SUGGESTED READINGS

Gerteis M, Edgman-Levitan S, Daley J, eds. *Through the Patient's Eyes: Understanding and Promoting Patient-Centered Care.* San Francisco: Jossey-Bass; 1993.

Lorig K, Holman H, Sobel D, Gonzalez V. *Living a Healthy Life with Chronic Conditions: Self Management of Heart Disease, Arthritis, Stroke, Diabetes, Asthma, Bronchitis,*

Emphysema and Others. Palo Alto, CA: Bull Publishing Co; 1994.

Meichenbaum D, Turk D. *Facilitating Treatment Adherence: A Practitioner's Guidebook.* New York: Plenum Press; 1987.

Miller W, Rollnick S. *Motivational Interviewing: Preparing People to Change Addictive Behavior.* New York: Guilford Press; 1991.

Prochaska J, Norcross J, DiClemente C. *Changing for Good.* New York: Avon Books; 1994.

Seligman M. *Learned Optimism.* New York: Alfred A. Knopf; 1990.

Snyder C. *The Psychology of Hope: You Can Get There from Here.* New York: Free Press; 1994.

Vella J. *Learning to Listen, Learning to Teach: The Power of Dialogue in Educating Adults.* San Francisco: Jossey-Bass, Publishers; 1994.

NANCY W. SPANGLER is president of Spangler Associates, a Kansas City consulting company that specializes in health promotion, demand management, and patient education. She brings 20 years of health care experience to the enhancement of patient behavior change. Previously, she was a corporate health promotion specialist for Saint Luke's Health System in Kansas City, and she has worked with the consulting group Wendy Fink Associates in the Boston area.

Part XIV

Complementary and Alternative Medicine

In the United States, a large number of individuals seek out and receive care from nontraditional providers. The desire for this type of care is even more prevalent overseas. Managed health care organizations have recently begun to address this consumer desire, as well as to slowly incorporate some elements of alternative care into their basic medical management programs. This is an area rife with controversy; a controversy that will not be settled here. What follows in Part XIV is a broad and rational discussion of these services, and how many managed health care plans and providers are incorporating them into their other best medical practices.

CHAPTER 41

Complementary and Alternative Medicine

Alan Dumoff

Chapter Outline

- Growth in Alternative Practices
- The Modalities
- Prevention and Wellness
- Efficacy of CAM Approaches
- Growth in Professional Development
- Growth in Coverage
- Structuring CAM Caregiving
- Understanding CAM Philosophy: Guidance for Inclusion in MCO Settings
- Conclusion

GROWTH IN ALTERNATIVE PRACTICES

The past decade has seen accelerating growth in the public and professional recognition of complementary and alternative medical (CAM)

The editors of this book recognize that there are some readers who will not be receptive and some who will be very receptive to the information in this chapter. While all medical practitioners have their own opinions about complementary and alternative medicine, there is a clear desire on the part of many recipients of medical care for these services. In addition, many managed care organizations are including access to at least some of these modalities in their care management programs.

approaches to health care as an important ingredient in health and wellness. The contributions of alternative approaches such as acupuncture, herbal remedies, and homeopathy; the role of proper nutrition in healing illness as well as maintaining health; the effect of lifestyle on modern ailments; and the role of patient attitude and responsibility toward their own health has been more fully acknowledged. This growing interest is due both to the successes of alternative approaches and a recognition of the limitations of conventional medicine.

While still termed "alternative," many of these approaches have become significant parts of our health care system, and consumer demand for alternative health care practitioners has grown dramatically over recent decades. According to an oft-quoted study by David Eisenberg of Harvard Medical School, one third of adults used some form of unconventional therapy during 1990; of these, one third did so by visiting an unconventional or alternative practitioner.[1] More recent studies have found that as many as 50% of patients have had some alternative medicine experience.[2] One of several surprises in Eisenberg's study was the conclusion that patients made more ambulatory visits to practitioners of unconventional therapy than to primary care physicians.[1] The study also found that out-of-pocket expenditures for the services of unconventional practitioners were comparable to that of out-of-pocket expenditures for hospitalization,[1] reflecting a surprisingly strong willingness on the part of consumers to invest in such treatment. Over 65 medical schools, including Harvard, Yale, Cornell, and many others, are offering courses in alternative medical practices. This patient interest in alternative medicine has also been reflected in a great deal of media attention. Examples include *The Heart of Healing,* which aired on TBS in 1993, and magazine articles (often cover stories) that have appeared in *Life, US News & World Report, Nation, Newsweek, Time,* and *Discover.* A number of magazines for a lay audience devoted to this topic are available, including the *Alternative Medicine Digest, Natural Health,* and *Herbs for Health.*

The National Institutes of Health (NIH) has played an increasing, somewhat controversial role in the recognition of CAM practices. The Office of Alternative Medicine (OAM), established within NIH in 1992, is charged with furthering the investigation of CAM treatments by searching out and documenting the range of promising approaches, designing appropriate methodologies, issuing grants as part of a new commitment to research the effectiveness of alternative treatments, and creating a database of information about CAM methods and their effectiveness. Ten research centers have been established to investigate a number of issues, including chronic pain, lower back pain, musculoskeletal problems, diabetes, and human immunodeficiency virus (HIV; Table 41–1). The budget for the OAM has grown from $1.7 million in 1992 to an anticipated budget in 1998 of $20 million.

THE MODALITIES

CAM practitioners apply a great diversity of health care approaches, ranging from well-established, credentialed, and widely practiced methods to unique methods supported by little research and few proponents. Answering the demand for CAM services and accessing the best range of available treatments require examination of a smorgasbord of offerings such as acupuncture, Ayurvedic medicine, chiropractic, herbal medicine, homeopathy, massage and other body therapies, mind-body approaches, naturopathy, and nutritional counseling. The CAM community also includes the services of holistic physicians, who offer a spectrum of modalities also reflecting a range of treatments, from the well-documented to the controversial. These approaches include testing for environmental sensitivities, nutritional treatments for an array of illnesses, chelation therapy for cardiovascular disease, osteopathic adjustments, and a host of other nonstandard medical offerings.

In addition to bringing other traditions or techniques to bear, holistic practitioners adopt a systems view of health that views wellness as arising from a balance of the multiple, complex systems making up the body, mind, and spirit of the patient. Whether looking from the perspective of traditional Chinese medicine or naturopathy, this systems view examines signs and symptoms using a wide inquiry for interactions between multiple levels of functioning, with an emphasis on the use of low-tech, noninvasive natural treatments where possible. The demand for such whole care is a reaction to both the fragmented approach to medicine arising from intensely specialized care and the feeling of caring and positive outcomes many patients have experienced from whole care.

One of the strengths of the CAM community is its diversity of approaches and treatments. This diversity is a challenge for managed care organizations (MCOs) moving toward including CAM practices. Generally considered to encompass all those approaches not taught in Western medical schools, CAM practices include everything from Chinese herbs to hypnotherapy, spinal adjustments to intravenous (IV) vitamins—all under the same rubric.

These approaches, nonetheless, generally do share some common philosophical tenets. In addition to focusing on systems approaches more than on linear decision making, CAM practices are often patient centered, ascribe primary responsibility to the patient rather than to a professional, use low-technology, involve few inva-

Table 41–1 The 10 NIH OAM Centers

Center	Research Focus
Center for the Study of Complementary and Alternative Therapies, University of Virginia School of Nursing, Charlottesville, VA	Pain management, both acute and chronic
Center for Research in Alternative and Complementary Medicine in Stroke and Related Neurological Disorders, Kessler Institute for Rehabilitation, West Orange, NJ	Stroke, brain injury, and spinal cord injury
The Alternative Medicine Research Center for Cancer, University of Texas Health Sciences Center, Houston, TX	Assessing the state of the science for widely used, potentially promising biopharmacologic/herbal/natural CAM therapies
The Center for Complementary and Alternative Medicine Research in Women's Health, Columbia University College of Physicians and Surgeons, New York, NY	Women's health
The Center to Assess Alternative Therapies for Chronic Illness, Beth Israel Hospital/Harvard Medical School, Boston, MA	Low back pain, ischemic heart disease, the use of CAM in managed care settings, legal/professional liability issues, and development of medical education programs
The Bastyr University AIDS Research Center, Seattle, WA	Collecting information on and describing the use of CAM therapies in treating HIV and acquired immune deficiency syndrome (AIDS); screening and evaluating these therapies; and providing support, funding, and technical assistance to researchers in this area
The Center for Addiction and Alternative Medicine Research, Minneapolis, MN	Studying the efficacy of CAM modalities for the treatment of substance abuse
The Center for Complementary and Alternative Medicine Research in Asthma, Allergy, and Immunology, University of California—Davis, Davis, CA	Priority CAM modalities for the treatment of asthma are acupuncture, botanicals, homeopathy, mind-body therapies, and nutrition
The Center for Alternative Medicine Pain Research and Evaluation, University of Maryland School of Medicine, Baltimore, MD	Evaluation of the scientific foundation for CAM therapies for musculoskeletal pain and rigorous investigation of the efficacy, safety, and cost-effectiveness of alternative therapies for pain, initially in the areas of acupuncture, mind-body techniques, and homeopathy treatments
The Complementary and Alternative Medicine Program at Stanford, Stanford University, Palo Alto, CA	Identifies CAM therapies that are likely to prevent or manage disability and frailty and to improve physical function and quality of life among the elderly

Source: Reprinted from Office of Alternative Medicine, National Institutes of Health.

sive procedures, and place an emphasis on the importance of attitude and spiritual orientation. These similar tenets can be treated differently, however, by various CAM professions. One area common to most CAM practices is the recognition of the interrelationship of mind and body. There is a considerable range of opinion within the CAM community about the nature of that relationship and how to affect it.

MCOs seeking to include CAM practices in their offerings need to carefully consider the underlying philosophies as well as the available research regarding efficacy. The philosophical underpinnings of CAM practices have direct effect on patient flow, utilization patterns, time management, billing, and other aspects of practice management. Bringing acupuncture into a setting to provide pain management as a technical component misrepresents acupuncture as targeted toward symptom relief, when acupuncturists view it as a complete system of care that relieves pain by addressing core issues presented by the patient. Following are brief descriptions of some relatively well-established CAM practices.

Acupuncture

Community acceptance of acupuncture has grown dramatically in the last 25 years. Acupuncture has moved from outright rejection by the medical establishment to approval in 1996 by the Food and Drug Administration (FDA) for the general use of acupuncture needles as a medical device, placing them in the same class as scalpels and syringes. This supplanted the FDA's long-held posture that these needles, which had been used for thousands of years in China, were experimental medical devices.

There has been a considerable amount of research done into the efficacy of acupuncture.[3] An NIH consensus panel convened in November 1997 and concluded that there is clear evidence that acupuncture is effective in the treatment of nausea caused by chemotherapeutic agents, surgical anesthesia, or pregnancy, and for pain following dental surgery. The panel also concluded that there was some evidence that acupuncture is useful for conditions such as menstrual cramps, fibromyalgia, drug addiction, stroke, and headache. The NIH consensus panel noted that acupuncture has proven to be remarkably safe with far fewer side effects than many well-established medical approaches.

Oriental medicine, of which acupuncture is but one approach, recognizes the rhythms of the day and the seasons and works to encourage an unobstructed and balanced flow of the life force within these rhythms. Acupuncture views health as arising from the unobstructed flow of energy, through a system of meridians mapped across the body. Needles, pressure, or heat from burning an herb known as moxa are used to balance and encourage the flow of energy. The treatment points on the meridians are often placed in distant and seemingly unrelated areas to the site of a patient's symptoms, which is part of the basis for the skepticism and misunderstanding about acupuncture. Meridians link tissues that were contiguous in embryonic development, a phenomenon that creates channels that account for the communication of referred pain; acupuncture recognizes this same phenomenon and has clinical experience that such connections can have a referred effect. The market for acupuncture services is significant. In 1993, the FDA estimated that $500 million was spent for acupuncture treatments in the United States by over a million patients a year. There are approximately 9 to 12 million acupuncture visits per year.[4]

Clinical experience suggests that the inclusion of acupuncture in an MCO creates an opportunity for many patients to resolve health issues that they were unable to resolve through biomedicine. In addition, acupuncturists as team members can assist in managing postsurgical or chemotherapy-induced nausea, drug detox, pain management, and many other conditions.

Chiropractic

Chiropractic involves the relief of musculoskeletal pain and dysfunction through the manual manipulation of the spine. It is particularly effective for neck and back pain, but it appears to have usefulness for a wider variety of ailments. Many chiropractors, for example, perform adjustments of the wrist that can be useful in the treatment of carpal tunnel syndrome, or adjustments to treat pain emanating from the ribs.

Chiropractic has become so well established that some consider chiropractic to be a mainstream rather than an alternative modality. The number of visits to chiropractors in the United States is growing. While there have been significant disputes between the American Medical Association (AMA) and the chiropractic profession, the AMA now includes chiropractors in its review committees for the establishment of Current Procedural Terminology (CPT) coding appropriate to chiropractic care.

Chiropractic has been a covered benefit for the past decade. In many MCOs and other settings, chiropractors can provide excellent services for patients who in the past would have been referred to physical therapists. Because chiropractors generally treat musculoskeletal and soft tissue problems, chiropractic linkages are generally to family physicians, orthopaedists, and physical medicine specialists. Chiropractors can be an early part of differential diagnosis where musculoskeletal and soft tissue issues are present, and they have the capacity to resolve back pain and related complaints without surgical interventions or lengthy recuperative periods. Chiropractors can also contribute in the physical rehabilitation department. In a medical setting, chiropractors can provide improved services, because they have access to much more sophisticated imaging techniques. Some chiropractic techniques require a hospital setting because they involve manipulation while the patient is anesthetized.

Herbal Therapies

Many herbs are becoming well known and respected for their medicinal effects, a view that has been long held in Europe. Ginkgo biloba, an herb used for Alzheimer's disease, senility, and memory loss[5–7] and which appears to have numerous cardiovascular benefits, is the largest selling prescription drug in Germany. Most over-the-counter (OTC) categories in Germany are led by herbal products. Since 1993, all German medical students have been taught natural therapies and tested for this knowledge on their medical boards.[8]

Saw palmetto has been found to be effective in benign prostatic hyperplasia, with some studies showing improvement for as many as 90% of patients compared to 57% for Proscar, the primary prescription drug.[8] There are persuasive bodies of research documenting the efficacy of St. John's Wort for depression,[9] feverfew for migraine,[10–12] licorice for ulcers[13–17] and as an anti-inflammatory (though one must be aware of licorice's ability to increase blood pressure),[18–20] valerian for anxiety,[21,22] garlic for cholesterol reduction and immune support,[23,24] cranberries for urinary tract infections,[25–27] and echinacea for stimulation of the immune system,[28] particularly against upper respiratory viral infections.

Most herbs used for healing purposes come from a long history of traditional use, with extensive anecdotal safety as well as efficacy data supporting such use. Recently, the American Herbal Pharmacopeia has been launched, which is developing monographs about the proper uses and documented efficacies of a variety of herbs. These monographs, similar to those used to guide the regulation and use of OTC drugs, will assist practitioners by providing reliable sources of information about the use of medicinal herbs. The US Pharmacopeia has begun developing herbal monographs as well.

Herbal remedies provide MCO patients with a significant addition to the list of traditional pharmaceutical products. As the regulatory process recognizes, botanical products are often considered safer, with less serious adverse reactions, than pharmaceutically developed drugs.

Homeopathy

Homeopathy is the use of extremely dilute substances that, if used in significant quantity, would create the same symptom complex for which people are seeking treatment. Homeopathic remedies were determined by giving biologically active doses to volunteers, and then noting the symptom pictures that emerged. With the knowledge gained from these "provings," minute doses of these same remedies are used to treat presentations that approximate those revealed by the proving. Given this empirical method, homeopaths are known for the extensive nature of their interviews, covering a wide array of seemingly unrelated facts that assist in the selection of the proper remedy.

While this is similar in concept to the approach that led to immune stimulation via vaccination, homeopathy is controversial because the amounts used are so minute there is doubt whether any of the substance even remains in the remedies. Homeopaths rest their practice on their empirical experience of effectiveness. Current thinking is that the remedies may work by conveying information that is spread throughout the remedy by the manner in which it is prepared. This information makes changes in the complex homeostatic processes of the body. While such effects may seem farfetched to some people, there has been interesting research demonstrating them. One study, for example, showed that known reactions by basophils exposed in vitro to therapeutic does of immunoglobulin E antiserum could be replicated by exposure to homeopathic levels of the antiserum.[29]

Homeopathy plays a central role in European health care, with many French and German doctors prescribing homeopathic remedies. A meta-analysis of 105 controlled clinical studies of homeopathic medicines found that 75% showed a positive result.[30]

Massage/Somatic Practices

Massage is the use of soft tissue techniques to assist the body in achieving a relaxation response, as well as to directly assist the body in resolving musculoskeletal injuries or imbalances. Chronic headaches, arthritis, chronic pain, and many other conditions can be responsive to massage. Massage recognizes the mind-body connection directly: muscular tension reflects psychological distress, and muscular relaxation reduces pain and anxiety.

Massage and bodywork encompass a wide variety of specialized techniques. Lymphedema, a serious postsurgical complication without effective conventional treatment, is responsive to manual lymph drainage techniques. Poor body mechanics can aggravate, if not cause, serious joint conditions, spinal problems, tension headaches, and other ills. The chronic misalignments that come from such conditions can be approached with deep tissue work, such as rolfing, movement reeducation such as Feldenkrais, or through trigger point release, such as neuromuscular techniques. Massage has been used in hospitals for some time to assist bed-bound patients. Massage has much more to offer MCO patients, as it can be used with focused therapeutic effect for many conditions.

Mind-Body Medicine

The extent that psychosocial factors influence medical status and care is slowly achieving greater recognition. From the effect of attitude on the immune system to family dysfunction as a concomitant of organic problems, mind-body interventions recognize the need to explore and improve psychosocial functioning as a core part of health care. Mind-body interventions include various psychotherapies, hypnosis and guided imagery, group support, bioenergetics, and a variety of other approaches. Most CAM practices recognize and work with the interwoven nature of mind and body in some fashion.

The popularity of mind-body medicine may arise in part because allopathic medicine's theoretical view of the body as distinct from the mind has limited the attention given to the realities of its patients' psychosocial life and its effect on health. Alternative, complementary, and allied professions are more directly responsive to these needs.

It is not simply that nursing and social work, for example, are caring professions. It is also that the whole view taken by these professions has allowed the development of broader understanding of the role of psychosocial functioning on organic illness. Therapies that focus on energetics, such as acupuncture, bioenergetics, and homeopathy, have developed a sophisticated view of the interaction between emotional experience and organic response as reflections of common processes. Medicine has begun to shift its emphasis, placing increasing recognition on the importance of attitude on somatic health, including the acceptance of interventions such as psychoneuroimmunology and family interventions.

Biomedicine's approach to mind-body interactions has spawned some of its own difficulties with patients who overuse health services. Patients with problems medicine has not yet learned to diagnose, or whose problems do not fit within its biomedical paradigm, are presumed to be acting psychosomatically, even where no psychological mechanism is seen. Many of these patients have conditions that a CAM system of care would recognize. This misdiagnosis often makes the patients responsible for psychologically creating their conditions, with the resulting diagnosis of psychosomatic disorder that is too often disempowering and prematurely ends the search for the true etiology. This search ends with a prescription for a major tranquilizer rather than a treatment responsive to the unseen organic or psychosocial situation.

MCOs can benefit from approaches that assist patients in taking a positive approach toward their own healing, with a recognition of how management of stress affects well-being. Problems with overutilization and compliance are also potentially more manageable using mind-body and other CAM approaches.

PREVENTION AND WELLNESS

One characteristic most CAM practices share is a belief that impending illness manifests itself earlier than that recognized through biomedicine's morphology. CAM practitioners also believe that they have a role to play in encouraging wellness, a state of vitality beyond the mere absence of disease. This broader focus attracts many people to CAM practices.

Modern medicine has come to recognize that this era is marked by the existence of preventable chronic illnesses that are not easily managed once they become diagnostically symptomatic. Yet the Centers for Disease Control and Prevention (CDC) notes that the budget for prevention is approximately 0.07% of the total health care budget in the United States.[31] MCOs have a stated agenda of promoting wellness, though it is often commented that short subscriber enrollment has proven a disincentive for pouring resources into prevention. CAM services provide healthy nutrition and a balancing of energies and address other underlying health functions; they often combine prevention, early detection, and disease treatment in a seamless whole.

EFFICACY OF CAM APPROACHES

CAM may be effective in treating a wide variety of conditions, including the biggest killers, heart disease and cancer. CAM practices may also be effective in treating chronic illnesses that exact great cost in lost work, such as low back pain, fibromyalgia, and chronic fatigue syndrome. In one survey, US pharmacists, who are in a unique place to observe patient response to health care, reported substantial belief in the efficacy of many CAM practices.[8] Acupuncture was considered useful by 84%, chiropractic by 73%, hypnosis by 66%, herbal remedies by 43%, and homeopathic remedies by 27%.[8] The following very brief discussion highlights only a fraction of the evidence regarding the efficacy of CAM approaches.

Heart Disease

While the medical community has remained skeptical about the value of nutritional and other CAM interventions in patient treatment, many physicians themselves employ preventive treatments in their own lives. A wide range of nutritional supplements have been linked to cardiac health, including magnesium[32,33] and B vitamins.[34–36]

A controversial treatment used by many holistic physicians for coronary heart disease is IV chelation therapy. The research is not clear,[37] but chelation therapy may have an important role to play as a nonsurgical treatment. Changes from chelation may prove to be more permanent than coronary grafts, half of which reocclude within 5 to 7 years, as the underlying etiology of the disease is not managed in this surgical approach.[38]

Nutritional medicine plays an important role, not only in reducing fat intake, but in the use of magnesium and other metabolic agents that reduce hypertension and improve heart function. Acupuncture can contribute by reducing blood pressure through vascular dilation. Dean Ornish's Heart Disease Reversal Program has shown that lifestyle training can reverse cardiovascular disease.[38]

Low Back Pain

Chiropractic, acupuncture, bodywork and massage, and even nutritional interventions have all been shown to make significant contributions in the treatment of lower back pain. The Agency for Health Care Policy and Research guidelines for lower back pain list chiropractic as among the first two preferred options for treatment.[39] Metastudies have shown that chiropractic is more effective than any other approach in resolving lower back pain.[40] Acupuncture has also been shown to be effective for lower back pain, returning to work intransigent cases that conventional treatment had not resolved.[41]

Diabetes

Diabetes, a topic covered in detail in Chapter 29, reflects a complex systemic illness that encompasses a variety of metabolic pathways affected by the loss of insulin production. Natural medicine approaches to this disease include vitamin and mineral supplementation, including glucose tolerance factor (GTF) chromium, vanadele sulfate, niacin, and potassium.[42] Naturopathic remedies, such as Gymnema Sylvestre extract, are reported to cause decreased blood glucose and increased serum insulin, with a concomitant reduction in insulin needs.[42]

GROWTH IN PROFESSIONAL DEVELOPMENT

Licensure and Certification

Inclusion of a profession in managed care settings requires a certain level of professional development. Of primary concern is licensure, followed by recognized private certification programs that allow the MCO to assure patients and partners that it is providing quality care.

Chiropractic is the most widespread alternative approach, having been licensed in all 50 states and the District of Columbia since 1974. Chiropractic is so pervasive that it is no longer clearly an alternative approach. The independent practice of acupuncture is currently licensed in 31 states and in the District of Columbia; 12 additional states allow acupuncture to be practiced in some circumstances under medical supervision. Michigan, Missouri, and North Carolina allow nonphysician acupuncturists to work under the supervision of a physician, but there are no provisions to regulate them. Acupuncture may be performed by medical physicians in most of the remaining states. Physicians may not practice acupuncture in Georgia. Massage therapy is a licensed profession in 25 states and the District of Columbia. Naturopathy is currently licensed or otherwise allowed in 12 states and the District of Columbia.

Beyond licensure, MCO efforts to meet quality assurance standards for medical practitioners generally include an expectation that a practitioner will be board certified. In medicine, over 150 boards offer such specialty credentials. Only 24 of these boards are recognized by the American Board of Medical Specialties (ABMS); the remaining Boards range from the respected to those that engender some skepticism.

A number of boards have evolved to support the efforts of physicians practicing certain forms of holistic medicine. These boards include the American Academy of Environmental Medicine (for physicians addressing multiple chemical sensitivity) and the American College for the Advancement of Medicine (for physicians addressing cardiovascular disease with chelation). CAM has been moving forward on other fronts as well. The American Public Health Association now has an active section devoted to alternative medicine as well as a section devoted to chiropractic care.

The professional development of CAM, even in the well-established profession of chiropractic, is not as sophisticated as professional development in biomedicine. However, many of these professions have achieved significant professional development. The profession of acupuncture, for example, has recognized bodies that credential and discipline members and accredit its schools. The National Commission for the Certification of Acupuncture and Oriental Medicine (NCCAOM), established in 1984, developed and administers the national certification examination to acupuncturists qualified by training or experience. (The commission recently changed its name. It was formerly known as the National Commission for the Certification of Acupuncture.) Of the jurisdictions that license acupuncturists, 27 rely in whole or in part on the NCCAOM examination. This examination process includes a written exam and a practical examination of point location skills and of clean needle technique. Successful applicants may report that they are an NCCAOM diplomate. The NCCAOM and its examination are recognized by the US Department of Education, and the NCCAOM provides a forum for disciplinary review of any complaints that are filed. The NCCAOM has also developed an examination in Chinese herbology, and certificates have been issued for this specialty.

The development of accredited educational bodies also reflects the quality of training and the existence of some standardization of care. There are nearly 100 schools of acupuncture in the United States. These schools can receive curriculum development assistance from the Council of Colleges of Acupuncture and Oriental Medicine; 29 schools are accredited or in candidacy review by the National Accreditation Commission for Schools and Colleges of Acupuncture and Oriental Medicine. Graduation from an accredited school and state licensure are sufficient to demonstrate a quality education and right to practice; NCCAOM diplomate status is an added qualification an MCO may choose to require.

GROWTH IN COVERAGE

MCOs and health plans first began to offer some coverage for CAM services in the mid-1980s, when Prudential began offering products covering acupuncture for the management of some pain conditions and for anesthesia under some circumstances. MCOs are increasingly recognizing the medical and financial value of including alternative modalities in their health plans. American Western Life Insurance Company has a wellness plan that covers a wide variety of such care. Blue Cross of Washington and Alaska conducted a pilot project in which 1,000 of its subscribers enrolled in a supplemental plan, "AlternaPath." Members were given access to herbalists, naturopaths, homeopaths, acupuncturists, and other practitioners. Demand was so great that the 1,000 slots were filled before the program was even advertised.

Other MCOs and health plans are providing coverage for specific alternative treatments. Mutual of Omaha has been sending heart patients through a program of intense dietary change developed by Dean Ornish, because of evidence that the $5,000 fee will save up to $58,000 in fees for bypass surgery, angioplasty, and medical services for heart attacks.[38] The Harvard Community Health Plan provides a mind-body relaxation course for its membership.[43]

State mandates for coverage of CAM benefits are evolving. Forty-one states require insurers to reimburse for chiropractic services, while seven states have some mandate for reimbursement for acupuncture.[43,44] Forty-six percent of MCOs currently cover some chiropractic services.[43,44] Federal programs, as the most conservative payers, have not generally reimbursed such care. Medicare expressly considers acupuncture to be a noncovered service. A small percentage of insurance companies cover acupuncture. Landmark Healthcare reported in 1996 that 58% of the MCOs contacted in 13 states would offer some form of complementary medicine within 2 years.[45]

STRUCTURING CAM CAREGIVING

The primary task for an MCO wishing to respond to its consumers' demand for CAM care is to determine how it will fashion the role CAM practitioners will play and the access its subscribers will have to these practitioners. This raises two sets of questions:

1. What clinical involvement will CAM practitioners have? For what conditions will they see patients? What route of referral, consultation, or team collaboration will patients use to access CAM practitioners?
2. How will the cost of CAM practitioners be managed? How will utilization be kept at manageable levels?

While proper utilization review and benefit design is critical, MCOs developing CAM programs must understand the nature of CAM clinical methods before seriously addressing how clinical decision making can best integrate biomedical and CAM approaches. Methods that combine biomedicine and CAM to create best practices have the potential to offer cost-effective treatments for the chronic conditions that are placing MCOs at significant risk as well as provide a sought-after benefit to members without such chronic diseases.

However, much of the currently developed care delivery that integrates biomedical and CAM approaches, particularly in managed care settings, has merely created access to independent CAM practices through discounted fee-for-service networks or riders allowing for some limited CAM benefits. Legitimate concerns about overutilization have limited the full participation of CAM practitioners in MCO clinical settings or in plan benefits. The potential for integrated care has yet to be fully realized.

The concern about overutilization arises in part because case management and coordination of services among medical and CAM practitioners are not yet well developed. MCOs have little historical experience and lack the knowledge about CAM practices to provide such case management services. The CAM community, often practicing in solo or small independent practices on a self-pay basis, also has very limited clinical and practice management experience from which it can work easily within the constraints faced by MCOs.

As a result of these barriers, current MCO offerings create limited access to CAM practitioners. Such access fails to assist patients in making choices among the smorgasbord of available approaches. Patients need guidance in choosing among all available options and in responsibly integrating biomedical and CAM approaches to their health situations. Without such coordination, MCOs face the financial risk that CAM services will simply become add-ons that increase cost rather than cost-effectiveness. Achieving the cost-efficiencies available through CAM offerings requires learning how to best match patients to practitioners. This requires gaining the confidence in CAM to forgo some conventional services when CAM services are more appropriately provided, and learning how to use these new services to reduce the need for conventional services. Garnering cost savings with desired outcomes also demands learning how to efficiently allow for collaboration given the time pressures in the practice of medicine. To meet these challenges, MCOs must explore the nature and potential that clinical integration has to offer.

Even where an MCO allows patients to access CAM practitioners under its benefits program, patients still must navigate a bewildering array of reactions to their presenting symptoms. Exhibit 41–1 provides a simple example of the different responses a patient presenting with fatigue syndrome might encounter.

Integration: The Benefits of True Collaboration

The promise of integrated care is deeper than merely creating access; cross-fertilization among the various health approaches has the potential to not only coordinate a larger repertoire of diagnostic impressions and treatments, but create significant developments in the theory and practice of health care.

As a first goal, integrating the complete spectrum of care can allow patients to be more competently matched to the full range of available care. The demands of existing practice structures make it difficult for medical specialists to integrate care among themselves, let alone to effectively and knowledgeably involve CAM practitioners. In addition to making all diagnostic tools available, integrated care allows health care providers to combine approaches not available in any other setting, for more positive results. For example, to help heal trauma, acupuncture and homeopathic remedies such as arnica could be used in conjunction with conventional treatment after accidental trauma or surgery. A nutritionist and behavioral social worker are best trained to help a heart patient make necessary dietary changes.

At the most basic level, for example, a legitimate understanding of when patients with back problems should be seen by a chiropractor and when an orthopaedic surgeon should be involved could save much suffering and economic loss, given that even an extensive course of chiropractic care costs in the range of $500 to $2,000, while a laminectomy costs approximately $20,000. Conversely, an effective matching program would assist chiropractic patients who truly are appropriate surgical candidates to get such care. Another example with significant economic impact is Dean Ornish's program for cardiovascular patients, which reduced annual average expenditures for patients from $12,276 to between $6,000 and $7,500.[38]

Bedell-Logan Billing Systems, a national billing service established in 1990 that provides claims service and negotiations with payers of care for CAM providers, has been collecting cost data, given its requirement that providers send their notes along with the superbill in order to verify the claim. A preliminary check into its database of 8,000 records for patients complaining of lower back pain revealed that the average cost per episode for patients who saw a massage therapist was approximately $1,800; for an acupuncturist, $1,500; and for a chiropractor, $1,200 (Bedell-Logan Billing Systems, unpublished data, 1997). Those patients, however, who combined care and saw more than one modality for their episode of pain, spent a combined total of only $800.

We may determine that any significant illness involves dimensions of functioning greater than a single modality of care can recognize. Clinical experience with patients viewed through both Western knowledge and the Chinese understanding of the interaction between organ systems, for example, may enable an understanding neither approach can achieve alone. An example would be the alternative approaches to cancer, autoim-

Exhibit 41–1 Examples of Clinical Exchanges

Presenting Complaint: Fatigue Syndrome

Traditional medical physician: You don't have hypoglycemia, despite what you read in *Sugar Blues*. It's widely overdiagnosed. Just eat a better diet and get some exercise and you'll be just fine.

Holistic physician: Let's check your thyroid and cortisol levels, and do a hair analysis and check your cell salt levels.

Nutritionist: You probably have a form of hypoglycemia. Take GTF chromium and B-complex vitamins.

Acupuncturist: You have an inner wind injury and a deficient spleen.

mune, and infectious diseases that work to support the immune system rather than to develop magic bullets targeting specific antigens. When the value in such approaches is recognized, the immunosupportive effects of acupuncture, Chinese herbs, homeopathy, and other approaches must be responsibly integrated into care.

Team Care and the Role of MCOs in Managing Care

One of the visions that brought MCOs into being was the need to effectively manage care to assist patients in obtaining high-quality, cost-effective treatments. Due to market pressures, the goal of MCOs now must be to obtain cost-effective, high-quality outcomes by learning how to best match patients to the most appropriate treatments from the outset—a goal best met by an inclusive team approach to care. One solution is thus in the nature of the practice setting itself. Administratively, managed care is a secondary system, put in place to manage the cost failures that occur when practice settings encourage excessive services. MCOs' strained response to this problem has been to shift responsibility for care management to a secondary, administrative organization, because the practitioners are not properly managing the care themselves. An integrated practice structure has a major role to play; it provides a method for the clinicians to make more cost-effective choices themselves.

Integrated teams that include CAM practitioners place practitioners who treat similar presenting issues in "managed competition" with each other. This can offer economic advantages. For a massage therapist, rather than a physical therapist, to treat a patient, the massage therapist must demonstrate greater competency and potential cost-effectiveness than the physical therapist. This managed competition requires the professionals working with a patient to balance considerations of efficacy, safety, and cost. Particularly where teams are in risk-sharing clinical settings, it is in each practitioner's self-interest to have cost-effective care given by the appropriate team member. Properly structured diverse teams provide counterbalance, allowing the return of patient care decisions to the practitioners with reduced concern that practitioner-generated demand will fuel medical inflation.

It is important to note that whole care has become a valued goal for medical care, and it is often touted as what many physicians and alternative practices provide. Yet truly whole care can occur only within a practice and theoretical framework in which the various helping practices contribute their perspective toward a view of the whole. Just because CAM methods come from an alternative tradition does not qualify them as whole care. The daily sorting through of cases by professionals of varying perspectives in a clinical setting sets the stage for whole care to occur. While collaboration in medical settings often refers to "diagnose and refer" for consultation, a true collaborative model allows professionals to develop a common perspective to address the physiologic, psychosocial, energetic, and structural aspects of their patients' functioning.[46]

Just as diagnosis can be improved by the interaction of diverse diagnostic viewpoints, so can treatment. This is not only because the broader diagnostic lens brings with it additional, potentially more focused treatments, but also because differing treatments for Western medical diagnoses will be available. A patient with carpal tunnel syndrome, for example, can be given an inexpensive and noninvasive course of chiropractic adjustment prior to determining the need for surgery. High cholesterol can be assisted with a nutritional intervention prior to the use of antihypercholesterolemic medications.

Physician Acceptance

While it may seem odd at first, clinical integration offers one of the keys to physician acceptance of CAM practitioners as part of the caregiving system. It has been a primary concern of physicians, for example, that some patients may be deterred from seeking appropriate medical treatment because they seek only alternative methods. While the evidence suggests that this is rarely the case, serious cardiac, cancerous, infectious, and other conditions could potentially be missed because a patient sees only an alternative practitioner. Further, growing proof of the validity of some alternative approaches should not sweep all of these varied methods into accepted practice. The fact that psychoneuroimmunology is gaining clinical support, for example, does not imply that psychic surgery is valid. A discerning approach is clearly vital.

Since most patients seeing CAM practitioners in practice settings outside the institutional health system do not inform their physicians,[1] team practice provides the potential for much better communication among all concerned. If a patient is taking St. John's Wort for depression, for example, a physician about to prescribe Prozac for that patient should know about it so he or she can address potential interactions.

Where physicians and CAM practitioners work in unison, coordination of care becomes a real possibility. Such teamwork ensures that fears of quackery can be greatly minimized because integrated settings work to eliminate extended treatment without evaluation, the use of unknown and untested formulas, the abandonment of conventional medical involvement, and the refusal to share information with the physician.

Gatekeeping

In MCOs that use it, gatekeeping has two tasks. First, gatekeeping helps to triage cases, determining which services can enter the gate. This function, generally performed by a primary care physician, directs patients to particular types of practitioners. Even with inclusive benefit design, this critical function will determine patient access to CAM care. The second task, generally performed as a utilization review function, is to determine whether the gate should open to certain practitioners' treatments, determining whether a practitioner's services are medically necessary for the patient. When an MCO is integrating CAM practitioners, both these aspects of gatekeeping should be considered.

Utilization Review and Medical Necessity

Utilization review (UR) is problematic for MCOs that make CAM services available; frequently, the medical staff may not understand or believe in the medical necessity of CAM services. While triage/case management is best served by those cross-trained in a variety of approaches or by a diverse team, once a patient is under the care of a particular type of practitioner, the need for that practitioner's care should be assessed according to the standards for that type of practitioner.

This is initially addressed by ensuring that the same CAM practitioners represented in the delivery team are represented on the UR team. From a care perspective, only those in a profession know the standards of care and understand the semantics and charting methods for that profession. From a legal perspective, it is well settled that malpractice standards are set by the individual professions, a standard increasingly followed by the trend to establish a state regulatory board for each profession rather than regulate CAM professions under the medical board. UR should reflect this same development.

It is important to recognize that the methods of professions can be very different, even if they have an appearance of similarity. The standard of care for chiropractic X-rays, for example, is that they be taken with the patient standing; the recumbent back X-rays often taken in medical settings do not serve these chiropractic requirements, and it is thus valid for a chiropractor to take his or her own weight-bearing X-rays if the medical X-rays were recumbent. Semantics can create significant confusion as well. For example, the acupuncture meridian called the "spleen" is, in some schools of thought, more closely allied with pancreatic function than the spleen. These practice issues, and the overarching understanding of standards of care, can come only from those trained in the profession being reviewed.

Adapting UR to CAM practices also requires cognizance of philosophical and practice differences. CAM practitioners' decision trees, including those of holistic physicians, require spending significantly more time with their patients than biomedically oriented physicians do; the CAM practitioner seeks to uncover deeper underlying etiologies spanning multiple systems, and this process takes time. Another difference is that many CAM practices are empirical, in that the reaction to treatment is itself diagnostic; a best effort is applied, the situation reassessed, and then treatment altered as indicated. CAM practitioners spend more time not only at intake but on an ongoing basis as they assess changes in their patients.

Controlling Overutilization

CAM services in MCO settings currently are either offered as discounted fee-for-service access to a panel of practitioners, as actual coverage under a rider, or as specialists whose access is controlled through gatekeeping mechanisms. Most of the experience to date has involved the creation of CAM panels that can be accessed at a discount as a rider benefit, which is the least integrated approach to the inclusion of CAM modalities. One of the primary reasons for limiting plan offerings to discounted access is that inclusion as a policy benefit requires actuarial data that has not yet been adequately developed. Expected utilization by consumers, and the benefits in health status improvement such visits yield, are not well documented. In addition to this lack of data, the use of CAM services for both wellness and illness makes utilization control difficult. Massage therapy, for example, has many benefits for musculoskeletal injuries but can also be used to reduce stress as part of a wellness program. A health plan may wish to provide massage therapy for injuries but would understandably conclude that massage for wellness is not economically viable. This issue is similar to that faced by MCOs in determining mental health benefits. There are clearly cases in which mental health services have been utilized for self-actualization or personal growth. Whether such services are truly needed has been the subject of much UR activity.

Data about the effect of mental health benefits on overall utilization may be suggestive of what future data will show about CAM benefits. There are numerous studies demonstrating that the inclusion of mental health benefits results in a reduction in overall utilization; the combined claim payments for medical and mental health services in such plans is lower than the medical claims paid out in plans providing only medical services.[47,48] This result should not be surprising, as approximately 80% of visits to primary care practitioners are for presenting conditions in which a mental health component, such as a life issue, anxiety, or psychosomatic complaint, is the primary reason for the visit.[49] The reduction in medical service utilization when mental health services are offered occurs partly because of the high consumption of services by high-utilizing patients in need of such care. Medical gatekeepers, such as internists and family physicians, are not well equipped to recognize and treat such conditions. Referrals to mental health professionals within a plan are often a more cost-effective response, not only because mental health professionals are less cost-intensive but because these approaches are often more appropriate to the presenting issues.

CAM services may well demonstrate these same efficiencies by providing more appropriate services for some conditions. CAM approaches, which include techniques that address interactions among body, mind, and spirit and energetic imbalances that are not recognized in Western medicine, have much to offer patients with anxiety and psychosomatic issues. Musculoskeletal pain, chronic fatigue and related conditions, and a host of other conditions may be better served by acupuncture, chiropractic, medical nutritional interventions, and other CAM approaches than by Western medicine. While the research questions raised by integrating as diverse a field as CAM into MCOs are more complex than those raised by the inclusion of mental health services in MCOs, the issue is currently being studied. No results are available at the time this chapter is being written.

As the early experiences of MCOs, health plans, and medical institutions integrating some form of CAM care generate outcome data, MCOs will be in a better position to target the practitioners and the benefits they wish to include. Data emerging from the OAM, which include currently available data as well as original off-campus research, will provide an increasingly strong data set for projections of efficacy. There is already a surprisingly strong body of literature about the efficacy of many CAM approaches.[3,50]

UNDERSTANDING CAM PHILOSOPHY: GUIDANCE FOR INCLUSION IN MCO SETTINGS

A guiding philosophy of most CAM practitioners is that spending the time to understand and work with a patient at the outset is a wise investment too often unmet in the pressures of medical practice settings. MCOs designing CAM services should recognize that they are generally time-intensive, and that efforts to unduly restrict time will be counterproductive; CAM services are effective partly because of their time-intensive care.

A corollary of holism is that CAM practitioners each approach patients from the unique perspective of their CAM tradition. While an acupuncturist can provide relief from pain, an acupuncturist cannot be relegated to the role of pain management on prescription from a physician. The physician may be motivated to make a referral due to a patient's pain, but the acupuncturist will see the patient as a whole and will base the diagnosis and treatment upon the patient's presentation as viewed through the acupuncturist's training. Just because pain may be alleviated as a consequence of treatment does not make acupuncturists simply technicians who administer an agent to reduce pain. The relegation of social workers, who have much to offer in primary treatment, to discharge planners in hospital settings is a analogous situation; CAM practitioners will be poorly utilized and not perform to their potential if program design attempts to unduly constrain their practice. Most CAM practitioners function from their independent viewpoint, rather than simply exercising their tools as technical components for the physician. This is not to say that practitioners cannot integrate into medical settings, but that the design of patient flow should allow for the full range of the CAM practitioners' work.

A principal difference between biomedical and CAM approaches is the methodology by which knowledge is gained and evaluated. Biomedicine values prospective, randomized, and controlled double-blind studies as the gold standard of developing knowledge. CAM approaches have generally grown from the empirical experience of clinical efforts. Highly individualized care does not fit well with double-blind methodology. Methodologies need to fit the question being raised. Pair-matched demographic studies comparing CAM or integrated approaches, as one example, have much to teach. The most useful starting point to address this issue, however, may be to recognize that the differences in reliance on research are not as marked as they are often made out to be. It has been argued that biomedicine is largely based on untested treatments that are accepted because they meet the expectations of medical science, and it has been estimated that as much as 80% of biomedical treatments have not been verified by the standard aspired to by Western researchers.[51] A large number of prescriptions, for example, are for off-label uses of drugs that have not been subjected to such studies but are known anecdotally to work.

From a pragmatic perspective, outcome studies are probably the most critical research to be done on the efficacy of CAM care. MCOs have a primary role to play in this research, because CAM practices integrated into MCO offerings are tracked as part of the MCO's overall outcome research.

CONCLUSION

The CAM community is rich and diverse in its offerings. The rapid professional growth and research regarding the efficacy of many CAM practices make them viable for inclusion in MCO offerings, where CAM providers will create opportunities for improved patient care. MCOs should allow for truly integrated care in which the best clinical options are responsibly selected from among all the available approaches to care—biomedical and alternative. MCOs have a critical role to play in learning how to develop practice structures and clinical management tools to assist practitioners and patients in using approaches from the full spectrum of care.

REFERENCES

1. Eisenberg D. Unconventional medicine in the United States: prevalence, costs, and patterns of use. *N Engl J Med.* 1993;329(4):246–252.
2. Elder N, Gillerist A, Minz R. Use of alternative health care by family practice patients. *Arch Fam Med.* 1997;6:181–184.
3. Birch S, Hammerschlag R. *Acupuncture Efficacy: A Compendium of Controlled Clinical Studies.* Tarrytown, NY: National Academy of Acupuncture and Oriental Medicine; 1996.
4. Lytle C. *An Overview of Acupuncture.* Rockville, MD: Center for Devices and Radiological Health, US Department of Health and Human Services, Public Health Service, Food and Drug Administration; 1993.
5. Kleijnen J. Ginkgo biloba for cerebral insufficiency. *Br J Clin Pharmacol.* 1992;34:352–358.
6. Kleijnen J. Ginkgo biloba. *Lancet.* 1992;340:1136–1139.
7. Hofferberth B. The efficacy of EGb 761 in patients with senile dementia of the Alzheimer type: a double-blind, placebo-controlled study on different levels of investigation. *Hum Psychopharmacol.* 1994;9:215–222.
8. Ullman D. The mainstreaming of alternative medicine. *Healthcare Forum J.* Nov/Dec 1993:24–30.
9. Ernst E. St. John's Wort, an antidepressant? A systematic, criteria-based review. *Phytomedicine.* 1995;2(1):67–71.
10. Johnson E, Kadam N, Hylands D, Hylands P. Efficacy of feverfew as prophylactic treatment of migraine. *Br Med J.* 1985;291:569–573.
11. Murphy J, Heptinstall S, Mitchell J. Randomized double-blind placebo-controlled trial of feverfew in migraine prevention. *Lancet.* 1988:189–192.
12. Awang DU. Herbal medicine: feverfew. *Can Pharm J.* 1989;122:266–270.
13. Doll R, Hill ID. Clinical trial of a triterpenoid liquorice compound in gastric and duodenal ulcer. *Lancet.* 1962;2:1166–1167.
14. Turpie AG, Runcie J, Thomson TJ. Clinical trial of deglycyrrhizinized liquorice in gastric ulcer. *Gut.* 1969;10:299–302.
15. Tewari S, Wilson A. Deglycyrrhizinated liquorice in duodenal ulcer. *Practitioner.* 1973;210:820–823.
16. Cliff J, Milton-Thomson G. A double-blind trial of carbenoxolone sodium capsules in the treatment of duodenal ulcer. *Gut.* 1970;11:167–170.
17. Amure B. Clinical study of duogastrone in the treatment of duodenal ulcers. *Gut.* 1970;11:171–175.
18. Farese R, Biglieri E, Shackleton C, Irony I, Gomez-Fonter R. Licorice-induced hypermineralocorticoidism. *N Engl J Med.* 1991;325(17):1223–1227.
19. Epstein M, Espiner EA, Donald RA, Hughes H. Effect of eating liquorice on the renin-angiotensin aldosterone axis in normal subjects. *Br Med J.* 1977;1:488–490.
20. Bannister B. Cardiac arrest due to liquorice-induced hypokalaemia. *Br Med J.* 1977;2:738–739.
21. Leathwood P, Chauffard F. Aqueous extract of valerian root improves sleep quality in man. *Pharmacol Biochem Behav.* 1982;17:65–71.
22. Lindahl O, Lindwall L. Double-blind study of a valerian preparation. *Pharmacol Biochem Behav.* 1989;32:1065–1066.
23. Phelps S. Garlic supplementation and lipoprotein oxidation susceptibility. *Lipids.* 1993;28(5):475–477.
24. Warshafsky S, Kramer R, Sivak S. Effect of garlic on total serum cholesterol: a meta-analysis. *Ann Intern Med.* 1993;119:599–605.
25. Sobota A. Inhibition of bacterial adherence by cranberry juice: potential use for the treatment of urinary tract infections. *J Urol.* 1984;131:1013–1016.
26. Avorn J, Minane M, Gurwitz J, et al. Reduction of bacteriuria and pyuria after ingestion of cranberry juice. *JAMA.* 1994;271(10):751–754.
27. Ofek I, Goldhan J, Zafriri D, et al. Anti-escherichia coli adhesion activity of cranberry and blueberry juices. *N Engl J Med.* 1991;324(22):1599.
28. German Ministry of Health. *Echinacea Purpurea Lead.* Commission E. Monographs for Phytomedicines. Bonn, Germany: German Ministry of Health; 1989.
29. Davenas E, Beauvais F, Amara J, et al. Human basophil degranulation triggered by very dilute antiserum against IgE. *Nature.* 1988;333:816–818.

30. Kleijnen J, Knipschild P, et al. Clinical trials of homeopathy. *Br Med J.* 1992;302:316–323.
31. Resources and priorities for chronic disease prevention and control. *Morbidity Mortality Weekly Rep.* 1997;46(13):286–287.
32. Brodsky M, Orlou M, Caparelli E, et al. Magnesium therapy in new-onset atrial fibrillation. *Am J Cardiol.* 1994;73:1227–1229.
33. England M, Gordon G, Salem M, Chernow B. Magnesium administration and dysrhythmias after cardiac surgery. *JAMA.* 1992;268:2395–2402.
34. Stampfer M, Malinow M, Willett W, et al. A prospective study of plasma homocysteine and risk of myocardial infarction in US physicians. *JAMA.* 1992;286:877–881.
35. Israelsson B, Brattstrom L, Hultberg B. Homocysteine and myocardial infarction. *Atherosclerosis.* 1988;71:227–233.
36. Coull B, Malinow M, Beamer N, et al. Elevated plasma homocysteine concentration as a possible independent risk factor for stroke. *Stroke.* 1990;21:572–576.
37. Grier M, Meyers D. So much writing, so little science: a review of 37 years of literature on edetate sodium chelation therapy. *Ann Pharmacol.* 1993;27:1504–1509.
38. Smith V. *First Clinical Results Show Effectiveness of Ornish Heart Disease Reversal Program.* Mutual of Omaha Press Release, 1997.
39. Bigos S, Davis G. *Acute Low Back Problems in Adults.* Clinical Practice Guidelines #14. Rockville, MD: US Department of Health and Human Services, Public Health Service, Agency for Health Care Policy and Research; 1994.
40. Anderson R, Meeker W, Wirick B, et al. A meta-analysis of clinical trials of spinal manipulations. *J Manipulative Physiol Ther.* 1992;15(3):181–194.
41. Gunn C, Milbrandt W, Little A, Masm K. Dry needling of muscle motor points for chronic low back pain. *Spine.* 1980;5:279–291.
42. Pizzorno J, Murray M, eds. *Textbook of Natural Medicine.* Seattle, WA: John Bastyr College Publications; 1992.
43. Health insurers embrace eye-of-newt therapy. *Wall Street Journal.* January 30, 1995:B1.
44. Firshein J. Picture alternative medicine in the mainstream. *Business Health.* April 1995:32.
45. Edlin M. Changing their ways to keep up with the times. *Managed Healthcare.* 1997;6(7):14–18.
46. James G. *Making Managed Care Work: Strategies for Local Market Dominance.* Chicago, IL: Irwin Professional Publishing; 1997.
47. Jones KR, Vischi TR. Impact of alcohol, drug abuse and mental health treatment on medical care utilization: a review of the research literature. *Med Care.* 1979;17:1–82
48. Reed L, Myers E, Scheidemandel P. *Health Insurance and Psychiatric Care: Utilization and Cost.* Washington, DC: The American Psychiatric Association; 1972.
49. US Department of Health and Human Services. *1993 National Hospital Ambulatory Medical Care Survey.* Washington, DC: US Department of Health and Human Services; 1996.
50. Fugh-Berman, A. *Alternative Medicine—What Works: A Comprehensive, Easy-to-Read Review of Technology Assessment.* Baltimore: Williams & Wilkins; 1997.
51. Office of Technology Assessment. *Assessing the Efficacy and Safety of Medical Technologies.* Washington, DC: Office of Technology Assessment, US Congress; 1978.

ALAN DUMOFF, JD, MSW, is the executive director of LifeTree Medical Center and an attorney specializing in the needs of unconventional physicians and providers. A former acting director of the National Commission for the Certification of Acupuncturists, he assists physicians and providers with insurance, regulatory, and disciplinary issues. Mr. Dumoff successfully lobbied for changes protecting alternative medicine in the recent health reform legislation passed by Congress as well as a law licensing massage therapists in the District of Columbia. Mr. Dumoff publishes on the legal aspects of alternative care, and co-edits a legal column in *Alternative/Complementary Therapies*.

CHAPTER 42

Structure for CAM Integration

John Weeks

Chapter Outline

- Introduction
- Motivators for CAM Integration and Coverage
- Challenges to CAM Integration
- Credentialing
- Selecting and Defining the CAM Benefit
- Discounted CAM Services Through Credentialed Networks
- The CAM Rider
- Conclusion

INTRODUCTION

From the perspectives of the users and providers of complementary and alternative medicine (CAM), the potential applications

---

The editors of this book recognize that there are some readers who will not be receptive and some who will be very receptive to the information in this chapter. While all medical practitioners have their own opinions about complementary and alternative medicine, there is a clear desire on the part of many recipients of medical care for these services. In addition, many managed care organizations are including access to at least some of these modalities in their care management programs.

and value of this field of services are as broad as those of conventional medicine. CAM users and providers apply their interventions and approaches in pediatrics and in gerontology, in outpatient clinics and in tertiary care settings. They work with acute situations and with chronic complaints, with psychosomatic issues and as adjunctive support for complex surgeries. Practitioners may serve their patients as primary care providers or as specialists. The movement is framed by advocates as a "paradigm shift" in medicine, or a different way of viewing health and illness. Therefore, CAM interventions to assist a person toward health may be applied across the spectrum of care settings.

The movement for CAM integration reflects this diversity of applications. This chapter provides an overview of the principal challenges associated with CAM integration as well as some of the contexts in which CAM integration is being explored. The focus is on the two leading models:

1. delivery of CAM services through credentialed networks of CAM providers
2. creation of clinics in which conventional and CAM services are integrated

The chapter begins with an exploration of the distinct institutional missions in health care entities that are embracing some form of CAM integration. This leads into a discussion of the variety of meanings that "CAM integration" may have to a payer or delivery system. The opportunities and risks associated with specific integration choices are noted. Case studies are provided that explore some of the most significant initiatives and issues in greater detail. Finally, some comments are offered about directions the integration movement may take in the near future.

MOTIVATORS FOR CAM INTEGRATION AND COVERAGE

Motivation for developing CAM products may be simply summarized as the three M's: mission (of the organization), mandates, and marketplace.

Mission

Leaders of some health care systems, particularly organizations founded by religious groups, come to the integration process through an abiding respect for the spiritual component in health care. Holistic or whole-person approaches to the delivery of medicine, such as those promoted by CAM advocates, may be viewed as potentially aligned with this perspective. Some philosophic underpinnings of the CAM movement may be comfortably embraced by these leaders. These include an interest in patient-centered care, patient empowerment, education for behavior change, and the role of life choices and stress in the manifestation and exacerbation of disease. The CAM movement's critical perspective toward medical delivery that rests primarily on pharmaceutical and surgical interventions may also be viewed as an expression of frustration with a disease-based model, according to Corrine Bayley, senior vice president of St. Joseph's Healthcare in Orange, California (personal communication, September 1997), and Sister Diana Bader, formerly with the Sisters of Providence Health System in Seattle, Washington (personal communication, August 1996).

Such leaders may champion CAM initiatives within the system. Programs or therapies that focus on the body-mind—or spiritual—connection may be viewed as particularly valuable areas for exploration. This philosophical openness may create a belief that exploration of appropriate CAM integration, or even responding to member interest in CAM, may also help the system meet additional requirements of its mission. CAM may be viewed as potentially delivering more cost-effective care that creates greater health in the population served.

Mandates

Behind the other two motivators—mandates and marketplace—is the health care stakeholder, widely acknowledged as the driver in the integration process: the CAM consumer. In the case of mandates, consumer interest expresses itself through laws passed by state legislators. While CAM provider organizations are often the economic interests behind these legislative campaigns, such lobbying is usually buoyed by letter writing in which CAM patients are asked to contact their legislators.

By 1997, 41 states had some kind of mandate to cover chiropractic services, 8 for acupuncture, 3 for services of naturopathic physicians, and 1 for massage practitioners.[1] The substance of these mandates varies widely. Mandates may, for example

- only cover workers' compensation
- require or allow primary care referral
- be limited to a few conditions
- apply only to insurance products and not to managed care organizations
- give plans additional utilization management authority

The passage of such mandates during the 20 years prior to the current era of CAM integration has given some plans a minimal level of familiarity with various CAM provider services. As will be seen, plans may also have initiated relationships, particularly with chiropractic management organizations, that may serve them well when they expand their CAM benefit offerings.

One of the most important of these mandates was a 1995 act of the Washington State legislature that required all of the state's health plans to include "every category of provider" as of January of the following year. The experience of Washington's plans with such groups as acupuncturists, naturopaths, licensed midwives, and massage practitioners has provided the nationwide CAM integration process with its first widespread experience and outcomes. Some are reported in the case study of Group Health Cooperative of Puget Sound in Appendix 42–A.

Marketplace

The individual user of CAM services is the dominant force behind CAM integration activity. The lesson for some health plans in the 1993 data on use of "unconventional medicine" among American consumers was that meeting this interest could give them an advantage in the market. These plans often engaged their own local market surveys in order to test whether the Eisenberg data applied in their service area or among their members. Table 42–1 describes some outcomes of a variety of surveys engaged by individual plans in efforts to clarify interest among their members or potential members.

The marketing opportunity represented by this consumer interest is expressed by plans in a variety of ways:

Table 42–1 Plan or Delivery Systems Surveys on Use of CAM Practitioners

Surveyor	Year	Market	Features of Survey	Percentage Seeing Alternative Provider
Eisenberg et al	1990	National	Phone survey of residents	10 (in 1 year)
The Alternare Group	1994	Portland, OR	Phone survey of residents	35 (in 2 years)
Seattle–King County Department of Public Health	1995	King County, WA	Survey of clientele in public health clinics who saw naturopathic physicians, chiropractors, acupuncturists	19 (in 1 year)
Oxford Health Plans	1995–1996	CT, NY, NJ	Phone survey of 750 plan members	33 (in 2 years)
Unified Physicians of Washington	1996	Seattle, WA	Survey at a University District Women's Clinic	56 (in 1 year)
Presbyterian Healthcare System	1996	NM	Phone survey of residents	33 (in 1 year)

Courtesy of John Weeks/Integration Strategies, Seattle, Washington.

- marketplace differentiation to attract new enrollees
- enrollment of members who appear to have relatively healthy lifestyles and may therefore be low utilizers of more costly services
- efforts to attract populations, such as Asian or Hispanic populations, that may value CAM approaches such as acupuncture or herbal medicine

In markets where a major health plan has already created and publicized a CAM product, some plans develop CAM products as defensive measures. Here the interest is in retaining enrollees. By 1997, this force was in evident in California, the upper Midwest, New England, and the Northwest. In each region, consumer interest in CAM is viewed as particularly high.

Other Motivators

While marketplace and member interest dominate in prompting CAM activity, once an investigation commences, other aspects of an organization's mission frequently come into consideration. These include a desire to create more effective and cost-effective care, and to stimulate healthy practices among the population served. Once the process is engaged and internally publicized, individuals within the plan may step into leadership roles. For instance, physician surveys have shown that a significant percentage of physicians believe that better CAM integration may lead to more effective or cost-effective care.[2] Plans generally discover that certain members of their executive teams, or family members, have quietly been using CAM and developing a belief that the system's health care would be enhanced by exploration of CAM practices.[3]

Such interest among physicians may be expected to grow. By 1997, nearly a third of conventional medical schools offered at least an overview course on CAM. Many medical schools began sponsoring continuing education programs through which physicians can receive continuing education credits for courses on CAM approaches. A variety of research is under way under the aegis of the National Institutes of Health's Office of Alternative Medicine. All of these factors, as well as the public's growing acceptance of CAM, suggest that a new generation of physicians can be expected to be both more friendly toward, and more knowledgeable about, CAM therapies.

CHALLENGES TO CAM INTEGRATION

These perceptions of potential benefits and the forces behind the CAM integration momentum noted above encounter numerous countervailing influences. Chief among these are

- costs concerns and lack of actuarial data
- research limits
- lack of CAM standards and templates
- reluctance of plans to investigate CAM benefits
- "paradigm issues" in integration
- bilateral ignorance and prejudice

These items are discussed in more detail below.

Cost Concerns and Lack of Actuarial Data

Little information is available on the customary costs of delivering CAM benefits to populations. Even less is readily available that looks at whether the CAM approaches are an add-on to or a replacement for conventional interventions and associated costs. This uncertainty may be compounded by the expectation of an upward trend in health care costs forecast for 1998–2000, which may be viewed as a disincentive to adding new benefits of any kind. Some CAM providers, however, view the end of the era of cost cutting through stringent utilization management and discounted fees as an opportunity to focus attention on what they believe to be more fundamental issues about the nature of routine medical care.

Research Limits

For most conventional providers, conversation about what CAM approaches should be covered, and for which conditions, frequently unfolds around questions regarding scientific evidence. The perspective holds that only after CAM has successfully passed through rigorous technology assessment processes and has been deemed medically necessary should CAM therapies be covered. The same procedures and criteria used to evaluate traditional approaches to patient care should be applied to nontraditional approaches, without a higher standard or a lower standard. In such a view, the valued scientific periodicals are often limited to peer-reviewed journals published in the United States. Given this condition, few CAM interventions have yet garnered the requisite research support to allow for coverage. A representative position on CAM coverage following these guidelines is offered in Table 42–2.

CAM advocates respond to this criticism with an apology for the low level of research that exists. The elements of the apology are as follows:

- *Nonpatentable nature of most CAM therapies.* Most CAM therapies and agents—whether mind-body interventions, acupuncture, massage, botanical medicines, vitamins, minerals, or enzymes—are not patentable. Little private incentive exists to fund research. The US government and private foundations have only recently begun to view CAM as a legitimate area for research.
- *More research exists than is usually acknowledged.* Advocates argue that a significant amount of research to shape benefit decisions is available. Leading areas are

Table 42–2 Prudential Healthcare: Status of Technology Assessment and Coverage Status of Alternative Medicine Benefits

Treatment	Formal Technology Assessment Performed?	Coverage Status
Acupuncture	Yes	Certain number of chronic pain syndromes
Ayurvedic medicine	No	No
Biofeedback	Yes	"With some limitations"
Chelation therapy	Yes	Bona fide heavy metal poisoning only
Chiropractic	Yes	Limited to contractual agreements
Environmental medicine	Yes	No
Herbal medicine	No	No
Light box therapy	Yes	Seasonal affective disorder only
Massage therapy	No	Part of physical therapy; limited to short-term physical therapy
Naturopathy	No	No
Oxygen therapy	No	No
Therapeutic diet	Yes	For inherited metabolic disorders only (like phenylketonuria)

Note: A review by the US Health Care Financing Administration of best practices in managed care determined that Prudential's tech assessment process was among the best.

Courtesy of John Weeks/Integration Strategies, Seattle, Washington.

body-mind approaches, certain botanical and therapeutic nutrition interventions, touch therapies, and the use of homeopathics. Plans must be willing to access new journals, especially those from abroad, particularly from Europe, where CAM approaches are more widely integrated and studied.
- *The placebo-controlled, single-agent trial does not fit many CAM interventions.* The whole-person approach frequently utilizes protocols that are multiagent and individualized and therefore are hard to measure by the gold standard.
- *Studies must be longitudinal and are therefore more costly.*

The CAM provider will also assert that a requirement that CAM therapies meet rigid technology assessment criteria before being accepted for coverage means that CAM therapies are being held to a higher standard than conventional therapies.[4] Many conventional therapies and treatments are continuing in use and continue to be covered, despite not being held to the standards of evidence-based medicine.

Lack of CAM Standards and Templates

The relatively recent opportunity for integration of CAM providers and therapies means that few standards for management have been developed and even fewer analyzed. Few algorithms, even speculative ones, exist for integrating CAM into conventional case management. Evidence-based algorithms are virtually nonexistent. Most plans and business entities that are developing such templates tend to view them as proprietary. Published literature on CAM management practices is just beginning to develop. (Additional issues on CAM standards are examined in the section on credentialing, below.)

Reluctance of Plans To Investigate CAM Benefits

Most plans that are embracing CAM integration initiatives do not view CAM as a core part of doing business. CAM is looked upon as an ancillary, market-driven addition to basic medical services. CAM approaches and providers are not involved in plans' chief clinical undertakings (discussed throughout this book) in areas such as disease management, development of specialty services teams, limits on costs of tertiary care, and even patient education and health promotion initiatives. Plan resources generally are not directed to exploration of appropriate integration.

In addition, tremendous energy is being spent by health systems in re-engineering care, merging information systems with new partners, and other substantive requirements of participating in a rapidly shifting health care environment. These conditions often make it difficult for leading plan personnel to devote adequate time to take more than a cursory look at the role CAM may have in their efforts to deliver more effective and cost-effective care. This hindrance to integration is explored further in the section on the CAM rider, below.

Paradigm Issues in Integration

CAM providers will assert that their approach to patient care reflects a health-creating rather than symptom-suppressing or disease-managing approach. Data suggest that interest in more wellness-oriented approaches to conditions is one factor that has moved consumers toward wanting CAM.

CAM providers assert their need to spend more time with patients than conventional practitioners do. CAM providers focus essentially on primary prevention, targeting removal of the causal factors in the health problem rather than alleviating symptoms, which has been Western medicine's focus in the past. CAM providers believe it is inappropriate to expect them to successfully treat patients in the same time frame and with the same patterns of evaluation and management codes used by other medical specialists.

Bilateral Ignorance and Prejudice

An unusual issue in CAM integration (which is generally not a part of discussion of medical management) is the importance of acknowledging and addressing some of the historic polarization between conventional and CAM providers if optimal integration of CAM services is to be discovered and developed.

Most conventional providers currently in practice, as well as medical directors for plans, were trained in an era when CAM was viewed as fraud and quackery, or, at best, as a heightening of the placebo effect. Yet these same providers and directors may now be asked to serve as gatekeepers controlling patient access to services about which the providers know little and in which they often do not believe. Conventional providers may find it difficult to believe that there are bodies of valuable knowledge that were not part of their medical training. They tend to frame the integration exchange as divided into scientific medicine and unscientific practices, although each of the characterizations has a shadow of falsehood. Such framing polarizes discussion.

Conventional providers may feel even more conflicted when they realize that some of their patients are probably using CAM therapies or providers. (A national study commissioned by Landmark Healthcare in Sacramento, California, and made public in January 1998 concluded that 42% of the 1,500 nationally sampled interviewees had used alternative medicine in the previous year.)[5] The patients may know more about CAM therapies than the providers do. Providers may be aware that members of the CAM community sometimes make sweeping judgments that question the value of conventional provider practices. Conventional providers may look upon the relatively relaxed, time-intensive treatment of CAM providers with some envy, certain that they too could please their patients if their managed care contracts allowed such extensive patient contact. The context can create a defensiveness that hinders the ability to find common ground.

For their part, CAM providers may view conventional medical practices from polarized perspectives. They may boldly assert the relative value of their approaches, then quietly add that such approaches may not work if patients fail to comply with demanding behavioral change protocols. CAM providers may fail to appreciate that their self-selecting, cash-paying patients create an unusually positive climate for caregiving—that the payment of cash assists the placebo response. They may point at the prevalence of self-limiting conditions as evidence of the need for reform of more aggressive pharmaceutical approaches offered by conventional providers, while accepting self-limiting conditions in their own practices as evidence of successful treatment. To build up their own position, they may tear down the value of conventional services. They may envy the income of conventional providers.

This historic and cultural rift suggests that developing optimal relationships between CAM providers and conventional providers will require attention to developing relationships through which the polarization may be diminished. Relationship building is particularly important in an environment in which a gatekeeper may determine a patient's access to CAM services.

CREDENTIALING

One core distinction in viewing CAM integration is whether the focus is on integrating individual CAM therapies, such as a botanical remedy or a type of massage, or on a specific type of CAM provider. From the perspective of the distinct CAM professionals—acupuncturists, naturopaths, and massage practitioners—the past 25 years may be seen as a long campaign to set up credentials. They worked to strengthen schools and educational standards, establish credentialing agencies and standardized exams, and to expand licensing. (For the chiropractors, this work was principally done prior to this period.)

Table 42–3 shows the status of these core standards for the leading CAM professions. In states where these professions are licensed, the core credentialing standards of licensing, passage of an examination, and ability to purchase malpractice coverage are essentially in order.

Despite the progress in establishing standards, considerable challenges remain. Multistate plans must be aware that the scope of practice for these provider categories may differ. For instance, acupuncturists in some states are authorized to order laboratory tests while in others they may be forbidden from assigning a Western diagnosis to a patient. Naturopaths in one state may have broad prescriptive rights or be allowed to perform acupuncture under their naturopathic license. In certain jurisdictions, CAM practitioners may be able to use the title "physician." The CAM professions face the challenge of standardizing their scope of practice across jurisdictions. Such efforts may be charged with significant philosophic differences among providers. In addition, CAM practitioners may show substantial variation in the nature of the services they offer. Exhibit 42–1 describes such differences.

In states where these providers are not licensed, the status of some of these professionals, from a credentialing perspective, appears to be equivocal. First, plans must be aware that, without standards, some individuals will practice without having achieved the professional standards represented by Table 42–3. Some delivery systems are comfortable working with such providers when they are directly supervised by licensed physicians. However, state laws in some jurisdictions expressly forbid such practices. In such a situation, one strategy for guaranteeing a level of competency is to require that the practitioner has passed the profession's national exam. Alternatively, the practitioner may be required to have secured and to maintain a license in a state that does license the provider type. The National Committee for Quality Assurance has not established standards in this arena, except for chiropractic care.

Restrictive Strategies of Some Plans

The integration of CAM and traditional services is, depending on a person's perspective, either more *rich* with diversity or *fraught* with diversity, than even the individual practice styles listed in Exhibit 42–1. Some health plans that credential complementary providers have established additional, restrictive standards to cull a subset from the group of available providers. These additional credentialing criteria are then

Table 42–3 Development of Standards by the Complementary Professions

Profession	Accrediting Agency Established	US Department of Education Recognition	Recognized Schools	Standardized National Exam Created	State Regulation*	Malpractice Insurance
Acupuncture	1982	1990		1982	33 states	Early 1980s
Chiropractic	1971	1974	16	1963	50 states	
Massage	1982	No		1994	26 states	1993
Midwifery**	1990s	Planning under way	First school accredited 1995	First certification exam 1994	18 states	Off and on since 1980s
Naturopathy	1978	1987	4	1986	11 states	1988

*For chiropractors and naturopathic physicians, this category uniformly represents licensing statutes; for acupuncture, massage, and midwifery, it represents a mixture of licensing, certification, and registration.
**This is European-style, direct-entry midwifery.

Courtesy of John Weeks/Integration Strategies, Seattle, Washington.

Exhibit 42–1 What You See and What You Get: Some Distinctions Between Category and Practice with CAM Providers

What you see	Alternative Medical Doctor	Licensed Naturopathic Physician	Licensed Acupuncturist	Licensed Massage Therapist	Licensed Chiropractor
What you get	• Strong belief in behavioral health interventions	• General practitioner of natural medicine	• Only uses needles	• Occupational health specialist	• Only adjusts the spine
	• Uses natural agents sometimes in place of conventional pharmaceuticals	• Classical homeopath	• Works as an Oriental medical doctor	• Rolfer	• Diagnoses using laboratory methods
	• Sees self as a naturopath, using broad scope of natural therapies	• Explorer of diverse experimental, energy medicine modalities	• Occupational health specialist	• Also provides nutritional counseling and homeopathic consultation	• General practitioner of natural medicine
	• Took acupuncture course for physicians	• Practice dominated by physical medicine approaches	• Certificated both in acupuncture and in Chinese herbs	• Colon therapist	• Uses various natural modalities but cannot do laboratory diagnosis
	• Experiments with exotic injectable natural agents	• Similar to primary care physician but uses natural agents	• Specializes in pain management	• Mainly deep tissue work	• Strong interest in homeopathy
				• Only uses Swedish technique	

Courtesy of John Weeks/Integration Strategies, Seattle, Washington.

directed at ensuring that the CAM providers are comfortable working in a collaborative fashion with the conventional medical community. Examples include the following:

- continuing education beyond that which may be required for licensing
- evidence that the CAM provider has working relationships with conventional medical professionals
- a minimum number of years of practice, especially in lieu of a residency
- evidence that one or more medical professionals will agree to consult when patient

needs are beyond the scope of the CAM provider's practice or the provider's legal ability, such as hospital admissions

One interesting example of special criteria is the Regence Blue Shield Washington strategy relative to naturopathic physicians. Regence allows naturopathic physicians to act either as primary care physicians (PCPs) or as specialists. Those who wish to be in the Regence network as PCPs are required to show, in their application, that they (1) are willing to perform immunizations, (2) have plans for 24-hour coverage, and (3) have a relationship with a conventional physician (MD or doctor of osteopathy) who will handle hospital admissions for them. (No Washington State hospitals allow naturopaths to admit patients.) Naturopathic physicians who do not meet these criteria but met the other Regence credentialing requirements, can be listed as specialists who are available only on referral.

Finding Good CAM Providers Who Are Prepared for Participation

Credentialing processes may also encounter informal barriers. CAM providers are often not prepared for participation in managed care from the perspective of capital (malpractice, office staff, computers, etc) or experience. Most are extremely unfamiliar with health insurance, much less with managed care. CAM providers typically desire more education about referral procedures, utilization management, insurance procedures, capitation, medical recordkeeping, medical necessity, technology assessment processes, and the role of the gatekeeper. Plans should educate these providers upon bringing them into networks.

Another useful strategy is an elaborate provider preselection process. The plan or network may request information on typical billing rates, most frequently seen conditions or codes utilized, number of patients, number of support staff, use of computers for office management, and comfort with the integration processes. Plans may also begin by finding a few trusted providers, or consultants familiar with the CAM profession, then build a network based on their expertise.

Credentialing Conventional Providers Who Use CAM Therapies

Credentialing processes are paradoxical for medical doctors and other conventionally trained and licensed medical professionals who use complementary methods. On the surface—with licensing in all 50 states and very similar scopes of practice nationwide—it would seem that these providers would easily meet core standards. If the intent of credentialing is to ensure that providers meet standards *for the delivery of CAM*, the picture shifts.

- *Medical education.* Most conventional medical, nursing, physician assistant, and dietetics educational programs do not include complementary therapeutics in their core curriculum, or as electives. Clinical training is virtually nonexistent.
- *Licensing examination.* Conventional providers are not tested in these skill areas as part of their examination process prior to attaining licenses.
- *Malpractice insurance.* Malpractice insurance carriers typically offer policies with the expectation that conventional providers will practice within the community standard of care. Most complementary approaches are outside this standard and therefore may not be covered by the provider's policy. Some policies that specifically cover alternative methods are available, however.

Currently, most alternative medical doctors gain their education in CAM through a nonstandardized composite of lectures, books, tapes, conferences, collegial relationships, and clinical experimentation. A medical doctor may be exceptionally well skilled in one or more complementary therapies. Objective, verifiable standards for medical education, licensing, and examination in CAM—the backbone of managed care credentialing—are virtually nonexistent. Thus, the conventionally trained categories of providers with which the health plan is familiar and may be most comfortable are often the least qualified, from a credentialing standpoint, to provide complementary services.

The recent growth in education programs in complementary medicine inside conventional medical schools and nursing schools may eventually lead to development of traditional credentialing standards. Courses on specific areas of CAM that offer continuing education credits through, or in partnership with, academic medical centers begin to fill the gap. The standout example is acupuncture training offered through the University of California at Los Angeles. However, neither standardization of these programs nor inclusion of a standardized complementary medicine section in licensing examinations is expected soon.

No accrediting agencies for managed care have put standards for the delivery of complementary therapeutics to a credentialing test. Therefore, no clarity on the leniency these agencies might show has been established. Until the conventional medical professions establish verifiable standards for credentialing, intermediate steps may fill the void.

- Request full documentation of all complementary education, including the curriculum vitae of the teaching faculty.
- Investigate the extent to which the education offered included a clinical component.
- Request information on any education that has led to a certificate of completion or that led to an examination.
- Request information on the status, if any, the certificate program has achieved with an independent review organization.
- Request evidence that the provider's malpractice carrier is aware of the provider's complementary practices and will cover these services.

Credentialing Unregulated Providers

A subset of CAM services is frequently provided by individuals who have no accredited health care training but who have undertaken to educate themselves, sometimes extensively, in one or more complementary medicine modalities. Included in this category are lay homeopaths; herbalists; bodyworkers; yoga, qigong, and tai chi instructors; and nutritional counselors.

Health plan accreditation standards would not appear to allow such individuals to provide services for an accredited health plan. There is some flexibility here—perhaps because the potential for harm is believed to be low. Some integrated clinics may offer such services under the aegis of a medical doctor. In addition, some plans will offer some, at least, of these services as part of health education or wellness and not clinical services. Case 1 in Appendix 42–A looks at a program for offering qigong, a traditional Chinese movement and relaxation therapy, through an unlicensed provider.

SELECTING AND DEFINING THE CAM BENEFIT

Insurance companies and managed care organizations are sometimes compared with automobiles. The marketing director is said to have a foot on the gas while the chief financial officer's foot is slammed on the brake. The car's direction, meantime, is guided by the actuary who, basing decisions on historic data, is looking out the back window.

This story comes up in CAM discussions because organized medicine in the United States does not yet have much experience with developing, pricing, offering, and managing CAM benefits. The actuary tends to side with the chief financial officer: *Put on the brakes!* To move ahead with CAM, the actuary has to take a leap of faith. The following is a discussion of the array of benefits now emerging.

DISCOUNTED CAM SERVICES THROUGH CREDENTIALED NETWORKS

One direction some plans and purchasers take, given the dearth of actuarial data, is to offer members value-added services that do not put them at any risk. In this model, plans develop programs for services that are not in the benefit plan, then offer them to their members at a discount. Such programs have been developed in recent years around conventional treatments, such as eye care or cosmetic surgery, and are now an easy niche for CAM services. In this model, the plan creates, or contracts with, a network of providers who agree to give the plan's members a discount, usually of 10% to 30%. In some of these programs, licensed categories of providers may be formally credentialed, with independent verification, as a selling point for the value of the network to the member. Plans may use this approach for a range of services, from licensed CAM providers such as acupuncturists and naturopaths, to fitness centers, stress management programs, and even healthy-eating restaurants.

This strategy is viewed as win-win-win for the parties involved.

- The plan gains a new feature without added risk.
- The member gets a discount on CAM, as well as some reassurance that the provider meets a credentialing standard.
- By being included on a plan's provider list, the CAM provider gains some recognition that may increase his or her business.

In addition, if the plan sets up appropriate mechanisms for capturing data, it can establish a baseline from which to better estimate the actual cost of offering a CAM benefit.

THE CAM RIDER

The dominant trend in integrating CAM providers is to offer services through a benefit rider. The largest interest is in offering chiropractic, then acupuncture, followed by services of naturopathic physicians in those states where naturopathic doctors are licensed. Some plans are also looking at offering services of massage practitioners in CAM riders. Plans view the new CAM benefit as they have viewed behavioral health. Some believe there may be a high potential for overutilization because of the nature of the services offered and because the plan may not have internal competency in the new services area. Therefore, the services may benefit from specialized management skills and are frequently carved out to specialty management firms.

Some characteristics of CAM riders have included the following:

- generally offered only to groups (21 or more, 51 or more, etc) in order to limit adverse selection
- allow direct access without referral from a physician for a limited benefit (either a total dollar figure, typically $500 to $2,000, or annual number of visits, typically 12 to 20)
- a higher than usual copay, perhaps up to 50%

Exhibit 42–2 provides an overview of a benefit structure and plan price for an acupuncture insurance product that began to be successfully offered to group purchasers in mid-1997. A health maintenance organization's (HMO's) model for the rider, in the context of a more global approach to CAM services, is offered in Exhibit 42–3.

Exhibit 42–2 Monthly Charges for AcupuncturePlus Policy

Plan A5-40

$5 copay, 40 visits per year, $300 herbal max per year

Employee only	$ 5.75
Employee + spouse	$10.00
Employee + child(ren)	$11.45
Employee + family	$14.00

Plan A5-20

$5 copay, 40 visits per year, $200 herbal max per year

Employee only	$ 5.25
Employee + spouse	$ 9.50
Employee + child(ren)	$11.00
Employee + family	$12.95

Plan A10-40

$10 copay, 30 visits per year, $250 herbal max per year

Employee only	$ 4.75
Employee + spouse	$ 8.75
Employee + child(ren)	$10.05
Employee + family	$11.65

Courtesy of AcupuncturePlus, Milpitas, California.

Exhibit 42–3 Characteristics of Oxford Health Plans' Initial Alternative Medicine Program

Limitations/Copay	**Options**
	• Copay of $10, $15, or $20
	• Maximum at $2,000, $3,000, or $5,000
Cost	Price as a supplement of 2% to 3% added to premium
Provider fees	Schedule not released; expected to be at a discounted rate
Target market	Large group clients
Excluded market	Individuals, to protect against expected adverse selection
Patient access	• Direct to the initial categories (see below)
	• No primary care physician referral required
Provider groups	• Initially chiropractors, naturopathic physicians, and acupuncturists
	• Second phase adds clinical nutritionists, registered dietitians, licensed massage practitioners, yoga instructors
Core credentialing criteria	• Licensed in state of practice
	• Graduate of a fully accredited professional training program
	• At least 2 years of clinical experience
	• Ongoing continuing education credits required (unspecified number)
	• Proper malpractice insurance (unspecified levels)
	• On-site visits may be required
Numbers of providers	• 500 to 1,000 by the end of 1996
	• 2,000 by the end of 1997
Market research	• Poll of 750 members revealed that 35% had used an alternative provider in the previous 2 years
	• Poll of large employers showed that 75% were interested in the product
Research and outcomes	Partner with David Eisenberg at Harvard University
Internal operations and management	• 12-member department
	• Advisory boards for chiropractors, naturopathic physicians, and acupuncturists
	• Leading practitioner in each discipline chairs board
Natural medicinals	Available at a discounted rate through a health plan mail-order service
Member self-care	• Natural health educational materials (books, tapes, videos, etc) available via discounted mail-order service
	• Facilitated access to on-line information on alternative medicine and self-care
Special programs	Educational seminars on menopause and senior citizen health concerns to start; others to follow

Courtesy of John Weeks/Integration Strategies, Seattle, Washington.

Plans may not only model their benefits on their experience with chiropractic, but also contract for these new CAM services through the same businesses with which they contract to manage their chiropractic benefits. A number of the leading chiropractic managed care organizations have credentialed networks of acupuncturists, massage practitioners, or naturopathic physicians. Some chiropractic managed care organizations originated the business plan, some merged with acupuncture networks, and, in a growing number of cases, the chiropractic managed care organization was asked to move into the new field by a purchaser that was looking to expand its CAM rider offerings. The chiropractic-plus model for developing other CAM riders is attractive to some health plans. The plans can deal with companies with which they are familiar and that they trust. In doing so, the plans limit the need for outsourcing to additional parties.

For the provider of acupuncture, massage, or naturopathic services, the model may be acceptable merely because these professions, as a rule, have neither the infrastructure nor the capital to create their own networks or independent practitioner associations. These financial constraints effectively mean that newer categories of CAM providers will be joining networks developed by venture capitalists.

The Limits of a Rider as an "Integrated" Model

For many plans, riders are an exceptional way to begin offering CAM benefits. Once the plan has experience in this context of diminished risk, it can, if it so chooses, begin to consider CAM as a part of a core benefit in which fewer limits on consumer use are required. In addition, for the consumer who may have historically had insurance that covered only conventional care, and who paid out of pocket for CAM, the rider will create a form of economic integration in the consumer's health care experience. The rider may also be created in a way that allows the consumer to directly access the CAM provider, without going through the referral from a conventional physician. Consumers may not need to face any known or anticipated conflicts their conventional provider may have over their decision to seek CAM. In these ways, the acupuncture, chiropractic, or other CAM benefit that is purchased through a rider may feel more "integrated" to the customer.

However, from the perspectives of the payment and the delivery of care, the rider is an essentially nonintegrated product.

- The rider is usually not clinically integrated, since often no referral or reporting is required.
- The rider is not economically integrated, as payment for the services comes out of a separate fund, the additional per member per month (PMPM) or per employee per month (PEPM) payment of the rider.
- The rider is frequently not organizationally integrated, because the benefit is often "carved out" to a specialty organization.

Unless organizations develop policies to mediate against these nonintegration tendencies, the following can be viewed as expected side effects of using the rider as a mechanism for offering CAM services:

- Neither conventional nor CAM providers, because they may be in separate organizations, will have substantial organizational incentives to learn to work closely and understand when CAM is most appropriate.
- If the outside contractor does a good job, CAM will not receive much internal attention.
- The leadership of the health plan will have little reason to assess whether CAM actually *replaces* or limits conventional services—and thus might be best considered as a core benefit—or is merely an add-on benefit, and thus reasonably paid for by additional fees.

Interestingly, CAM providers and many CAM consumers believe that better integration of CAM will lead to more cost-effective treatment. They believe that CAM methods can help the health care system toward a more fundamental health-oriented focus that they believe is true reform. However, the side effects listed above suggest that the rider may limit the extent to which the health care payment and delivery system discovers and optimizes the role of CAM in delivery of effective and cost-effective care.

CAM Services as Core Benefits

Some purchasers and HMOs are including CAM as a core benefit. Most of this activity is in Washington State; it began under mandate but was maintained despite a federal judge's decision that effectively revoked the mandate in May 1997.[6] California-based Lifeguard Healthcare began offering acupuncture as a value-added benefit, at no additional cost, in the spring of 1997.

The first data from an HMO experience that may confirm the value of offering at least some CAM benefits without additional costs was developed by Alternare of Washington, a CAM network, for its client, Group Health Cooperative of Puget Sound (Group Health). In a survey by Alternare of Group Health members who used the services of acupuncturists, naturopathic physicians, and massage practitioners under the HMO's managed CAM programs, 49% of respondents said they believed that their use of these providers reduced their use of their "conventional team."[7] Roughly 55% responded that they believed their use of prescriptions drugs had declined.[7] Interestingly, 66% of the patients of naturopathic physicians, who often prescribe natural agents such as botanical medicines or nutrients in lieu of conventional pharmacy, reported diminished use of conventional drugs.[7] These data suggest that, in the short term at least, services are perceived as an add-on for some patients (complementary medicine) and a replacement (alternative medicine) for others.

In markets where offering CAM services through a rider is commonplace, rolling CAM into core benefit design will be a logical way for a plan to distinguish itself among consumers who are interested in the CAM benefit.

Other Forms of Limited Benefits

Coverage of CAM can also be restricted to specific programs that target specific conditions. An insurer, for instance, may cover a multifaceted, integrated program for managing a major costly condition, such as coronary artery disease or diabetes. Under this model, a defined program is covered, or partially covered, by a third party. Some integrated clinics associated with academic medical centers appear to favor this approach, which offers CAM as an additional specialist service. Rather than using credentialed providers from distinct CAM professions, the services tend to be provided by, or overseen by, conventionally trained providers who have learned additional CAM therapies.

For the health plan that seeks to develop CAM benefits but finds that insufficient data are available to support its conventional technology assessment, the following strategies may be useful:

- Develop panels of providers, with relevant CAM professionals to provide guidance.
- Request information on research from state and national professional associations.
- Review research that has been published abroad but not in the United States.
- Request information from advisors and their respective professions on the leading conditions seen in their practices and where they believe their services can be most useful.
- Consider surveying a sample of CAM providers to gather additional information.

CONCLUSION

By early 1998, the movement to cover and integrate various CAM modalities and provider types was underway in a multitude of delivery settings and payment structures. Because consumers have driven the movement, most of the activity has focused on responding to consumer interest. Few organizations have investigated the extent to which health care in the United States may be more effectively and cost-effectively delivered through better CAM integration. Investigating this important issue requires bringing CAM providers into a plan's leading clinical initiatives, such as the development of care pathways and disease management programs. Some plans and delivery systems may decide to proactively recommend that their members use CAM services rather than conventional services. Only then will the plan and the mainstream system begin to be fully joined with the consumer in promoting a systematic approach to optimally integrated care.

REFERENCES

1. Pelletier K, Marie A, Krasner MA, Haskell WL. Current trends in the integration and reimbursement of complementary and alternative medicine by managed care, insurance carriers, and hospital providers. *Am J Health Promotion.* 1997;12(2):112–123.
2. Weeks J, Layton R. Integration as community organizing: toward a model for optimizing relationships between networks of conventional and alternative providers. *Integrative Med.* 1997;1(1):15–25.
3. Weeks J. Operational issues in incorporating complementary and alternative therapies and providers in benefit plans and managed care organizations. Presented at Complementary and Alternative Medicine: Issues Impacting Coverage Decisions; October 9, 1996; Tucson, AZ.
4. Jonas W. The complementary medicine and alternative health practices movement (CMAHP): an overview. Presented at Complementary Medicine and Alternative Health Practices: A New Paradigm for Improving Health Status for Medically Underserved Populations; September 25, 1997; Rockville, MD.
5. Landmark Healthcare. *The Landmark Report on Public Perceptions of Alternative Care.* Sacramento, CA: Landmark Healthcare; January 1998.
6. Weeks J. ERISA suit guts mandate: what's next? *Alternative Med Integration Coverage.* July 1997: 1–2.
7. Weeks J. First retrospective member survey on HMO-defined CAM benefits: alternate survey suggests high satisfaction, possible cost savings. *Alternative Med Integration Coverage.* February 1998:1–5.

ADDITIONAL RESOURCES

Complementary and alternative medicine: issues impacting coverage decisions. Executive summary and presented papers available through the NIH Office of Alternative Medicine Clearinghouse, Silver Spring, MD; October 1996.

Duggan R. Complementary medicine: transforming influence or footnote to history? *Alternative Ther Health Med.* 1995;1(2):28–33.

Eisenberg D. Advising patients who seek alternative medical therapies. *Ann Intern Med.* 1997;127(1):61–69.

Jonas W, Levin J, eds. *Textbook of Complementary and Alternative Medicine.* Baltimore, MD: Williams & Wilkins; 1998.

Weeks J. Managed care meets alternative medicine: reflections on overcoming the polarization. *Alternative Complementary Ther.* February 1997:37–41.

Integrating Complementary and Alternative Medicine into Managed Care. Tapes of 2-day seminar offered by Institute for International Research, October 7–8, 1996; New York; (1–800–999–3123).

Other tapes developed by the National Managed Health Care Congress (1–888–882–2500).

JOHN WEEKS, founder and principal of Integration Strategies for Natural Healthcare, consults nationally in development of integrated products and services. His clients in CAM integration have included HMOs, physician networks, hospitals, complementary provider organizations, integrated clinics, purchasers, and diverse government agencies such as the Washington State Office of the Insurance Commissioner, US Bureau of Primary Health Care, and the Arizona Department of Health. Previously, Mr. Weeks served for 10 years in a variety of leadership roles in the maturation of the alternative professions. He writes and speaks widely on coverage issues, including serving as executive editor for and producing *Alternative Medicine Integration and Coverage,* a monthly newsletter devoted to practical information for those engaged in the integration process.

Appendix 42–A

Case Studies

The following case studies are offered to explore some of the issues raised by the business of CAM integration and coverage in greater detail. Case 1 explores efforts to weave CAM into health promotion and chronic disease care. Case 2 discusses the process and early outcomes of the pioneering work of Group Health Cooperative of Puget Sound in offering CAM through a credentialed network of CAM providers. Case 3 investigates the leading alternative setting for delivering CAM, the integrated clinic in which conventional and CAM services are offered side by side.

CASE 1: INTEGRATING GROUP–DELIVERED CAM PROGRAMS INTO CONVENTIONAL AND INDIVIDUALIZED CAM SERVICES—KAISER NORTHERN CALIFORNIA*

One of the first areas where CAM approaches began to be available in managed care is through member education and health promotion programs. A variety of self-care techniques that originally flourished outside the mainstream began to be offered in this environment. Examples are tai chi, qigong, yoga, meditation, acupressure, and the relaxation response training developed by Herbert Benson and associates at Harvard. The programs are viewed as potentially beneficial in the areas of stress reduction, increased activity, and patient empowerment.

In 1996, Kaiser Permanente in Northern California began developing a program that seeks to better integrate these services into care delivery for interested members. Early results suggest that these programs are building better, more empowered patients, as well as helping with the bottom line. The principle behind this program—mixing group delivery of CAM programs with individual delivery of services—may prove to be applicable to diverse care alternatives as well as conventional services.

The program has two distinct origins. Kaiser wished to appropriately manage costs and utilization of its new acupuncture benefits. The HMO's region also sought to optimize the use of group-delivered CAM programs as adjuncts to their conventional medical services.

Kaiser was increasingly offering acupuncture, mainly for chronic pain conditions. While much of the alternative provider community claims to promote self-care, Kaiser's physician leaders knew that acupuncture, in itself, did not necessarily have any more self-care in it than many

---

*This case study is courtesy of John Weeks/Integration Strategies, Seattle, Washington.

conventional procedures do. "You've got to cover basic issues of wellness or you're still in a Band-Aid process," noted Lee Ballance, chief of pain management and alternative medicine for Kaiser's Vallejo, California, medical center. He adds, "You're creating external treatment without internal change."

Acupuncture: A "Secondary" Treatment in Chinese Medicine

In traditional Chinese medicine (TCM), acupuncture is viewed as a secondary modality that supports the primary modalities such as qigong and tai chi. Qigong is considered a healing art. Tai chi is a martial art. Each works on the principles of energy, life force (qi), meridians, points, and balance through which acupuncture and acupressure work. Kaiser began to encourage members to take acupressure or qigong with their acupuncture. In some clinics, these programs are actually *required* prior to acceptance as a patient for acupuncture treatment. Explains Ballance, "We want to give them the skills before they are 'done to.' We begin to remove the anxiety of believing that all help comes from the outside. It's an attempt to internalize the healer."

Learning Traditional Chinese Medicine Principles and Self-Care in a Group Setting

During introductory sessions—generally two sessions, each of 1 to 3 hours—Kaiser members learn about the TCM way of viewing sickness and health. They also learn self-care techniques. Informal data gathered at Kaiser Vallejo suggested that nearly three in four of the members who were first referred for classes prior to receiving acupuncture later decided that they did not need the acupuncture treatment. Kaiser also views the programs as a way to effectively expand a limited benefit. The expansion of the benefit may be felt by the member both as a clinical outcome and as increased satisfaction.

Linking CAM Self-Care with Conventional Services

The other source of the Kaiser exploration was a decision to attempt to better integrate physician education and member education programs. For example, as the HMO discovered, members might be learning to value the practice of qigong, but members' physicians might still be in the dark. The region chose to give interested physicians an opportunity to learn about, and experience, some CAM self-care techniques in the hope that the health promotion programs would be better utilized in their patient care.

The experiment appears to be beneficial but is producing interesting teaching challenges for the community instructors retained to offer services. The usual clientele for community qigong classes, for instance, are already relatively self-motivated and healthy. Kaiser members referred by physicians, nurses, psychologists, and physical therapists are often overweight, older, unconditioned, and sometimes, physically disabled. They may be neither health conscious nor particularly well motivated.

The classes revised their structure.

- They reduced class size—from 30 to 40, to 15 to 20 participants.
- They added more personalized attention and more verbal communication.
- They developed more of a medical focus.
- They allowed for many variations in individual ability to do the exercises (at any time, some participants may be doing the exercises sitting down or lying down, and others may be taking a break).
- They tried to ensure that the class was felt to be a safe place for any person to explore the CAM method.

Subjective Reports: Clients Getting in Touch with Themselves

While Kaiser has developed no formal outcomes, subjective reports on the qigong program from clients and instructors include the following:

- Probably 3 out of 20 clients have fibromyalgia. Many seem to find qigong useful in getting energy flowing.
- Some clients find they can sleep better than they have in a long while.
- Participants are becoming more aware of their bodies. According to one instructor, "People who've been out of touch with their bodies are waking up."
- The experience is negative for some. Those who simply want a problem fixed are often frustrated.
- Qigong will sometimes "rile up a condition" and seem to make it worse, according to an instructor who believes that some members may not "wish to face the hurt or pain involved in getting in touch."
- Physicians like the closer integration as an expanded tool in their repertoire.

While not strictly a benefit of membership in Kaiser, the classes are subsidized. The charge to members is generally priced at $4 to $5 per contact hour. The price charged to nonmembers is 150% of that charged to members.

CASE 2: MANAGING CAM BENEFITS THROUGH CREDENTIALING PROVIDER NETWORKS—GROUP HEALTH COOPERATIVE OF PUGET SOUND*

Of any HMO in the United States, Group Health Cooperative of Puget Sound (Group Health) has the most extensive experience in offering a wide array of CAM services through credentialed networks of CAM providers, coupled with a willingness to share its process and outcomes. Group Health is a staff model that developed as a cooperative in structure. It is the dominant HMO presence in its service area of Western Washington, with over 500,000 covered lives. (Group Health recently combined with Kaiser Permanente—somewhat less than a full merger, but clearly more than an affiliation—and now operates as part of Kaiser.)

*This case study is courtesy of John Weeks/Integration Strategies, Seattle, Washington.

Group Health began formal exploration of CAM in 1994 for two principal reasons. The cooperative knew that members were interested in alternatives. As far back as 1986, some members pushed coverage of some complementary services onto the agenda of Group Health's annual meeting. In a subsequent vote, roughly one fourth of the voting members chose to vote against the published position of the cooperative's medical leaders and ask that services of naturopathic physicians be included among the HMO's offerings. While a minority, the vote signified a substantial member interest, particularly in a time in which the idea of such coverage was not even on the radar screen of the broader health care system.

Group Health's entrance into the field was also prompted by the health reform climate in Washington State. Under a sweeping "managed competition" reform measure passed by the state's Democrat-controlled legislature in 1993, the state's health plans were required to include in their service delivery every category of provider that was licensed by the state. This meant massage practitioners, acupuncturists, licensed midwives, and naturopathic physicians, as well as the chiropractic services that the HMO already offered via an outside chiropractic network. A new legislature controlled by Republicans gutted the sweeping 1993 reform measure but kept the "every category" clause.

Process of Benefit Development

Group Health began its investigative process in 1994. The HMO set up an internal, 12-member task force headed by Simeon Rubenstein, vice president for corporate health. Representatives of the CAM professions and CAM educational institutions were invited to present in person and provide written materials. Key questions included the following:

- Would the services be targeted toward specific clinical entities (such as obstetrics or gynecology)?
- How would the profession interact with the HMO's guidelines and technology assessment committees?

- What sources of published data on research would the profession recommend?
- For which conditions does evidence suggest that CAM services should be covered?
- Would these providers practice independently or be integrated into the organization?
- What joint areas would be most valuable for outcomes study?

Initial recommendations, reported a year later, were that chiropractic services should be available under specific practice guidelines; services of the state's licensed midwives would be covered and a network credentialed; massage would be offered on a limited basis through the HMO's physical therapy department; acupuncture would be available only as part of focused research; and, while naturopathy would continue to be explored, it would not be covered initially. The task force stressed that these offerings were anticipated to be part of an evolving process.

In 1995, Group Health began to support its initiative by offering focused educational sessions on CAM issues for its physicians.

1996 Utilization Plan for Acupuncture, Naturopathy, and Massage

The 1996 utilization plan unveiled by Group Health was substantially different from the task force's recommendations. A part of the evolution was due to regulatory pressure on all plans to find ways to include every category of provider and to offer the services as a core benefit, with no additional costs to the purchaser or member, rather than as a rider. However, the program has important characteristics that helped the HMO manage the use and costs of CAM services.

- Members must have referrals from their primary care providers.
- Approved CAM services are based on limited numbers of visits.
- CAM services are approved for only certain conditions.
- A network of credentialed CAM providers offer these services.

The HMO chose to manage the benefit by contracting with an outside provider network, the Alternare Group, for credentialing, billing, and some additional service. In addition, the HMO established an office that included a nurse as alternative care coordinator and a part-time clinical director for alternative medicine, Laura Patton. Table 42–A–1 is Group Health's initial alternative provider grid.

First Year Experience

Patton reported the HMO's early experience at a meeting of the American Association of Health Plans in June 1997. Table 42–A–2 provides information on which of the conditions selected by Group Health were most often approved for referral. Other findings were the following:

- The biggest problem with utilization, from the health plan perspective, was in the area of massage services; the plan has since helped develop a special program to help massage practitioners to understand and work in a managed care arena.
- The initial sense is that acupuncture and naturopathic services were helpful to at least some users, employed treatments limited in duration, and were worth further exploration, including a possible expansion of covered services.
- Utilization was less than expected. It grew toward the end of the first year, but it will not, in Patton's words, "break the bank."
- Lack of CAM understanding among Group Health providers probably limited referrals.

The importance of the Group Health experience in the exploratory process of CAM integration and coverage is this: The first substantial HMO in the nation to report its initial experience with CAM integration and coverage has given the process a cautious vote of confidence. On May 2, 1997, when a federal judge held that the state mandate was preempted by federal statute, Group Health immediately sent out a press release affirming that it would voluntarily continue its CAM offerings.

Table 42–A–1 Leading Conditions for Referral (1996–1997) in Group Health's CAM Program (January 1, 1996)

	Acupuncture	Massage Therapy	Naturopathy
Authorization required?	Yes	Yes	Yes
Diagnoses and clinical conditions that are covered	• Myofascial pain syndrome • Fibromyalgia • Chronic pain (neck and back) • Dysmenorrhea • Chronic headaches, including migraine and stress • Pain secondary to metastatic disease • Neuropathic pain • Chronic arthritis	• Lymphedema where traditional therapy has failed • Part of rehab benefit where expected to produce sustainable functional improvement in 60 days and to only cover for an acute precipitating event • Not covered for recreational, sedative, or palliative reasons	• Premenstrual syndrome • Menopausal symptoms • Chronic fatigue • Chronic arthritis • Chronic irritable bowel syndrome • Fibromyalgia
Visit limits	• 3 visits and then review by PCP or alternative care coordinator (this was later changed to 6 to 8 visits) • Treatment plan within 120 days of first visit • Treatment summary 30 days after third visit	• All visits within 60 days and may occur simultaneously with a physical therapy program and then reviewed by PCP and alternative care coordinator • Treatment plan within 10 days of first visit • Treatment summary 30 days after sixth visit	• 3 visits and then reviewed by PCP and alternative care coordinator • Treatment plan within 10 days of first visit • Treatment summary 30 days after third visit
Ancillary services (lab, pharmacy, X-ray)	• Ordered via PCP	• Ordered via PCP	• To only listed labs • Urged to get laboratory information from Group Health labs • Excludes NTX • Pharmacy subscription must be obtained via PCP • No coverage for botanical, herbs, vitamins, food supplements • All X-ray, electrocardiogram, ultrasounds, procedures (scoping), allergy testing, and injections at Group Health

Courtesy of Group Health Cooperative of Puget Sound, Seattle, Washington.

Table 42-A-2 Relative Rates of Utilization for Selected CAM Conditions

Acupuncture (%)		Massage (%)		Naturopathy (%)	
Myalgia	27	Myalgia	63	Menopause	35
Lumbago	24	Cervicalgia	18	Arthritis	17
Migraines	18	Lumbago	13	Irritable bowel syndrome	14
Cervicalgia	13	Spasms	2	Myalgia	14
Joint pain	7	Joint pain	2	Premenstrual syndrome	10
Neuritis	5	Migraine	1	Malaise and fatigue	9
Rheumatoid arthritis	4	Other	1		
Dysmenorrhea	2				
Cancer (adjunctive)	1				
Total*	101		100		99

*Variations from 100 are because of rounding.

Courtesy of Group Health Cooperative of Puget Sound, Seattle, Washington.

CASE 3: DEVELOPING CAM THROUGH AN INTEGRATED CLINIC— AMERICAN CENTERS FOR HEALTH AND MEDICINE*

American Centers for Health and Medicine (ACHM) offers a model for delivering CAM through an integrated clinic that offers both conventional medicine and CAM. The ACHM mission is to develop a financially viable model for integration, to demonstrate the value of integration with other elements of the continuum of care, and to create a model that is replicable.

Beginning in 1996, ACHM began to be financially supported by Catholic Healthcare West (CHW), an affiliation of Catholic health care systems in Western states. The replicability of ACHM's model is expected to be first tested by other partners in the CHW network, with at least two CHW systems in California expecting to develop ACHM centers in 1998. ACHM also anticipates partnering with other health care systems that are not in the CHW fold.

Arizona Center for Health and Medicine in Phoenix, Arizona, the venture's anchor clinic, was founded in 1994 and opened its doors a year later. Unlike most outpatient clinics, the physical space of this 10,000-square-foot center was designed around fluid, holistic principles of architecture. Features include curved walls, plants, a Zen rock garden in the waiting area, and full-spectrum lighting.

Providers, Services, Conditions, Demographics

ACHM is an MD/DO-centered model. Conventionally trained physicians provide clinical leadership. They offer conventional medical services and therapies, as well as CAM services. CAM services, however, may be provided by physicians or by ancillary providers under their supervision. These may be conventional mid-level providers or professionals from distinct CAM professions, such as massage practitioners, acupuncturists, and naturopaths (in states where naturopaths are licensed). The initial model does not include chiropractors, as adjustments and physical manipulation are offered by the clinic's osteopaths.

The center's core CAM services are acupuncture, botanical medicine, homeopathy, osteopathic manipulation, and body-mind techniques. Other CAM services are therapeutic massage, touch therapy, Feldenkrais and Trager, tai chi, guided imagery, and a form of music therapy. The reasons for office calls, in order of frequency, are back or joint pain, upper respiratory problems, chronic fatigue, sport injuries, mi-

---

*This case study is courtesy of John Weeks/Integration Strategies, Seattle, Washington.

graine, preventive care, stress, and hypertension. One special service is a general assessment based on alternative medicine principles.

Patient demographics for ACHM are similar to those in a conventional outpatient practice, although the patients have substantially higher than average education. Two thirds of the patients are women. A third have a college degree, and another third have some college education. One fourth of the patients are over 50 years of age, and 57% are between the ages of 21 and 50.

Networks and Adjunct Clinics

In the ACHM model in Phoenix, the anchor clinic is in the center of a network of other relationships. These relationships are developed and valued as sources of referrals and as part of a strategy for meeting the geographic reach ACHM must offer to develop its long-term payment strategy, described further below, of taking global capitation. The relationship layers, some of which are contractual, include

- smaller satellite clinics, with somewhat more focused service offerings (a second clinic was opened in Scottsdale in late 1997 with a third scheduled in the Phoenix area in 1998)
- a standard primary care clinic in which one physician is interested in alternatives
- credentialed MD/DO network of conventional physicians who are skilled in providing at least one CAM therapy, such as acupuncture or homeopathy
- selected networks of CAM providers from distinct professions, such as massage therapists, acupuncturists, and naturopaths
- wellness-based providers, such as health food stores, spas, and health clubs

ACHM's mission is not merely to offer a few adjunctive CAM services. Rather, the effort includes what chief executive officer Phyllis Biedess calls "carrying the culture of CAM—the mindset and the philosophy for total integration of care, for the patient, the individual practitioner and for the center itself." One part of this mission is evident in ACHM's offerings of various self-care tools to help patients take charge of their health. These tools include books, tapes, botanicals, and a lending library.

Administrative Challenges and Payment Strategy

When different paradigms of medicine meet, organizations can face serious administrative challenges. Biedess calls the administrative model "one-off administration." As compared with a conventional clinic:

- Patient scheduling is more varied, given the range of services and the various time allotments for evaluation and management.
- Receptionists need specialized training, because they must answer far more questions and provide a much greater amount of education for patients or prospective patients, on site or on the telephone, about clinical options and available therapies.
- CAM-oriented physicians are likely to have little or no understanding of managed care billing.
- CAM-oriented physicians tend to be independent thinkers who have been outside any system, much less one of managed care, and therefore pose unusual personnel management challenges.

ACHM's initial payment strategy was to position the clinic as a PCP inside the managed care context. The MD/DO providers are all physicians who are credentialed into managed care networks and accept discounted fee-for-service. In the first year, managed care firms made 85% of payments to the anchor clinic, with just 15% of payments made out of pocket.

ACHM's payment strategy has subsequently shifted in three ways. First, ACHM realized that a substantial clientele existed that would pay out of pocket for the unique services the clinic was offering in its marketplace. By late 1997, the portion of payments that were paid directly by patients had increased to 25%. Marketing began to help shape this trend.

Second, ACHM realized that it might increase business if it positioned the clinic as a specialty provider. Some specialty referrals were already for physical therapy, notably osteopathic manipulation. But others were for the clinic's uniquely integrated services. The center received referrals from community providers for difficult cases. ACHM learned that the specialist role was one with which the conventional provider community was most comfortable. "We realize that we were more than PCPs—what I call 'specialist light,'" Biedess states. In addition, employer groups showed interest in specially designed programs for key, costly conditions. The center began focusing on developing its role in case management.

Third, ACHM began positioning itself for its desired position: taking global capitation. Early utilization data supports the concept. Data that had not been adjusted for case mix showed that patients are more expensive on the front end but potentially cheaper overall. The center's patients average 4.7 visits a year. The relatively time-intensive care means that ACHM providers see only one half to one third of the patients a conventional PCP sees in a day. But patient costs were found to be relatively light downstream, with just 11% of patients referred to outside specialists and 19 hospital days per 1,000 patients. The addition of the two clinics in the greater Phoenix area is expected to allow ACHM to begin to accept global capitation from some geographically defined employee groups.

Other Issues

ACHM views its relationship with its payers as a process in which the managed care firm must take a broader view than requiring authorization for every service, given the complex nature of the typical whole-person treatment at the center. The payer is asked to begin focusing on how to offer *health* care, to focus on primary prevention and integration, rather than simply responding to disease processes. ACHM has also found that standard billing systems cannot support more complex strategies. In addition, ACHM believes that the cost structure on patient care cannot be shifted in just a few months. ACHM estimates that its health-oriented services require at least 3 years to make full economic sense. Yet most purchasers aren't signing long-term agreements.

Since 1995, representatives of over three dozen health care systems have toured ACHM in order to glean ideas for their own ventures. Yet ACHM's personnel argue that there is no single answer to how to best integrate CAM. They acknowledge that while for some the uncertainty is scary, for them the challenge is infused with the excitement of creating new ways to deliver high-quality, cost-effective care.

PART XV

Clinical Managed Care in Government Programs

The two largest government programs are Medicare and Medicaid. There are other programs, such as the military health system, the public health system, Veterans Affairs, and others. When considering size, cost, and effect on society, the top two programs are Medicare and Medicaid. While many of the best practices described in this book apply equally to members of these programs as to other populations, there are certain attributes of these programs that medical managers need to be aware of. Superior results are possible if special attention is given to the needs of individuals in these programs.

Chapter 43

Medicaid Managed Care

Donna M. Henderson

Chapter Outline

- Introduction
- What Is Medicaid?
- Medicaid Enrollment and Expenditures
- Barriers to Care for Medicaid Beneficiaries
- Preventive Care and Medicaid Beneficiaries
- Health Risk Factors for Medicaid Beneficiaries
- Medicaid Managed Care Initiatives
- Capitation Rates for Medicaid Managed Care
- Characteristics of an Effective Medicaid Managed Care Plan
- Successful Interventions for Improving Member Access and Compliance
- Conclusion

INTRODUCTION

Medicaid managed care has developed in response to increasing pressure to control state and federal Medicaid spending. The major goals of the initiative are to control this spending and to improve access to care for Medicaid beneficiaries. Enrollment in Medicaid managed care is rising rapidly. In 1991, almost 10% of Medicaid beneficiaries were enrolled in managed care plans. By 1994 that rate had increased to 23%. In 1996, 40% of all Medicaid beneficiaries were enrolled in managed care plans (Table 43–1).[1] Currently, virtually all states are pursuing some version of managed care for their Medicaid population.[2]

WHAT IS MEDICAID?

Medicaid is a publicly financed, means-tested entitlement program authorized in 1965 by Title XIX of the Social Security Act. The program, designed to provide health care and long-term care to low-income individuals, is financed by state and federal governments and is administered by the states. State Medicaid programs that meet federal eligibility and benefit guidelines receive federal matching funds based on the state's per capita income.

Poverty does not automatically qualify a person for Medicaid. In 1995, about 34% of American families with annual incomes of less than $14,000 and 28% of families with annual incomes between $14,000 and $24,999 lacked health care coverage (Table 43–2).[3]

To qualify for Medicaid, potential enrollees must meet income guidelines and must belong to an eligible beneficiary category. Federal guidelines mandate Medicaid coverage for specified groups of people. These mandated groups include, but are not limited to, the following:

Table 43–1 Medicaid Managed Care Trends

Year	Total Medicaid Population	Volume of Medicaid Managed Care	Percent of Medicaid Managed Care
1991	28,280,000	2,696,397	9.53
1992	30,926,390	3,634,516	11.75
1993	33,430,051	4,808,951	14.39
1994	33,634,000	7,794,250	23.17
1995	33,373,000	9,800,000	29.37
1996	33,241,147	13,330,119	40.10

Source: Reprinted from *Medicaid National Summary Statistics,* 1997, Health Care Financing Administration.

- recipients of Aid to Families with Dependent Children (AFDC)
- recipients of Supplemental Security Income (SSI)
- infants born to Medicaid-eligible pregnant women
- children under 6 and pregnant women who meet the state's AFDC financial requirements or whose family income is at or below 133% of the federal poverty level
- recipients of adoption assistance and foster care under Title IV-E of the Social Security Act
- certain Medicare beneficiaries[4]

The federal government also mandates a minimum benefits package for Medicaid beneficiaries. The mandated services include

- inpatient and outpatient hospital
- physician, nurse-midwife, and pediatric and family nurse practitioner
- medical and surgical dentistry
- laboratory and X-ray
- nursing facility for individuals aged 21 or older
- home health
- early and periodic screening, diagnosis, and treatment (EPSDT) for individuals under age 21
- family planning services and supplies
- rural health clinics and federally qualified health centers[5]

In addition to the above, states have the option (but are not required) to provide Medicaid coverage for other "categorically needy" or "medically needy" groups. These optional groups share characteristics of the mandatory groups, but the eligibility criteria are somewhat more liberally defined.[4] If a state chooses to provide Medicaid benefits to the medically needy, the federal government mandates a minimum set of services (eg, prenatal care and delivery services for pregnant women) to be delivered to that population.[5]

States may offer specified additional services (eg, prescription drugs, prosthetic devices) to their Medicaid enrollees and still receive federal matching funds.[5] Because of the latitude granted in establishing benefit structures and income thresholds, there are large variations in the structure of Medicaid programs among the states.

Table 43–2 Health Care Coverage for Persons Under 65 Years of Age

Annual Family Income: 1995	Percent of Population		
	Private Insurance (%)	Medicaid (%)	No Insurance (%)
Less than $14,000	24.3	40.8	33.5
$14,000–$24,999	55.7	13.6	28.0
$25,000–$34,999	75.4	4.8	17.2
$35,000–$49,999	87.7	2.4	8.3
$50,000 or more	93.6	0.7	4.6

Source: Reprinted from *Health, United States, 1996–97 and Injury Chart Book,* 1997, National Center for Health Statistics.

Table 43-3 Medicaid Recipients and Program Payments

Fiscal Year	Recipients (Millions)	Program Payments (Billions)
1987	23.1	$ 47.7
1988	22.9	$ 51.6
1989	23.5	$ 58.0
1990	25.3	$ 68.7
1991	28.3	$ 90.5
1992	31.2	$115.9
1993	33.4	$125.8
1994	35.1	$137.6
1995	36.3	$151.8

Source: Reprinted from *Medicaid National Summary Statistics,* 1997, Health Care Financing Administration.

Table 43-4 Medicaid Recipients and Vendor Payments by Basis of Eligibility

Basis of Eligibility: Fiscal Year 1995	Percent of Medicaid Population	Percent of Medicaid Expenditures
Aged, blind, and disabled	27	72
Children under 21	47	15
Adults in FDC	21	11
Other and unknown	4	2

Source: Reprinted from *Medicaid National Summary Statistics,* 1997, Health Care Financing Administration.

MEDICAID ENROLLMENT AND EXPENDITURES

As shown in Table 43-3, between the years 1987 and 1995, Medicaid enrollment rose from 23.1 million to 36.3 million, an increase of 57%. During that same interval, Medicaid spending more than tripled. In 1995, total expenditures for the Medicaid program exceeded $151 billion.[6]

Medicaid finances 13% of all US health care spending[7] and helps to finance health care for more than 10% of Americans.[3] The program pays for about one third of all births and one half of all nursing home care in this country.[5] In 1995, 37% of children under age 5 and 20% of children between the ages of 6 and 14 were covered by Medicaid.[8]

As shown in Table 43-4, 47% of Medicaid beneficiaries are children under 21 years of age;[9] 24% are less than 6 years old.[10] Twenty-one percent of the enrollees are adults in low-income families.[9] While children under 21 and adults in AFDC families make up 68% of the Medicaid population, they account for only 26% of the program's total expenditures. The aged, blind, and disabled make up 27% of the beneficiaries, but they account for 72% of the expenditures.[9] Almost one third of Americans over the age of 85 receive Medicaid benefits.[5] Sixty-eight percent of all US nursing home residents receive Medicaid.[11] Table 43-5 breaks out Medicaid recipients by age group, showing the percentage of total Medicaid expenditures accounted for by each age group.

Uneducated, unmarried females with children are especially likely to require government health care support. Federal statistics[12] for the 24-month interval from 1991 through 1992 demonstrated that 25.8% of American females with no spouse

Table 43-5 Medicaid Recipients and Vendor Payments by Age of Recipients

Age in Years: Fiscal Year 1995	Percent of Medicaid Population	Percent of Medicaid Expenditures
0–5	24	10
6–14	19	6
15–20	9	6
21–44	24	27
45–64	8	16
65–74	5	8
75–84	4	12
85 and over	3	13
Unknown	5	1

Source: Reprinted from *Medicaid National Summary Statistics,* 1997, Health Care Financing Administration.

and at least one child under age 18 lived below the poverty line. In an analysis of 10,875 live births between 1991 and 1995,[13] the Centers for Disease Control and Prevention (CDC) identified the lack of a high school education as a powerful predictor of a pregnant woman's potential to require Medicaid. In the CDC's sample, over 70% of mothers with no high school education or graduate equivalency diploma (GED) received Medicaid (Table 43–6).[13] Sixteen percent of all American women are covered by Medicaid as compared to only 10% of males.[14] Fifty-nine percent of all Medicaid recipients are female.[15]

Thirty-five percent of Medicaid dollars are paid to nursing facilities, mental hospitals, and intermediate care facilities (ICFs) for the mentally retarded. General hospitals and outpatient hospital services account for another 28%. Home health vendors receive only 8% of the total dollars paid (Table 43–7).

Table 43–6 Women Age 15–44 Who Had a Live Birth in 1991–1995

Characteristic	Percent with Medicaid
No high school education or graduate equivalency diploma (GED)	70.3
High school education or GED	33.4
Some college, no bachelor's degree	18.5
Bachelor's degree or higher	5.4
Non-Hispanic black	62.0
Hispanic	56.3
Non-Hispanic other	25.5
Non-Hispanic white	23.0

Source: Reprinted from *Live Birth in 1991–95/ Method of Payment,* 1997, US Centers for Disease Control and Prevention.

Table 43–7 Medicaid Vendor Payments by Type of Service

Type of Service: 1995	Medicaid Payments (Billions)	Percent of Medicaid Expenditures
Nursing facilities	$29.1	24
General hospital	$26.3	22
ICF mentally retarded	$10.4	9
Prescribed drugs	$ 9.8	8
Home health	$ 9.4	8
Physician services	$ 7.4	6
Outpatient hospital	$ 6.6	6
Clinic services	$ 4.3	4
Mental hospital	$ 2.5	2
Lab and X-ray	$ 1.2	1
EPSDT	$ 1.2	1
Dental services	$ 1.0	1
Other practitioners	$ 1.0	1
Family planning	$ 0.5	0
Rural health clinic	$ 0.2	0
Other and unknown	$ 9.3	8

Source: Reprinted from *Medicaid National Summary Statistics,* 1997, Health Care Financing Administration.

BARRIERS TO CARE FOR MEDICAID BENEFICIARIES

Medicaid beneficiaries encounter significant barriers to access of the health care system. They are twice as likely as their privately insured counterparts to receive care in an institutional setting,[16] to travel at least 60 minutes to their site of care, and to wait at least 60 minutes after arriving at their site of care.[17] Factors that contribute to their limited access to health care include

- inadequate access to timely primary care[18]
- lack of physician participation[16,17,19,20]
- discontinuous primary care utilization patterns[18,19]
- reduced access to office-based physician care[17–19]
- lack of preventive care[20]
- limited access to specialty care[17,18]
- reduced access to "adapted" care (ie, care that addresses special needs arising out of chronic illness and physical, mental, and developmental delays)[18]

St. Peter et al[19] found that only 52% of poor children have a physician's office as their usual source of care. They noted that Medicaid coverage "only slightly improved poor children's access to physicians' offices."[19(p2762)] Their research also demonstrated that children whose usual source of routine care was a community clinic rather than a physician's office were 10 times more likely to go to another facility for their sick care and almost 5 times more likely to receive their sick care in an emergency department.

Medicaid beneficiaries often experience great difficulty finding providers willing to accept Medicaid as a payment source. Only about one third of US physicians participate fully in Medicaid. Approximately one third limit the number of Medicaid patients they will see. Five percent report that they will not accept any new Medicaid patients. One fourth report they will not accept Medicaid at all.[16] From 1987 to 1990, fewer than 50% of obstetricians and gynecologists in the United States participated in the Medicaid program. Many low-income communities lack an adequate supply and/or distribution of health providers. Seventy percent of US counties (predominately in inner cities, rural areas, and the South) are defined as medically underserved.[1]

PREVENTIVE CARE AND MEDICAID BENEFICIARIES

Three of the most significant and cost-effective public health programs that have contributed to improved maternal and child health are immunization programs, lead abatement efforts, and nutritional supplementation through the Women's, Infant's, and Children's (WIC) program.[18] Immunization rates are good markers for primary care in general. Compared with children who are immunized, children who are not immunized are 11.8 times more likely not to be screened for anemia, 8.7 times more likely not to be screened for lead, and 2.8 times more likely not to be screened for tuberculosis.[21] Recent research has demonstrated inadequate rates of immunization among the poor: During 1989 and 1990, the Los Angeles measles epidemic was concentrated among low-income, minority preschool children.[22] In 1991, 75% of the sample of unvaccinated children in New York City who contracted measles were on Medicaid.[21]

State Medicaid policies have contributed to a declining number of pediatricians who will provide immunization services. In 1992, the Children's Defense Fund found that no state paid the usual, customary, and reasonable charge for all four childhood vaccines. Several states actually reimbursed physicians for immunization services at a rate less than the cost of the vaccine alone.[14] Wood et al have concluded that without financial incentives to encourage private physicians and health maintenance organizations (HMOs) to provide immunizations to inner-city children, managed care is unlikely to improve immunization rates.[23]

HEALTH RISK FACTORS FOR MEDICAID BENEFICIARIES

When compared to those with higher incomes, low-income Americans have 1.5 times the rate of neonatal mortality and twice the rate of low-birthweight deliveries.[17] Approximately 15% of children enrolled in Medicaid have a chronic health condition.[24] Ireys et al found that approximately 10% of the beneficiaries in the Washington State Medicaid program between the ages of 0 and 18 years had one of eight chronic conditions.[24] The 10% of children with these eight chronic health conditions accounted for 70% of expenditures for the population[24]:

1. asthma
2. cerebral palsy
3. chronic respiratory disease
4. cystic fibrosis
5. diabetes
6. muscular dystrophy
7. neoplasms, malignant
8. spina bifida

Newacheck et al[25] report that children with chronic conditions causing limitations in their usual activities are twice as likely to be hospitalized, consume twice as many physician services, and use six times as many nonphysician professional services as children without activity-limiting chronic conditions.

MEDICAID MANAGED CARE INITIATIVES

To establish a Medicaid managed care program, states must obtain one of two types of waivers from HCFA.[26,27] (1) Section 1115 research and demonstration waivers allow states to undertake statewide managed care projects that do not meet federally mandated statutory requirements. Many of these demonstration Medicaid projects (eg, TennCare) extend coverage to low-income individuals and families that are not eligible for Medicaid. (2) Section 1915(b) freedom-of-choice waivers allow states to implement managed care plans that require mandatory managed care enrollment, or to implement managed care in only part of a state or for only certain categories of beneficiaries.

Managed care plans can serve Medicaid beneficiaries through three types of contracts: risk, cost, and health care prepayment plans.[27]

1. *Full-risk plans.* Such plans are capitated and are paid a fixed per member per month (PMPM) fee. They assume full financial risk for providing all medically necessary health care services. Examples of this type of plan are an HMO or a health insuring organization (HIO).
2. *Limited-risk prepaid health plans (PHPs).* Under this arrangement, organizations contract on a prepaid, capitated risk basis to provide services that are not risk-comprehensive (eg, ambulatory care), or they contract on a nonrisk basis.
3. *Fee-for-service primary care case management (PCCM).* In these plans, providers, usually primary care physicians, are delegated the responsibility to act as "gatekeepers." The providers contract directly with the state, they do not assume financial risk, and they are paid for medical care on a fee-for-service basis. They also receive a monthly per patient case management fee.

Of the 511 Medicaid managed care plans identified in June 1996, 46% were state-plan-defined HMOs, 22.3% were federally qualified (ie, full-risk) HMOs, 17.4% were PHPs, and 11.5% were PCCMs.[1]

CAPITATION RATES FOR MEDICAID MANAGED CARE

One goal of Medicaid managed care is to establish a network of primary care providers for Medicaid beneficiaries. The success of that goal depends on the adequacy of capitation rates.[22] Historically, provider payments for Medicaid services have been substantially below market rates. In 1990, Medicaid payments to office-based physicians were 66% of Medicare's prevailing rate and approximately 55% of the rate of private payers.[25] The American Medical Association (AMA) reports that in 1991, hospitals recouped only 82 cents for each dollar of Medicaid costs.[16] In 1994, Medicaid paid physicians, on average, about 73% of Medicare's payments and 47% of the amount paid by private payers.[17]

Capitation rates for Medicaid managed care providers are also low. Often, plans serving Medicaid populations cannot set their capitation rates independently.[28] Although rate setting is nominally a negotiated process, in many cases

Medicaid agencies set rates independently of the plans. Often, Medicaid capitation rates are determined by applying a discount to average fee-for-service Medicaid expenditures by "comparable" populations.[28] Currently, managed care capitation rates are said to be below commercial rates in all states.[22] Gorgan has reported that "the main reason cited by providers for lack of Medicaid participation is inadequate fees."[29(p831)] Siverstein and Kirkman-Liff report that among Medicaid physician providers "reimbursement appears to be a primary determinant in both participation and satisfaction."[30(p361)]

Many Medicaid programs mandate services that are not offered by the majority of managed care plans (eg, dental care, transportation to physicians' offices). The combination of poor Medicaid reimbursement levels and a high-risk population has made securing risk-sharing agreements with physicians extremely difficult.[20]

CHARACTERISTICS OF AN EFFECTIVE MEDICAID MANAGED CARE PLAN

Medicaid beneficiaries are a culturally diverse group that includes children, single parents, disabled individuals, and the elderly—the only characteristic the individuals share is poverty.[16] According to the Kaiser Family Foundation, "non-elderly families on Medicaid are disproportionately likely to be headed by young adults with low educational attainment who live alone or with other family members who are equally stressed by poverty."[20(p63)]

An analysis by the Kaiser Foundation identified the following essential components of an effective delivery system for low-income patients:

- Outreach is ongoing and, in some cases, intensive and personalized.
- Services are comprehensive, including medical and nonmedical components such as basic medical care, nutritional services, psychological counseling, substance abuse counseling and treatment, communitywide programs to identify and reduce the transmission of disease, and enhanced services tailored to the specific needs of the population (eg, social services, transportation, and parent employment programs).
- Preventive services, primary care, and prenatal care are provided with no deductibles or copays.
- Services are coordinated; multiple services are located at one site, or accessible referral networks are developed.
- Case management is utilized.
- Services are readily available and accessible. Facilities are easily reached and, ideally, located in the neighborhood in which they are needed. Hours are flexible. Mid-level professionals and lay staff are utilized to extend service capacity. Translation services are provided, or the plan employs multicultural and bilingual staff.[18]

The Kaiser report goes on to state that reimbursement strategies must be designed to support the above initiatives.

- Provider payments and incentives should include rates that are reasonably close to those paid by the private market or to actual costs.
- Reimbursement rates for midlevel professionals should provide an incentive to service low-income women and children.
- The plan should implement payment incentives for providers who deliver timely preventive and primary care.
- Provider reimbursement policies should favor those who are able to deliver a broad array of services.
- The plan should strive to contract with providers that have a proven track record in serving low-income women and children.
- Providers should be required to coordinate care.[18]

Gold et al have identified 10 strategies that increase the potential for success in structuring managed care plans for Medicaid beneficiaries.

1. Invest in effective enrollment procedures; anticipate confusion and questions.
2. Emphasize education about the system for both enrollees and providers.
3. Build a well-developed oversight system to minimize problems and monitor performance.
4. Build managed care strategies that are sensitive to the configuration of existing plans and providers and to the experience they have had in accepting risk for medical delivery.
5. Allow sufficient time for implementation and system development.
6. Invest in administrative structures and assume they will cost, rather than save, money, at least in the short term.
7. Pay special attention to policies and procedures for the chronically ill.
8. Set rates that are sensitive to the populations enrolled in the plan and the costs associated with treating them.
9. Minimize extensive and rapid eligibility turnover.
10. Set objectives that are realistic.[22]

Witek and Hostage have concluded that cost savings in Medicaid managed care plans are generated from three sources: discounted rates accepted by providers, decreased utilization of emergency services, and reductions in inpatient care.[20] Other cost-effective strategies they have identified include the following:

- Develop a tightly knit network of providers selected on the basis of their cost-effectiveness.
- Share financial risk among providers using payment mechanisms such as capitation.
- Implement strong disincentives so that out-of-network utilization by beneficiaries is minimized.
- Provide incentives to beneficiaries for healthy behavior, such as primary care and preventive care.
- Include clinical guidelines in the utilization management plan.[20]

SUCCESSFUL INTERVENTIONS FOR IMPROVING MEMBER ACCESS AND COMPLIANCE

A number of key principles have been found to characterize care delivery programs that succeed at improving access and compliance for low-income populations. These include creative and continuous outreach to the eligible population, provision of a comprehensive set of medical and nonmedical social support services, case management or similar strategies to coordinate services and promote access to care, efforts to make services more accessible to clients, and efforts to ensure adequate availability of providers and staff to deliver service.[18]

Various programs aimed at improving access and compliance for low-income populations are described in detail by the Kaiser Family Health Foundation. These programs include the following:

- *Alabama's Medicaid Maternity Waiver Program.* Pregnant women were required to receive prenatal care from a designated primary care provider or subcontractor. Once assigned to a provider, women could obtain services from or through only that provider. The primary care providers were responsible for locating, coordinating, and monitoring all pregnancy-related care on behalf of enrollees. An independent evaluation found that participants in the program started prenatal care earlier and were more likely to have an adequate number of prenatal visits. Participants were also less likely to receive routine ambulatory care in emergency departments and had a lower Caesarean section rate.
- *California's Comprehensive Perinatal Services Program (CPSP).* Under the umbrella of the CPSP program, pregnant women received enhanced prenatal care including nutritional counseling and support, health education, and psychosocial interventions. CPSP clients who received "full care" had a 4.7% rate of low-birthweight infants, compared to a 7% rate among a control group who did not receive the services.

- *Illinois's Parents Too Soon.* The program funded a broad array of health, social service, and educational programs aimed at reducing the incidence of teen pregnancy, improving birth outcomes among teen mothers, and improving teenage mothers' ability to cope with parenthood. Outcomes of the program included reduced rates of low-birthweight infants and improved rates of prenatal care.
- *North Carolina's Baby Love Program.* A statewide network of Medicaid maternity care coordinators provided comprehensive prenatal care and infant health services to all of the state's 100 counties. In addition to more traditional case management interventions, the program included public education campaigns with a toll-free telephone number and mass-media messages. When compared to data for women on Medicaid who participated in the program, the women who did not receive the services had a 21% higher low-birthweight rate, a 62% higher very low-birthweight rate, and a 23% higher infant mortality rate. Researchers estimated that for $1 spent on the program, Medicaid saved $2 in medical costs for newborns up to 60 days old.[18]

Another program that has been found to improve access and compliance includes the Philadelphia-based High Tech, Soft Touch immunization program developed by Mercy Health Plan for members of a Medicaid managed care organization.[31] Utilizing a combination of electronic claims tracking and home visits by registered nurses and paraprofessionals, program managers estimate that 46% of their targeted enrollees received an immunization within 60 days of the home visit.

CONCLUSION

The Medicaid population has significant and definable differences from the non-Medicaid population, and these differences must be recognized and addressed. By understanding the differences and using that understanding to manage care in a way better suited to the Medicaid population, improved outcomes and financial results will be more likely to occur.

REFERENCES

1. Health Care Financing Administration. Medicaid national summary statistics. Table 11: National summary of Medicaid managed care programs and enrollment. http://www.hcfa.gov/medicaid/trends1.htm; accessed February 1998.
2. Health Care Financing Administration. Medicaid managed care state enrollment. http://www.hcfa.gov/medicaid/pntrtn3.htm; accessed February 1998.
3. National Center for Health Statistics. *Health, United States, 1996–97 and injury chart book.* Hyattsville, MD: National Center for Health Statistics; 1997.
4. Health Care Financing Administration. Medicaid eligibility. http://www.hcfa.gov/medicaid/meligib.htm; accessed February 1998.
5. Health Care Financing Administration. Medicaid services. http://www.hcfa.gov/medicaid/mservice.htm; accessed February 1998.
6. Health Care Financing Administration. Medicaid national summary statistics. Table 1: Medicaid recipients, vendor, medical assistance and administrative payments. http://www.hcfa.gov/medicaid/195.htm; accessed February 1998.
7. Henry J Kaiser Family Foundation. *Medicaid Facts.* Washington, DC: Henry J Kaiser Family Foundation; 1995.
8. Health Care Financing Administration. Medicaid national summary statistics. Table 9: Medicaid recipients as a percentage of population by age. http://www.hcfa.gov/medicaid/005.htm; accessed February 1998.
9. Health Care Financing Administration. Medicaid national summary statistics. Table 3: Medicaid recipients and vendor payments by basis of eligibility. http://www.hcfa.gov/medicaid/395.htm; accessed February 1998.
10. Health Care Financing Administration. Medicaid national summary statistics. Table 6: Medicaid recipients and vendor participation by age. http://www.hcfa.gov/medicaid/695.htm; accessed February 1998.
11. Health Care Financing Administration. The Medicaid program. http://www.hcfa.gov/medicaid/mcdsta95.htm; accessed February 1998.
12. Bureau of the Census. Poverty dynamics: 1991 to 1993. http://www.census.gov/hhes/poverty/povdynam/pov91t2.html; accessed November 1997.

13. Abma JC, Chandra A, Mosher WD, Peterson L, Piccinino L. Fertility, family planning, and women's health: new data from the 1995 National Survey of Family Growth. *Vital Health Stat.* 1997;23:19.
14. Health Care Financing Administration. Medicaid national summary statistics. Table 10: Medicaid recipients as a percentage of population by sex. http://www.hcfa.gov/medicaid/1095.htm; accessed February 1998.
15. Health Care Financing Administration. Medicaid national summary statistics. Table 7: Medicaid recipients and vendor payments by sex. http://www.hcfa.gov/medicaid/795.htm; accessed February 1998.
16. Rowland D, Salganicoff A. Commentary: lessons from Medicaid—improving access to office-based care for the low-income population. *Am J Public Health.* 1994;84(4):550–552.
17. Henry J Kaiser Family Foundation. *Policy Brief: Access to Care: Is Health Insurance Enough?* Washington, DC: Henry J Kaiser Family Foundation; 1995.
18. Henry J Kaiser Family Foundation. *Elements of Effective Health Service Delivery for the Low-Income Population: Background Papers.* Washington, DC: Henry J Kaiser Family Foundation; 1993.
19. St. Peter RF, Newacheck PW, Halfon N. Access to care for poor children: separate and unequal? *JAMA.* 1992;267(20):2760–2764.
20. Witek JE, Hostage JL. Medicaid managed care: problems and promises. *J Ambulatory Care Manage.* 1994;17(1):61–69.
21. Fairbrother G, Friedman S, DuMont KA, Lobach KS. Markers for primary care: missed opportunities to immunize and screen for lead and tuberculosis by private physicians serving large numbers of inner-city Medicaid-eligible children. *Pediatr.* 1996;97(6):785–790.
22. Gold M, Sparer M, Chu K. Medicaid managed care: lessons from five states. *Health Aff.* Fall 1996:153–166.
23. Wood D, Halfon N, Sherbourne C, Grabowsky M. Access to infant immunizations for poor inner-city families: what is the impact of managed care? *J Health Care Poor Underserved.* 1994;5(2):113–123.
24. Ireys HT, Anderson GF, Shaffert TJ, Neff JM. Expenditures for care of children with chronic illnesses enrolled in the Washington State Medicaid program, fiscal year 1993. *Pediatr.* 1997;100(2):197–204.
25. Newacheck PW, Hughes DC, Stoddard JJ, Halfon N. Children with chronic illness and Medicaid managed care. *Pediatr.* 1994;100(93):497–500.
26. Health Care Financing Administration. Managed care in Medicare and Medicaid. http://www.hcfa.gov/facts/f960900.htm; accessed February 1998.
27. Henry J Kaiser Family Foundation. *Medicaid Facts: Medicaid and Managed Care.* Washington, DC: Henry J Kaiser Family Foundation; 1996.
28. Buchanan J, Lindsey P, Leibowitz A, Davies A. HMOs for Medicaid: the road to financial independence is often poorly paved. *J Health Politics Policy Law.* 1992;17(1):71–96.
29. Gorgan CM. The Medicaid managed care policy consensus for welfare recipients: a reflection of traditional welfare concerns. *J Health Politics Policy Law.* 1997;22(3):815–838.
30. Siverstein G, Kirkman-Liff B. Physician participation in Medicaid managed care. *Soc Sci Med.* 1995;41(3):355–363.
31. Kennedy KM, Browngoehl K. A "high tech," "soft touch" immunization program for members of a Medicaid managed care organization. *HMO Practice.* 1994;8(3):115–125.

DONNA M. HENDERSON, RN, is director of resource and case management at Alexian Brothers Hospital in San Jose, California. She has over 20 years of experience in the health care industry. Her experience has included health care administration, the development and implementation of case management systems, and a nationwide health care consulting practice in acute care and managed care environments. She has been a guest lecturer at numerous educational and professional organizations.

CHAPTER 44

Medical Management in the Medicare Population

Rita Petty Manninen and Barry K. Baines

Chapter Outline

- Introduction
- Unique Characteristics of Medicare Managed Care
- Conceptual Model for Program Development in Managed Care
- Managing Acute Care
- Population Management
- Where To Start in Developing a Medicare Managed Care Program
- Conclusion

INTRODUCTION

Medicare enrollees compose about 12% of the nation's population, yet they utilize 19.6% of all personal health care expenditures.[1] With the aging of the baby boom generation and increases in life span, the senior population will continue to grow as a proportion of the US population. It is estimated that by 2050, one in four Americans will be 65 years of age or older.[2] In preparation for this future, our government is exploring various options to control the rising costs of Medicare. Most of these options include some form of managed care, and the health care industry is responding: the percent of Medicare enrollees enrolled in health maintenance organizations (HMOs) doubled between 1983 and 1993, from 3.5% to 7%, and continues to increase rapidly.[3] Provider service organizations (PSOs) are poised to take advantage of direct contracting with the Health Care Financing Agency (HCFA) for its vertically integrated health systems.[4] While there is opportunity in this market, there are also significant risks if the health system does not recognize the unique challenges of caring for seniors and develop clinical and operational systems to support seniors' needs.

In this chapter we review some of the characteristics of seniors that make them a challenging population to manage. Then we will describe programs that can be implemented, some of which are vital to effective and successful care management of this population.

UNIQUE CHARACTERISTICS OF MEDICARE MANAGED CARE

Effect of the Aging Process on Health Care Utilization

As our bodies age, they are less able to adapt to change. The healing process is slower. For this reason, a senior having an acute illness, such as pneumonia or a fracture, will need a longer (and thus more costly) period of recovery than a younger person. To control the costs of long hospitalizations, it becomes increasingly important to consider alternative venues of care for the senior. These venues would offer programs more specific to seniors' needs.

Incidence of Chronic Diseases

In 1994, nearly 40% of seniors not living in nursing homes had a chronic condition that limited their daily activity. A quarter of these seniors were limited to such a degree that they were unable to perform activities of independent living, such as bathing, shopping, dressing, and eating. Sixty-nine percent of seniors have multiple chronic conditions, increasing their risk of personal burden and their use of health care resources.[2] Group Health Cooperative of Puget Sound, an HMO serving 400,000 persons in western Washington State, recently published an analysis of its chronic care costs. It found that the average annual cost of an enrollee without a chronic condition was $924. This compared to $2,346 for the enrollee with one chronic condition, and $7,019 for the enrollee with multiple chronic conditions.[5] As the baby boom generation ages, the percentage of the population with chronic conditions, and therefore higher health care costs, will increase.

In the past, the US health care system attended predominantly to acute diseases with short-term, quick fixes. But the health care system must change its focus. Management of chronic diseases requires a dramatic transformation of systems to provide ongoing monitoring and support and to recognize early warning signs and prevent costly exacerbations of illness.

Polypharmacy

With this incidence of chronic disease and comorbidity, it is no surprise that seniors take more medications than younger people. In a 1995 survey of seniors in Minneapolis/St. Paul, 40% reported taking three or more prescription medications daily. Among seniors 75 years old and above, this figure increased to 54%.[6] It is estimated that as many as 10% of hospitalizations for seniors are related to adverse drug reactions. Once hospitalized, the senior has a 25% chance of being the victim of an adverse drug reaction.[7]

Focus on Functional Capabilities

As previously mentioned, 40% of seniors residing in the community have some limitation on their daily activities due to chronic illness. As a result, care provided at all points of the continuum must focus on maintaining optimal functional level. An example of primary prevention of functional decline would be a program of moderate physical activity to slow the progression of arthritis, cardiac disease, pulmonary disease, and complications of diabetes, thus minimizing health care costs. Secondary prevention focuses on minimizing the effects of an acute episode. Even short episodes of bed rest can result in deconditioning, decreased flexibility, orthostatic hypotension (which can predispose the senior to falls), and decreased lung capacity with risk of atelectasis.[8]

Mental Health Issues

More than 10% of the seniors (age 65 and older) in the United States have Alzheimer's disease. In addition, it is estimated that between 25% and 45% of those over the age of 85 have severe dementia, including Alzheimer's disease. Alzheimer's disease and dementia impose a substantial medical, social, psychological, and financial burden on patients and their families. They also create an additional challenge in monitoring and treating their other medical conditions, whether patients are in the home, nursing home, or hospital setting.[9]

Depression is also common in the elderly and has been associated with increased mortality,[10] morbidity,[11] and health care costs.[12] Yet depression continues to be underdiagnosed. One study found that 16% of seniors in one HMO showed signs of depression, indicated by a score of 11 or more on a common screening tool, the Geriatric

Depression Scale. Yet only half of these seniors had any indication of signs of depression documented in their medical record.[13]

Dependence on Caregivers

With a decline in functional abilities, whether physical or cognitive, temporary or permanent, the senior must turn to others for assistance. Caregivers are often vital in helping the senior with activities of daily living, including meal preparation, taking medications as prescribed, and transportation to the clinic. Thus, the caregiver becomes a vital extension of the patient. The medical team must assess and address the needs of the caregiver as well as those of the patient.

CONCEPTUAL MODEL FOR PROGRAM DEVELOPMENT IN MANAGED CARE

Medicare managed care organizations receive a fixed monthly payment for the care of the individual senior. The managed care organization is then at risk for providing all necessary Medicare services, as opposed to billing for each service, as is done in the traditional fee-for-service payment approach. This new capitated payment structure allows the provider the opportunity to restructure services provided to better meet the unique needs of the senior.

It is unfortunate that managed care organizations are developing a reputation (deserved or not) for valuing the financial outcomes of care above the clinical needs of the individual. This is, of course, a shortsighted approach. To be successful in a competitive market, a managed care organization needs satisfied customers. This requires a balanced approach to the clinical needs of the patient and the financial needs of the organization.

At HealthPartners, an HMO in Minneapolis, Minnesota, a conceptual model referred to as the "three worlds view" has been developed to assist in maintaining a balanced approach. This conceptual model reminds us that health care systems operate simultaneously in three worlds: clinical, operational, and financial. Each world has its own language and culture, uses different processes, and looks for different outcomes. Although this framework applies to managed care in general, it is an important concept in planning for seniors. Table 44–1 outlines this conceptual model.

The value of this conceptual framework is that it applies to care planning for the individual patient as well as program development. The medical team first decides what care the patient

Table 44–1 The Three Worlds of a Health Care Organization

	Clinical	Operational	Financial
Basic questions	What care is called for?	What will it take to accomplish care?	How will care utilize resources?
	Is it high quality?	Is it well executed?	Is it a good value?
Object	Unfolding casework	Systems	Numbers
Process	Actions by clinicians and patients	Operations	Accounting
Outcome	Achievement of health goals	Production	Bottom line
Standard	Technical and service quality and elegance	Efficiency and facility	Price and value

Source: Reprinted with permission from A Putman, Organizations, *Advances in Descriptive Psychology*, Vol 5, pp 11–46, © 1990, Jessica Kingsley.

needs (clinical), then decides in what setting this care can be offered in the most cost-effective way (financial), and then considers whether the systems are in place for implementation of this plan (operational).

To develop Medicare managed care programs, then, one needs to identify the care needs of the senior population (clinical), develop programs and resources in the right setting to cost-effectively manage that care (financial), then effectively implement those programs (operational). For programs to be effective there must be an alignment of financial incentives with the desired clinical and operational outcomes.

Contractual relationships and physician incentive programs must encourage appropriate care. Fee-for-service Medicare provides incentive for more services. In capitation, there needs to be an incentive for appropriate care, not minimal care. If needed services are not provided, there is a risk of missed diagnoses, complications, or dissatisfied members, all of which will cost more in the long run.

Access to Data

In order to monitor the financial success of programs and to determine where to focus programs, analysis is done to find out where capitated dollars are being spent (eg, primary care, acute care, skilled nursing facility, referrals, out-of-area care). Benchmarks are obtained from other organizations in order to select the greatest opportunities for savings.

Regulatory Issues

Although capitation allows a great deal of freedom, Medicare managed care is highly regulated. There are specific regulations on how seniors are to be informed of their rights of appeal, should there be a denial of coverage of health services, and strict regulations regarding marketing processes and materials. There must be a very close working relationship among the clinical, marketing, and regulatory (ie, government programs) areas when working with Medicare managed care.

Integration of the Continuum of Care

Relative to the rest of the population, seniors use a disproportionate share of health care dollars. Also, they use health care services in various venues. Chronic disease management increases the need to provide care across the entire continuum—to manage disease from prevention through acute stages, exacerbations, and maintenance. The continuum can be viewed as an inverted pyramid, as in Figure 44–1. The greatest proportion of care is received in the outpatient setting, shown in the base of the triangle. As we move along the triangle to subacute care and acute care, the cost of care increases, but the number of members involved decreases. It is not unusual to find that 20% of members utilize 80% of the resources. To control costs, it is important to

1. Identify which members are likely to be the high utilizers of health care services.
2. Develop systems and programs to decrease the cost of episodes of care.

Seniors utilize services throughout the continuum. Figure 44–2, adapted from a model by Thomas von Sternberg, shows the venues of care for seniors, potential pathways they follow as they navigate the system, and key personnel involved in facilitating their movement along the pathway. In the following pages, we will provide some examples for managing care and costs in a variety of venues.

MANAGING ACUTE CARE

Since hospitalization has the most expensive unit cost in health care, it is important for an organization to establish the target of acute care hospital days/1,000 patients necessary to break even with the capitated payment received in its region of the country. The challenge then is to design systems to achieve and maintain this target. Decreas-

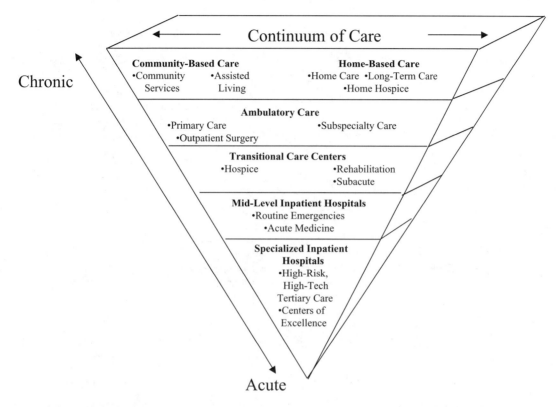

Figure 44–1 Health Care Delivery Model. *Source:* Adapted with permission from SZ Nelson et al, An Integrated Continuum of Care, *HMO Practice,* Vol 9, No 1, pp 40–43, © 1995.

ing the number of acute care hospital days/1,000 patients can be done in one of two ways: decrease admissions or decrease length of stay.

Tools for Managing Acute Admissions

Many admissions come through the emergency department. Imperative to minimizing admissions is having emergency department staff members who are knowledgeable about geriatric clinical issues and senior resources. Access to an observation unit where the patient can be evaluated and stabilized over a few hours can help minimize unnecessary admissions.

Other methods for managing admissions rely on closer outpatient management of patients with chronic conditions. The goal is to identify exacerbations earlier in order to avoid the need for an acute admission. This will be discussed later in the chapter.

Tools for Managing Acute Length of Stay

To decrease length of stay, organizations can employ various approaches, including using inpatient case managers and concurrent review, critical pathways, ACE (acute care for the elderly; not to be confused with angiotensin converting enzyme inhibitors) units, or access to subacute units.

Extended Care Pathways

Critical pathways have become a common tool used by hospitals to reduce length of stay. A critical pathway is a set of policies, procedures,

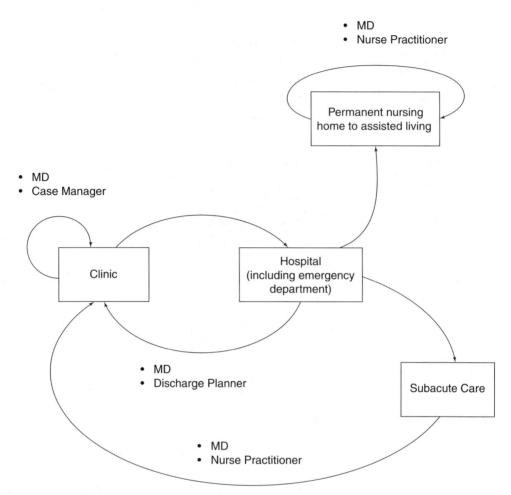

Figure 44–2 Clinical Pathways—Venues for Management. *Source:* Adapted with permission from T von Sternberg, Screening and Managing the Frail Elderly: The Advantages of Managed Care, *Concepts in Geriatric Managed Care,* Vol 2, No 8, pp 4 and 8–18.

or guidelines that have been assigned to a timeline in order to achieve a standardized, multidisciplinary approach to an individual with a specific diagnosis (see Chapter 18). An extended care pathway takes this same concept and expands it across multiple venues, thus providing standards to facilitate smooth transitions across the continuum of care.[14] When developing critical pathways, it is best to start with those diagnostic groups that represent the highest cost or most frequent admissions. It is also best to start with a diagnosis that is relatively easy to standardize; surgical procedures are usually easiest, followed by medical diagnosis, and then psychiatric diagnosis. Creating a pathway requires benchmarking, both externally and internally, to create an interdisciplinary best practice, then creating a timeline for efficiently implementing this best practice. The result is a system in which the default is the best practice from both a clinical and financial perspective. Yet the pathway of individual patients can and should be adjusted according to their individual needs, just as a guideline is. In developing pathways, organizations should not simply take a pathway created elsewhere and implement it in a new facility.

Usually there is some adaptation needed to match the pathway to operational systems in the new facility. Gaining input from the team that will be implementing the pathway will help ensure their support for its successful implementation.

Because seniors often utilize several venues during one episode of care, the extended care pathway becomes a valuable tool. HealthPartners has developed the joint replacement pathway, an example of an extended care pathway. It begins when the patient is scheduled for surgery and ends with the 6-week postoperative visit to the surgeon and after outpatient therapies are completed. The act of scheduling the patient for surgery triggers an invitation to a preoperative class, held 1 to 2 weeks before surgery. In this class, patients learn what to expect during their hospitalization and are taught strengthening exercises to perform preoperatively that will hasten their postoperative recovery. At the preoperative class, representatives of the nursing and therapy departments assess the patients to predict whether they are likely to return home directly from the hospital or be among the 35% who will require a longer rehabilitative stay in a transitional care unit. After admission to the hospital, patients follow the identified pathway of discharge to home on postoperative day 4, or transfer to transitional care on postoperative day 3, with the pathway continuing for an additional 6 days.

ACE Units

Most hospitals are structured to have patients of similar diagnosis clustered on separate units staffed by nurses that specialize in these diagnoses. The University Hospitals of Cleveland developed the concept of the ACE unit. These general medical units are designed to foster the independent functioning of seniors. The focus of care is more interdisciplinary, incorporating pharmacy reviews, geriatric assessments by nurses, psychosocial assessment by social workers, and daily team meetings to review patient progress. Family conferences are held to discuss discharge options. These units are set up to decrease iatrogenic illness among this population, improve functional level, and decrease readmission rate.[15]

Evaluation shows that ACE units are successful at achieving these outcomes. Patients randomly selected for treatment in the ACE unit in Cleveland had a 90-day readmission rate that is 4.4% less than the rate for the control group (36.7% vs 41.1%) and were more likely to improve in functioning in activities of daily living (34% vs 24%). Although the average cost per day was slightly higher for those in the ACE unit, this cost was more than offset by the decrease in length of stay (7.5 vs 8.4 days). Improving clinical outcomes while at the same time reducing overall costs is an outcome all can agree on![16]

For pathways, or any other inpatient programs, to be effective, there must be some method of monitoring inpatient stays to ensure that each day in the hospital is necessary and to assist the physician in identifying viable alternatives to inpatient care. Collecting data is useless unless managers know how to use it. At HealthPartners, we have inpatient nurse case managers, called care coordination specialists, who work with the attending physicians and handle both concurrent review and discharge planning. Care coordinators consider the care of each patient from the clinical, financial, and operational perspectives. By working with the physician, patient, and family, they identify alternatives to the hospital level of care (when appropriate) and facilitate implementation of the discharge plan. In the concurrent review role, they identify data on nonacute inpatient days. These data are reviewed on a regular basis to identify recurring problems that can be improved (such as delays in care because services are not available on a weekend).

Transitional/Subacute Care

An additional way to decrease hospital days is to provide an alternative, such as subacute care. HealthPartners has contracted with selected skilled nursing facilities to create a network of transitional care centers (TCCs) that offer subacute nursing and rehabilitative care. These facilities have a higher nurse:patient ratio than the typical nursing home, and most nurses at these facilities are registered nurses with hospital experience. TCCs accept admissions 24 hours a day, 7 days per week. Therapy is available 7 days per week. In addition, HealthPartners provides a nurse practitioner on site 3 to 5 days per week. This practitioner functions both as the primary provider and care coordinator. A geriatrician makes rounds twice weekly with the nurse practitioner—first in interdisciplinary team rounds, then seeing each patient. The nurse practitioner oversees development of the patient's discharge plan and authorizes resources necessary for the plan to succeed. He or she also communicates with the patient's primary physician in the clinic on a weekly basis, and at discharge, to ensure a smooth transition to the next level of care.

In some cases, patients may be ready for admission directly to a subacute unit, thus avoiding a hospital stay entirely. In our experience, the 3-day acute stay required by Medicare to qualify for coverage in a nursing home often results in unnecessary hospital days. Thus, we frequently waive this requirement, and approve coverage in the nursing home after only 1 to 2 days in the hospital. We will also cover the costs of a nursing home stay for an admission directly from the emergency department if patients have an acute change in their medical condition that would otherwise require hospitalization.[17]

The key to the success of this program is the collaborative relationship with these facilities. HealthPartners directs a volume of patients to a facility and provides easy access to the medical team, in exchange for collaboration on protocols and processes to achieve good outcomes. We meet with each facility on a regular basis to review outcomes (utilization, patient satisfaction, and readmission to the hospital from the TCC and within 30 days of discharge). Admission to transitional care is by definition an indication of frailty in older persons. For that reason, we use this venue of traditional care to focus on advance directive discussions and make referrals to case management for those who appear to be at high risk for readmission to the hospital or transitional care in the future.

Nursing Home or Assisted Living

HCFA pays a higher capitation for the senior residing in the nursing home, recognizing that this institutionalized population is more frail and thus at greater risk of utilizing health care dollars. However, good management of this population can result in improved clinical outcomes as well as decreased costs. Keys to success include the following:

- Hire nurse practitioners to team with physicians in management of the nursing home patients. It has been noted that patients followed by a nurse practitioner/physician team tend to receive more attention and achieve better clinical outcomes than patients followed by only a physician.[18] This closer attention also results in cost savings. When Fallon Community Health Plan hired geriatric nurse practitioners to team with physicians caring for nursing home patients, the health plan decided to study their effect from a cost benefit perspective. When comparing the nursing home practice of the nurse practitioner/physician teams to the nursing home practice of physicians alone, they found that pharmacy costs and covered skilled nursing days increased slightly, but this was more than offset: the number of hospital days decreased by 34%, and the number of emergency department visits dropped 37%.[19] Overall, the plan measured a 42% reduction in the cost of care for the patients followed by the teams, as compared to those followed by the physicians alone.[19]

- Focus on advance directives. Many nursing home residents would prefer not to be sent to the hospital unless absolutely necessary. Yet in most states, nursing homes do not qualify for increased reimbursement unless the patient has been hospitalized. Facilities cannot provide adequate staffing to respond

to increased needs without increased reimbursement. Again, the incentives must be aligned.
- Provide support services to the nursing facility. Contracting with vendors to provide such support services as portable X-ray, ultrasound, intravenous therapy, venipuncture, and laboratory work can allow the nursing home to provide care for patients without sending them to the hospital. Bringing services to the patient, rather than sending the patient to the services, is easier for the patient and often less costly for the health care plan.

Assisted living facilities are providing services to increasingly frail seniors. For these seniors, transportation to the clinic can become a huge barrier. Therefore, it would appear that assigning nurse practitioners to care for seniors in assisted living facilities would be as beneficial as it has been in the nursing home setting. As of January 1998, HCFA will reimburse nurse practitioners for visits made in the home setting, such as assisted living facilities, thus allowing this expansion of their service.

Outpatient/Clinic Care

Seniors can be a challenge for physicians in the clinic setting. Fifteen minutes (the amount of time allotted for the typical clinic appointment) is usually inadequate for assessing the needs of the patient with multiple chronic conditions. The patient's already complex situation is often compounded with multiple psychosocial issues, which the physician may feel inadequately prepared to address. Our current medical practices are organized to respond to patients' acute and urgent needs, not their chronic needs. Responding to seniors with chronic illness requires restructuring outpatient care. Effective interventions in improving outcomes for chronically ill tend to fall in one of four areas.[20]

1. *Use of protocols.* Protocols imply population-based care, meaning development and implementation of a plan for the care of all patients with specific clinical needs. Protocols for chronic diseases require ongoing monitoring to identify signs of exacerbation early and to maintain the disease within a stable range. Protocols for various chronic diseases serve as guidelines for monitoring. To be effective, these protocols need to be incorporated into regular clinic visits.[20] Computer triggering systems can be of immense help here. For example, guidelines for preventive care may include frequency of mammograms, immunizations, or A1c tests. Another example of protocols may be the use of screening tools prior to an appointment. At HealthPartners, it has been useful to have seniors annually complete a Mini Mental Status Exam, Geriatric Depression Scale, and a nutrition screening tool while waiting to see a physician. A brief review of these screening tools by the physician provides comprehensive information about the patient that could otherwise be easily overlooked.

2. *Focus on patient education and self-care.* Patients and their families need to take responsibility for the patients' care. Studies have shown that successful outcomes in the management of chronic illness are directly correlated with the patient's confidence about managing the disease. Patient education, in conjunction with peer-led support groups, can be very effective in achieving positive outcomes. At Kaiser's Cooperative Health Care Clinics for chronically ill older HMO members in Denver, for instance, patients with high health service utilization and one or more chronic conditions are invited to attend group clinics, which meet monthly and last about 2 hours. They begin with an educational session. Topics are chosen by the participants and may include fall prevention, home safety assessment, anatomy and physiology, skills for coping with chronic disease, or health care benefits. Following the educational program, patients meet with the nurse, then their physician, and any of the other profes-

sionals they need to see (pharmacist, social work, nutritionist, etc). Patient medical records are available for referral and documentation. Other members of the group are socializing during this time—an important aspect of the success of this program. A couple of appointment slots are held for those who require a physical exam, although these are often not needed. When they are, the nurse has already assessed needs and concerns and documented them in the chart. These group clinics substitute for the patient's routine physician appointments. Over the 2-hour period, the physician has seen about 20 patients, more than could have been scheduled in the same period otherwise, yet patients feel as if they have each spent more than an hour with their physician. Patient satisfaction with this program has been high. Kaiser in Denver initially documented $14.79 per member per month cost savings after initiation of this program.[21] Patients have increased confidence in the care of their chronic illness. At HealthPartners, compliance has improved using this model with a group of diabetics.

3. *Redesign of practice systems and provider roles.* In some programs, nurses monitor the chronically ill, consulting the physician only when the assessment falls outside the parameters of the protocol and intervention is needed. An example is the congestive heart failure (CHF) program developed at St. Louis University.[22] Patients hospitalized with a diagnosis of CHF are referred to this program. Nurses and a dietitian provide patients with education on the physiology of the disease and how to manage it, including modifying their diet, exercising, and monitoring their weight and symptoms of exacerbation such as dyspnea and edema. A self-care plan is developed for the patient, in collaboration with the physician. Patients learn to use parameters based on symptom changes to decide when to contact their physicians. A nurse telephones patients regularly to assess their status, provide encouragement, and answer questions. Following initiation of the program, there was a 60% decrease in readmissions to the hospital within 90 days of discharge for these patients.[22] This use of nurses was a change in practice. The use of telemedicine was also unique. It is another strategy that would not be reimbursed under traditional fee-for-service Medicare but makes sense under capitation.

4. *Access to expertise.* Patients value having a single source of care, and evidence supports the health and economic advantages of continuous primary care. Seniors should identify a primary physician, and systems need to be arranged so those patients can access their primary physician as needed. Physicians need access to experts, but referring patients to specialists can result in fragmented care. Better yet is a system that allows physicians the ability to contact specialists to review a case without referring the patient. (This system requires some financial arrangement with the specialists, such as a retainer fee.) One very valuable resource for the primary care physician is a pharmacist with expertise in geriatrics. Several managed care organizations have recognized the value of making pharmacists available to counsel patients on multiple medications to assess their understanding of their medications, compliance, and potential side effects, and then make recommendations for changes to simplify the regimen and minimize adverse outcomes.[23] Access to geropsychiatry services is another valuable resource. Although primary care physicians treat most mental illness in seniors,[13] formal and informal access to geropsychiatry consultation is believed to improve treatment outcomes.

The complexity of geriatric patients' medical conditions, compounded by psychosocial issues, can make treating seniors difficult for primary physicians. One avenue to support the primary physician is the ability to refer to a geriatric assessment clinic. Reasons for referrals include cognitive difficulties, caregiver burnout, depression, falls, and need for a home safety assessment or placement. Once the patient is referred, a geriatric social worker visits the patient and caregiver in the home. Following this, the patient and caregiver go to the geriatric assessment clinic, where a nurse interviews and assesses the patient using several common screening tools, including the Mini Mental Status Exam and the Geriatric Depression Scale. Next, the social worker meets with the caregiver while the geriatrician examines the patient. The providers, patient, and family then meet together to discuss the results of the assessment and recommendations. The primary physician receives a consultation report, and the nurse and social worker follow up with the patient and caregiver to facilitate follow through with recommendations.[24]

Referral Costs and Subspecialists

Attention to referral costs and use of subspecialists is an important issue in Medicare managed care. A well-managed referral process results in enhanced patient access within the medical care system and ensures that

- Services provided are medically necessary.
- Care is given by providers with the necessary expertise.
- Care is provided in the appropriate setting.
- Referral data can be collected to understand the needs of each provider.

Referral management driven by the primary physician is a common model that can provide cost-effective medical services and ensure appropriate levels of quality care (see Chapter 20 for an in-depth discussion of this). Such a referral process must support the primary care physician without being overly burdensome or resulting in micro-management of the providers. This can be accomplished by

- Establishing common referral requirements that can be authorized by the primary care physician.
- Creating a referral authorization system that identifies the procedures and services requiring prior authorization by someone other than the primary care physician (eg, referrals to out-of-plan hospitals or specialists, experimental procedures).

After-Hours Care

Like people of all ages, seniors do not plan their illnesses around a clinic's operating hours. To control costs, there must be an effective system for after-hours management of care. At HealthPartners in Minneapolis, a 24-hour nurse triage service is available to answer questions for patients and direct them to the appropriate site of care. Nurses refer to computerized protocols for screening and assessment and to guidelines for conditions that are to be treated at home or referred to urgent care, the emergency department, or the on-call physician. See Chapter 11 for further discussion of this topic.

POPULATION MANAGEMENT

Thus far the general strategies for improved management of the senior population have been discussed. However, the most important key to success is identifying those seniors whose care will be the most costly, and then focusing on improving the outcomes and controlling the costs of this population.

Screening for High-Risk Seniors

Over the past few years, there has been significant research on screening tools to identify those at risk of future utilization of health care services (see Part I). One tool recently receiving national attention is the "Pra plus" tool developed at the University of Minnesota. This validated tool uses nine questions, and weighs the answers to predict the senior's risk of using hospital and emergency department services in the coming year. Additional questions provide information but are not used in risk calculation.[25]

Screening alone, however, is of little value without a plan for reducing the risk of those potential high utilizers. All seniors need to have a primary care physician. Those identified as being at moderate risk should be referred to preventive programs to maintain their health. High-risk members should be referred to a case management program.

Case Management

Case management (see Chapter 17) has been defined by the Case Management Society of America as "the collaborative process which assesses, plans, implements, coordinates, monitors, and evaluates options and services to meet an individual's health needs through communication and available resources to promote quality and cost-effective outcomes."[26] This definition encompasses a wide range of activities. We previously discussed the value of hospital "case managers" who work in collaboration with the physician and patient to both manage the costs of the hospitalization and coordinate a discharge plan that will continue the patient's recovery. This same concept can be applied in any setting of care. However, those members at high risk require a case management plan that coordinates care throughout the continuum.

Disease management programs (see Part XI) usually span the continuum and focus on protocols and pathways to manage the care with a specific disease (such as the CHF protocol discussed earlier in this chapter). Because most seniors have several chronic diseases, they frequently do not fit neatly into one disease management program. Seniors with comorbidities are more likely to use a disproportionate share of health care costs. The focus turns to preventing "frailty," defined by Buchner and Wagner as "the state of reduced physiologic reserve associated with increased susceptibility to disability."[27]

Models of case management for seniors vary widely. We have found that an integrated, multidisciplinary approach, utilizing both nurses and social workers, is most effective in our system. The case manager works closely with the primary care physician to assess facets of the patients' health care, including their understanding of their disease, their understanding of and ability to access needed services including medical care, and their adaptation to their illness. The case managers then create a plan of care collaboratively with the other members of the health care team to meet the patient's needs and facilitate its implementation. This may include educating patients regarding their disease, providing information or tools to access needed care, discussing advance directives, and monitoring for exacerbations in their conditions. The volume of patients identified as "high risk" can be controlled by the definition of the "cutoff" point; most organizations target their case management programs to the 3% to 5% of the population identified as the highest risk.[24] Case manager load also varies, depending on the degree of involvement in a case. For the type of involvement described above, we have found an active case load of about 50 patients to be reasonable.

WHERE TO START IN DEVELOPING A MEDICARE MANAGED CARE PROGRAM

Blend of Fee for Service and Capitation

The transition into Medicare managed care will in most cases involve a significant shift in the reimbursement model for care (ie, fee for service to capitation). The financial incentives of these two methodologies are at opposite ends of the spectrum. The fee-for-service model rewards increased volume of services and procedures, while the capitation model rewards minimizing unnecessary services.

Moving straight from a fee-for-service environment to a fully capitated risk environment is a recipe for disaster. For that reason, it is best to move to capitation in stages. This can be accomplished by including the following steps:

- teaching providers the fundamentals of managed care so that there is an understanding of the link between appropriate resource utilization and financial rewards
- building an integrated care system that can manage global capitation
- providing a "safety net" for providers as they learn the intricacies of managed care and risk sharing
  - starting with a reduced fee schedule or withhold program
  - using shadow capitation reports so providers can compare results of the two models
- transitioning to a global capitation methodology over a period of 5 years
- implementing an actuarially sound risk adjustment to reflect the difference in illness burden for providers

Where To Focus Your Energies First

Acute care utilizes a large percentage of Medicare managed care costs. Thus, managing hospitalization costs is clearly the highest leverage area. Benchmarking admission and length of stay data for various diagnoses will reveal opportunities for initial focus. Major strategies, as previously discussed, will include

- creating a system to avoid unnecessary admissions (eg, nurse triage and urgent care)
- optimizing hospital discharge planning and hospital case management
- developing options for moving patients to a less intense, less costly "step-down" or subacute unit as quickly as possible
- using pathways and guidelines for improving efficiencies in management of common conditions

In the outpatient arena, the high-leverage starting point is to screen new enrollees and then include those identified as high risk in a case management program. The number of case managers can be expanded as the program grows.

CONCLUSION

It is clear that the senior population requires an approach to care management that addresses the unique aspects of that population. It is not optimal to simply use a care management program that is appropriate for a nonsenior or commercial population and apply it to Medicare members. The Medicare-focused program will yield better outcomes and greater cost-effectiveness.

REFERENCES

1. Levit K, Lazenby H, Braden B. National health spending trends in 1996. *Health Aff.* 1998;17(1):35–51.
2. Freudenheim D. *Chronic Care in America: A 21st Century Challenge*. Princeton, NJ: Institute for Health and Aging; 1996.
3. US Department of Health and Human Services. *Health Care Financing Review: 1995 Statistical Supplement*. Baltimore, MD: US Department of Health and Human Services; 1997.
4. Does your PSO have what it takes to direct-contract? *Public Sector Contracting Rep.* 1997;3(9):129–133.
5. Fishman P. Chronic care costs in managed care. *Health Aff.* 1997;16(3):239–247.
6. Hauber F. *1995 Survey of Older Minnesotans: Results for the Twin City Metropolitan Area*. St. Paul, MN: Metropolitan Area Agency on Aging, Inc; 1996.
7. Kane R, Ouslander JG, Abrass IB. *Essentials of Clinical Geriatrics*. New York: McGraw-Hill Information Services Co; 1989.
8. Gorbien M, Bishop J, Beers MH, et al. Iatrogenic illness in hospitalized elderly people. *J Am Geriatr Soc*. 1992; 40:1031–1042.
9. Rice D, Fox P, Max W, et al. The economic burden of Alzheimer's disease care. *Health Aff.* 1993;12(2): 164–176.
10. Hendrie HC, Crossett JHW. An overview of depression in the elderly. *Psychiatr Ann.* 1990;20:64–70.
11. Coulehan JL, Schulberg HC, Block MR, Janowsky JE,

Arena VC. Depressive symptomatology and medical comorbidity in a primary care clinic. *Int J Psychiatr Med.* 1990;20(4):335–347.
12. Broadhead WE, Blazer DG, George LK, Tse CK. Depression, disability days, and days lost from work in a prospective epidemiologic survey. *JAMA.* 1990;264: 2524–2528.
13. Garrard J, Rolnick SJ, Nitz NM, et al. Clinical detection of depression among community-based elderly people with self-reported symptoms of depression. *J Gerontol A Biol Sci Med Sci.* 1998;53(2):M92–M101.
14. National Chronic Care Consortium. *Conceptualizing, Implementing, and Evaluating Extended Care Pathways.* Bloomington, MN: National Chronic Care Consortium; 1995.
15. Palmer R, Landefeld CS, Kresevic D, Kowal J. A medical unit for the acute care of the elderly. *J Am Geriatr Soc.* 1994;42:545–554.
16. Covinski KE, King JT, Quinn LM, et al. Do acute care for elders units increase hospital costs? A cost analysis using the hospital perspective. *J Am Geriatr Soc.* 1997;45(6):729–734.
17. von Sternberg T, Hepburn K, Cibuzar P, et al. Post-hospital sub-acute care: an example of a managed care model. *J Am Geriatr Soc.* 1997;45(1):87–91.
18. Kane RL, Garrard J, Buchanan JL, et al. Improving primary care in nursing homes. *J Am Geriatr Soc.* 1991;45(4):359–367.
19. Burl J, Bonner A, Rao M. Demonstration of the cost-effectiveness of nurse practitioner/physician teams in long-term care facilities. *HMO Practice.* December 1994:157–161.
20. Wagner EH, Austin BT, Von Korff M. Improving outcomes in chronic illness. *Managed Care Q.* 1996; 4(2):12–25.
21. Beck A, Scott J, Williams P, et al. A randomized trial of group outpatient visits for chronically ill older HMO members: the cooperative health care clinic. *J Am Geriatr Soc.* 1997;45:543–549.
22. Rich MW. A multidisciplinary intervention to prevent the readmission of elderly patients with congestive heart failure. *N Engl J Med.* 1995;333:1190–1195.
23. Kramer A, Fox P, Morgenstern N. Geriatric care approaches in health maintenance organizations. *J Am Geriatr Soc.* 1992;40:1055–1067.
24. von Sternberg T. Screening and managing the frail elderly: the advantages of managed care. *Curr Concepts Geriatr Managed Care.* 1996;2(8):4,8–18.
25. Pacala J, Boult C, Boult L. Predictive validity of a questionnaire that identifies older persons at risk for hospital admissions. *J Am Geriatr Soc.* 1995;43:374–377.
26. Case Management Society of America. *Standards of Practice for Case Management.* Little Rock, AR: Case Management Society of America; 1995.
27. Buchner DM, Wagner E. Preventing frail health. *Clin Geriatr Med.* 1992;8(1):1–17.

RITA PETTY MANNINEN, RN, MPH, MBA, is manager of geriatrics programs for HealthPartners health maintenance organization in Minneapolis, Minnesota, where she has responsibility for clinical program development and evaluation for the Medicare managed care program. Her areas of expertise are quality improvement processes, case management, and program evaluation. She received her MPH and MBA from the University of Minnesota.

BARRY K. BAINES, MD, is the associate medical director for centralized patient care services within HealthPartners. Trained as a family physician, Dr. Baines provides overall leadership for the delivery of comprehensive geriatric services across the continuum of care for the HealthPartners Medical Group. He also serves as medical director for two Medicare-certified home health care agencies and for a Medicare-certified home-based hospice program within the HealthPartners system. He also provides medical management consulting services through the HealthPartners Ventures division.

Glossary of Terms and Acronyms

AAHP—American Association of Health Plans. It was formed by the merger of GHAA and AMCRA in 1995 and is the leading trade association for managed care plans.

AAPCC—Adjusted average per capita cost. The HCFA's best estimate of the amount of money it costs to care for Medicare recipients under fee-for-service Medicare in a given area. The AAPCC is made up of 142 different rate cells; 140 of them are factored for age, sex, Medicaid eligibility, institutional status, working aged (individuals who are old enough for Medicare but who are still working full time and retain private health insurance), and whether a person has both Part A and Part B of Medicare. The two remaining cells are for individuals with end-stage renal disease.

Accrete—The term used by HCFA for the process of adding new Medicare enrollees to a plan. Also see Delete.

Accrual—The amount of money that is set aside to cover expenses. The accrual is the plan's best estimate of what those expenses are and (for medical expenses) is based on a combination of data from the authorization system, the claims system, the lag studies, and the plan's prior history.

ACG—Ambulatory care group. ACGs are a method of categorizing outpatient episodes. There are 51 mutually exclusive ACGs, which are based on resource use over time, and modified by principal diagnosis, age, and sex. Also see ADG and APG.

ACR—Adjusted community rate. Used by HMOs and CMPs with Medicare risk contracts. A calculation of what premium the plan would charge for providing exactly the Medicare-covered benefits to a group account adjusted to allow for the greater intensity and frequency of utilization by Medicare recipients. The ACR includes the normal profit of a for-profit HMO or CMP. The ACR may be equal to or lower than the APR (see below) but can never exceed it.

Actuarial assumptions—The assumptions that an actuary uses in calculating the expected costs and revenues of the plan. Examples include utilization rates, age and sex mix of enrollees, and cost for medical services.

ADG—Ambulatory diagnostic group. ADGs are a method of categorizing outpatient episodes. There are 34 possible ADGs. Also see ACG and APG.

This glossary is adapted from PR Kongstvedt, *The Managed Health Care Handbook*, 3rd ed, PR Kongstvedt, ed, pp 987–1004, © 1996, Aspen Publishers, Inc.

Adverse selection—The problem of attracting members who are sicker than the general population (specifically, members who are sicker than was anticipated when the budget for medical costs was developed).

AHCPR—The Agency for Health Care Policy and Research.

ALOS—Average length of stay.

Alternative medicine—See CAM.

AMCRA—American Managed Care and Review Association. A trade association that represented managed indemnity plans, PPOs, MCOs, and HMOs. Merged with GHAA (see below) in 1995 to form the American Association of Health Plans (AAHP).

APG—Ambulatory patient group. A reimbursement methodology developed by 3M Health Information Systems for the HCFA, which has still not implemented them at the time this book was written (though some commercial MCOs have). APGs are to outpatient procedures what DRGs are to inpatient days. APGs provide for a fixed reimbursement to an institution for outpatient procedures or visits and incorporate data regarding the reason for the visit and patient data. APGs prevent unbundling of ancillary services. Also see ACG and ADG.

APR—Average payment rate. The amount of money that the HCFA could conceivably pay an HMO or CMP for services to Medicare recipients under a risk contract. The figure is derived from the AAPCC for the service area adjusted for the enrollment characteristics that the plan would expect to have. The payment to the plan, the ACR, can never be higher than the APR, but it may be less.

ASO—Administrative services only. A contract between an insurance company and a self-funded plan where the insurance company performs administrative services only and does not assume any risk. Services usually include claims processing but may include other services such as actuarial analysis, utilization review, and so forth. Also see ERISA.

Assignment of benefits—The payment of medical benefits directly to a provider of care rather than to a member. Generally requires either a contract between the health plan and the provider, or a written release from the subscriber to the provider allowing the provider to bill the health plan.

AWP—Average wholesale price. Commonly used in pharmacy contracting, the AWP is generally determined through reference to a common source of information.

AWP—Any willing provider. This is a form of state law that requires an MCO to accept any provider willing to meet the terms and conditions in the MCO's contract, whether the MCO wants or needs that provider or not. Considered to be an expensive form of anti–managed care legislation.

Balance billing—The practice of a provider billing a patient for all charges not paid for by the insurance plan, even if those charges are above the plan's UCR or are considered medically unnecessary. Managed care plans and service plans generally prohibit providers from balance billing except for allowed copays, coinsurance, and deductibles. Such prohibition against balance billing may even extend to the plan's failure to pay at all (eg, because of bankruptcy).

CAM—Complementary and alternative medicine. This is a general term that covers treatment modalities other that traditional allopathic medicine. Examples include acupuncture, chiropractic medicine, homeopathy, and various forms of "natural healing."

Capitation—A set amount of money received or paid out; it is based on membership rather than on services delivered and usually is expressed in units of PMPM. May vary because of such factors as age and sex of the enrolled member.

Carve-out—Refers to a set of medical services that are "carved out" of the basic arrangement. In terms of plan benefits, may refer to a set of benefits that are carved out and contracted for separately; for example, mental health/substance abuse services may be separated from basic medical and surgical services. May also refer to carving out a set of services from a basic capitation rate with a provider (for example, capitating for cardiac care, but carving out cardiac surgery and paying case rates for that).

Case management—A method of managing the provision of health care to members with high-cost medical conditions. The goal is to coordinate the care so as to improve continuity and quality of care as well as lower costs. This generally is a dedicated function of the utilization management department. When focused solely on high-cost inpatient cases, case management may be referred to as large case management or catastrophic case management.

Case mix—Refers to the mix of illness and severity of cases for a provider.

Certificate of coverage—Refers to the document that a plan must provide to members to show evidence that they have coverage and to give basic information about that coverage. Required under state regulations.

CHAMPUS—Civilian Health and Medical Program of the Uniformed Services. The federal program providing health care coverage to families of military personnel, military retirees, certain spouses and dependents of such personnel, and certain others.

Chest pain unit—The term used to describe a specialized unit, usually either in or associated with the emergency department. The purpose of the chest pain unit is to rapidly identify an evolving cardiac event and initiate treatment as early as possible in order to decrease morbidity and mortality. The other (lesser) primary value of the unit is to rapidly identify chest pain that is noncardiac in origin so as to avoid unnecessary hospitalization. Other terms that may be used include chest pain emergency room, chest pain evaluation unit, short-stay ED critical care unit, and ED monitored observation beds.

Churning—The practice of a provider seeing a patient more often than is medically necessary, primarily to increase revenue through an increased number of services. Churning may also apply to any performance-based reimbursement system where there is a heavy emphasis on productivity (in other words, rewarding a provider for seeing a high volume of patients whether through fee-for-service or through an appraisal system that pays a bonus for productivity).

Closed panel—A managed care plan that contracts with physicians on an exclusive basis for services and does not allow those physicians to see patients for another managed care organization. Examples include staff and group model HMOs. Could apply to a large private medical group that contracts with an HMO.

CMP—Competitive medical plan. A federal designation that allows a health plan to obtain eligibility to receive a Medicare risk contract without having to obtain qualification as an HMO. Requirements for eligibility are somewhat less restrictive than they are for an HMO.

COA—Certificate of authority. The state-issued operating license for an HMO.

COB—Coordination of benefits. An agreement that uses language developed by the National Association of Insurance Commissioners and prevents double payment for services when a subscriber has coverage from two or more sources. For example, a husband may have Blue Cross Blue Shield through work, and the wife may have elected an HMO through her place of employment. The agreement gives the order for what organization has primary responsibility for payment and what organization has secondary responsibility for payment.

COBRA—Consolidated Omnibus Budget Reconciliation Act. A portion of COBRA requires employers to offer the opportunity for terminated employees to purchase continuation of health care coverage under the group's medical plan (also see Conversion). Another portion eases a Medicare recipient's ability to disenroll from an HMO or CMP with a Medicare risk contract.

Coinsurance—A provision in a member's coverage that limits the amount of coverage by the plan to a certain percentage, commonly 80%. Any additional costs are paid by the member out of pocket.

Commission—The money paid to a sales representative, broker, or other type of sales agent for selling the health plan. May be a flat amount of money or a percentage of the premium.

Community rating—The rating methodology required of federally qualified HMOs and of HMOs under the laws of many states, and indemnity plans under certain circumstances. The HMO must obtain the same amount of money per member for all members in the plan. Community rating does allow for variability by allowing the HMO to factor in differences for age, sex, mix (average contract size), and industry factors; not all factors are necessarily allowed under state laws, however. Such techniques are referred to as community rating by class and adjusted community rating. See also Experience rating.

CON—Certificate of need. The requirement that a health care organization obtain permission from an oversight agency before making changes. Generally applies only to facilities or facility-based services.

Concurrent review—Refers to utilization management that takes place during the provision of services. Almost exclusively applied to inpatient hospital stays.

Contract year—The 12-month period that a contract for services is in force. Not necessarily tied to a calendar year.

Contributory plan—A group health plan in which the employees must contribute a certain amount toward the premium cost, with the employer paying the rest.

Conversion—The conversion of a member covered under a group master contract to coverage under an individual contract. This is offered to subscribers who lose their group coverage (for example, through job loss, death of a working spouse, and so forth) and who are ineligible for coverage under another group contract (also see COBRA).

Cookbook medicine—A pejorative term for medical guidelines; the term is used by physicians and others who object to such guidelines. The main complaint behind the term is that the practice of medicine requires a far greater degree of flexibility than do other activities, such as making cookies, for the simple reason that human bodies and human diseases are highly complex. This is a valid point, though there are clearly many conditions where adherence to clinical guidelines improves quality and outcomes, while simultaneously lowering costs.

Copayment—That portion of a claim or medical expense that a member must pay out of pocket. Usually a fixed amount, such as $5 in many HMOs.

Corporate Practice of Medicine Acts or Statutes—State laws that prohibit a physician from working for a corporation; in other words, physicians can work for only themselves or another physician. A corporation cannot practice medicine. Often created through the effort on the part of certain members of the medical community to prevent physicians from working directly for managed care plans or hospitals.

Cost sharing—Any form of coverage in which the member pays some portion of the cost of providing services. Usual forms of cost sharing include deductibles, coinsurance, and copayments.

Cost shifting—When a provider cannot cover the cost of providing services under the reimbursement received, the provider raises the prices to other payers to cover that portion of the cost.

CPT-4—Current Procedural Terminology, 4th Edition. A set of five-digit codes that apply to medical services delivered. Frequently used for billing by professionals (also see HCPCS).

Credentialing—Most commonly, this term refers to obtaining and reviewing the documentation of professional providers. Such documentation includes licensure, certifications, insurance, evidence of malpractice insurance, malpractice history, and so forth. Generally includes both reviewing information provided by the provider as well as verification that the information is correct and complete. A much less frequent use of the term applies to closed panels and medical groups and refers to obtaining hospital privileges and other privileges to practice medicine.

Critical paths—Defined pathways of clinical care that provide for the greatest efficiency of care at the greatest quality. As science and medicine evolve, critical paths are updated.

Custodial care—Care provided to an individual that focuses primarily on the basic activities of living. May be medical or nonmedical, but the care is not meant to be curative or as a form of medical treatment, and it is often lifelong. Rarely covered by any form of group health insurance or HMO.

CVO—Credentialing verification organization. This is an independent organization that performs primary verification of a professional provider's credentials. The managed care organization may then rely on that verification rather than asking the provider to furnish credentials independently. This lowers the cost and hassle of credentialing. NCQA has issued certification standards for CVOs.

CWW—Clinic without walls. See Group practice without walls.

Date of service—Refers to the date that medical services were rendered. Usually different from the date a claim is submitted.

DAW—Dispense as written. The instruction from a physician to a pharmacist to dispense a brand-name pharmaceutical rather than a generic substitution.

Days per thousand—A standard unit of measurement of utilization. Refers to an annualized use of the hospital or other institutional care. It is the number of hospital days that are used in a year for each 1,000 covered lives.

DCG—Diagnostic care group. A new methodology commissioned by the HCFA to look at how to adjust prospective payments based on retrospective severity. This system, which was still not finalized or implemented as this book was being written, looks at ICD-9-CM diagnoses and sorts them iteratively until the patient is classified into one of more than 100 DCGs that are then to be used to compensate a risk-bearing Medicare MCO or PSO.

Death spiral—An insurance term that refers to a vicious spiral of high premium rates and adverse selection, generally in a free-choice environment (typically, an insurance company or health plan in an account with multiple other plans, or a plan offering coverage to potential members who have alternative choices, such as through an association). One plan, often the indemnity plan competing with managed care plans, ends up having such high, and always rising, premium rates that the only members who stay with the plan are those whose medical costs are so high (or who cannot change because of provider loyalty or benefits restrictions such as pre-existing conditions) that they far exceed any possible premium revenue. Called the death spiral because the losses from underwriting mount faster than the premiums can ever recover, and the account eventually terminates coverage, leaving the carrier in a permanent loss position.

Deductible—That portion of a subscriber's (or member's) health care expenses that must be paid out of pocket before any insurance coverage applies, commonly $100 to $300. Common in insurance plans and PPOs, but uncommon in HMOs. May apply only to the out-of-network portion of a point-of-service plan. May also apply only to one portion of the plan coverage (for example, there may be a deductible for pharmacy services but not for anything else).

Delete—The term used by HCFA for the process of removing Medicare enrollees from a plan. Also see Accrete.

Dependent—A member who is covered by virtue of a family relationship with the member who has the health plan coverage. For example, one person has health insurance or an HMO through work, and that individual's spouse and children, the dependents, also have coverage under that contract.

DHMO—Dental health maintenance organization. An HMO organized strictly to provide dental benefits.

Direct contracting—A term describing a provider or integrated health care delivery system contracting directly with employers rather than through an insurance company or managed care organization. A superficially attractive option that occasionally works when the employer is large enough. Not to be confused with direct contract model (see below).

Direct contract model—A managed care health plan that contracts directly with private practice physicians in the community, rather than through an intermediary such as an IPA or a medical group. A common type of model in open panel HMOs.

Discharge planning—That part of utilization management that is concerned with arranging for care or medical needs to facilitate discharge from the hospital.

Disease management—The process of intensively managing a particular disease. This differs from large case management in that it goes well beyond a given case in the hospital, or an acute exacerbation of a condition. Disease management encompasses all settings of care and places a heavy emphasis on prevention and maintenance. Similar to case management, but more focused on a defined set of diseases.

Disenrollment—The process of termination of coverage. Voluntary termination would include a member quitting because he or she simply wants out. Involuntary termination would include leaving the plan because of changing jobs. A rare and serious form of involuntary disenrollment is when the plan terminates a member's coverage against the member's will. This is usually only allowed (under state and federal laws) for gross offenses such as fraud, abuse, nonpayment of premium or copayments, or a demonstrated inability to comply with recommended treatment plans.

DME—Durable medical equipment. Medical equipment that is not disposable (ie, is used repeatedly) and is only related to care for a medical condition. Examples would include wheelchairs, home hospital beds, and so forth. An area of increasing expense, particularly in conjunction with case management.

Dread disease policy—A peculiar and uncommon type of health insurance that covers only a specific and frightening type of illness, such as cancer.

DRG—Diagnosis-related group. A statistical system of classifying any inpatient stay into groups for purposes of payment. DRGs may be primary or secondary, and an outlier classification also exists. This is the form of reimbursement that HCFA uses to pay hospitals for Medicare recipients. Also used by a few states for all payers and by many private health plans (usually non-HMO) for contracting purposes.

DSM-IV—*Diagnostic and Statistical Manual of Mental Disorders*, 4th Edition. The manual used to provide a diagnostic coding system for mental and substance abuse disorders. Far different from ICD-9-CM.

Dual choice—Sometimes referred to as Section 1310 or mandating. That portion of the federal HMO regulations that requires any employer with 25 or more employees that reside in an HMO's service area, pays minimum wage, and offers health coverage to offer a federally qualified HMO as well. The HMO must request it. This provision "sunseted" in 1995.

Dual option—The offering of both an HMO and a traditional insurance plan by one carrier.

Duplicate claims—When the same claim is submitted more than once, usually because payment hasn't been received quickly. Can lead to duplicate payments and incorrect data in the claims file.

DUR—Drug utilization review.

EAP—Employee assistance program. A program that a company puts into effect for its employees to provide them with help in dealing with personal problems such as alcohol or drug abuse, mental health or stress issues, and so forth.

ED—Emergency department. That location or department in a hospital or other institutional facility that is focused on caring for acutely ill or injured patients. In earlier times, this was often a room or set of rooms, hence the older designation emergency room, or ER. These days, at least in busy urban and suburban hospitals, volume is high, physicians are specially trained and certified in emergency care, and emergency care is provided in not a room but an entire department.

Effective date—The day that health plan coverage goes into effect, or is modified.

Eligibility—When an individual is eligible for coverage under a plan. Also used to determine when an individual is no longer eligible for coverage (for example, a dependent child reaches a certain age and is no longer eligible for coverage under his or her parent's health plan).

ELOS—Estimated length of stay.

Encounter—An outpatient or ambulatory visit by a member to a provider. Applies primarily to physician office visits but may encompass other types of encounters as well. In fee-for-service plans, an encounter also generates a claim. In capitated plans, the encounter is still the visit, but no claim is generated.

Enrollee—An individual enrolled in a managed health care plan. Usually applies to the subscribers or people who have the coverage in the first place rather than to their dependents, but the term is not always used that precisely.

EOB—Explanation of benefits (statement). A statement mailed to a member or covered insured explaining how and why a claim was or was not paid; the Medicare version is called an EOMB (also see ERISA).

EPO—Exclusive provider organization. An EPO may be similar to an HMO in that it may use primary physicians as gatekeepers, capitate providers, have a limited provider panel, use an authorization system, and so on. Some EPOs do not use a primary care model. It is referred to as exclusive because the member must remain within the network to receive any benefits. EPOs are generally regulated under insurance statutes rather than HMO regulations. Not allowed in many states that maintain that EPOs are really HMOs.

Equity model—A term applied to a form of for-profit vertically integrated health care delivery system in which the physicians are owners.

ER—Emergency room. See ED.

ERISA—Employee Retirement Income Security Act. One provision of this Act allows self-funded plans to avoid paying premium taxes, complying with state-mandated benefits, or otherwise complying with state laws and regulations regarding insurance, even when insurance companies and managed care plans that stand risk for medical costs must do so. Another provision requires that plans and insurance companies provide an EOB statement to a member or covered insured in the event of a denial of a claim, explaining why the claim was denied and informing the individual of his or her rights of appeal. Numerous other provisions in ERISA are very important for a managed care organization to know.

Evidence of insurability—The form that documents whether an individual is eligible for health plan coverage when the individual does not enroll through an open enrollment period. For example, if an employee wants to change health plans in the middle of a contract year, the new health plan may require evidence of insurability (often both a questionnaire and a medical exam) to ensure that it will not be accepting adverse risk.

Experience rating—The method of setting premium rates based on the actual health care costs of a group or groups.

Extra-contractual benefits—Health care benefits beyond what the member's actual policy covers. These benefits are provided by a plan in order to reduce utilization. For example, a plan may not provide coverage for a hospital bed at home, but it is more cost-effective for the plan to provide such a bed than to keep admitting a member to the hospital.

FAR—Federal Acquisition Regulations. The regulations applied to the federal government's acquisition of services, including health care services (also see FEHBARS).

Fast track ED—A pathway in the ED allowing minor ailments to be managed quickly, at lower cost, often by nonphysician practitioners.

Favored nations discount—A contractual agreement between a provider and a payer stating that the provider will automatically give the payer the provider's best discount.

Federal qualification—Applies to HMOs and CMPs. It means that the HMO or CMP meets federal standards regarding benefits, financial solvency, rating methods, marketing, member services, health care delivery systems, and other standards. An HMO or CMP must apply for federal qualification and be examined by the OMC, including an on-site review. Federal qualification does place some restrictions on how a plan operates but also allows it to enter the Medicare and FEHBP markets in an expedited way. Federal qualification is voluntary and not required to enter the market.

Fee schedule—May also be referred to as fee maximums or as a fee allowance schedule. A listing of the maximum fee that a health plan will pay for a certain service, based on CPT billing codes.

FEHBARS—Federal Employee Health Benefit Acquisition Regulations. The regulations applied to OPM's purchase of health care benefits programs for federal employees.

FEHBP—Federal Employee Health Benefits Program. The program that provides health benefits to federal employees. See OPM.

FFS—Fee for service. A patient sees a provider, then the provider bills the health plan or patient and gets paid based on that bill.

Flexible benefit plan—When an employer allows employees to choose a variety of options in benefits up to a certain total amount. Employees then can tailor their benefits packages, considering health coverage, life insurance, child care, and so forth, to optimize benefits for their particular needs.

Formulary—A listing of drugs that a physician may prescribe. The physician is requested or required to use only formulary drugs unless there is a valid medical reason to use a nonformulary drug.

Foundation—A not-for-profit form of integrated health care delivery system. The foundation model is usually formed in response to tax laws that affect not-for-profit hospitals, or in response to states with laws prohibiting the corporate practice of medicine (see Corporate Practice of Medicine Acts or Statutes). The foundation purchases both the tangible and intangible assets of a physician's practice. The physicians then form a medical group that contracts with the foundation on an exclusive basis for services to patients seen through the foundation.

FPP—Faculty practice plan. A form of group practice organized around a teaching program. It may be a single group encompassing all the physicians providing services to patients at the teaching hospital and clinics, or it may be multiple groups drawn along specialty lines (for example, psychiatry, cardiology, or surgery).

Fraudandabuse—Fraud and abuse, used in reality as if it were a single word. This term has its roots in a description applied to fraud and/or abuse by health care providers or intermediaries in the provision of services to Medicare and Medicaid beneficiaries. Fraudandabuse has taken on a generic meaning applied to any form of perceived skullduggery on the part of a provider or health plan doing business with the government. See also Waste, Fraud, and Abuse.

FTE—Full-time equivalent. The equivalent of one full-time employee. For example, two part-time employees are 0.5 FTE each, for a total of 1 FTE.

Full capitation—A loose term used to refer to a physician group or organization receiving capitation for all professional expenses, not just for the services provided by members of that organization or group; does not include capitation for institutional services (see global capitation). The group is then responsible for subcapitating or otherwise reimbursing other physicians for services to its members.

Gatekeeper—An informal, though widely used term that refers to a primary care case management model health plan. In this model, all care from providers other than the primary care physician, except for true emergencies, must be authorized by the primary care physician before care is rendered. This is a predominant feature of almost all HMOs.

Generic drug—A drug that is equivalent to a brand-name drug, but usually less expensive. Most managed care organizations that provide drug benefits cover generic drugs, but may require a member to pay the difference in cost between a generic drug and a brand-name drug or pay a higher copay, unless there is no generic equivalent.

GHAA—Group Health Association of America. See AAHP.

Global capitation—The term used when an organization receives capitation for all medical services, including institutional and professional.

Group—The members that are covered by virtue of receiving health plan coverage at a single company.

Group model HMO—An HMO that contracts with a medical group for the provision of health care services. The relationship between the HMO and the medical group is generally very close, although there are wide variations in the relative independence of the group from the HMO. A form of closed panel health plan.

Group practice—The American Medical Association defines group practice as three or more physicians who deliver patient care, make joint use of equipment and personnel, and divide income by a prearranged formula.

Group practice without walls (GPWW)—A group practice in which the members of the group come together legally but continue to practice in private offices scattered throughout the service area. Sometimes called a clinic without walls (CWW).

HCFA—Health Care Financing Administration. The federal agency that oversees all aspects of health financing for Medicare and also oversees the OMC.

HCFA-1500—A claims form used by professionals to bill for services. Required by Medicare and generally used by private insurance companies and managed care plans.

HCPCS—HCFA Common Procedural Coding System. A set of codes used by Medicare that describes services and procedures. HCPCS includes CPT codes but also has codes for services not included in CPT such as DME and ambulance. While HCPCS is nationally defined, there is provision for local use of certain codes.

HCPP—Health care prepayment plan. HCPP is a form of cost contract between HCFA and a medical group to provide professional services, but it does not cover Part A institutional services. HCFA intends to eliminate this program in the near future.

Health care—The term is generally used to refer to the services that a health care professional or institution provides (for example, services from a physician, at a hospital, from a physical therapist, and so forth); this definition of health care is used when discussing care management. There is a broader definition, however, that encompasses services from nontraditional providers, and more important, the health care that individuals self-administer (which is actually the majority of health care). When individuals use the broad sense of the term health care, they frequently use medical care to refer to what is considered the narrow meaning noted above.

Health risk appraisals—Instruments designed to elicit or compile information about the health risk of any given individual. Initially these tools were fairly uniform, but recently they have become quite specialized and targeted toward populations with distinctive risk profiles (for example, Medicare, Medicaid, underserved, commercial, and other groups).

HEDIS—Health Plan Employer Data and Information Set. Developed by NCQA with considerable input from the employer community and the managed care community, HEDIS is an ever-evolving set of data reporting standards. HEDIS is designed to provide some standardization in performance reporting for financial, utilization, membership, and clinical data so that employers and others can compare performance between plans.

HIPAA—Health Insurance Portability and Accountability Act. Enacted in 1997, this Act creates a rather vaguely worded set of requirements that allow for insurance portability (ie, the ability to keep health insurance even if people move or change jobs), guaranteed issue of all health insurance products to small groups (but only if they have met requirements for prior continuous coverage) and mental health parity (ie, the dollar limits on mental health coverage cannot be less than those for medical coverage). The Act is silent, however, about the issues of differential visit limitations, differential coinsurance requirements, or restrictions on networks for mental health coverage. Enforcement of HIPAA has been unresolved.

HMO—Health maintenance organization. The definition of an HMO has changed substantially. Originally, an HMO was defined as a prepaid organization that provided health care to voluntarily enrolled members in return for a preset amount of money on a PMPM basis. With the increase in self-insured business, or with financial arrangements that do not rely on prepayment, that definition is no longer accurate. Now the definition needs to encompass two possibilities: a licensed health plan (licensed as an HMO, that is) that places at least some of the providers at risk for medical expenses, and a health plan that utilizes designated (usually primary care) physicians as gatekeepers (although there are some HMOs that do not). Many in the field use MCO, a more flexible term.

Hospitalist—A physician who concentrates solely on hospitalized patients. In an MCO or medical group, this physician may specialize in hospital care, or the duties may be undertaken on a rotating basis. This model allows the other physicians to concentrate on outpatient care, while the hospitalist focuses on the care of all the plan's or group's patients in the hospital.

IBNR—Incurred but not reported. The amount of money that the plan had better accrue for medical expenses that it knows nothing about yet. These are medical expenses that the authorization system has not captured and for which claims have not yet hit the door. More than any other factors, unexpected IBNRs have torpedoed some managed care plans.

ICD-9-CM—International Classification of Diseases, 9th Edition, Clinical Modification. The classification of disease by diagnosis codified into six-digit numbers. The ICD-10 uses alphanumeric codes.

IDFN—See IDS.

IDFS—See IDS.

IDN—See IDS.

IDS—Integrated delivery system; also referred to as an integrated health care delivery system. Other acronyms with the same meaning are IDN (integrated delivery network), IDFS (integrated delivery and financing system), and IDFN (integrated delivery and financing network). An IDS is an organized system of health care providers that span a broad range of health care services. Although there is no clear definition of an IDS, in its full flower an IDS should be able to access the market on a broad basis, optimize cost and clinical outcomes, accept and manage a full range of financial arrangements to provide a set of defined benefits to a defined population, align financial incentives of the participants (including physicians), and operate under a cohesive management structure. See also Equity model, Foundation, IHO, IPA, MSO, PHO, and Staff model HMO.

IHO—Integrated healthcare organization. An IDS that is predominantly owned by physicians. This term is not used very often.

IPA—Independent practice association. An organization that has a contract with a managed care plan to deliver services in return for a single capitation rate. The IPA in turn contracts with individual providers to provide the services either on a capitation basis or on a fee-for-service basis. The typical IPA encompasses all specialties, but an IPA can be solely for primary care, or may be single specialty. An IPA may also be the PO (physician organization) part of a PHO.

Joint Commission—Joint Commission on Accreditation of Healthcare Organizations. A not-for-profit organization that performs accreditation reviews primarily on hospitals, other institutional facilities, and outpatient facilities. Most managed care plans require any hospital under contract to be accredited by the Joint Commission. The Joint Commission has also begun to accredit MCOs and IDSs.

Lag study—A report that tells managers how old the claims are that are being processed and how much is paid out each month (both for that month and for any earlier months, by month) and compares these to the amount of money that was accrued for expenses each month. A powerful tool used to determine whether the plan's reserves are adequate to meet all expenses. Plans that fail to perform lag studies properly may find themselves staring into the abyss.

Law of small numbers—The notion that predictions that are based on large numbers (eg, a population of 2 million lives) have little relevance when the numbers are small (eg, 100 lives); then, chance plays a far more important role.

Line of business—A health plan (for example, an HMO, EPO, or PPO) that is set up as a line of business within another, larger organization, usually an insurance company. This legally differentiates it from a freestanding company or a company set up as a subsidiary. It may also refer to a unique product type (for example, Medicaid) within a health plan.

LOS—Length of stay.

Loss ratio—See Medical loss ratio.

MAC—Maximum allowable charge (or cost). The maximum, although not the minimum, that a vendor may charge for something. This term is often used in pharmacy contracting; a related term, used in conjunction with professional fees, is fee maximum.

Managed health care—A regrettably nebulous term. At the very least, managed health care is a system of health care delivery that tries to manage the cost of health care, the quality of that health care, and access to that care. Common denominators include a panel of contracted providers that is less than the entire universe of available providers, some type of limitations on benefits to subscribers who use noncontracted providers (unless authorized to do so), and some type of authorization system. Managed health care is actually a spectrum of systems, ranging from so-called managed indemnity, through PPOs, POS, open panel HMOs, closed panel HMOs, IDSs, and PSOs.

Mandated benefits—Benefits that a health plan is required to provide by law. This is generally used to refer to benefits above and beyond routine insurance-type benefits, and it generally applies at the state level (where there is high variability from state to state). Common examples include in vitro fertilization, defined days of inpatient mental health or substance abuse treatment, and other treatments for special conditions. Self-funded plans are exempt from mandated benefits under ERISA.

Master group contract—The actual contract between a health plan and a group that purchases coverage. The master group contract provides specific terms of coverage, rights, and responsibilities of both parties.

Maximum out-of-pocket cost—The largest amount of money a member will ever need to pay for covered services during a contract year. The maximum out-of-pocket cost includes deductibles and coinsurance. Once this limit is reached, the health plan pays for all services up to the maximum level of coverage. Applies mostly to non-HMO plans such as indemnity plans, PPOs, and POS plans.

MCE—Medical care evaluation. A component of a quality assurance program that looks at the process of medical care.

MCO—Managed care organization. A generic term applied to a managed care plan. Some people prefer it to the term HMO because it encompasses plans that do not conform exactly to the strict definition of an HMO (although that definition has itself loosened considerably). May also apply to a PPO, EPO, IDS, PSO, or OWA.

Medical loss ratio—The ratio between the cost to deliver medical care and the amount of money that was taken in by a plan. Insurance companies often have a medical loss ratio of 92% or more; tightly managed HMOs may have medical loss ratios of 75% to 85%, although the overhead (or administrative cost ratio) is concomitantly higher. The medical loss ratio is dependent on the amount of money brought in as well as the cost of delivering care; thus, if the rates are too low, the ratio may be high, even though the actual cost of delivering care is not really out of line.

Medical policy—Refers to the policies of a health plan regarding what will be paid for as medical benefits. Routine medical policy is linked to routine claims processing and may even be automated in the claims system; for example, the plan may pay only 50% of the fee of a second surgeon or may not pay for two surgical procedures done during one episode of anesthesia. This term also refers to how a plan approaches payment policies for experimental or investigational care, and payment for noncovered services in lieu of more expensive covered services.

Member—An individual covered under a managed care plan. May be either the subscriber or a dependent.

Member months—The total of all months that each member was covered. For example, if a plan had 10,000 members in January and 12,000 members in February, the total member months for the year to date as of March 1 would be 22,000.

MeSH—Medical staff-hospital organization. An archaic term. See PHO.

MET—Multiple employer trust. See MEWA.

MEWA—Multiple employer welfare association. A group of employers that band together to purchase or provide group health insurance, often through a self-funded approach to avoid state mandates and insurance regulation. ERISA provides for scant, if any, regulation of such entities. Many MEWAs have enabled small employers to obtain cost-effective health coverage, but some MEWAs have not had the financial resources to withstand the risk of medical costs and have failed, leaving the members without insurance or recourse. In some states, MEWAs and METs are no longer legal.

MIS—Management information system. The common term for the computer hardware and software that provides the support for managing the plan.

Mixed model—A managed care plan that mixes two or more types of delivery systems. This has traditionally been used to describe an HMO that has both closed panel and open panel delivery systems.

MLP—Midlevel practitioner. Physician's assistants, clinical nurse practitioners, nurse midwives, and the like. Nonphysicians who deliver medical care, generally under the supervision of a physician but for less cost.

MSO—Management service organization. A form of integrated health delivery system. Sometimes similar to a service bureau (see below), the MSO often actually purchases certain hard assets of a physician's practice, and then provides services to that physician at fair market rates. MSOs are usually formed as a means to contract more effectively with managed care organizations, although their simple creation does not guarantee success.

Multispecialty group—A medical group made up of different specialty physicians. May or may not include primary care.

NAHMOR—National Association of HMO Regulators.

NAIC—National Association of Insurance Commissioners.

NCQA—National Committee on Quality Assurance. A not-for-profit organization that performs quality-oriented accreditation reviews on HMOs and similar types of managed care plans. NCQA also accredits CVOs and develops HEDIS standards.

NDC—National drug code. The national classification system for identifying prescription drugs.

Network model HMO—A health plan that contracts with multiple physician groups to deliver health care to members. Generally limited to large single or multispecialty groups. Distinguished from group model plans that contract with a single medical group, IPAs that contract through an intermediary, and direct contract model plans that contract with individual physicians in the community.

No brainer—A term used to describe a decision so obvious that one doesn't need to engage one's brain in order to make the right choice. Not to be confused with a description of any figure in authority who *just does not get it*.

Nonpar—Short for nonparticipating. Refers to a provider that does not have a contract with the health plan.

OBRA—Omnibus Budget Reconciliation Act. What Congress calls the many annual tax and budget reconciliation acts. Most of these acts contain language important to managed care, generally in the Medicare market segment.

Observation unit—A treatment room, usually adjacent to the ED, where rapid evaluation and stabilization of a medical problem can be managed, resulting in discharge of the patient to home or, if necessary, admission of the patient to the hospital. Chest pain units are examples of observation units.

OMC—Office of Managed Care. The latest name for the federal agency that oversees federal qualification and compliance for HMOs and eligibility for CMPs and PSOs. Its former names were HMOS (Health Maintenance Organization Service), OHMO (Office of Health Maintenance Organizations), OPHC (Office of Prepaid Health Care), and Office of Prepaid Health Care Operations and Oversight (OPHCOO). Once part of the Public Health Service, the OMC and most of its predecessors are now part of the HCFA.

Open enrollment period—The period when an employee may change health plans; usually occurs once per year. A general rule is that most managed care plans will have around half their membership up for open enrollment in the fall for an effective date of January 1. A special form of open enrollment is still law in some states. This yearly open enrollment requires an HMO to accept any individual applicant (ie, one not coming in through an employer group) for coverage, regardless of health status. Such special open enrollments usually occur for 1 month each year. Many Blue Cross Blue Shield plans have similar open enrollments for indemnity products.

Open panel HMO—A managed care plan that contracts (either directly or indirectly) with private physicians to deliver care in their own offices. Examples would include a direct contract HMO and an IPA.

OPL—Other party liability. See COB.

OPM—Office of Personnel Management. The federal agency that administers the FEHBP. This is the agency with which a managed care plan contracts to provide coverage for federal employees.

Outlier—Something that is well outside of an expected range. May refer to providers who are using medical resources at a much higher rate than their peers, or to a case in a hospital that is far more expensive than anticipated, or in fact to anything at all that is significantly more or less than expected.

OWA—Other weird arrangement. A general acronym that applies to any new and bizarre managed care plan that has thought up a novel twist.

Package pricing—Also referred to as bundled pricing. An MCO pays an organization a single fee for all inpatient, outpatient, and professional expenses associated with a procedure, including preadmission and postdischarge care. Common procedures that use this form of pricing include cardiac bypass surgery and transplants.

Par provider—Shorthand term for participating provider (ie, one who has signed an agreement with a plan to provide services). May apply to professional or institutional providers.

PAS norms—The common term for Professional Activity Study results of the Commission on Professional and Hospital Activities. Broken out by region; the Western region has the lowest average LOS, so it tends to be used most often to set an estimated LOS. (Available as *LOS: Length of Stay by Diagnosis*, published by CPHA publications, Ann Arbor, MI.)

PCCM—Primary care case manager. This acronym is used in Medicaid managed care programs to describe when a state designates PCPs as case managers to function as gatekeepers but reimburses those PCPs using traditional Medicaid fee for service, as well as paying the PCP a nominal management fee, such as $2 to $5 PMPM.

PCP—Primary care physician. Generally applies to internists, pediatricians, family physicians, and general practitioners and occasionally to obstetrician/gynecologists.

PEPM—Per employee per month. Like PMPM, but moves the unit up to the level of the employee or subscriber, rather than measuring based on all members (subscribers plus dependents).

Per diem reimbursement—Reimbursement of an institution, usually a hospital, based on a set rate per day rather than on charges. Per diem reimbursement can be varied by service (for example, medical/surgical, obstetrics, mental health, and intensive care) or can be uniform regardless of intensity of services.

PHO—Physician-hospital organization. These are legal (or perhaps informal) organizations that bond hospitals and the attending medical staff. Frequently developed for the purpose of contracting with managed care plans. A PHO may be open to any member of the staff who applies or may be closed to staff members who fail to qualify (or who are part of an already overrepresented specialty).

PMG—Primary medical group. A group practice made up of primary care physicians, although some may have obstetrician/gynecologists as well.

PMPM—Per member per month. Specifically applies to a revenue or cost for each enrolled member each month.

PMPY—Per member per year. The same as PMPM but based on a year.

POD—Pool of doctors. This refers to the plan's grouping physicians into units smaller than the entire panel, but larger than individual practices. Typical PODs have between 10 and 30 physicians. Often used for performance measurement and compensation. The POD is often not a legal entity but just a grouping.

POS—Point of service. A plan where members do not have to choose how to receive services until they need them. The most common use of the term applies to a plan that enrolls each member in both an HMO (or HMO-like) system and an indemnity plan. Occasionally referred to as an HMO swing-out plan, an out-of-plan benefits rider to an HMO, or a primary care PPO. These plans provide a difference in benefits (for example, 100% coverage rather than 70%) depending on whether the member chooses to use the plan (including its providers and in compliance with the authorization system) or go outside the plan for services. Dual choice refers to an HMO-like plan with an indemnity plan, and triple choice refers to the addition of a PPO to the dual choice. An archaic but still valid definition applies to a simple PPO, where members receive coverage at a greater level if they use preferred providers (albeit without a gatekeeper system) than if they choose not to do so.

PPA—Preferred provider arrangement. Same as a PPO but sometimes used to refer to a somewhat looser type of plan in which the payer (ie, the employer) makes the arrangement rather than the providers. This is an archaic and seldomly used term.

PPM—Physician practice management company. An organization that manages physician's practices and in most cases either owns the practices outright or has rights to purchase them in the future. PPMs concentrate only on physicians, and not on hospitals, although some PPMs have also branched into joint ventures with hospitals and insurers. Many PPMs are publicly traded.

PPO—Preferred provider organization. A plan that contracts with independent providers at a discount for services. The panel is limited in size and usually has some type of utilization review system associated with it. A PPO may be risk bearing, like an insurance company, or may be non–risk bearing, like a physician-sponsored PPO that markets itself to insurance companies or self-insured companies via an access fee.

PPS—Prospective payment system. A generic term applied to a reimbursement system that pays prospectively rather than on the basis of charges. Generally, it is used only to refer to hospital reimbursement and applied only to DRGs, but it may encompass other methodologies as well.

Precertification—Also known as preadmission certification, preadmission review, and precert. The process of obtaining certification or authorization from the health plan for routine hospital admissions (inpatient or outpatient). Often involves appropriateness review against criteria and assignment of length of stay. Failure to obtain precertification often results in a financial penalty to either the provider or the subscriber.

Pre-existing condition—A medical condition for which a member has received treatment during a specified period of time prior to becoming covered under a health plan. May affect whether treatments for that condition will be covered under certain types of health plans.

Preventive care—Health care that is aimed at preventing complications of existing diseases or preventing the occurrence of a disease.

Private inurement—What happens when a not-for-profit business operates in such a way as to provide more than incidental financial gain to a private individual; for example, if a not-for-profit hospital pays too much money for a physician's practice, or fails to charge fair market rates for services provided to a physician. An Internal Revenue Service no-no.

PRO—Peer review organization. An organization charged with reviewing quality and cost for Medicare. Established under TEFRA. Generally operates at the state level.

Prospective review—Reviewing the need for medical care before the care is rendered. Also see Precertification.

Provider—The generic term used to refer to anyone providing medical services. In fact, it may even be used to refer to any entity that provides medical services, such as a hospital. Most often, however, it is used to refer to physicians. How physicians migrated from being called physicians to being called providers is not very clear, and the term is certainly not embraced by physicians, but it is a term in general use, including in this book.

Prudent layperson—See Reasonable layperson standard.

PSA—Professional services agreement. A contract between a physician or medical group and an IDS or MCO for the provision of medical services. Not to be confused with prostate surface antigen, a screening blood test for prostate cancer.

PSN—See PSO.

PSO—Provider-sponsored organization. Occasionally, the acronym is defined as provider service organization. Also referred to as a provider-sponsored network (PSN). A network developed by providers, whether as a vertically integrated IDS with both physicians and hospitals, or a physician-only network. Formed to contract directly with Medicare.

PTMPY—Per thousand members per year. A common way of reporting utilization. The most common example is hospital utilization, expressed as days per 1,000 members per year.

QA or QM—Quality assurance (older term) or quality management (newer term).

Rate—The amount of money that a group or individual must pay to the health plan for coverage. Usually a monthly fee. Rating refers to the health plan's developing those rates.

RBRVS—Resource-based relative value scale. This is a relative value scale developed for HCFA for use by Medicare. The RBRVS assigns relative values to each CPT code for services on the basis of the resources related to the procedure rather than simply on the basis of historic trends. The practical effect has been to lower reimbursement for procedural services (eg, cardiac surgery) and to raise reimbursement for cognitive services (eg, office visits).

Reasonable layperson standard—This means that the judgment of a reasonable nonclinician should be applied in determining if a service is warranted or not. This standard is almost always focused on the use of emergency or urgent care, when a layperson has good reason to believe that a medical problem must be addressed immediately, even if a trained provider may not feel that it was urgent. The specific language most often used, and addressed directly in the Balanced Budget Act of 1997 as pertaining to Medicare and Medicaid recipients, is: "Health plans should provide payment when a consumer presents to an emergency department with acute symptoms of sufficient severity—including severe pain—such that a 'prudent layperson' could reasonably expect the absence of medical attention to result in placing health in serious jeopardy, serious impairment to bodily functions, or serious dysfunction of any bodily organ or part."

Reinsurance—Insurance purchased by a health plan to protect it against extremely high cost cases. Also see Stop loss.

Reserves—The amount of money that a health plan puts aside to cover health care costs. May apply to anticipated costs such as IBNRs, or may apply to money that the plan does not expect to have to use to pay for current medical claims but keeps as a cushion against future adverse health care costs.

Retrospective review—Reviewing health care costs after the care has been rendered. There are several forms of retrospective review. One form looks at individual claims for medical necessity, billing errors, or fraud. Another form looks at patterns of costs, rather than individual cases.

Risk contract—Also known as a Medicare risk contract. A contract between an HMO, CMP, or PSO and HCFA to provide services to Medicare beneficiaries under which the health plan receives a fixed monthly payment for enrolled Medicare members, and then must provide all services on an at-risk basis.

Risk management—Management activities aimed at lowering an organization's legal and financial exposures, especially to lawsuits.

SCP—Specialty care physician. A physician who is not a PCP.

Second opinion—An opinion obtained from a physician regarding the necessity for a treatment that has been recommended by another physician. May be required by some health plans for certain high-cost cases such as cardiac surgery.

Self-care—The series of steps "lay" individuals take to assess and treat an illness or injury, typically without the benefit of higher levels of training in the theory or science of medicine and with little or no consultation with a medical professional.

Self-insured or self-funded plan—A health plan where the risk for medical cost is assumed by the company rather than an insurance company or managed care plan. Under ERISA, self-funded plans are exempt from state laws and regulations such as premium taxes and mandatory benefits. Self-funded plans often contract with insurance companies or third-party administrators to administer the benefits. See also ASO.

Sentinel effect—A name for a phenomenon that occurs when people know that their behavior is being observed: their behavior changes, often in the direction the observer is looking for. This effect can explain why utilization management systems and profiling systems often lead to reductions in utilization before much intervention even takes place, simply because the providers know that someone is watching.

Service area—The geographic area where an HMO provides access to primary care. The service area is usually specifically designated by the regulators (state or federal), and the HMO is prohibited from marketing outside of the service area. May be defined by county or by ZIP Code. It is possible for an HMO to have more than one service area and for the service areas to either be contiguous (ie, they border each other) or noncontiguous (ie, there is a geographic gap between the service areas).

Service bureau—A weak form of integrated delivery system in which a hospital (or other organization) provides services to a physician's practice in return for a fair market price. Service bureaus may also try to negotiate with managed care plans but generally are not considered effective negotiating mechanisms.

Service plan—A health insurance plan that has direct contracts with providers but is not necessarily a managed care plan. The archetypal (and virtually only) service plans are Blue Cross and Blue Shield plans. The contract applies to direct billing of the plan by providers (rather than billing of the member), a provision for direct payment of the provider (rather than reimbursement of the member), a requirement that the provider accept the plan's determination of UCR and not balance bill the member in excess of that amount, and a range of other terms. May or may not address issues of utilization and quality.

Shadow pricing—The practice of setting premium rates at a level just below the competition's rates, whether or not those rates can be justified. In other words, the premium rates could actually be lower, but to maximize profit the rates are raised to a level that will remain attractive but result in greater revenue. This practice is generally considered unethical and, in the case of community rating, possibly illegal.

SHMO—Social health maintenance organization. An HMO that goes beyond the medical care needs of its membership to address their social needs as well. A relatively rare form of HMO.

Shoebox effect—When an indemnity-type benefits plan has a deductible, there may be beneficiaries who save up their receipts to file for reimbursement at a later time (ie, save them in a shoebox). Those receipts then get lost, or the beneficiary never sends them in, so the insurance company never has to pay.

Single point of entry—A relatively new term that means that an individual uses the same system to access both group health medical benefits and benefits for work-related medical conditions.

SMG—Specialty medical group. A medical group made up predominantly of specialty physicians. May be a single specialty group or a multispecialty group.

Specialty network manager—A term used to describe a single specialist (or perhaps a specialist organization) that accepts capitation to manage a single specialty. Specialty services are supplied by many different specialty physicians, but the network manager has the responsibility for managing access and cost and is at economic risk. A relatively uncommon model as this text is being written.

Staff model HMO—An HMO that employs providers directly and has those providers see members in the HMO's own facilities. A form of closed-panel HMO. A different use of this term is sometimes applied to vertically integrated health care delivery systems that employ physicians but in which the system is not licensed as an HMO.

Stop loss—A form of reinsurance that provides protection for medical expenses above a certain limit, generally on a year-by-year basis. This may apply to an entire health plan or to any single component. For example, the health plan may have stop loss reinsurance for cases that exceed $100,000. After a case hits $100,000, the plan receives 80% of expenses in excess of $100,000 back from the reinsurance company for the rest of the year. Another example would be the plan providing a stop loss to participating physicians for referral expenses over $2,500. When a case exceeds that amount in a single year, the plan no longer deducts those costs from the physician's referral pool for the remainder of the year.

Subacute care facility—A health facility that is a step down from an acute care hospital. May be a nursing home, or a facility that provides medical care but not surgical or emergency care. However, a subacute care facility is a step up from the conventional skilled nursing facility intensity of services; it offers intravenous medications and registered nurses around the clock.

Subrogation—The contractual right of a health plan to recover payments made to a member for health care costs after that member has received such payment for damages in a legal action.

Subscribers—Members who have health plan coverage by virtue of being eligible on their own behalf, rather than as a dependent.

Sutton's law—"Go where the money is!" Attributed to the Depression-era bank robber Willy Sutton, who, when asked why he robbed banks, replied "That's where the money is." Sutton apparently denies ever having made that statement. In any event, it is a good law to use when determining what needs attention in a managed care plan.

TAT—Turnaround time. The amount of time it takes a health plan to process and pay a claim from the time it arrives.

TEFRA—Tax Equity and Fiscal Responsibility Act. One key provision of this Act prohibits employers and health plans from requiring full-time employees between the ages of 65 and 69 to use Medicare rather than the group health plan. Another key provision codified Medicare risk contracts for HMOs and CMPs.

Termination date—The day that health plan coverage is no longer in effect.

Time loss management—The application of managed care techniques to workers' compensation treatments for injuries or illnesses in order to reduce the amount of time lost on the job by the affected employee.

Total capitation—See Global capitation.

TPA—Third-party administrator. A firm that performs administrative functions (for example, claims processing, membership, and the like) for a self-funded plan or a start-up managed care plan (also see ASO).

Triage—The process of sorting out requests for services by members into those who need to be seen right away, those who can wait a little while, and those whose problems can be handled with advice over the phone.

Triple option—The offering of an HMO, a PPO, and a traditional insurance plan by one carrier.

Twenty-four-hour care—An ill-defined term that essentially means that health care is provided 24 hours per day, regardless of the financing mechanism; applies primarily to the convergence of group health, workers' compensation, and industrial health, all under managed care.

UB-92—The common claim form used by hospitals to bill for services. Some managed care plans demand greater detail than is available on the UB-92, requiring the hospitals to send additional itemized bills.

UCR—Usual, customary, or reasonable. A method of profiling prevailing fees in an area and reimbursing providers on the basis of that profile. One archaic method is to average all fees and choose the 80th or 90th percentile, although in this era a plan will usually use another method to determine what is reasonable. Sometimes this term is used synonymously with fee allowance schedule when the fee allowance schedule is set relatively high.

Unbundling—The practice of a provider billing for multiple components of service that were previously included in a single fee. For example, if dressings and instruments were included in a fee for a minor procedure, the fee for the procedure remains the same but there are now additional charges for the dressings and instruments.

Underwriting—In one definition, this refers to bearing the risk for something (ie, a policy is underwritten by an insurance company). In another definition, this refers to the analysis of a group that is done to determine rates and benefits, or to determine whether the group should be offered coverage at all. A related definition refers to health screening of each applicant for insurance and refusing to provide coverage for pre-existing conditions.

Upcoding—The practice of a provider billing for a procedure that pays better than the service actually performed. For example, an office visit that would normally be reimbursed at $45 is coded as one that is reimbursed at $53.

URAC—Utilization Review Accreditation Commission. A not-for-profit organization that performs reviews on external utilization review agencies (freestanding companies, utilization management departments of insurance companies, or utilization management departments of managed care plans). Its sole focus is managed indemnity and PPOs, not HMOs or similar types of plans. States often require certification by URAC for a utilization management organization to operate.

URO—Utilization review organization. A freestanding organization that does nothing but UR (utilization review), usually on a remote basis, using the telephone and paper correspondence. It may be independent or may be part of another company such as an insurance company that sells UR services on a stand-alone basis.

Waste, fraud, and abuse—This troika is used to name greedy and sometimes illegal behavior on the part of either providers or health plans. The term is usually used by the government but may be used by private purchasers of health care benefits. See also Fraudandabuse.

Workers' compensation—A form of social insurance provided through property–casualty insurers. Workers' compensation provides medical benefits and replacement of lost wages that result from injuries or illnesses that arise from the workplace; in turn, the employee cannot normally sue the employer unless true negligence exists. Workers' compensation has undergone dramatic increases in cost as group health has shifted into managed care, resulting in workers' compensation carriers adopting managed care approaches. Workers' compensation is often heavily regulated under state laws that are significantly different than those used for group health insurance, and it is often the subject of intense negotiation between management and organized labor. See also Time loss management and Twenty-four-hour care.

Wraparound plan—Term commonly used to refer to insurance or health plan coverage for co-pays and deductibles that are not covered under a member's base plan. This is often used for Medicare.

Zero down—The practice of a medical group or provider system distributing all of the capital surplus in a health plan or group to the members of the group, rather than retaining any capital or reinvesting it in the group or plan.

Index

A

Accountability, in office service management, 247–248
Accreditation, of subacute care provider, 291–292
ACE inhibitors, in congestive heart failure management, 356
ACE unit, for Medicare managed care, 629–633
ACHM. *See* American Centers for Health and Medicine
Activity/precedent table format, in critical path approach, 227–228
Actuarial data, lack of, in alternative medicine, 590
Acupuncture, use of, 572
Acute inpatient care, 151–217
Administrative costs, medical costs, distinguished, 153
Advanced care management. *See* Medical management
Advice services, nursing, 117–124
    call center
        efficiency of, 120
        size of, 119–120
    clinical knowledge systems, 120–121
    developments in, 119–120
    historical incentives, 117–119
    process engineering and, 121–122
    technology in, 121
After-hours care, Medicare, 633
Aging population. *See* Elderly
Alternative medicine, 567–610
    actuarial data, lack of, 590
    case studies, 603–610
    cost, 590
    coverage, growth in, 577–578
    credentialing, 593–597
    defining benefit, 597
    diabetes, 576
    discounted services, through credentialed networks, 597–598
    efficacy of, 575–576
    growth in, 569–570
    heart disease, 575–576
    integration of, 579–580, 588–593
        American Centers for Health and Medicine, 608–610
        gatekeeping, 581–582
            philosophy of, 583
            utilization review, 581–582
        Group Health Cooperative of Puget Sound, 605–608
        Kaiser Northern California, 603–605
        paradigm issues, 592
        physician acceptance, 580–581
        team care, 580
    low back pain, 576
    modalities, 570–575
        acupuncture, 572
        chiropractic, 572–573
        herbal therapies, 573
        homeopathy, 573–574
        massage/somatic practices, 574
        mind-body medicine, 574–575
    overutilization, controlling, 582–583
    prevention, 575
    professional development, 576–577
        certification, 576–577
        licensure, 576–577
    rider, 598–601
        limits of, 600–601
    standards, 592
    structuring, 578–583
    wellness, 575
Ambulatory care, 239–266
    assessment of practice, 10–11
    clinical outcomes measurement, 498–500
    guidelines, 261–266
        financial risk management, 265
        guideline products, in ambulatory care, 263–265
        products, 263–265
American Centers for Health and Medicine, alternative medicine integration, 608–610

Ancillary services, 307–336
  authority to authorize, limits on, 313
  contracting, 313–315
  data capture and, 311
  financial incentives for, 311
  physician-owned, 310–311
  reimbursement for, 313–315
  services authorized, limits on, 313
Assessment, of health risk, 19–34
Assisted living, in Medicare managed care, 630–631
Asthma disease management, 377–395
  asthma workshops, 390
  barriers to implementation, 393–394
  buddy system, 390
  co-case management, 388
  complications of, 378–379
  epidemiology, 378
  industry alternatives to, 392–393
  manageability, 379
  Medicaid education, 390
  member education, materials for, 388–389
  Oxford Health Plan components, 380–385
    case management, 384
    continuous quality improvement, 385
    education
      member, 381–382
      provider, 382–383
    network development, 383–384
    outcomes, evaluation of, 385
    patient empowerment, 381
    technological support, 384–385
    treatment guidelines, 382
  patient identification, 386–387
    durable medical equipment request, 387
    field outreach, 387
    Medicaid welcome call, 387
    Medicare high-risk assessment, 387
    member profile, 387
    member referral, 386
    pharmacy data, 386
    physician referral, 386
    utilization episode, 386
  patient stratification, 387
  program objectives, 379–380
  progress, tracking of, 390–392
  self-management resources, 389–390
  treatment, 379
Audit, pharmaceutical services, 330
Authority, to authorize, limits on, ancillary services and, 313
Authorization for clinical services, 249–260
  authorization system reports, 258–259
  categories of authorization, 253–255
    concurrent, 253–254
    denial, 254–255
    pended, 254
    prospective, 253
    retrospective, 254
    subauthorization, 255

  claims payment, 252
  concurrent, 253–254
  data
    capture, methods for, 257–258
    elements, 256
  electronic authorization systems, 258
  issuance, methods for, 257–258
  non-physician-based authorization systems, 260
  open access HMOs, 259
  paper-based authorization systems, 257
  point of service, 252–253
  specialty physician-based authorization systems, 260
  staffing, 255–256
  telephone-based authorization systems, 257–258
Authorization in medical-surgical utilization, 158

B

Back pain, alternative medicine in, 576
Behavioral factors, pregnancy prevention, 91–92
Behavioral health care, 407–432
  benefit plan design, 417–419
    coverage limits, 417
    disorders, types of, 418
    incentives, 419
    levels of care, 417
    providers, types of, 418
    treatment, types of, 418
  channeling mechanisms, 420–422
  continuum of care, 412
  data systems, 427–429
  integrated delivery systems, provider structures for, 423–425
  mental health case manager, as gatekeepers, 421–422
  methods of treatment, 411–412
    crisis intervention, 412
    goal-directed psychotherapy, 412
    psychiatric hospitalization, alternatives to, 411
    restrictive treatment for substance abuse, alternatives to, 411–412
  objectives of treatment, 409
  provider networks, 422–423
    selection criteria, 422–423
    size, scope of, 422
  public/private systems integration, 429–430
  quality assurance, 425–427
    external quality assurance monitoring, 426–427
      inservice training, 427
      staff qualifications, 426
      utilization criteria, 426
    network providers, 425–426
    outcomes measurement, 427
    problem identification, 427
    provider credentialing, 427
    utilization review/case management, 425
  strategic approaches, 409–410
  substance abuse case manager, as gatekeepers, 421–422
  treatment principles, 408–412

treatment services, 413–417
  basic mental health services, 413–414
  dual diagnosis, 414–415
  paradigmatic shifts, 415–417
  substance abuse services, 413
 utilization management, 419–420
  case management, 419–420
  utilization review, 419
Behavioral/motivational activities, of patient, 190
Beliefs, effect of, on change, 552
Benchmarking, in medical management, 11–12
"Best-of-class" standards, in quality management, 445–446
Biological needs, defining, 63–65
Budget development, hospice, 302–303

C

Call center, in nurse advice service
 efficiency of, 120
 size of, 119–120
Cardiac nurses, for congestive heart failure management, 355–356
Cardiologists, role of, in congestive heart failure management, 356
Care management. *See* Medical management
Carve-out accommodation, vendors, provider profiling, 531
Case management
 assessing data, 192–193
 case management reports, 205
 concurrent review, case management reports, 205
 equipment providers, talking with, 197
 monitoring, 199–200
 process of, 192–200
 second opinion exam, 196–197
Case manager role, 187–217
 24-hour coverage programs, 215
 claims management, 213–214
 community resources, talking with, 198
 coordinating, 199–200
 cost benefit analysis reports, 214–215
 disease management, 215–216
 evaluating plan, 200
 family, talking with, 196
 gathering data, 192–193
 independent medical exam, 196–197
 indicators for, 205–212
 initial assessment, 193
 on-site versus telephone-based, 190–191
 patient, talking with, 194–195
 patient profile, 188–190
  behavioral/motivational activities, 190
  financial activities, 189–190
  medical activities, 189
  vocational activities, 190
 payer, obtaining approval from, 199
 planning, 198
 preadmission review, case management reports, 205
 referral source, talking with, 193–194

 reporting, 198–199
 service providers, talking with, 197
 timing of, 213
 treating physician, talking with, 196
 utilization review, 200–205
 wellness programs, 215
 work format, 192–200
Case mix, adjusting for, in provider profiling, 527–528
Certificate of coverage, pharmaceutical services, 319–320
Certification, in alternative therapies, 576–577
Cessation of smoking. *See* Smoking cessation
Change, organizational, process of, in medical management, 10–11
Chemical dependency services, 407–432
 benefit plan design, 417–419
  coverage limits, 417
  disorders, types of, 418
  incentives, 419
  levels of care, 417
  providers, types of, 418
  treatment, types of, 418
 channeling mechanisms, 420–422
 continuum of care, 412
 data systems, 427–429
 integrated delivery systems, provider structures for, 423–425
 methods of treatment, 411–412
  crisis intervention, 412
  goal-directed psychotherapy, 412
  restrictive treatment for substance abuse, alternatives to, 411–412
 objectives of treatment, 409
 provider networks, 422–423
  selection criteria, 422–423
  size, scope of, 422
 public/private systems integration, 429–430
 quality assurance, 425–427
  external quality assurance monitoring, 426–427
   inservice training, 427
   staff qualifications, 426
   utilization criteria, 426
  network providers, 425–426
  outcomes measurement, 427
  problem identification, 427
  provider credentialing, 427
  utilization review/case management, 425
 strategic approaches, 409–410
 substance abuse case manager, as gatekeepers, 421–422
 treatment principles, 408–412
 treatment services, 413–417
 utilization management, 419–420
  case management, 419–420
  utilization review, 419
Chest pain center, 139–150
 chest pain unit, 141–143
 defined, 140–141
 development of, 148–149
 economic benefits, 146–147

management of
    change in, 140
    traditional, 139–140
observation program, 143
outreach program, 143
quality management program, 144–146
Chiropractic care, 572–573
Claims adjudication
    electronic, in pharmaceutical services, 325
    in pharmaceutical services, 324
Claims management, case manager role, 213–214
Clinical knowledge systems, in nurse advice service, 120–121
Clinical outcome
    management of, 501–510
        clinical processes
            characterization of, 502–504
            components of, 501–502
            processes of care, clinical outcomes, relation, 504–509
        measurement of, 461–477, 479–500
            ambulatory care, 498–500
            control charts, 487–489
            data integration, 489–492
            databases, 485–487
            risk-adjusted functional status, 493–498
        with medical management, 501–510
Clinical preventive services, 39
Clinical processes
    characterization of, 502–504
    components of, 501–502
Clinical quality, measurement, 433–510
Clinical staff, subacute care, 293
Clinician office service management, 241–248
    accountability, 247–248
    collaboratives, 245–247
    points of engagement, 241–242
    practice guideline
        development, 242–245
        program, 242–243
    trust in, 248
Clinician's office, medical management in, 241–248
Closed panel managed care organization, 321–322
Collaboratives, in office service management, 245–247
Collection of data, in critical path approach, 223
Community-based hospice care, 302
Community programs, 40–42
    for managed care, 39
    prevention in, 39, 40–42
Community resources, case manager role with, 198
Companions, in home health care, 275
Compensation, for specialty physicians, 161
Complementary and alternative medicine, 567–610
    actuarial data, lack of, 590
    case studies, 603–610
    cost, 590
    coverage, growth in, 577–578
    credentialing, 593–597
    defining benefit, 597
    diabetes, 576
    discounted services, through credentialed networks, 597–598
    efficacy of, 575–576
    growth in, 569–570
    heart disease, 575–576
    integration of, 579–580, 588–593
        American Centers for Health and Medicine, 608–610
        gatekeeping, 581–582
            philosophy of, 583
            utilization review, 581–582
        Group Health Cooperative of Puget Sound, 605–608
        Kaiser Northern California, 603–605
        paradigm issues, 592
        physician acceptance, 580–581
        team care, 580
    low back pain, 576
    modalities, 570–575
        acupuncture, 572
        chiropractic, 572–573
        herbal therapies, 573
        homeopathy, 573–574
        massage/somatic practices, 574
        mind-body medicine, 574–575
    overutilization, controlling, 582–583
    prevention, 575
    professional development, 576–577
        certification, 576–577
        licensure, 576–577
    rider, 598–601
        limits of, 600–601
    standards, 592
    structuring, 578–583
    wellness, 575
Components of medical management
    advanced, 15–17
        elements beyond, 16–17
        infrastructure, 16
    integration of, 4–6
Concurrent authorization, for clinical services, 253–254
Concurrent review, institutional, 166–172
    assignment of length of stay, 166
    communications, 171–172
    daily review of utilization, 172
    discharge planning, 168–169
    hospitalist model, 170–171
    medical director's responsibilities, 171
    primary care physician responsibilities, 169–170
    specialist physician responsibilities, 170
    utilization management nurse, 166–168
Congestive heart failure disease management, 349–362
    ACE inhibitors, 356
    acute care, 358
    cardiac nurses, 355–356
    cardiologists, role of, 356
    care continuum, 350–351
    confirmation, 353
    cost benefit analysis, 360

education, 356–357
evaluation, 359–360
  internal measurement, 360
  process/outcome of care, 359–360
  quality of life, 359
  satisfaction, 360
home visits, 357
incentives, 358–359
interventions, 354–355
outpatient clinic, 358
population-based identification, 351–353
prioritization, 353–354
rehabilitation, 358
stratification, 353–354
telemonitoring, 357
validation, 353
Consumer education, quality management and, 455–456
Continuum process, extended, in medical management, assessment of, 10–11
Contraception, 94
Contracting, for ancillary services, 313–315
Control charts, in measurement of clinical outcomes, 487–489
Core competencies, medical management and, 339–347
Cost benefit analysis
  congestive heart failure management, 360
  reports, case manager role, 214–215
Costs
  in alternative medicine, 590
  of drugs, 318
  economic concept of, in disease management, 397–398
  pharmaceutical services, 323–324
  referral, Medicare managed care, 633
  in subacute care, 294
Credentialing, in alternative medicine, 593–597
Crisis intervention, in behavioral health care, 412
Critical path approach, 219–237
  activity/precedent table format, 227–228
  alternatives formats, 227–228
  best practices, determination of, 223–224
  current practices, challenging, 222
  data, collection of, 223
  developing, 223–226
  diagnosis, 223
  environment for, 221–223
    champions, 222
    external environment, 222
    urgency to change, 222
  floats, 233
  flowcharts, 223, 228
  Gantt chart format, 228
  multidisciplinary team, 223
  outcomes, identification of, 224
  patient care objectives, defining, 224–225
  resource formats, 228–233
  sample uses, 227–228
  scope of, 223
  slack time data, 233
  standardization, versus independence, 222–223
  uses of, overview, 220–221
Cultural needs, defining, 65–66
Cultural sensitivity, 72

D

Daily log, in hospital utilization report, 517–519
Data, use of, 39, 511–532
  actuarial, lack of, in alternative medicine, 590
  case manager role in gathering, 192–193
  collection of, in critical path approach, 223
  focus of, 516–517
    geographically related center, 516–517
    health center, 516–517
    physician, individual, 517
    plan average, 516
    practice association, individual, 516–517
    premium source group, 517
    provider organization, 516–517
    service type, 517
    vendor type, 517
  hospital utilization report, 517–520
    daily log, 517–519
    monthly summary, 519
  medical-surgical utilization and, 156–157
  outpatient utilization, 520–522
  patient, hospice care, 298–299
  provider profiling, 522–523
    feedback, 523
    focused utilization management, 523
    incorporation, other data, 522–523
  requirements for using, 513–516
    data characteristics, 513–516
    format, 515
    reports, 515–516
    tools, use with, 515
    user needs, 515
  service type, 517
Data capture
  ancillary services and, 311
  for authorization, methods, 257–258
Data integration, in measurement of clinical outcomes, 489–492
Data tools, for prevention in clinical setting, 50–51
Databases, in measurement of clinical outcomes, 485–487
Defining benefit, in alternative medicine, 597
Delegated self-care, 105–109
Demographic shifts, and demand for home health care, 272
Denial of authorization, for clinical services, 254–255
Diabetes
  alternative medicine in, 576
  disease management, 363–376
    changes necessary, 371–374
      within health care system, 371–372
      within health care team, 372
      for patient, 372–374

foot care, 368
future developments, 374–375
identification, 365
patient education, 368
population-based approach, 364–371
progress, tracking of, 369–371
retinal screening, 368
vital statistics, 368
Dieticians, in home health care, 275
Disease management, 337–432. *See also under* specific disease
barriers to, 341
benefits of, 401–403
economic, 397–406
business plan, 342
case study, 345–346
core competencies, 339–347
costs, 403–405
defined, 339
drivers for, 341
economic study designs, 401
effectiveness of, studies, 404–405
evaluation issues, 398–401
program survey, 342–344
Disease prevention. *See* Prevention
Drug dependency services, 407–432
benefit plan design, 417–419
coverage limits, 417
disorders, types of, 418
incentives, 419
levels of care, 417
providers, types of, 418
treatment, types of, 418
channeling mechanisms, 420–422
continuum of care, 412
data systems, 427–429
integrated delivery systems, provider structures for, 423–425
methods of treatment, 411–412
crisis intervention, 412
goal-directed psychotherapy, 412
restrictive treatment for substance abuse, alternatives to, 411–412
objectives of treatment, 409
provider networks, 422–423
selection criteria, 422–423
size, scope of, 422
public/private systems integration, 429–430
quality assurance, 425–427
external quality assurance monitoring, 426–427
inservice training, 427
staff qualifications, 426
utilization criteria, 426
network providers, 425–426
outcomes measurement, 427
problem identification, 427
provider credentialing, 427
utilization review/case management, 425
strategic approaches, 409–410
substance abuse case manager, as gatekeepers, 421–422
treatment principles, 408–412
treatment services, 413–417
utilization management, 419–420
case management, 419–420
utilization review, 419
Drug formulary, in pharmaceutical services, 331

E

Economic study designs, in disease management, 401
Education
in congestive heart failure management, 356–357
pregnancy prevention and, 93–94
Elderly
aging process, Medicare managed care, 623–624
chronic diseases, incidence of, 624
dependence on caregivers, 625
functional capabilities, 624
mental health illness, 624–625
polypharmacy, 624
high-risk, Medicare screening, 633–634
Electronic authorization systems, 258
Electronic claims adjudication, in pharmaceutical services, 325
Eligibility verification, pharmaceutical services, 325
Emergency department
fast track, 135–150
design of, 137
location, 137
observation unit, 135–136
processes, 137
schedule, 137
staffing, 136
triage, 131–132
transfer, 129–131
Emergency services, 125–150. *See also* Emergency department
efficient use of, 127–134
emergency department, triage, 129–132
transfer, 129–131
triage, 131–132
site
for continuing care, 133
for immediate care, 132–133
staff selection
for continuing care, 133
for immediate care, 132–133
triage
emergency department, 129–132
prehospital, 128–129
Enabling technologies, in self-care, 111
Enrollment data, pharmaceutical services, 325
Episodes of care, in provider profiling, 527

Ethics, in hospice care, 300
Evaluation
    in disease management, 398–401
    of health risk appraisal instrument, 32–33
Extended care facility, hospice affiliated with, 302
Extended continuum process, medical management, assessment of, 10–11

F

Family, case manager role with, 196
Fast track emergency department, 135–150
Feedback, in quality management, 449–451
Financial activities, in patient profile, 189–190
Financial risk management, in ambulatory procedures, 265
Financing home health care, 277–278
Flowchart
    in critical path approach, 223
    network format, 228
Foot care, in diabetes management, 368
Formal, versus informal caregivers, demand for home health care and, 272–273
Future developments, in medical management, overview, 7–8

G

Gantt chart format, in critical path approach, 228
Gatekeeping, in alternative medicine, 581–582
    philosophy of, 583
    utilization review, 581–582
Government programs, 611–636. *See also under* specific program
    as provider of pharmaceutical benefit, 323
Group, constitution of, in provider profiling, 529
Group Health Cooperative of Puget Sound, alternative medicine integration, 605–608

H

Habit-based health risk appraisals, 23
Health advisory services, 97–124
Health center data, 516–517
Health data systems
    in managed care, 39
    for prevention, 39
Health risk appraisal, 19–34
    instrument for, 29–34
        evaluation of, 32–33
        individuals surveyed, 31
        methodology, 31, 32
        rationale for, 29–31
        response, 32
        timing, 32
    models, 22–24
        habit-based, 23
        risk-based, 22–23
        utilization-based, 23–24
    target populations, 25–26
    technologies, 24–25
Heart disease, alternative medicine in, 575–576
HEDIS 3.0 production
    vendors, provider profiling, 531
Herbal therapies, 573
High-risk behaviors, preventive programs for, 75–96
History of home health care, 270
Home health care, 269–280
    advanced clinical practices in, 280
    as alternative to acute care hospitalization, 174–175
    defined, 270
    demand for, predictors of, 271–273
        demographic shifts, 272
        formal, versus informal caregivers, 272–273
        hospital system shrinkage, 272
    financing, 277–278
    history of, 270
    infusion services, 273
    medical equipment, supplies, 273
    nursing services, traditional, 273
    professional disciplines, 274–275
        companions, 275
        dieticians, 275
        home health aides, 275
        homemakers, 275
        medical social workers, 274
        nurses, 274
        occupational therapists, 274
        physical therapies, 274
        physicians, 274–275
        respiratory therapists, 274
        speech language pathologists, 274
        volunteers, 275
    quality management, 279–280
    regulation of, 275–277, 278–279
    respiratory services, 273–274
Home visits, congestive heart failure management, 357
Homemakers, in home health care, 275
Homeopathy, 573–574
Hospice care, 295–305
    as alternative to acute care hospitalization, 174
    budget development, 302–303
    community-based, 302
    extended care facility, affiliated with, 302
    financing, 297–298
    freestanding, 301
    future developments in, 304–305
    growth in, 296
    growth projections, 299
    hospital-based, 301–302
    hospitalist model, service, 301–302
    managed care, 297–298
    medical coverage, 297
    Medicare benefit, 297

organization of, 296–297
patient data, 298–299
philosophy of, 295
policy issues, 300–301
  care provision, 301
  ethics, 300
  legal issues, 300–301
program development, 301–302
reimbursement, 297–298
size of industry, 298–299
skilled nursing facility, affiliated with, 302
specialty programs, 304
  pediatric hospice programs, 304
  Zen Hospice Project Residence Program, 304
structure, 296–297
Hospital-based hospice care, 301–302
Hospital-based processes, medical management, assessment of, 10
Hospital system shrinkage, demand for home health care and, 272
Hospital utilization report, 517–520
  daily log, 517–519
  monthly summary, 519
Hospitalist model
  in hospice care, 301–302
  inpatient care management, 179–185
    clinical outcomes, 181–182
    community physicians, 182–183
    continuum of care, 183
    hospitalist model, 179–181
    pitfalls of, 183–184
    recruiting hospitalists, 184
HRA. *See* Health risk appraisal
Humana program, member behavior change, 561–564
  materials, 563
  opinion, effect on, 563–564
  participation data, 563
  patient changes, 563
  program effect, 563

I

ICSI. *See* Institute for Clinical Systems Integration
Immigrant population, clinical preventive services, 63–73
  biological needs, defining, 63–65
  commitment, fostering of, 69
  community assessment, 67
  contact, 66–67
  cultural needs, defining, 65–66
  cultural sensitivity, 72
  development of program, 67–68
  interpretation of behaviors, 70–72
  nurses, role of, 69–70
  program design, 67–68
  progress evaluation, 69
Implementation, staged, in medical management, 13

IMPROVE Project, learning research trial, 50
Indemnity insurance plans, as provider of pharmaceutical benefit, 322–323
Independent medical exam, case manager role, 196–197
Information. *See* Data
Infrastructure, 16
  design of, 10–11
Infusion services, home care, 273
Ingredient cost, in pharmaceutical services, 326–329
  drug formularies, 327–329
  flat rate, 327
  generic drug policy, 326–327
  rebates, 329
  volume purchasing, 329
  wholesale price discounts, 327
Initial assessment, case manager role, 193
Inpatient care, acute, 151–217
Institute for Clinical Systems Integration, 49–50
Institutional utilization management, 161–176
  acute care hospitalization, alternatives to, 172–175
    home health care, 174–175
    hospice care, 174
    outpatient procedure units, 174
    step-down units, 174
    subacute care, 173–174
  concurrent review, 166–172
    assignment of length of stay, 166
    communications, 171–172
    daily review of utilization, 172
    discharge planning, 168–169
    hospitalist model, 170–171
    medical director's responsibilities, 171
    primary care physician responsibilities, 169–170
    specialist physician responsibilities, 170
    utilization management nurse, 166–168
  formulas, 162
  large case management, 175–176
  measurements, 162–163
  prospective review, 164–166
    mandatory outpatient surgery, 165–166
    preadmission testing, 165
    precertification, 164–165
  retrospective review, 172
    claims review, 172
    pattern review, 172
Interactive voice response system, use of in smoking cessation, 87–88
Internet, use of in smoking cessation, 86
Interpretation of behaviors, with immigrant population, 70–72

K

Kaiser Northern California, alternative medicine integration, 603–605
Knowledge systems, clinical, in nurse advice service, 120–121

L

Large case management, by specialty physicians, 161
Leadership
 in managed care, 39–40
Legal issues, in hospice care, 300–301
Licensure, in alternative therapies, 576–577
Location, of emergency department, 137
Long-term care hospitals, as provider of subacute care, 288
Long-term planning, in medical management, 12–13
Low back pain, alternative medicine in, 576

M

Marketing techniques, use of in smoking cessation, 81–85
 duration, 81
 frequency, 81
 intensity, 81
 pricing, 84–85
 resource optimization, 81–84
 segmentation, 81–84
Massage, 574
Measurement
 of clinical outcomes, 461–477, 479–500
  control charts, 487–489
  data integration, 489–492
  databases, 485–487
  domains, 461–462
  goals, 462–463
  process, 463–476
  risk-adjusted functional status, 493–498
 of clinical quality, 433–510
Medicaid
 asthma disease management, 390
 managed care, 613–622
  barriers to care, 616–617
  capitation rates, 618–619
  compliance, improvement, 620–621
  defined, 613–614
  effective plan, characteristics of, 619–620
  enrollment, 615–616
  expenditures, 615–616
  health risk factors, 617–618
  initiatives, 618
  member access, improvement, 620–621
  preventive care, 617
 pharmaceutical service benefit, 323
 vendors, provider profiling, 530
Medical costs, administrative costs, distinguished, 153
Medical equipment, supplies, for home health care, 273
Medical informatics, medical-surgical utilization and, 155
Medical management
 advanced, 1–17
 asthma, 377–395
 case management, 187–217
 characteristics of, 6
 clinical outcome with, 501–510
 in clinician's office, 241–248
 components, integration of, 4–6
 congestive heart failure, 349–362
 core competencies, 339–347
 diabetes, 363–376
 elements beyond, 16–17
 establishment of, 9–13
  ambulatory practice, assessment of, 10–11
  benchmarking, 11–12
  current state assessment, 9–11
  extended continuum process, assessment of, 10–11
  future state design, 11–12
  hospital-based processes, assessment of, 10
  implementation, staged, 13
  infrastructure design, 10–11
  long-term plan, 12–13
  mission, 9–11
  model, construction of, 12–13
  organizational change process, assessment of, 10–11
  vision, 9–11
 future issues in, overview, 7–8
 infrastructure, 16
 investment, return on, 397–406
 in Medicare population, 623–636
 nurse advice services in, 122–123
 overview, 1–14
 physician, role of, 8–9
 prevention in, 37–38
 quality control, 435–459
 use of data in, 513–524
Medical social workers, in home health care, 274
Medical-surgical utilization, 153–177
 administrative costs, medical costs, distinguished, 153
 authorization system, 158
 compensation, for specialty physicians, 161
 consulting providers, selection of, 158
 data, 156–157
 demand management, 154–156
  health risk appraisal, 155–156
  medical consumerism program, 154
  medical informatics, 155
  nurse advice lines, 154
  preventive services, 155–156
  self-care program, 154
  shared decision-making programs, 154–155
 financial incentives for specialty physicians, 161
 institutional utilization management, 161–176
  acute care hospitalization, alternatives to, 172–175
   home health care, 174–175
   hospice care, 174
   intermediate nursing facilities, 173–174
   outpatient procedure units, 174
   skilled nursing facilities, 173–174
   step-down units, 174
   subacute care, 173–174
  concurrent review, 166–172
   assignment of length of stay, 166

communications, 171–172
daily review of utilization, 172
discharge planning, 168–169
follow-up, 168–169
hospitalist model, 170–171
medical director's responsibilities, 171
primary care physician responsibilities, 169–170
specialist physician responsibilities, 170
utilization management nurse, 166–168
formulas, 162
large case management, 175–176
measurements, 162–163
prospective review, 164–166
mandatory outpatient surgery, 165–166
preadmission testing, 165
precertification, 164–165
same-day surgery, 165
retrospective review, 172
claims review, 172
pattern review, 172
large case management by specialty physicians, 161
referral providers, selection of, 158
self-referrals by members, 161
specialty physician services, control of, 158–160
reasons for referral, review of, 160
secondary referrals, prohibition of, 159–160
single visit authorization, 158–159
specialty physician utilization management, 156–161
Medicare
benefit, hospice care, 297
managed care, 623–636
acute care, 626–633
ACE unit, 629–633
assisted living, 630–631
nursing home, 630–631
outpatient care, 631–633
transitional care, 629–630
admissions, 627
after-hours care, 633
extended care pathways, 627–629
length of stay, 627
referral costs, 633
aging process, health care utilization and, 623–624
chronic diseases, incidence of, 624
dependence on caregivers, 625
functional capabilities, 624
mental health illness, 624–625
polypharmacy, 624
characteristics of, 623–625
development of program, 634–635
fee, blend of, for service, capitation, 634–635
population management, 633–634
case management, 634
high-risk elderly, screening for, 633–634
program development model, 625–626
continuum of care, 626

data, access to, 626
regulatory issues, 626
referral costs, 633
subspecialists, 633
population, medical management, 623–636
vendors, provider profiling, 530
Medications. *See* Pharmaceutical services
Member behavior change, 549–565
beliefs, effect of, 552
Humana program, 561–564
materials, 563
opinion, effect on, 563–564
participation data, 563
patient changes, 563
program effect, 563
models for, 553–558
community systems, 554
patient-provider models, 554–556
relapse, 556–557
stepped model, 556
system-based models, 553–554
worksite model, 557–558
readiness to change, 550–551
tools, 558–561
communications, 558
reinforcers, 558–561
action plans, 559
contracts, 559
incentives, 560–561
reminder systems, 559
rewards, 560–561
tracking methods, 558–559
social support, 561–562
coaching, 561
enlisting, 561
Mental health case manager, 421–422
Mind-body medicine, 574–575
Mission, in medical management, 9–11
Model
health risk appraisal, 22–24
habit-based, 23
risk-based, 22–23
utilization-based, 23–24
hospitalist, 170–171, 179–185
clinical outcomes, 181–182
community physicians, 182–183
service, 301–302
inpatient care, 179–185
medical management
advanced, construction of, 12–13
construction of, 12–13
modern quality management program, process, 439–456
for patient behaviors, 553–558
primary care physician, 170
program development in managed care, 625–626
risk-adjustment, for clinical indicators, 466–469
rounding physician, or hospitalist, 170–171

Monthly summary, in hospital utilization report, 519
Motivational activities, of patient, 190
Multidisciplinary team, in critical path approach, 223

N

Non-physician-based authorization systems, 260
Nurse advice services, 117–124
   call center
      efficiency, 120
      size, 119–120
   clinical knowledge systems, 120–121
   developments in, 119–120
   historical incentives, 117–119
   medical-surgical utilization and, 154
   process engineering and, 121–122
   technology in, 121
Nursing home, Medicare managed care, 630–631
Nursing services
   in home health care, 273, 274
   in preventive services, 69–70

O

Observation unit, for emergency department, 135–136
Occupational therapists, in home health care, 274
Office service management, 241–248
   accountability, 247–248
   collaboratives, 245–247
   points of engagement, 241–242
   practice guideline
      development, 242, 243–245
      program, 242–243
   trust in, 248
Organizational change process, in medical management, assessment of, 10–11
Outcomes, measurement of
   clinical, 461–477
   subacute care, 293–294
Outpatient clinic, for congestive heart failure management, 358
Outpatient procedure units, as alternative to acute care hospitalization, 174
Outpatient utilization data, 520–522
Outreach program, 55–62
   for chest pain center, 143
   population health cycle, 56–57
Oxford Health Plan, asthma disease management
   components, 380–385
   case management, 384
   continuous quality improvement, 385
   education
      member, 381–382
      provider, 382–383
   network development, 383–384
   outcomes, evaluation of, 385
   patient empowerment, 381

   technological support, 384–385
   treatment guidelines, 382

P

Paper-based authorization systems, 257
Paradigm issues, in integration of alternative medicine, 592
Patient, case manager role with, 194–195
Patient care objectives, defining, in critical path approach, 224–225
Patient data, hospice care, 298–299
Patient education, in diabetes management, 368
Patient profile, 188–190
   behavioral/motivational activities, 190
   financial activities, 189–190
   medical activities, 189
Payer, obtaining approval from, case manager role, 199
Pediatric hospice programs, 304
Peer review, quality management and, 436–438
Pended authorization, for clinical services, 254
Pharmaceutical services, 317–336
   audits, 330
   benefit
      components of, 321
      design of, 324
      Medicaid, 323
      receipt of, 320–321
   certificate of coverage, 319–320
   claims adjudication, 324
   costs, 318, 320, 323–324
   electronic claims adjudication, 325
   eligibility verification, 325
   enrollment data, 325
   ingredient cost, 326–329
      drug formularies, 327–329
      flat rate, 327
      generic drug policy, 326–327
      rebates, 329
      volume purchasing, 329
      wholesale price discounts, 327
   organization expectations, 333
   outcomes data in, 336
   partial pay, 320–321
      coinsurance, 321
      copayment, 320
      deductibles, 320–321
   pharmacy provider networks, 325–326
   point-of-service review, 333
   providers, 321–323
      closed panel managed care organization, 321–322
      government programs, 323
      indemnity insurance plans, 322–323
      independent practice association, 322
      Medicaid, 323
      networks, 325–326
      open panel managed care organization, 322
      preferred provider organization, 322

staff-insured benefits, 323
staff model, 321–322
quality control, 330–333
  outcomes management, 332
  patient expectations, 332–333
  therapeutics, 331–332
    community standards, 332
    drug formulary, 331
    step therapy, 331–332
  utilization review, 329–330, 333–334
Philosophy
  of alternative medicine, 583
  of hospice care, 295
Physical therapies, in home health care, 274
Physician
  role of, in medical management, 8–9
  self-care, 101
    obstacles, 101–103
Physician acceptance, of alternative medicine, 580–581
Physician behavior, 535–548
  autonomy issues, 536–537
  changing, approach to, 540–541
    goals, 540
    individual physician
      discipline, 544–546
      sanctions, 544–546
      stepwise approach, 543
    programmatic approaches, 541–543
      clinical protocols, 542–543
      continuing medical education, 541
      data, 541–542
      feedback, 541–542
      practice guidelines, 542–543
    rewards, versus sanctions, 540–541
  competing plans, differentiation among, 539–540
  control, 536–537
    of patient care, 537
    of quality, 537
    of where care received, 536–537
  economics, 539
  insurance function of plan, 538
  modification of, 536–540
  role conflict, 537–538
Physician data, 517
Physician-owned ancillary services, 310–311
Plan average data, 516
Point-of-service review, pharmaceutical services, 333
Policy issues, in hospice care, 300–301
  care provision, 301
  ethics, 300
  legal issues, 300–301
Population-based programs
  in managed care, 39
  for prevention, 39
Population health cycle, outreach, 56–57
Post-acute care settings, 267–305

Practice association data, 516–517
Practice guideline, development of, in office service management, 242
Preadmission review, case management reports, case manager role, 205
Preferred provider organization, as provider of pharmaceutical benefit, 322
Pregnancy prevention, 91–96
  behavioral factors, 91–92
  contraception, 94
  education, 93–94
  health plan, 91
  public health agencies, role of, 92–93
  reimbursement policies, 94–95
  religion, impact of, 95–96
  risks of pregnancy, 94
  service coverage, 94–95
Premium source group data, 517
Preventive services, 37–43
  in clinical setting, 39, 45–53
    data tool, 50–51
    Institute for Clinical Systems Integration, 49–50
    primary, versus secondary prevention, 51–52
    Project IMPROVE, 50
  community programs, 39, 40–42
  disease prevention activities, typology of, 39
  health promotion activities, typology of, 39
  high-risk behaviors, 75–96
  to immigrant population, 63–73
  leadership, 39–40
  Medicaid, 617
  medical-surgical utilization and, 155–156
  population-based programs, 39
  primary, 35–73
    versus secondary prevention, 51–52
  public policy, 39, 42
  rationale, 37–39
  to underserved population, 63–73
Process engineering, in nurse advice service, 121–122
Project IMPROVE, 50
  learning research trial, 50
Prospective review
  institutional
    mandatory outpatient surgery, 165–166
    preadmission testing, 165
    precertification, 164–165
    utilization management, 164–166
Provider organization data, 516–517
Provider profiling, 525–532
  case mix, adjusting for, 527–528
  data, 522–523
    feedback, 523
    focused utilization management, 523
    incorporation, other data, 522–523
  episodes of care, 527
  group, constitution of, 529

linkages, 529
measures, 526–527
results, comparing, 529–530
severity, adjusting for, 527–528
specialty of physician, 528–529
vendor, 530–531
    carve-out accommodation, 531
    comprehensibility, 530
    HEDIS 3.0 production, 531
    independent validity, 531
    Medicaid, 530
    Medicare, 530
    point of service, 530
    prioritization of services, 531
Psychiatric health care, 407–432
    benefit plan design, 417–419
        coverage limits, 417
        disorders, types of, 418
        incentives, 419
        levels of care, 417
        providers, types of, 418
        treatment, types of, 418
    channeling mechanisms, 420–422
    continuum of care, 412
    data systems, 427–429
    integrated delivery systems, provider structures for, 423–425
    mental health case manager, as gatekeepers, 421–422
    methods of treatment, 411–412
        crisis intervention, 412
        goal-directed psychotherapy, 412
        psychiatric hospitalization, alternatives to, 411
        restrictive treatment for substance abuse, alternatives to, 411–412
    objectives of treatment, 409
    provider networks, 422–423
        selection criteria, 422–423
        size, scope of, 422
    public/private systems integration, 429–430
    quality assurance, 425–427
        external quality assurance monitoring, 426–427
            inservice training, 427
            staff qualifications, 426
            utilization criteria, 426
        network providers, 425–426
        outcomes measurement, 427
        problem identification, 427
        provider credentialing, 427
        utilization review/case management, 425
    strategic approaches, 409–410
    substance abuse case manager, as gatekeepers, 421–422
    treatment principles, 408–412
    treatment services, 413–417
        basic mental health services, 413–414
        dual diagnosis, 414–415
        paradigmatic shifts, 415–417
        substance abuse services, 413
    utilization management, 419–420
        case management, 419–420
        utilization review, 419
Psychiatric hospitalization, alternatives to, 411
Psychotherapy, goal-directed, 412
Public health agencies, role of, in pregnancy prevention, 92–93
Public policy
    initiatives
        in managed care, 42
        prevention issues, 42
    in managed care, 39
    prevention issues, 39

Q

Quality assurance
    in behavioral health care, 425–427
    quality management, distinguished, 435–438
Quality improvement teams, 455
Quality management, 435–459
    agenda for, 456
    appropriateness evaluation, 436–438
    "best-of-class" standards, 445–446
    case management, 454
    in chest pain center, 144–146
    components of program, 438–439
    consumer education, 455–456
    feedback, 449–451
    in home health care, 279–280
    indicators, defined, 447–448
    outcome criteria, 436
    peer review, 436–438
    performance expectations, 448
        compared, 448–449
    in pharmaceutical services, 330–333
        outcomes management, 332
        patient expectations, 332–333
        therapeutics, 331–332
            community standards, 332
            drug formulary, 331
            step therapy, 331–332
    practice guidelines, 453–454
    process criteria, 436
    process model, 439–456
    profiling, 449–450
    quality assurance, distinguished, 435–438
    quality improvement teams, 455
    report cards, 450–451
    structure criteria, 435–436
Quality of life, congestive heart failure management, 359

R

Readiness to change, effect of, 550–551
Recruiting hospitalists, 184
Referral costs, Medicare managed care, 633

Referral providers, selection of, in medical-surgical utilization, 158
Referral source, talking with, case manager role, 193–194
Regulation of home health care, 275–279
Rehabilitation, congestive heart failure management, 358
Reinforcers, for member behavior change, 558–561
    action plans, 559
    contracts, 559
    incentives, 560–561
    reminder systems, 559
    rewards, 560–561
    tools, 558–561
    tracking methods, 558–559
Religion, impact of, on pregnancy prevention, 95–96
Report cards, for quality management, 450–451
Resource optimization, in smoking cessation, 81–84
Respiratory services, home care, 273–274
Respiratory therapists, in home health care, 274
Response, to health risk appraisal results, 32
Retinal screening, diabetes management, 368
Retrospective review, institutional, 172
    claims review, 172
    pattern review, 172
Risk-based health risk appraisals, 22–23

S

Schedule, of emergency department, 137
Secondary prevention. *See also* Prevention
Segmentation, in smoking cessation, 81–84
Self-care, 97–124
    benefits of, 100–101
    contact management, 109–110
    delegated, 105–109
    domains of care, 103–104
    enabling technologies, 111
    historical perspective, 100–101
    medical-surgical utilization and, 154
    as part of standard practice, 104–105
    physician involvement in, 101
    physician obstacles, 101–103
    in standard practice, 104–105
Self-management resources, asthma disease management, 389–390
Seniors. *See* Elderly
Sensitivity, cultural, 72
Service providers, talking with, case manager role, 197
Shared decision-making programs, 154–155
Skilled nursing facility
    freestanding, as provider of subacute care, 287–288
    hospice affiliated with, 302
    hospital-based, as provider of subacute care, 286–287
Slack time data, in critical path approach, 233
Smoking cessation, 77–90
    cost issues, 88
    interactive voice response system, 87–88
    Internet, 86
    larger populations, approaches to, 79–81
    marketing techniques in, 81–85
        duration, 81
        frequency, 81
        intensity, and duration, 81
        pricing, 84–85
        resource optimization, 81–84
        segmentation, 81–84
    print, 86–87
    state of art in, 78–79
    technology, use of, 85–88
    telephone call centers, 87
Social support, member behavior change and, 561–562
    coaching, 561
    enlisting, 561
Somatic practices, 574
Specialty hospital-based subacute care, 288–289
Specialty of physician, in provider profiling, 528–529
Specialty physician-based authorization systems, 260
Specialty physician services
    compensation, 161
    control of, 158–160
        reasons for referral, review of, 160
        secondary referrals, prohibition of, 159–160
        single visit authorization, 158–159
    large case management by, 161
    utilization management, 156–161
Speech language pathologists, in home health care, 274
Staff-insured benefits, as provider of pharmaceutical benefit, 323
Staffing
    for continuing emergency care, 133
    for immediate emergency care, 132–133, 136
Staged implementation, in medical management, 13
Standards, in alternative medicine, 592
Step-down units, as alternative to acute care hospitalization, 174
Subacute care, 283–294
    as alternative to acute care hospitalization, 173–174
    categories of, 283–284
    within continuum of care, 289–290
    defined, 283
    patients, 284–286
    payment for, 290–291
    providers, 286–289
        long-term care hospitals, 288
        selection of, 291–294
            accreditation, 291–292
            case management, 293
            clinical staff, 293
            cost-effectiveness, 294
            outcome measurement system, 293–294
            programs of care, 292–293
        skilled nursing facility
            freestanding, 287–288
            hospital-based, 286–287
        specialty hospital-based subacute, 288–289

Subauthorization, for clinical services, 255
Subspecialists, in Medicare managed care, 633
Substance abuse, restrictive treatment for, alternatives to, 411–412

T

Target populations, health risk appraisal, 25–26
Technology
   for health risk appraisal, 24–25
   in nurse advice service, 121
Telemonitoring, in congestive heart failure management, 357
Telephone-based authorization systems, 257–258
Telephone call centers, use of in smoking cessation, 87
Templates, in alternative medicine, 592
Timing, use of health risk appraisal instrument, 32
Transitional care for elderly, Medicare managed care, 629–630
Triage
   emergency department, 129–132
      transfer, 129–131
   prehospital, 128–129
Trust, in office service management, 248
Typology
   disease prevention activities, 39
   health promotion activities, 39

U

Underserved population, clinical preventive services, 63–73
   biological needs, defining, 63–65
   commitment, fostering of, 69
   community assessment, 67
   contact, 66–67
   cultural needs, defining, 65–66
   cultural sensitivity, 72
   development of program, 67–68
   interpretation of behaviors, 70–72
   nurses, role of, 69–70
   program design, 67–68
   progress evaluation, 69
Use of data, in medical management, 513–524
Utilization-based health risk appraisals, 23–24
Utilization management, institutional, 161–176
   acute care hospitalization, alternatives to, 172–175
   formulas, 162
   large case management, 175–176
   measurements, 162–163
   prospective review, 164–166
      precertification, 164–165
Utilization review, 329–330, 333–334

V

Vendors
   data, use of, 517
   provider profiling, 530–531
      carve-out accommodation, 531
      comprehensibility, 530
      HEDIS 3.0 production, 531
      independent validity, 531
      point of service, 530
      prioritization of services, 531
Vision, in medical management, 9–11
Vocational activities, in patient profile, 190
Voice response system, interactive, use of in smoking cessation, 87–88
Volunteers, in home health care, 275

W

Wellness programs, case manager role in, 215

Z

Zen Hospice Project Residence Program, 304

About the Editors

PETER R. KONGSTVEDT, MD, FACP, is a partner in the Washington, DC, office of Ernst & Young LLP. He is responsible for both leading and assisting consulting engagements in managed care strategy and operations. In addition to being a director of the firm's managed care group, he serves as one of the firm's thought leaders. He is a frequent lecturer and writer in managed health care. Dr. Kongstvedt has extensive experience in managed care, particularly in the health maintenance organization industry. He has served as chief executive officer of several large health maintenance organizations, as chief operating officer of a large insurer and managed care company, as regional officer of a large insurer, and in many other operating positions in the managed health care industry. He has also served on a number of state and national health care policy and strategy committees.

Dr. Kongstvedt is a licensed physician and board-certified internist. He received his undergraduate and medical degree from the University of Wisconsin. He is a Fellow in the American College of Physicians and a member of a number of professional societies. He is the editor and principal author of *The Managed Health Care Handbook,* 3rd Edition, a prize-winning book that is considered the leading text on managed care in the country; and of the *Essentials of Managed Health Care,* 2nd Edition, which is used in numerous academic programs.

DAVID W. PLOCHER, MD, is currently a partner with Ernst & Young LLP, serving as a national practice leader for managed care services. Dr. Plocher has 20 years of managed care experience, acquired partly in the Minneapolis market and also through working with a large managed care organization's 40 health maintenance organizations. With special interest in quality-driven selective contracting, he developed the first nationwide centers of excellence network for solid organ transplants in 1986 and for allogeneic bone marrow transplants in 1987. During the past 8 years with Ernst & Young, he has worked with self-insured employers and more recently with payers, physicians, and hospitals. Recent activities include working with integrated delivery systems on premium management, physician practice management, and advanced care management.

Dr. Plocher is a board-certified internist and a graduate of the University of Minnesota system, magna cum laude and Alpha Omega Alpha. He practiced medicine for 8 years at a tertiary care center in St. Paul, Minnesota.